TRAUMATIC STRESS

The Effects of Overwhelming Experience on Mind, Body, and Society

EDITED BY
Bessel A. van der Kolk
Alexander C. McFarlane
Lars Weisaeth

THE GUILFORD PRESS
New York   London

© 1996 The Guilford Press
A Division of Guilford Publications, Inc.
72 Spring Street, New York, NY 10012

Printed in the United States of America

This book is printed on acid-free paper.

Last digit is print number: 9   8   7

Library of Congress Cataloging-in-Publication Data

Traumatic stress : the effects of overwhelming experience on mind,
    body, and society / editors, Bessel A. van der Kolk, Alexander C.
    McFarlane, Lars Weisaeth.
        p.   cm.
    Includes bibliographical references and index.
    ISBN   1-57230-088-4
    1. Post-traumatic stress disorder.   2. Post-traumatic stress
disorder—Social aspects.   I. van der Kolk, Bessel A., 1943–
II. McFarlane, Alexander C.   III. Weisaeth, Lars.
RC552.P67T758   1996
616.85'21—dc20   96-10818
                                                           CIP

1003600141

This book is dedicated to Nelson Mandela and all those who, after having been hurt, work on transforming the trauma of others, rather than seeking oblivion or revenge.

Contributors

Petra G. Aarts, MA, National Institute for Victims of War, Utrecht, The Netherlands

Elizabeth A. Brett, PhD, Department of Psychiatry, Yale University School of Medicine, New Haven, Connecticut

Jonathon R. T. Davidson, MD, Department of Psychiatry, Duke University Medical Center, Durham, North Carolina

Giovanni de Girolamo, MD, Department of Mental Health, Azienda, USL, Bologna, Italy

Marten W. deVries, MD, Department of Psychiatry and Neuropsychology, Section of Social Psychiatry and Psychiatric Epidemiology, University of Limburg, Maastricht, The Netherlands

Edna B. Foa, PhD, Medical College of Pennsylvania, Philadelphia, Pennsylvania

Armen Goenjian, MD, Traumatic Psychiatry Program, Department of Psychiatry and Biobehavioral Sciences, University of California at Los Angeles, California

Thomas A. Grieger, MD, Department of Psychiatry, F. Edward Hebert School of Medicine, Uniformed Services University of the Health Sciences, Bethesda, Maryland

Danny G. Kaloupek, PhD, Department of Psychiatry, Tufts University School of Medicine; National Center for PTSD, Boston, Massachusetts

Terence M. Keane, PhD, National Center for Posttraumatic Stress Disorder, VA Medical Center, Boston, Massachusetts

Nathaniel Laror, MD, Ramat Chen Mental Health Clinic and Sackler School of Medicine, Tel Aviv University, Tel Aviv, Israel

Jacob D. Lindy, MD, Cincinnati Psychoanalytic Institute and Cincinnati University Department of Psychiatry, Cincinnati, Ohio

Charles R. Marmar, MD, Department of Psychiatry, University of California, San Francisco

James E. McCarroll, PhD, Department of Psychiatry, F. Edward Hebert School of Medicine, Uniformed Services University of the Health Sciences, Bethesda, Maryland

Alexander C. McFarlane, MD, DipPsychother, FRANZC, Queen Elizabeth Hospital, University of Adelaide, Australia

Lenore Meldrum, BEd, BPsych, Department of Psychiatry, University of Queensland, Mental Health Center, Royal Brisbane Hospital, Herston, Australia

Elana Newman, PhD, Department of Veterans Affairs, Boston VA Medical Center, National Center for Posttraumatic Stress Disorder, Boston, Massachusetts

Wybrand Op den Velde, MD, Department of Psychiatry, Saint Lucas Hospital, Amsterdam, The Netherlands

Roger K. Pitman, MD, Veterans Affairs Medical Center, Manchester, New Hampshire; Department of Psychiatry, Harvard Medical School, Boston, Massachusetts

Robert S. Pynoos, MD, Traumatic Psychiatry Program, Department of Psychiatry and Biobehavioral Sciences, University of California at Los Angeles, California

Beverley Raphael, PhD, Department of Psychiatry, Clinical Sciences Building, Royal Brisbane Hospital, Brisbane, Australia

Barbara Olasov Rothbaum, PhD, Emory University School of Medicine, Atlanta, Georgia

Linda S. Saunders, JD, New Hampshire Division of Mental Health and Development Services, Concord, New Hampshire

Arieh Y. Shalev, MD, Department of Psychiatry, Hadassah University Hospital, Jerusalem, Israel

Zahava Solomon, PhD, Medical Corp, Israeli Defense Forces, and Bob Shapell School of Social Work, Tel Aviv University, Tel Aviv, Israel

Landy F. Sparr, MD, VA Medical Center, Portland, Oregon; Department of Psychiatry, Oregon Health Sciences University, Portland, Oregon

Alan M. Steinberg, PhD, Traumatic Psychiatry Program, Department of Psychiatry and Biobehavioral Sciences, University of California at Los Angeles, California

Gordon J. Turnbull, MD, Traumatic Stress Treatment Unit, Ticehurst House Hospital, Ticehurst, Wadhurst, East Sussex, United Kingdom

Stuart Turner, MA, MD, FRCP, FRCPsych, The Traumatic Stress Clinic, Camden and Islington Community Health Services NHS Trust and University College, London, United Kingdom

Robert J. Ursano, MD, Department of Psychiatry, F. Edward Hebert School of Medicine, Uniformed Services University of the Health Sciences, Bethesda, Maryland

Onno van der Hart, PhD, Department of Psychology, University of Utrecht, The Netherlands

Bessel A. van der Kolk, MD, Department of Psychiatry, Harvard Medical School, Boston; HRI Trauma Center, Brookline, Massachusetts

Lars Weisaeth, MD, PhD, Department of Disaster Psychiatry, University of Oslo, Norway

John Wilson, PhD, Department of Psychiatry, Cleveland State University, Cleveland, Ohio

Preface

[This] subject (the traumatic neuroses) has been submitted to a
good deal of capriciousness in public interest. The public does not
sustain its interest, and neither does psychiatry. Hence these
conditions are not subject to continuous study, but only to periodic
efforts which cannot be characterized as very diligent. Though not
true in psychiatry generally, it is a deplorable fact that each
investigator who undertakes to study these conditions considers it
his sacred obligation to start from scratch and work at the problem
as if no one had ever done anything with it before.
                                        —KARDINER AND SPIEGEL (1947, p. 1)

The recognition of posttraumatic stress disorder (PTSD) as a formal diagnosis in the psychiatric nomenclature in 1980 has spawned a vast literature on the treatment of victims of many different sorts of trauma, and produced an explosion of scientific investigations into the ways people react to overwhelming experiences. It has been about 20 years since the contemporary scientific study of trauma began; the time seems ripe to attempt to synthesize what has been learned, and to delineate some of the dilemmas and challenges that lie ahead. To accomplish this, we have invited some of our most knowledgeable colleagues from around the world to participate in an effort to integrate our current knowledge about what we do and do not know about trauma, and to distill the research and clinical wisdom that have accumulated over these years.

Over the past 5 years this group has met (in various configurations and on numerous occasions) to present our data, discuss our research, and compare our impressions about the state of the field of traumatic stress. These discussions have always involved clinicians and researchers who are doing their work in different places around the globe, because the human response to trauma is universal. It involved people who represent many different theoretical and practical orientations, because the human response to trauma cannot be understood from one frame of mind alone.

The study of traumatic stress confronts clinicians and researchers alike with the need to approach their subject with a blend of objective science and an awareness of the sociopolitical contexts in which trauma is embedded. In this book we attempt to summarize the current state of knowledge about the effects of trauma on psychological, biological, and social systems, and to examine the interrelationships among these different realms. We then present a range of treatment options that have been developed for different trauma populations over the past two decades.

The acceptability of traumatic stress as a concept continues to be challenged by social and political dynamics, as well as by a variety of legitimate scientific considerations. For more than a century and a half, the recognition of the effects of trauma on individuals and on society has been marked by controversies. The study of trauma emerged from curiosity about whether the unexplainable physical symptoms seen in accident victims and in hysterics had biological or psychological causes. Because these patients claimed to be helpless, and because they suffered from strange symptoms that were susceptible to suggestion, they have always invited vehement disputes about the genuineness of their complaints; they have always been suspected of malingering and of suffering from "false memories" or "compensation neuroses."

The issue of memory has always been central to the study of trauma. Ever since psychiatrists and psychologists have devoted themselves to the study of trauma's impact on consciousness, they have noted that traumatic memories are stored in a state-dependent fashion, which may render them inaccessible to verbal recall for prolonged periods of time. When traumatic memories are dissociated from other life experiences and stored outside of ordinary awareness, they may be expressed in such seemingly incomprehensible symptoms as physical ailments, behavioral reenactments, and vivid sensory reliving experiences. The reenactment of trauma in personal and social relationships is a major source of shame for the victims and is a source of ongoing tragedy in society. The issue of dissociated experience also raises critical issues about responsibility, and about the mutual obligations between victims and society. Not being consciously aware of what one is reenacting makes it difficult to take responsibility for one's actions; it is difficult to be an effective human being when one feels helpless; and it is virtually impossible to trust in the rules, or to be guided by empathy, when one feels that one's life is being threatened.

The acceptance of PTSD as a diagnosis was closely related to the recognition of the effects of trauma in veterans of the Vietnam War. Following acute trauma, the relationships between patients' reactions and what led up to them can still be easily understood. In these individuals, the haunting memories of the trauma seem to be the paramount problem. However, over time, after patients develop their secondary adaptations to trauma, the connections between the patients' symptoms and their histories can become obscured. For example, the generalized affect dysregulation and constriction of ego functioning seen in almost all traumatized individuals are not easily pegged to particular life experiences. This issue becomes even more complex in people who were traumatized as children, because trauma early in the life cycle fundamentally affects the maturation of the systems in charge of the regulation of psychological and biological processes. The disruption of these self-regulatory processes makes these individuals vulnerable to develop chronic affect dysregulation, destructive behavior against self and others, learning disabilities, dissociative problems, somatization, and distortions in concepts about self and others.

This book is divided into six parts: (I) Background Issues and History; (II) Acute Reactions; (III) Adaptations to Trauma; (IV) Memory: Mechanisms and Processes; (V) Developmental, Social, and Cultural Issues; and (VI) Treatment. This book ends with a chapter on conclusions and future directions.

PART I. BACKGROUND ISSUES AND HISTORY

Chapter 1 examines the reaction to trauma as a process of adaptation over time. Rather than a unitary disorder consisting of separate clusters of symptoms, PTSD needs to be seen as the result of a complex interrelationship among psychological, biological, and social processes—one that varies, depending on the maturational level of the victim, as well as the length of time for which the person was exposed to the trauma. Central to understanding these processes is awareness of the nature of traumatic memory and its biological substrates. In this and many other chapters of this book, we explore various facets of the psychological and biological processes that lead to the dominance of the trauma in memory and to its maintenance over time. In Chapter 2, we discuss how the issue of responsibility, both individual and shared, is at the very core of how a society defines itself. We discuss how different societies have taken very different approaches to the question of whether the inescapably traumatic events that befall its members become a shared burden, morally and financially, or whether victims are held responsible for their own fate and left to fend for themselves. This opens up the issue of human rights: Do people have the right to expect support when their own resources are inadequate, or do they have to live with their suffering and not expect any particular compensation for their pain? Are people encouraged to attend to their pain (and learn from the past), or should they cultivate a "stiff upper lip," which does not allow them to reflect on the meaning of their experience? The resistances to the acknowledgment of trauma are explored, as are the price and the benefits of denial.

In Chapter 3, we discuss how the issues raised in Chapters 1 and 2 have been conceptualized over the past century and a half, and we examine the troubled relationship of the psychiatric profession with the idea that reality can profoundly and permanently alter people's psychology and biology. Mirroring the intrusions, confusion, and disbelief of victims whose lives are suddenly shattered by traumatic experiences, the psychiatric profession has periodically been fascinated by trauma, followed by stubborn disbelief about the relevance of patients' stories. Psychiatry has periodically suffered from marked amnesias, in which well-established knowledge was abruptly forgotten and the psychological impact of overwhelming experiences was ascribed to constitutional or intrapsychic factors alone. From the earliest involvement of psychiatry with traumatized patients, there have been vehement arguments: Is the etiology of these patients' complaints organic or psychological? Is trauma the event itself or its subjective interpretation? Does the trauma itself cause the disorder, or do preexisting vulnerabilities? Are these patients malingering and suffering from moral weakness, or do they suffer from an involuntary disintegration of the capacity to take charge of their lives? Should people examine their reactions to the trauma in order to overcome it, or should they be helped to ignore it and go on with their lives? The history of these arguments is summarized in this chapter, and the status of current knowledge is presented in the rest of the book.

PART II. ACUTE REACTIONS

The two chapters of Part II examine the progression from acute traumatic response to long-term outcome, taking into account issues of vulnerability, temperament, and adjustment. In response to acute trauma, people may experience a range of reactions, including dissociation. Acute stress disorder, a new category in the *Diagnostic and Statistical Manual of Mental Disorders* (DSM-IV), may or may not progress to full-blown PTSD. The symptoms of PTSD emerge as part of a longitudinal process of adjustment to the effects of trauma. These chapters examine the merits of the ongoing debate about whether PTSD is a normal or abnormal response to traumatic stress and about when clinicians should intervene. Furthermore, these chapters explore what we know about long-term effects of acute trauma, so that clinicians can more accurately predict eventual impairment and disability.

PART III. ADAPTATIONS TO TRAUMA

Part III begins with a chapter that delineates the background issues for the development of PTSD as a diagnostic category in DSM-III and DSM-IV. Since the placement of psychiatric problems within diagnostic systems determines how clinicians and investigators conceptualize the inner structure of a disorder, this raises the very important question of whether PTSD is most appropriately classified as an anxiety disorder. This chapter examines the rationale for establishing a separate axis for stress disorders in the DSM system of diagnostic classifications, which could include dissociative disorders, adjustment disorders, grief reactions, and a variety of characterological adaptations.

The next two chapters of this section—Chapter 7, on the nature of the stressor, and Chapter 8, on vulnerability and resilience—examine the interactions between external events and subjective response. In this regard, the meaning of the trauma, the physiological response, preexisting personality structures and experiences, and the degree of social support are all critical factors in a person's ultimate response to trauma. The stressor criterion defines who is and who is not included in the diagnosis, and hence this determines the prevalence of PTSD. Chapter 8 summarizes the epidemiological studies conducted to date, which emphasize the importance of traumatic stress as a public health issue. It further examines the relative importance of the traumatic event itself, in contrast to vulnerability or predisposing factors. The conclusion is that issues of predisposition and vulnerability may be more relevant to understanding recovery from acute symptomatology and the individual's long-term resilience than to understanding acute patterns of response to a stressor. Vulnerability factors may also define the patterns of comorbidity, which play an important role in chronic PTSD. Critical in these considerations is the emergence of chronic patterns of adaptation, in which lack of involvement in current reality, rather than preoccupation with the past, are the most pathological features.

Chapter 9, on the complex nature of adaptation to trauma, examines the intricate ways in which psychological and biological processes interact with development to produce a range of problems with self-regulation, attention, the ways people view themselves, and the ways they make their way in the world. Chronic trauma is associated with dissociative disorders, somatization, and a host of self-destructive behaviors (e.g., suicide attempts, self-mutilation, and eating disorders). In addition, trauma at different developmental levels has different effects on further personality development. This theme of complexity of adaptation continues in Chapter 10, which examines the biology of PTSD, including both hormonal and autonomic nervous system dimensions. Topics covered include the unusual patterns of cortisol, norepinephrine, and dopamine metabolite excretion; the role of the serotonergic and opioid systems; and receptor modification by processes such as kindling. This chapter also examines the involvement of central pathways involved in the integration of perception, memory, and arousal, as well as the impact of these central pathways on patterns of information processing in PTSD.

Part III concludes with a chapter on research methodology, which discusses the currently available diagnostic and assessment tools that are helpful in both clinical and research settings. There is often conflict between clinical realities and research paradigms in PTSD. Because of forensic as well as research issues, the problem of a valid and reliable diagnosis is of paramount importance. This question is given further relevance by the fact that a number of studies demonstrate low rates of PTSD in exposed populations. Whereas strict standards of diagnosis for PTSD are essential for good research, broader definitions may be helpful in clinical settings to assess the full extent of disability. Over time some people's PTSD may become subclinical, and yet it may continue to influence their level of functioning.

PART IV. MEMORY: MECHANISMS AND PROCESSES

Because it would be unethical to conduct laboratory experiments that are so overwhelming as to cause subjects to develop PTSD, research on the nature of traumatic memories needs to rely on reports of traumatized individuals, on biochemical challenge studies, and on inferences from animal investigations. Unfortunately, it has become common for experimental psychologists to make undue inferences from memories of ordinary events in the laboratory to memories of rapes, assaults, and murder. Chapter 12 describes that in recent years, research with traumatized individuals has been able to show that traumatic memories are qualitatively different from memories of ordinary events, and that amnesia coexists with vivid recollections. Brain imaging technologies have also made it possible to gain insights into the ways traumatic memories may be organized in the central nervous system. In Chapter 13, on information processing and dissociation in PTSD, we examine how trauma affects an individual's ability to perceive and integrate the overwhelming experience. Arousal and dissociative responses during the trauma lead to fragmentation of the experience. This chapter focuses both on the dissociative responses during traumatic experiences and on the continuing role of dissociation in subsequent adaptation, including the organization of experience in dissociated fragments of the self, such as occurs in dissociative identity disorder.

PART V. DEVELOPMENTAL, SOCIAL, AND CULTURAL ISSUES

Trauma and the Life Cycle

Trauma in childhood can disrupt normal developmental processes. Because of their dependence on their caregivers, their incomplete biological development, and their immature concepts of themselves and their surroundings, children have unique patterns of reaction and needs for intervention. Chapter 14 addresses the fluidity of children's schemata and the role of their caregivers in modifying the trauma response. On the other end of the life cycle, in the elderly, trauma has its own long-term impact: Recent research has shown that as external and internal resources diminish, trauma may renew its hold over people's psychology. Long-term studies of traumatized individuals show that although they may suffer from subclinical PTSD in middle age, memories of the trauma come once again to dominate their lives in senescence. Chapter 15 discusses adjustment in old age after an earlier trauma, such as concentration camp incarceration or combat experiences, as well as the issue of lack of flexibility or capacity to repair damage with increasing age.

Social and Cultural Issues

The history of PTSD has been intimately entwined with the ways legal systems have dealt with disability and pension entitlements. Legal systems have played a major role in defining how societies acknowledge the association between traumatic events and psychiatric symptomatology. Chapter 16 deals with the ways in which legal systems in North America, Europe, and Asia have approached these questions. Chapter 17 then explores the possible role of cultural issues in PTSD. Although this is an area that has received very little attention, the cultural context of the trauma is an important dimension because the meaning of trauma is often culturally specific, and the social and religious rituals surrounding loss and disaster have an important healing role in both individual and community trauma. This chapter also discusses the specific functions of social supports in minimizing the impact of trauma, and the protective role of attachment.

PART VI. TREATMENT

Well-controlled treatment studies are difficult to conduct, since there are always more variables that affect outcome than can be controlled. Nevertheless, PTSD research has provided some excellent treatment outcome studies from widely divergent theoretical orientations—cognitive-behavioral therapy, psychodynamic therapy, psychopharmacology and eye movement desensitization and reprocessing (EMDR). In actual practice, most clinicians use an eclectic approach, in which they must constantly reevaluate what is being accomplished. They must also continually evaluate what particular interventions are most effective for which trauma-related problems. For example, the core PTSD symptoms (intrusions, numbing, and hyperarousal), occupational disabilities, dissociative phenomena, and interpersonal problems and alienation may all need different approaches. Therefore, the treatment must in large part be derived from clinical judgment, and must draw from the available knowledge about the etiology and longitudinal course of this condition.

As we note in Chapter 18, the overall aim of therapy with traumatized patients is to help them move from being haunted by the past and interpreting subsequent emotionally arousing stimuli as a return of the trauma, to being present in the here and now, capable of responding to current exigencies to their fullest potential. In order to do that, people need to regain control over their emotional responses and place the trauma in the larger perspective of their lives—as a historical event (or series of events), that occurred at a particular time and in a particular place, and that can be expected not to recur if the traumatized individuals take charge of their lives. The key element in the psychotherapy of people with PTSD is the integration of the alien, the unacceptable, the terrifying, and the incomprehensible; the trauma must come to be "personalized" as an integrated aspect of one's personal history.

The therapeutic relationship with these patients is often the cornerstone of effective treatment. It tends to be extraordinarily complex, particularly since the interpersonal aspects of the trauma, such as mistrust, betrayal, dependency, love, and hate, tend to be replayed within the therapeutic dyad. Dealing with trauma in therapy confronts all participants with intense emotional experiences, ranging from helplessness to intense feelings of revenge, from vicarious traumatization to vicarious thrills.

The other chapters of this section examine specific therapeutic responses, starting with preventive strategies. The military and other emergency services have learned that it is possible to modify people's behavior during extremely stressful situations in such a way as to optimize their survival behaviors. The possibilities for preventing severe posttraumatic reactions have become a major focus of clinical efforts in the last decade, as described in Chapters 19 and 20. Critical incident stress debriefing has been proposed as a major vehicle for modifying the stress reactions of emergency service workers. Despite the strength of the advocacy for these services, there has been little systematic research examining their value. Much of the treatment literature about PTSD has focused on the management of acute patterns of distress or very chronic patterns of adjustment, such as those seen in Vietnam veterans. However, the increasing recognition of traumatic stress has led patients to present within weeks of the development of acute symptomatology. The absence of stable symptom patterns and extreme degrees of physiological hyperarousal at this stage mean that there are unique problems in the treatment of acute reactions; Chapter 21 describes these.

Of the various proposed therapies, the effects of cognitive-behavioral treatments have been most thoroughly examined, and these are discussed in Chapter 22. There is a growing body of systematic research demonstrating the ability of such treatments to assist in alleviating the broad range of PTSD symptoms. However, because uncontrolled exposure may have negative consequences, and since traumatized people with very high levels of avoidance are often most reluctant to expose themselves to their traumatic memories, there remain important questions about the necessary technical skills and timing for these forms of treatment.

The hyperarousal, sleep disturbances, and embeddedness in the trauma of patients with PTSD make effectve pharmacological treatment essential, as described in Chapter 23. During the last 5 years, a number of controlled trials have shown that some antidepressants and serotonin reuptake inhibitors can be quite helpful in providing symptomatic relief. The multiplicity of PTSD symptoms suggests that psychopharmacological interventions need to be targeted at specific subsets of symptoms.

Psychodynamic treatment has also made important contributions to the treatment of traumatized patients. Its most important contribution has been its focus on the understanding the subjective meaning of the traumatic event, and the process of (and barriers to) the integration of the experience with preexisting attitudes, beliefs, and psychological constructs. Chapter 24 provides a detailed description of psychodynamic treatment of PTSD.

The multidimensional nature of PTSD means that in clinical reality, a combination of several different approaches is often needed. Dealing with traumatized people often requires a staged process of treatment that is responsive to how much the victims can tolerate. The chronicity and severity of PTSD, and the reluctance of many victims to involve themselves in the treatment process, mean that various approaches to managing this condition need to be explored. The specific nature of the therapeutic relationship is often a critical variable in outcome. New treatments of PTSD are regularly proposed, and these deserve careful clinical trials to test their efficacy. All these factors are discussed in Chapter 25.

CONCLUSIONS AND FUTURE DIRECTIONS

The final chapter of the book integrates common themes and attempts to signal the future issues and directions of clinical care, service delivery, and research in the area of trauma. More than most areas of psychiatry, the field of trauma has reflected not only the established knowledge base of the discipline, but also a diverse range of social and political factors. The way victims of trauma are treated is often an indicator of society's general attitude to promoting the general welfare of its citizens. Much remains to be learned about how trauma affects people's capacity to regulate bodily homeostasis; how, years after the trauma has ceased, memories continue to dominate people's perceptions; and how victims can best be helped to reestablish control over their lives.

Many questions that have been explored in this book continue to be challenges for the future. How do the biological effects of trauma continue to affect people's capacity to think and make sense out of current experience? To what degree can psychological interventions reverse a disorder with such strong biological underpinnings? Do patients benefit from getting compensation payments, or does it impair their recovery? What is the role of predisposition, and what are the implications of preexisting vulnerabilities for treatment? To what degree is the essence of trauma the external reality or the internal processing of that event? Should treatment focus primarily on the trauma itself, on secondary adaptations, or on learning to pay attention to the here and now? Finally, possibly the most important questions that deserve intense study are these: What are the natural mechanisms that allow some individuals to face horrendous experiences and to go on? And what can we learn from them to help others do the same?

The past has shown how fragile existing knowledge can be, and how psychiatry is prone to become trapped in prevailing paradigms without being able to see their shortcomings. The unknown is the worst enemy of knowledge. This book is a body of work to be criticized and reacted against; only a critical reading will help us further define what we do not know, and determine the scope of future explorations.

REFERENCE

Kardiner, A., & Spiegel, H. (1947). *War stress and neurotic illness*. New York: Paul B. Hoeber.

Acknowledgments

The composition of a book that attempts to summarize the state of a scientific discipline at a particular moment in time involves thousands of lives and innumerable hours of collective devotion to a task that only intense commitment and deep affection between people can sustain. The intricate fabric of trust between patients and doctors, subjects and researchers, teachers and students, among colleagues, between husbands and wives, children and parents forms the glue for the creation of this piece of work. Since the development of this knowledge has entailed confrontation with the most horrible things that people can face, and the full extent of the cruelties that people can inflict on each other, this enterprise was bound to be accompanied by the entire spectrum of human emotions. Paradoxically, at the same time that we stared at abject misery, the exploration of trauma over the past 20 years has been so creative, startling, and rewarding an enterprise that the field of traumatic stress has been marked by an unusual spirit of cooperation and collegiality, in which professional and personal relationships have been dominated by a shared sense of wonder and excitement.

I want to acknowledge the following people without whom this work would not have been possible. The backbone of it all was the fantastic intellectual companionship and the unmitigated joy of working with Sandy McFarlane, executed in the far-flung places where we put the book together: from the pools of Bethesda to the Monte Rosa, and from the Wallabee reservation to the Salpêtrière. The International Society for Traumatic Stress Studies provided the forum for people from many different disciplines and from all parts of the world to share their experiences and to build a common knowledge base. Because of the time spent together, and the joy we have taken in one another's company, professional and personal roles have overlapped. Many close colleagues and friends contributed to this book, while others generously offered to review and critique it after the work was done. In Boston, the sense of discovery and wonder was mirrored in the by now retired Harvard Trauma Study Group; in which particularly Nina Fish Murray and Judith Herman opened up ways of looking at the world that I had never considered before, providing the intellectual and personal nurturance that for a short

xix

while made Boston for the study of trauma what Vienna once was for the composition of music. The support provided by these friendships made it possible to put into practice what Elvin Semrad and Leston Havens tried to teach me during my residency: that we have only one textbook, our patients.

My first two teachers were two Vietnam veterans born the same year that I was; one of whom refused to give up his nightmares, which he felt he needed to have in order to serve as a living memorial to his dead comrades, who otherwise would have died in vain; the other had virtual amnesia for many of his war experiences until the birth of his first child precipitated flashbacks of the children he failed to keep from dying in Vietnam. Their willingness to face their memories honestly, and their generosity in sharing their deepest horrors, fears, and shame, made me understand to what degree finishing the unfinished past can liberate people to be in the present. Their experiences prepared me for the lessons I subsequently learned from many other patients.

Since 1982 my professional home has been the Trauma Clinic, a small group of enthusiastic and underfunded people with a passion for understanding how children and adults can be helped to survive extreme experiences. Despite a series of catastrophic setbacks, we have survived as a devoted band of colleagues and friends. Hoping that the group will forgive me if I do not mention everybody by name, it would be impossible not to specifically thank Steven Krugman, Roslin Moore, Charlie Ducey, Glenn Saxe, Patti Levin, Kevin Becker, Liz Rice-Smith, Walter Penk, and Carrie Pekor. Perhaps my biggest stroke of luck has been a succession of amazing research assistants, the older ones of whom have gone on to distinguished careers of their own: Mary Coleman St. John, Mike Michaels (thanks to Roger Pitman, who told me that he was the man I was looking for), Rita Fisler, Jennifer Burbridge, and Joji Suzuki—whose fingerprints are all over this volume. Finally, I must thank Cliff Robinson and Roy Ettlinger, who saved us from extinction.

Like in the last book, it is necessary to stand still by the safe base—the members of my family, who simply have been there for me, and who in many different ways have been daily participants in this enterprise. From long discussions at the dinner table (sometimes involving various contributors to this book, and sometimes our teenage friends), to visits to strange places where we went to look at the ways people cope with the aftermath of trauma, to cooking dinners and making beds. In the meantime, we struggled with our own set of painful and scary challenges and grew closer while trying to go on. Hanna and Nicholas each have exemplified the life force in their own very different ways, and Betta has always believed in the value of what I was doing and encouraged me to speak the truth. After all these years, the poem that I sang the night I met you still holds true:

Meisje dat de innigheid der dingen mint,
je hebt geen taak te doen, geen woord te spreken,

je stil bewegend leven heeft
de wonderlijkheid der dromen van een kind.

Finally, I need to explain the dedication of this book. Just before we went to press, I had the great fortune to visit South Africa and to attend the inauguration of the Truth and Reconciliation Commission, which Nelson Mandela called to life in order to lay a secure foundation for a society with a history marked by hate and brutalization. Mandela became president of his country knowing trauma and the havoc it wreaks in people's souls. In articulating his vision of how his people should overcome their legacy of trauma, Mandela has put into action a program that is based on a hope for understanding, instead of vengeance; for reparation, rather than retaliation; for *ubuntu*, not victimization. Believing that only a True Memory Society can guarantee dignity, peace, and stability, Mandela, after 27 years of being imprisoned for his beliefs, proposes that before perpetrators can be forgiven, there first needs to be an honest accounting and a restoration of honor and dignity to victims; the facts need to be fully acknowledged in order to heal the wounds of the past. Only then can there be genuine forgiveness. Despite all the contrary lessons from history, we fervently hope that Mandela's dream will be fulfilled. We believe that the spirit of squarely facing the facts as a prelude to healing should guide both our clinical and our research work with victims of trauma and violence.

Bessel A. van der Kolk

Overt self-disclosure is not the intention of a book such as this, except in the acknowledgments section. The sentiments of obligation could easily lead to a listing of my academic pedigree and personal relationships. Yet the trauma field is one that depends on these relationships, because the sense of fascination and the perseverance required to complete and develop one's work do not have merely intellectual roots. An interest in trauma came to me early from my family. These included the stories of ship salvages and building coastal lifeboats that were part and parcel of my paternal grandfather's ship-building business, and the lingering shadow of Ypres and Passchendaele in the life of my maternal grandfather, who was a gunner in World War I. My father told stories of men dying in industrial accidents on the waterfront, and taught me about the sustaining pleasure of mastering fear in seamanship. When I was 16, my mother was left legally blind and mildly demented following a neurosurgical procedure—an affliction that she has survived with dignity and persistence. This experience has given me many moments to reflect on the nature of caring, intimacy, and numbing; it also influenced my choice of psychiatry as a profession.

My wife, Cate, has shared the chapters that follow, and has been the hard cover and binding to the loose leaves of my life. My children, James, David, and Anna, provide me with a great deal of pleasure, as well as insight into the struggle to master and contain the elements of life that buffet enthusiasm and hope.

(Indeed, the deprivations and rewards of living in a busy professional family sometimes constitute a microcosm of coping with trauma.) Then there are my friends, unnamed, who merge into my professional colleagues and mentors, many of whom are contributors to this book. Beverley Raphael, in particular, has encouraged me in this domain. I must also thank the many patients whose understated suffering and lives have provided an inspiration to understand.

This book has demanded a great deal of my staff. Tracy Air has mastered the transfer of files onto the Internet with uncomplaining skill, and Clara Bookless has devotedly maintained my research program. My secretary, Valda Doig, has tirelessly kept the world at bay when necessary and has acted as the organizer of my time and travels. Richard Barling also deserves a specific expression of thanks for his role in the early stages of the book. Finally, I must mention the scholarship, companionship, struggling, and wisdom of my fellow editors, and the encouragement and assistance of the staff at The Guilford Press, particularly Kitty Moore, Jodi Creditor, and Marie Sprayberry.

Alexander C. McFarlane

Contents

Truth, like love and sleep, resents
approaches that are too intense.
                                  —W. H. AUDEN

PART I

BACKGROUND ISSUES AND HISTORY

CHAPTER 1

The Black Hole of Trauma

BESSEL A. VAN DER KOLK
ALEXANDER C. McFARLANE

A stimulus impinging on the mind can be conceived as behaving like a ". . . raindrop land[ing] on a terrain of hills and valleys. The drop moves generally downhill until it ends up at the bottom of a nearby valley. The deeper the memory basin and the steeper the walls, the more likely the train of associations is likely to end up in it. In PTSD the traumatic event may be conceptualized as occupying . . . a Dead Sea of memory, into which all too many of the patient's associations inexorably flow" (Tank & Hopfield, 1987, p.106).

—As quoted in Pitman & Orr (1990, p. 469)

Experiencing trauma is an essential part of being human; history is written in blood. Although art and literature have always been preoccupied with how people cope with the inevitable tragedies of life, the large-scale scientific study of the effects of trauma on body and mind has had to wait till the latter part of this century—when the average life expectancy in the industrialized world is well above the Biblical three score and ten; when almost all children can be expected to outlive their parents; and when famine and epidemics no longer wipe out large sections of the population with the regularity that they once did.

Humans owe their ascendance in the animal kingdom to their extraordinary capacity to adapt. Throughout evolution humans have been exposed to terrible events; yet most people who are exposed to dreadful experiences survive without developing psychiatric disorders (see Chapters 4 and 7, this volume). Throughout history, some people have adapted to terrible life events with flexibility and creativity, while others have become fixated on the trauma and gone on to lead traumatized and traumatizing existences. Societies that have been massively traumatized have followed roughly similar patterns of adaptation and disintegration (e.g., Tuchman, 1978; Buruma, 1994; see Chapters 2 and 17, this volume). Many survivors seem to be able to transcend their trauma temporarily and harness their pain in acts of sublimated creation; for example, the writers and Holocaust survivors Jerzy Kosinski and Primo Levi seem to have done this, only to succumb to the despair of their memories in the end.

Despite the human capacity to survive and adapt, traumatic experiences can alter people's psychological, biological, and social equilibrium to such a degree that the memory of one particular event comes to taint all other experiences, spoiling appreciation of the present. This tyranny of the past interferes with the ability to pay attention to both new and familiar situations. When people come to concentrate selectively on reminders of their past, life tends to become colorless, and contemporary experience ceases to be a teacher. In much of the remainder of this book, we discuss what makes people vulnerable to developing such a fixation on trauma, and what can help them overcome it.

THE SYSTEMATIC STUDY OF TRAUMA

Since psychiatry has started to organize psychological problems in a diagnostic system that is based purely on their surface manifestations, it has, as a profession, increasingly lost interest in the workings of the mind and the mystery of medicine (Nemiah, 1995). Paradoxically, this has meant that the study of trauma has become the soul of psychiatry: The development of posttraumatic stress disorder (PTSD) as a diagnosis has created an organized framework for understanding how people's biology, conceptions of the world, and personalities are inextricably intertwined and shaped by experience. The PTSD diagnosis has reintroduced the notion that many "neurotic" symptoms are not the results of some mysterious, well-nigh inexplicable, genetically based irrationality, but of people's inability to come to terms with real experiences that have overwhelmed their capacity to cope.

In important ways, an experience does not really exist until it can be named and placed into larger categories. In Biblical mythology, Adam's first and main task in Paradise was to give names to the animals; the act of naming made him master over creation. The acceptance of the formal category of PTSD was a critical first step in making it possible to name the effects of overwhelming experiences on soma and psyche, and thus to open up the systematic investigation of how people come to be overwhelmed, how different people organize tragic experiences over time, and how their suffering can be alleviated. The recognition of PTSD as a legitimate psychiatric diagnosis has led to an explosion of scientific studies that have systematically examined many notions and popular prejudices about the effects of trauma.

Although there has been and continues to be concern about stigmatizing people with psychiatric labels in general, the diagnosis of PTSD seems to have been received by victims as a legitimization and validation of their psychic distress. Having a recognizable psychiatric disorder can help people make sense of what they are going through, instead of feeling "crazy" and forsaken. A diagnosis also bestows a sense of communality with other victims.

Essentially, the introduction of the PTSD diagnosis has opened a door to the scientific investigation of the nature of human suffering. Although much of human art and religion has always focused on expressing and understanding man's afflictions, science has paid scant attention to suffering as an object of study. Hitherto, science has generally categorized people's problems as discrete psychological or biological disorders—diseases without context, largely independent of the personal histories of the patients, their temperaments, or their environments. PTSD, then, serves as a model for correcting the decontextualized aspects of today's psychiatric nomenclature. It refocuses attention back on the living person instead of our overly concrete definitions of mental "disorders" as "things" in and of themselves, bringing us back to people's own experiences and the meaning which they assign to it (Nemiah, 1989).

PTSD has turned out to be a very common disorder. Exposure to extreme stress is widespread, and a substantial proportion of exposed individuals become symptomatic (see Chapter 8, this volume). A random survey of 1,245 American adolescents showed that 23% had been the victims of physical or sexual assaults, as well as witnesses of violence against others. One out of five of the exposed adolescents developed PTSD. This suggests that approximately 1.07 million U.S. teenagers currently suffer from PTSD (Kilpatrick, Saunders, Resnick, & Smith, 1995). Another survey (Elliot & Briere, 1995) found that 76% of American adults reported having been exposed to extreme stress. Nine percent of an urban population in a large North American city suffered from PTSD (Breslau & Davis, 1992), and approximately 20 years after the end of the Vietnam War, 15.2% of U.S. Vietnam theater veterans continued to suffer from PTSD (Kulka et al., 1990). The majority of psychiatric inpatients have consistently been found to have histories of severe (usually intrafamilial) trauma, and at least 15% meet diagnostic criteria for PTSD itself (Saxe et al., 1993). The available figures for the rest of the industrialized world are compatible with those of the United States. Outside of that world, no data are currently available.

Most people who have been exposed to traumatic stressors are somehow able to go on with their lives without becoming haunted by the memories of what has happened to them. That does not mean that the traumatic events go unnoticed. After exposure to a trauma, most people become preoccupied with the event; having involuntary intrusive memories is a normal way of responding to dreadful experiences. This repeated replaying of upsetting memories serves the function of modifying the emotions associated with the trauma, and in most cases creates a tolerance for the content of the memories (Horowitz,

1978). However, with the passage of time, some people are unable to integrate the awful experience and start developing the specific patterns of avoidance and hyperarousal that are associated with PTSD. What distinguishes people who develop PTSD from people who are merely temporarily stressed is that they start organizing their lives around the trauma. Thus, it is the persistence of intrusive and distressing recollections, and not the direct experience of the traumatic event itself, that actually drives the biological and psychological dimensions of PTSD (McFarlane, 1992; Creamer, Burgess, & Pattison, 1992). Although most people who suffer from PTSD have considerable interpersonal and occupational problems, the degree to which the symptoms of PTSD come to affect overall functioning varies a great deal from person to person.

The scientific study of suffering inevitably raises questions of causation, and with these, issues of blame and responsibility. Historically, doctors have highlighted predisposing vulnerability factors for developing PTSD, at the expense of recognizing the reality of their patients' experiences (see Chapter 3, this volume). This search for predisposing factors probably had its origins in the need to deny that all people can be stressed beyond endurance, rather than in solid scientific data; until very recently, such data were simply not available (see Chapters 7 and 8, this volume). When the issue of causation becomes a legitimate area of investigation, one is inevitably confronted with issues of man's inhumanity to man, with carelessness and callousness, with abrogation of responsibility, with manipulation, and with failures to protect. In short, the study of trauma confronts one with the best and the worst in human nature, and is bound to provoke a range of intense personal reactions in the people involved (Herman, 1992; Wilson & Lindy, 1994; Pearlman & Saakvitne, 1995; see also Chapters 24 and 25, this volume).

REALITY VERSUS NEUROSIS

Unlike other forms of psychological disorders, the core issue in trauma is reality: "It is indeed the truth of the traumatic experience that forms the center of its psychopathology; it is not a pathology of falsehood or displacement of meaning, but of history itself" (Caruth, 1995, p. 5). However, the critical element that makes an event traumatic is the subjective assessment by victims of how threatened and helpless they feel. So, although the reality of extraordinary events is at the core of PTSD, the meaning that victims attach to these events is as fundamental as the trauma itself. People's interpretations of the meaning of the trauma continue to evolve well after the trauma itself has ceased. This is well illustrated by a case of delayed PTSD reported by Kilpatrick et al. (1989): A woman who was raped did not develop PTSD symptoms until some months later, when she learned that her attacker had killed another rape victim. It was only when she received this information that she reinterpreted her rape as a life-threatening attack and developed full-blown PTSD.

This raises the question of how PTSD compares with the old notion of neurosis. Psychoanalysis held that the essence of neurosis is the pathological persistence of defense mechanisms employed to ward off unacceptable unconscious wishes and impulses. Over time, the ego is "hardened," defenses are consolidated, and "earlier conflict is transformed into chronic automatic modes of functioning . . . detached from the content of infantile conflict" (Shapiro, 1965, p. 7). "Once hardened, character continues to have a protective function. It 'binds' impulses in stable ways, limits flexibility, and constitutes an armor against the external world" (p. 8). Thus, the meaning that individuals cull out of the present depends on their prior experience and on the many subtle and indirect ways that their personal past has been incorporated into their current attitudes and beliefs. This can lead to a range of maladaptive responses in their current lives, to which "neurotics" keep responding as if they were reliving the past.

These notions about the nature of neurotic defense mechanisms are quite relevant in understanding how people adapt to trauma. All traumatized people develop their own peculiar defenses to cope with intrusive recollections and increased physiological arousal. Prior to the acceptance of the concepts of psychopathology that underpin PTSD, clinical thinking was dominated by the exclusive attention to secondary psychic elaborations, at the expense of paying attention to the realities that continue to drive these repetitions. The exploration of the fantasized elaborations of intrapsychic conflicts was seen as the sole purpose of the treatment of neuroses.

When people are traumatized, the choice of defenses is influenced by developmental stage, temperamental and contextual factors. Hence, the diagnosis of PTSD alone never fully captures the totality of people's suffering and the spectrum of adaptations that they engage in (see Chapter 9, this volume). However, even though psychodynamic psychiatry is invaluable in helping us understand the characterological adaptations to the memories of the trauma, the core issue in PTSD is that the primary symptoms are not symbolic, defensive, or driven by secondary gain. The core issue is the inability to integrate the reality of particular experiences, and the resulting repetitive replaying of the trauma in images, behaviors, feelings, physiological states, and interpersonal relationships. Thus, in dealing with traumatized people, it is critical to examine where they have become "stuck" and around which specific traumatic event(s) they have built their secondary psychic elaborations.

FIXATION ON THE TRAUMA

The posttraumatic syndrome is the result of a failure of time to heal all wounds. The memory of the trauma is not integrated and accepted as a part of one's personal past; instead, it comes to exist independently of previous schemata (i.e., it is dissociated). Some cognitive formulations of PTSD have proposed that a traumatic experience confronts an individual with experiences completely different from what he or she has been able to imagine before, and that this confrontation with the trauma radically shakes the individual's attitudes and beliefs (Janoff-Bulman, 1992). This may be true in some cases in which people encounter totally unexpected events or are confronted with aspects of the human capacity for evil that they had never before imagined. However, often trauma does not present a radically new experience, but rather confirms some belief that an individual has tried to evade. For many patients, what is most destructive about a traumatic event is that it confirms some long-feared belief, rather than presenting them with a novel incongruity.

Immediately after a traumatic event, almost all people suffer from intrusive thoughts about what has happened (McFarlane, 1992; Creamer et al., 1992; Joseph, Yule, & Williams, 1995). These intrusions help them either to learn from the experience and plan for restorative actions (accommodation), or to gradually accept what has happened and readjust their expectations (assimilation) (cf. Lindemann, 1944; Horowitz, 1978). One way or another, the passage of time modifies the ways in which the brain processes the trauma-related information. Either it is integrated in memory and stored as an unfortunate event belonging to the past, or the sensations and emotions belonging to the event start leading a life of their own. When people develop PTSD, the replaying of the trauma leads to sensitization; with every replay of the trauma, there is an increasing level of distress. In those individuals, the traumatic event, which started out as a social and interpersonal process, comes to have secondary biological consequences that are hard to reverse once they become entrenched (see Chapters 4 and 10, this volume). This new organization of experience is thought to be the result of iterative learning patterns, in which trauma-related memories become kindled; that is, repetitive exposure etches them more and more powerfully into the brain (van der Kolk & Greenberg, 1987; Post, 1992; McFarlane, Yehuda, & Clark, in press). These biological (mal)adaptations ultimately form the underpinnings of the remaining PTSD symptoms: problems with arousal, attention, and stimulus discrimination, and a host of psychological elaborations and defenses.

Ordinarily, memories of particular events are remembered as stories that change over time and that do not evoke intense emotions and sensations. In contrast, in PTSD the past is relived with an immediate sensory and emotional intensity that makes victims feel as if the event were occurring all over again (see Chapter 12, this volume). The "Grant Study," a longitudinal study of the psychological and physical health of 200 Harvard undergraduates who participated in World War II, is a good illustration of how people process traumatic events (Lee, Vaillant, Torrey, & Elder, 1995). When these men were reinterviewed about their experiences 45 years later, those who did not have PTSD had considerably altered their original accounts; the most intense horror of the events had been diluted. In contrast, time had not modified the memories of the minority of subjects who had developed PTSD. Thus, paradoxically, the ability to transform memory is the norm, whereas in PTSD the full brunt of an experience does not fade with time.

INFORMATION PROCESSING IN PTSD

There are six critical issues that affect how people with PTSD process information: (1) They experience persistent intrusions of memories related to the trauma, which interfere with attending to other incoming information; (2) they sometimes compulsively expose themselves to situations reminiscent of the trauma; (3) they actively attempt to avoid specific triggers of trauma-related emotions, and experience a generalized numbing of responsiveness; (4) they lose the ability to modulate their physiological responses to stress in general, which leads to a decreased capacity to utilize bodily signals as guides for action; (5) they suffer from generalized problems with attention, distractibility, and stimulus discrimination; and (6) they have alterations in their psychological defense mechanisms and in personal identity. This changes what new information is selected as relevant.

Intrusions

When Charcot (1887) first described traumatic memories over a century ago, he called them "parasites of the mind." Because people with PTSD have a fundamental impairment in the capacity to integrate traumatic experiences with other life events, their traumatic memories are often not coherent stories; they tend to consist of intense emotions or somatosensory impressions, which occur when the victims are aroused or exposed to reminders of the trauma (see Chapter 12). These intrusions of traumatic memories can take many different shapes: flashbacks; intense emotions, such as panic or rage; somatic sensations; nightmares; interpersonal reenactments; character styles; and pervasive life themes (Laub & Auerhahn, 1993). Years and even decades after the original trauma, victims claim that their reliving experiences are as vivid as when the trauma first occurred (van der Kolk & Fisler, 1995). Because of this timeless and unintegrated nature of traumatic memories, victims remain embedded in the trauma as a contemporary experience, instead of being able to accept it as something belonging to the past.

The personal meaning of the traumatic experience evolves over time, and often includes feelings of irretrievable loss, anger, betrayal, and helplessness. One of the serious complications that interferes with healing is that one particular event can activate other, long-forgotten memories of previous traumas, and create a "domino effect": A person who was not previously bothered by intrusive and distressing memories may, after exposure to yet another traumatic event, develop such memories of earlier experiences. For example, in an emergency medical technician who has witnessed many gruesome and horrifying events in the course of his or her career, one more dreadful event may trigger recollections of a host of previous experiences. Similarly, a sexual assault in adulthood may provoke long-forgotten memories of childhood abuse, and medical procedures in elderly concentration camp survivors may bring back memories to which the individuals may not have had access for decades.

Paradoxically, even though vivid elements of the trauma intrude insistently in the form of flashbacks and nightmares, many traumatized people have a great deal of difficulty relating precisely what has happened. People may experience sensory elements of the trauma without being able to make sense out of what they are feeling or seeing (van der Kolk & Fisler, 1995). One of the gravest symptoms of having been overwhelmed by a traumatic experience can be total amnesia. For example, describing the reactions to trauma in some Holocaust survivors, Henry Krystal noted that "no trace of registration of any kind is left in the psyche; instead, a void, a hole, is found" (Krystal, 1968).

Over time, the initial intrusive thoughts of the trauma may come to contaminate the individual's responses to a range of other cues and reinforce the selective dominance of the traumatic memory networks (Pitman & Orr, 1990; Pitman, Orr, & Shalev, 1993). Triggers for intrusive traumatic memories may become increasingly more subtle and generalized; what should be irrelevant stimuli may become reminders of the trauma. For example, a firefighter may not be able to wear a watch because this acts as a reminder of having to get to respond to sudden emergencies, or a combat veteran may become upset by the sound of rain because it suggests the monsoon season in Vietnam. This contrasts with more typical triggers that have an obvious connection to a traumatic memory, such as sexual situations for rape victims, or the sound of a firecracker (misinterpreted as the sound of gunfire) for war veterans.

We and our colleagues (van der Kolk & Ducey, 1989; McFarlane, Weber, & Clark, 1993), using two entirely different methodologies, were able to show that people who suffer from PTSD develop biased perception, so that they respond preferentially to trauma-related triggers at the expense of being able to attend to other perceptions. As a consequence, they have smaller repertoires of neutral or pleasurable internal and environmental sensations that could be restitutive and gratifying. This decreased attention to non-trauma-related stimuli adds further to the centrality of the trauma.

Compulsive Reexposure to the Trauma

One set of behaviors that is not mentioned in the diagnostic criteria for PTSD is the compulsive reexposure of some traumatized individuals to situations reminiscent of the trauma. This phenomenon can be seen in a wide range of traumatized populations. For example, combat soldiers may become mercenaries or join police SWAT teams; abused women may be attracted to men who mistreat them; sexually molested children may grow up to become prostitutes. Understanding this seemingly paradoxical phenomenon is of critical importance, because it could help to clarify many forms of social deviance and interpersonal misery. Freud (1920/1955) thought that the aim of such repetition is to gain mastery, but clinical experience shows that this rarely happens; instead, repetition causes further suffering for the victims and for the people around them (van der Kolk, 1989). In this reenactment of the trauma, an individual may play the role of either victimizer or victim.

1. *Harm to others.* Reenactment of victimization is a major cause of violence in society. Numerous studies have documented that many violent criminals were physically or sexually abused as children (e.g., Groth, 1979; Seghorn, Boucher, & Prentky, 1987). In a prospective study of 34 sexually molested boys, Burgess, Hartman, and McCormick (1987) found a link with drug abuse, juvenile delinquency, and criminal behavior within a few years after the abuse was first noticed. Dorothy Lewis and her colleagues (Lewis & Balla, 1976; Lewis et al., 1979) have also extensively documented the association between childhood abuse and subsequent victimization of others.

2. *Self-destructiveness.* Self-destructive acts are common in abused children. Studies consistently find a highly significant relationship between childhood sexual abuse and various forms of self-harm later in life, particularly suicide attempts, cutting, and self-starving (e.g., van der Kolk, Perry, & Herman, 1991). Clinical reports consistently show that most self-mutilators have childhood histories of physical or sexual abuse or repeated surgery (Graff & Mallin, 1967; Pattison & Kahan, 1983; Briere, 1988). Simpson and Porter (1981) sum up the consensus conclusion in stating that "self-destructive activities were not primarily related to conflict, guilt, and superego pressure, but to more primitive behavior patterns originating in painful encounters with hostile caretakers during the first years of life." (See Chapter 9 for a fuller discussion).

3. *Revictimization.* Many traumatized individuals continue to be revictimized. Rape victims are more likely to be raped again, and women who were physically or sexually abused as children are more likely to be abused as adults (van der Kolk, 1989). Victims of child sexual abuse are at high risk of becoming prostitutes (Finkelhor & Browne, 1984; Silbert & Pines, 1981). Diane Russell (1986), in her well-known study of incest's effects on the lives of women, found that few women made a conscious connection between their childhood victimization and their later drug abuse, prostitution, and suicide attempts. (Again, see Chapter 9 for more details.)

These phenomena are seldom understood by either victims or clinicians as repetitive reenactments of real events from the past. Understanding and remedying the fact that traumatized people tend to lead traumatizing and traumatized lives remain among the great challenges of psychiatry.

Avoiding and Numbing

Once traumatized individuals become haunted by intrusive reexperiences of their trauma, they generally start organizing their lives around avoiding having the emotions that these intrusions evoke (van der Kolk & Ducey, 1989). Avoidance may take many different forms, such as keeping away from reminders, ingesting drugs or alcohol in order to numb awareness of distressing emotional states, or utilizing dissociation to keep unpleasant experiences from conscious awareness. This avoidance of specific triggers is aggravated by a generalized numbing of responsiveness to a whole range of emotional aspects of life. Despite the fact that numbing and avoidance are lumped together in the *Diagnostic and Statistical Manual of Mental Disorders*, fourth edition (DSM-IV; American Psychiatric Association, 1994), numbing probably has a very different underlying pathophysiology from avoidance (e.g., van der Kolk et al., 1994). Studies of combat veterans (e.g., Kardiner, 1941), concentration camp survivors (Krystal, 1968), and other victim populations (Titchener, 1986) have described a gradual withdrawal and detachment from everyday activities. Krystal (1968) called this reaction "dead to the world," Kardiner (1941, p. 249) "a deterioration that is not dissimilar to that in schizophrenia," and Titchener (1986) "post-traumatic decline." Thus, many people with PTSD not only actively avoid emotional arousal, but experience a progressive decline and withdrawal, in which *any* stimulation (whether it is potentially pleasurable or aversive) provokes further detachment. To feel nothing seems to be better than feeling irritable and upset.

It would be an error to think of this detachment and withdrawal in PTSD either merely as a psychodynamic phenomenon, or as a deficit of certain neurotransmitters that can be "fixed" with the administration of neurotransmitter supplements (i.e., antidepressants or other psychopharmacological agents that stimulate the release of neurohormones; see Chapter 23, this volume). Roughly speaking, it seems that the chronic hyperarousal of PTSD depletes both the biological and the psychological resources needed to experience a wide variety of emotions (van der Kolk et al., 1985; Litz, 1992). McFarlane et al. (in press) have proposed that as intrusive memories come to dominate their thinking, people with PTSD become more and more sensitized to environmental stimuli that remind them of the trauma. Thus, over time, they become less and less responsive to various stimuli that are necessary for involvement in the present. They have proposed that this underresponsiveness leads to a series of changes in the central nervous system that are similar to the effects of prolonged sensory deprivation (see Chapter 10).

Litz et al. (1995) have proposed that the resulting failure to process emotional events fully leads to further physiological hyperarousal and to psychosomatic problems. Indeed, psychosomatic problems and emotional numbing in PTSD are intimately related (van der Kolk et al., in press). This line of investigation is further supported by the work of Pennebaker (1993) and others (e.g., Spiegel, 1992), which has shown that low levels of emotional expression lead to impairment of immune function and to an increase in physical illness.

Inability to Modulate Arousal

Although people with PTSD tend to deal with their environment through emotional constriction, their bodies continue to react to certain physical and emotional stimuli as if there were a continuing threat of annihilation; they suffer from hypervigilance, exaggerated startle response, and restlessness. Research has clearly established that people with PTSD suffer from conditioned autonomic arousal to trauma-related stimuli; however, evidence in recent years also suggests that many traumatized individuals suffer from extreme physiological arousal in response to a wide variety of stimuli (see Chapters 4 and 10).

People with PTSD tend to move immediately from stimulus to response without often realizing what makes them so upset. They tend to experience intense negative emotions (fear, anxiety, anger, and panic) in response to even minor stimuli; as a result, they either overreact and threaten others, or shut down and freeze. These hyperarousal phenomena represent complex psychological and biological processes, in which the continued anticipation of overwhelming threat seems to cause difficulties with attention and concentration. In turn, these difficulties give rise to distortions in information processing, including narrowing of attention onto sources of potential challenge or threat. Children and adults with such hyperarousal tend to experience sleep problems, both because they are unable to quiet themselves sufficiently to go to sleep, and because they deliberately wake themselves up in order to avoid having traumatic nightmares.

Perhaps the most distressing aspect of this hyperarousal is the generalization of threat. The world increasingly becomes an unsafe place: Innocuous sounds provoke an alerting startle response; trivial cues are perceived as indicators of danger. Ordinarily, autonomic arousal serves the very important function of alerting people to pay attention to potentially important situations. However, for persons who are chronically hyperaroused, the autonomic nervous system loses that function; the easy triggering of somatic stress reactions makes them unable to rely on their bodily sensations as an efficient warning system against impending threat. The persistent, irrelevant firing of warning signals causes physical sensations to lose their functions as signals of emotional states and, as a consequence, they stop serving as guides for action. Thus, like neutral environmental stimuli, normal physical sensations may take on a new and threatening significance. The person's own physiology becomes a source of fear.

The PTSD sufferers' inability to decipher messages from the autonomic nervous system interferes with their capacity to articulate how they are feeling (alexithymia) and makes them tend to react to their environment with either exaggerated or inhibited behaviors. After a traumatic experience, many people regress to earlier levels of coping with stress. In children, this may manifest itself as an inability to take care of themselves in such areas as feeding and toilet training; in adults, it is expressed in impulsive behavior, excessive dependence, and a loss of the capacity to make thoughtful, autonomous decisions.

Attention, Distractibility, and Stimulus Discrimination

Freud (1911/1959) described how, in order to function properly, people need to be able to define their needs, anticipate how to meet them, and plan for appropriate action. In order to do this, they first need to be able to consider a range of options without resorting to action—a capacity Freud called "thought as experimental action." People with PTSD seem to lose this capacity; they have problems fantasizing and playing with options. Studies both of traumatized children (e.g., Rieder & Cicchetti, 1989) and of traumatized adults (e.g., van der Kolk & Ducey, 1989) indicate that when traumatized people allow themselves to fantasize, this creates the danger of breaking down their barriers against being reminded of the trauma. In order to prevent this from happening, they become constricted and seem to organize their lives around *not* feeling and *not* considering options for the best ways of responding to emotionally arousing problems. Their problems with keeping thoughts in their minds without becoming aroused contribute greatly to their impulsivity.

People with PTSD have difficulty in sorting out relevant from irrelevant stimuli; they have problems ignoring what is unimportant and selecting only what is most relevant. Easily overstimulated, they compensate by shutting down. In a study using event-related potentials, McFarlane et al. (1993) were able to demonstrate these difficulties in stimulus discrimination (see Chapter 10 for details). The price of these problems is loss of involvement in ordinary, everyday life. This makes it even harder for these patients to get their minds off the trauma, and thus only increases the strength of their fixation on the trauma. As a result, the individuals lose the capacity to respond flexibly to their environment. This loss of flexibility may explain current findings of deficits in preservative learning and interference with the acquisition of new information (Bremner et al., 1993; Yehuda et al., 1995), as well as an inability to apply working memory to salient environmental stimuli (van der Kolk & Ducey, 1989; McFarlane et al., 1993).

Alterations in Defense Mechanisms and Changes in Personal Identity

In recent years, much has been written about trauma's effects on people's sense of themselves and their relationship to their environment (Cole & Putnam,

1992; Herman, 1992; Pearlman & Saakvitne, 1995). Reiker and Carmen (1986) have pointed out that "confrontations with violence challenge one's most basic assumptions about the self as invulnerable and intrinsically worthy, and about the world as orderly and just. After abuse, the victim's view of self and world can never be the same again: it must be reconstructed to incorporate the abuse experience" (p. 362). Of course, how old a person is when the trauma happens, and what the person's previous life experiences have been like, will profoundly affect his or her interpretation of the meaning of the trauma (van der Kolk & Fisler, 1994).

Many traumatized individuals, particularly children, tend to blame themselves for having been traumatized. Assuming responsibility for the trauma allows feelings of helplessness and vulnerability to be replaced with an illusion of potential control. Ironically, rape victims who blame themselves have a better prognosis than those who do not assume this false responsibility; it allows their locus of control to remain internal and prevents helplessness (Burgess & Holstrom, 1979). Traumatized children are even more likely to blame themselves: "The child needs to hold on to an image of the parent as good in order to deal with the intensity of fear and rage which is the effect of the tormenting experiences" (Reiker & Carmen, 1986, p. 368). In the context of these sorts of conflicts, defense mechanisms are activated that are designed to provide an accommodation with an intolerable reality (see Chapter 9).

The question of shame is critical to understanding the lack of self-regulation in trauma victims and the capacity of abused persons to become abusers. Trauma is usually accompanied by intense feelings of humiliation; to feel threatened, helpless, and out of control is a vital attack on the capacity to be able to count on oneself. Shame is the emotion related to having let oneself down. The shame that accompanies such personal violations as rape, torture, and abuse is so painful that it is frequently dissociated: Victims may be unaware of its presence, and yet it comes to dominate their interactions with the environment. Denial of one's own feelings of shame, as well as those of other people, opens the door for further abuse. Being sensitive to the shame in others is an essential protection against abusing one's fellow human beings, and it requires being in touch with one's own sense of shame. Similarly, not being in touch with one's own shame leaves one vulnerable to further abuse from others. The resulting disorganized patterns of engagement are commonly seen in traumatized people who suffer from borderline personality disorder, who need to be helped to understand how this perpetuates their getting hurt and their hurting others.

FIXATION ON THE DIAGNOSIS

Despite efforts to capture the essence of people's response to trauma, the PTSD diagnosis does not begin to describe the complexity of how people react to overwhelming experiences (see Chapter 9). The DSM's emphasis on phenom-enological diagnoses has resulted in a loss of interest in the way symptoms are interrelated and reflect subtle interactions between psychological and biological processes (Nemiah, 1995). Yet the same underlying psychopathology can have a range of symptomatic expressions. For example, when "hysteria" was first diagnosed and related to prior histories of trauma by Briquet in 1859, and subsequently by the school of the Salpêtrière under Charcot, posttraumatic symptoms were primarily expressed as conversion reactions and as psychoso-matic conditions (see Chapter 3). Those patterns seem to have persisted as the primary expressions of traumatic stress during World War I. Even though the same symptoms were described in combat soldiers during World War II, descriptions of soldiers at that time focused primarily on psychophysiological reactions and loss of impulse control. Descriptions of Vietnam veterans have focused on intrusive recollections and on characterological adaptations. Does this mean that the symptomatic expression of traumatic stress has changed in Western culture over time, or have clinicians focused on different aspects of the same syndrome during the past century and a half? Given the rather marked differences in vulnerability and symptoms among Vietnam combat soldiers belonging to different ethnic groups (Kulka et al., 1990), it is likely that the prevailing culture has a marked effect on the symptomatic expression of trau-matic stress.

The complexity of people's responses to trauma, and the comparative sim-plicity of the PTSD conceptualization, are illustrated by the recent rediscovery of the intimate association among trauma, dissociation, and somatization (van der Kolk et al., in press). Trauma can affect victims on every level of function-ing: biological, psychological, social, and spiritual. Conceptualized in terms of psychiatric diagnosis, this means that PTSD has a high rate of psychiatric comorbidity with mood, dissociative, and anxiety disorders; substance abuse; and character pathology (Green, Lindy, Grace, & Leonard, 1992; Davidson, Hughes, Blazer, & George, 1991; Kulka et al., 1990). The National Comorbidity Survey (Kessler, Bromet, & Nelson, in press) and the DSM-IV field trials for PTSD (van der Kolk, Roth, Pelcovitz, & Mandel, 1993) showed that people with simple diagnoses of PTSD were less likely to seek treatment than people who suffered from associated problems, such as depression, uncontrolled anger, and dissociation. As long as they can make meaning out of the trauma, victims often experience the symptoms of PTSD as natural reactions that do not re-quire professional help. For example, a study of Pearl Harbor survivors found they viewed their recurrent nightmares of the bombing as perfectly understand-able reactions to the terrible events they had witnessed on December 7, 1941. In their case, there never was a question about the validation of their experi-ence (Harel, Kahana, & Wilson, 1993).

Focusing solely on PTSD to describe what victims suffer from does not do justice to the complexity of what actually ails them. Excessive attention to the intrusion/numbing/arousal phenomena of PTSD may severely limit observations of how people react to trauma, and may thus interfere with appropriate treatment. The recognition of the profound personality changes that can follow childhood trauma or prolonged exposure in adults has been an important development, because these changes are major sources of distress and disability. This issue is beginning to be recognized by the inclusion of complex adaptations to trauma in the form of disturbed affect regulation, aggression against self and others, dissociative problems, somatization, and altered relationships with self and others in the "Associated Features and Disorders" section of the DSM-IV's entry on PTSD (American Psychiatric Association, 1994, p. 425).

TREATMENT IMPLICATIONS

Much remains to be learned about effective treatment of traumatic stress. Truly effective treatment would need to resolve the whole spectrum of posttraumatic problems discussed in this chapter: intrusions; compulsive reexposure; avoidance and numbing; hyperarousal; problems with attention, distractibility, and stimulus discrimination; altered perceptions of self and others; dissociation; and somatization. At this time, there have been no studies to show that effective intervention in one area will automatically have positive effects on the others as well. For example, there has been no research yet to show that improvement in intrusive reliving affects concentration, hyperarousal, and characterological problems. However, it is likely that effective treatment of one problem, such as physiological reactivity, will have widespread beneficial effects on the overall system, and can secondarily decrease intrusions, concentration problems, numbing, and the ways victims experience themselves and their surroundings.

Traumatized people often are incapable of finding flexible and adaptive solutions; the trauma keeps them rigidly fixated on the past, making them fight the last battle over and over again. However, since it is generally assumed that as long as memories of the trauma remain dissociated they will be expressed as psychiatric symptoms that will interfere with proper functioning, helping people avoid the past is not likely to resolve the effects of the trauma on their lives. Treatment needs to address the twin issues of helping patients (1) regain a sense of safety in their bodies and (2) complete the unfinished past. It is likely, though not proven, that attention to these two elements of treatment will alleviate most traumatic stress sequelae.

Clinicians need to be alert to the many ways in which past trauma determines current attitudes and perceptions. For example, one patient's frequent nightmares proved resistant to every intervention (including pharmacotherapy) until she moved to the third floor of a building she considered "safe," because it reminded her of the apartment of a loving aunt from her childhood. After the move, the nightmares spontaneously disappeared. Another example was a man whose wife died in an ambulance on the way to the hospital as he looked into her eyes; he only improved when he took the risk of continuing to look at, and not terminating a growing relationship with, a woman who could tolerate his sense of loss.

As noted above, the first task of treatment is for patients to regain a sense of safety in their bodies. For most individuals, this requires active engagement in challenges that can help them deal with issues of passivity and helplessness: play and exploration, artistic and creative pursuits, and some form of involvement with others. Assault victims often benefit from "model-mugging" programs, and physical challenges such as Outward Bound programs. Many women whose bodies have been violated report having been able to regain a sense of physical safety with the help of therapeutic massages (see Chapter 25).

The foundation of treatment is the safety of the therapeutic relationship. If treatment focuses prematurely on exploration of the past, this will exacerbate rather than relieve traumatic intrusions. Since most people with histories of psychological trauma suffer from a range of problems with information processing, fully effective treatment is likely to require a strategically staged, multimodal treatment approach, more thoroughly described in Part VI of this book. This includes overcoming (1) the patients' fear of confronting their helplessness and shame, (2) their fear of the traumatic memories, and (3) their fear of involvement with life itself (van der Hart, Steele, Boon, & Brown, 1993).

Because of these patients' problems in information processing, clinicians need to attend to and prioritize the critical treatment issues. Problems with somatization and affect dysregulation might be most usefully addressed by helping patients acquire skills that will help them to label and evaluate the meaning of sensations and affective states, to discriminate present from past, and to interpret social cues in the context of current realities rather than past events. Krystal (1978), Pennebaker (1993), and Nemiah (1991) have all discussed the critical importance of learning to identify and utilize emotions as signals, rather than as precipitants for fight-or-flight reactions. Pennebaker (1993), utilizing written accounts of traumatic personal experiences, has shown that verbalizing plays a critical role in maintaining physical and psychological health.

Kardiner (1941) described how some of his patients seemed able to "contain" the aftermath of the trauma in their symptoms, such as a hysterical paralysis of a limb. Some of his patients' anxiety and irritability appeared to be inversely proportional to their tendency toward conversion or dissociation. He recognized that some of the most depressed patients were the ones who possessed detailed recall of traumatic events, and that many of his less troubled patients who remembered little led more "ignorantly blissful" lives. Kardiner, with exemplary honesty, raised serious questions about the optimal treatment of patients presenting with dissociation or somatization. He questioned whether conscious awareness of a horrifying memory is always a preferable alternative to a bad back or fainting spells.

Merely uncovering memories is not enough; they need to be modified and transformed (i.e., placed in their proper context and reconstructed in a personally meaningful way). Thus, in therapy, memory paradoxically needs to become an act of creation rather than the static recording of events. Because the essence of the trauma is that it once confronted the victim with unacceptable reality, the patient needs to find a way of confronting the hidden secrets that no one, including the patient, wants to face (Langer, 1990). Like memories of ordinary events, the memory of the trauma needs to become merely a (often distorted) part of a patient's personal past. Exploring the trauma for its own sake has no therapeutic benefits unless it becomes attached to other experiences, such as feeling understood, being safe, feeling physically strong and capable, or being able to empathize with and help fellow sufferers.

The exploration of personal meaning of the trauma is critical; since patients cannot undo their past, giving it meaning is a central goal of therapy. It is important to deal with the existential issues evoked by the trauma, such as the role that victims feel they played in causing (or at least not preventing) the trauma, and the particular stance they took while they were in the middle of it. These personal attributions can have profound affects on whether victims see themselves as capable and worthy of having restorative experiences, and whether they consider themselves capable of being entrusted with responsibility, intimacy, and care.

We hope that the recognition of these complexities of people's adaptations to traumatic life experiences may lead to the further development and application of treatment approaches that can help integrate traumatic experiences as inevitable aspects of victims' lives, while helping with the secondary physiological and characterological adaptations that cause the trauma to remain a contemporary experience, instead of something that can be properly located in the past.

REFERENCES

American Psychiatric Association (1994). *Diagnostic and statistical manual of mental disorders* (4th ed.). Washington, DC: Author.

Bremner, D. J., Scott, T. M., Delaney, R. C., Southwick, S. M., Mason, J. W., Johnson, D. R., Innis, J. R., McCarthy, G., & Charney, D. S. (1993). Deficits in short-term memory in posttraumatic stress disorder. *American Journal of Psychiatry, 170,* 1015–1019.

Breslau, N., & Davis, G. C. (1992). Posttraumatic stress disorder in an urban population of young adults: Risk factors for chronicity. *American Journal of Psychiatry, 149,* 671–675.

Briere, J. (1988). Long-term clinical correlates of childhood sexual victimization. *Annals of the New York Academy of Science, 528,* 327–334.

Briquet, P. (1859). *Traité clinique et thérapeutique de l'hystérie.* Paris: Ballière.

Buruma, I. (1994). *The wages of guilt: Memories of war in Germany and Japan.* New York: Farrar, Strauss, and Giroux.

Burgess, A. W., Hartman, C. R., & McCormick, A. (1987). Abused to abuser: Antecedents of socially deviant behavior. *American Journal of Psychiatry, 144,* 1431–1436.

Burgess, A. W., & Holstrom, E. (1979). Adaptive strategies in recovery from rape. *American Journal of Psychiatry, 136,* 1278–1282.

Caruth, C. (Ed.). (1995). *Trauma and memory.* Baltimore: Johns Hopkins University Press.

Charcot, J. M. (1887). *Leçons sur les maladies du système nerveux faites à la Salpêtrière [Lessons on the illnesses of the nervous system held at the Salpêtrière]* (Vol. 3). Paris: Progrès Médical en A. Delahaye & E. Lecrosnie.

Cole, P., & Putnam, F. W. (1992). Effect of incest on self and social functioning: A developmental psychopathology perspective. *Journal of Consulting and Clinical Psychology,* 174–184.

Creamer, M., Burgess, P., & Pattison, P. (1992). Reactions to trauma: A cognitive processing model. *Journal of Abnormal Psychology, 101,* 452–459.

Davidson, J. R. T., Hughes, D., Blazer, D. G., & George, L. K. (1991). Post-traumatic stress disorder in the community: An epidemiological study. *Psychological Medicine, 21,* 713–721.

Elliot, D. M., & Briere, J. (1995). Posttraumatic stress associated with delayed recall of sexual abuse: A general population study. *Journal of Traumatic Stress, 8*(4), 629–648.

Finkelhor, D., & Browne, A. (1984). The traumatic impact of child sexual abuse: A conceptualization. *American Journal of Orthopsychiatry, 55,* 530–541.

Freud, S. (1955). Beyond the pleasure principle. In J. Strachey (Ed. and Trans.), *The standard edition of the complete psychological works of Sigmund Freud* (Vol. 18, pp. 3–64). London: Hogarth Press. (Original work published 1920)

Freud, S. (1958). Formulations on the two principles of mental functioning. In J. Strachey (Ed. and Trans.), *The standard edition of the complete psychological works of Sigmund Freud* (Vol. 12, pp. 23–226). London: Hogarth Press. (Original work published 1911)

Graff, H., & Mallin, R. (1967). The syndrome of wrist cutter. *American Journal of Psychiatry, 124,* 36–42.

Green, B. L., Lindy, J. D., Grace, M. C., & Leonard, A. C. (1992). Chronic posttraumatic stress disorder and diagnostic comorbidity in a disaster sample. *Journal of Nervous and Mental Disease, 180,* 70–76.

Groth, A. N. (1979). Sexual trauma in the life histories of sex offenders. *Victimology, 4,* 6–10.

Harel, A., Kahana, B., & Wilson, J. P. (1993). War and remembrance: The legacy of Pearl Harbor. In J. P. Wilson & B. Raphael (Eds.), *International handbook of traumatic stress syndromes* (pp. 263–274). New York: Plenum Press.

Herman, J. L. (1992). *Trauma and recovery.* New York: Basic Books.

Horowitz, M. (1978). *Stress response syndromes.* New York: Jason Aronson.

Janoff-Bulman, R. (1992). *Shattered assumptions: Towards a new psychology of trauma.* New York: Free Press.

Joseph, S., Yule, W., & Williams, R. (1995). Emotional processing in survivors of the *Jupiter* cruise ship disaster. *Behaviour Research and Therapy, 33,* 187–192.

Kardiner, A. (1941). *The traumatic neuroses of war.* New York: Hoeber.

Kessler, R. C., Bromet, E., & Nelson, C. B. (in press). *Posttraumatic stress disorder in the National Comorbidity Survey.*

Kilpatrick, D. G., Saunders, B. E., Amick-McMullan, A., Best, C. L., Veronen, L. J., & Resnick, H. S. (1989). Victim and crime factors associated with the development of crime-related post-traumatic stress disorder. *Behavior Therapy, 20,* 199–214.

Kilpatrick, D. G., Saunders, B. E., Resnick, H. S., & Smith, D. W. (1995). *The National Survey of Adolescents: Preliminary findings on lifetime prevalence of traumatic events and mental health correlates.* Manuscript submitted for publication.

Krystal, H. (Ed.). (1968). *Massive psychic trauma.* New York: International Universities Press.

Krystal, H. (1978). Trauma and affects. *Psychoanalytic Study of the Child, 33,* 81–116.

Kulka, R. A., Schlenger, W. E., Fairbank, J. A., Hough, R. L., Jordan, B. K., & Marmar, C. R. (1990). *Trauma and the Vietnam War generation: Report of findings from the National Vietnam Veterans Readjustment Study.* New York: Brunner/Mazel.

Langer, L. L. (1990). *Holocaust testimonies: The ruins of memory.* New Haven, CT: Yale University Press.

Laub, D., & Auerhahn, N. C. (1993). Knowing and not knowing massive psychic trauma: Forms of traumatic memory. *International Journal of Psycho-Analysis, 74,* 287–301.

Lee, K. A., Vaillant, G. E., Torrey, W. C., & Elder, G. H. (1995). A 50-year prospective study of the psychological sequelae of World War II combat. *American Journal of Psychiatry, 152*(4), 516–522.

Lewis, D. O., & Balla, D. (1976). *Delinquency and psychopathology.* New York: Grune & Stratton.

Lewis, D. O., Shanok, S. S., Pincus, J. H., & Glaser, G. H. (1979). Violent juvenile delinquency: Psychiatric, neurological, psychological and abuse factors. *Journal of the American Academy of Child Psychiatry, 18,* 307–319.

Lindemann, E. (1944). Symptomatology and management of acute grief. *American Journal of Psychiatry, 101,* 141–148.

Litz, B. T. (1992). Emotional numbing in combat-related post-traumatic stress disorder: A critical review and reformulation. *Clinical Psychology Review, 12,* 417–432.

Litz, B. T., Schlenger, W. E., Weathers, F. W., Fairbank, J. A., Caddell, J. M., & LaVange, L. M. (1995). *Predictors of emotional numbing in post-traumatic stress disorder.* Manuscript submitted for publication.

McFarlane, A. C. (1992). Avoidance and intrusion in posttraumatic stress disorder. *Journal of Nervous and Mental Disease, 180,* 258–262.

McFarlane, A. C., Weber, D. L., & Clark, C. R. (1993). Abnormal stimulus processing in posttraumatic stress disorder. *Biological Psychiatry, 34,* 311–320.

McFarlane, A. C., Yehuda, R., & Clark, C. R. (in press). The neural network theory of post-traumatic stress disorder. *Biological Psychiatry.*

Nemiah, J. C. (1989). Janet redivivus [editorial]. *American Journal of Psychiatry, 146,* 1527–1529.

Nemiah, J. C. (1991). Dissociation, conversion, and somatization. In A. Tasman & A. Goldfinger (Eds.), *American Psychiatric Press Review of psychiatry* (Vol. 10, pp. 248–260). Washington, DC: American Psychiatric Press.

Nemiah, J. C. (1995). Early concepts of trauma, dissociation and the unconscious: Their history and current implications. In D. Bremner & C. Marmar (Eds.), *Trauma, memory and dissociation*. Washington, DC: American Psychiatric Press.

Pattison, E. M., & Kahan, J. (1983). The deliberate self-harm syndrome. *American Journal of Psychiatry, 140,* 867–872.

Pearlman, L. A., & Saakvitne, K. W. (1995). *Trauma and the therapist.* New York: Norton.

Pennebaker, J. W. (1993). Putting stress into words: Health, linguistic, and therapeutic implications. *Behaviour Research and Therapy, 31*(6), 539–548.

Pitman, R. K., & Orr, S. (1990). The black hole of trauma. *Biological Psychiatry, 26,* 469–471.

Pitman, R. K., Orr, S., & Shalev, A. (1993). Once bitten, twice shy: Beyond the conditioning model of PTSD. *Biological Psychiatry, 33,* 145–146.

Post, R. M. (1992). Transduction of psychosocial stress into the neurobiology of recurrent affective disorder. *American Journal of Psychiatry, 149,* 999–1010.

Reiker, P. P., & Carmen, E. H. (1986). The victim-to-patient process: The disconfirmation and transformation of abuse. *American Journal of Orthopsychiatry, 56,* 360–370.

Rieder, C., & Cicchetti, D. (1989). An organizational perspective on cognitive control functioning and cognitive–affective balance in maltreated children. *Developmental Psychology, 25,* 482–493.

Russell, D. (1986). *The secret trauma.* New York: Basic Books.

Saxe, G. N., van der Kolk, B. A., Berkowitz, R., Chinman, G., Hall, K., Lieberg, G., & Schwartz, J. (1993). Dissociative disorders in psychiatric inpatients. *American Journal of Psychiatry, 150,* 1037–1042.

Seghorn, T. K., Boucher, R. J., & Prentky, R. A. (1987). Childhood sexual abuse in the lives of sexually aggressive offenders. *Journal of the American Academy of Child and Adolescent Psychiatry, 26,* 262–267.

Shapiro, D. (1965). *Neurotic styles.* New York: Basic Books.

Silbert, M. H., & Pines, A. M. (1981). Sexual child abuse as an antecedent to prostitution. *Bulletin of the Menninger Clinic, 45,* 428–438.

Simpson, C. A., & Porter, G. L. (1981). Self-mutilation in children and adolescents. *Bulletin of the Menninger Clinic, 45,* 428–438.

Spiegel, D. (1992). Effects of psychosocial support on patients with metastatic breast cancer. *Journal of Psychosocial Oncology, 10,* 113–120.

Tank, D. W., & Hopfield, J. J. (1987). Collective computation in neuronlike circuits. *Scientific American, 257,* 104–114.

Titchener, J. L. (1986). Post-traumatic decline: A consequence of unresolved destructive drives. In C. Figley (Ed.), *Trauma and its wake* (Vol. 2, pp. 5–19). New York: Brunner/Mazel.

Tuchman, B. (1978). *A distant mirror.* New York: Knopf.

van der Hart, O., Steele, K., Boon, S., & Brown, P. (1993). The treatment of traumatic memories: Synthesis, realization, and integration. *Dissociation, 6,* 162–180.

van der Kolk, B. A. (1989). The compulsion to repeat trauma: Revictimization, attachment and masochism. *Psychiatric Clinics of North America, 12,* 389–411.

van der Kolk, B. A., Dreyfuss, D., Michaels, M., Shera, D., Berkowitz, R., Fisler, R., & Saxe, G. (1994). Fluoxetine in posttraumatic stress disorder. *Journal of Clinical Psychiatry, 55*(12), 517–522.

van der Kolk, B. A., & Ducey, C. (1989). The psychological processing of traumatic experience: Rorschach patterns in PTSD. *Journal of Traumatic Stress*, 2(3), 259–274.

van der Kolk, B. A., & Fisler, R. (1994). Childhood abuse and neglect and loss of self-regulation. *Bulletin of the Menninger Clinic*, *58*, 145–168.

van der Kolk, B. A., & Fisler, R. (1995). Dissociation and the fragmentary nature of traumatic memories: Overview and exploratory study. *Journal of Traumatic Stress*, *9*, 505–525.

van der Kolk, B. A., Greenberg, M., Boyd, H., & Krystal, J. (1985). Inescapable shock, neurotransmitters, and addiction to trauma: Toward a psychobiology of post-traumatic stress. *Biological Psychiatry*, *20*, 314–325.

van der Kolk, B. A., Pelcovitz, D., Roth, S., Mandel, F. S., McFarlane, A. C., & Herman, J. L. (in press). Dissociation, affect dysregulation and somatization. *American Journal of Psychiatry*.

van der Kolk, B. A., Perry, C., & Herman, J. L. (1991). Childhood origins of self-destructive behavior. *American Journal of Psychiatry*, *148*, 1665–1671.

van der Kolk, B. A., Roth, S., Pelcovitz, D., & Mandel, F. (1993). *Disorders of extreme stress: Results of the DSM-IV Field Trials for PTSD*. Washington, DC: American Psychiatric Association.

Wilson, J. P., & Lindy, J. D. (Eds.). (1994). *Countertransference in the treatment of PTSD*. New York: Guilford Press.

Yehuda, R., Keefe, R. S. E., Harvey, P. D., Levengood, R. A., Gerber, D. K., Geni, J., & Siever, L. J. (1995). Learning and memory in combat veterans with posttraumatic stress disorder. *American Journal of Psychiatry*, *152*, 137–139.

CHAPTER 2

Trauma and Its Challenge to Society

ALEXANDER C. McFARLANE
BESSEL A. VAN DER KOLK

Shell shock. How many a brief bombardment had its long-delayed after-effect in the minds of these survivors. Not then was their evil hour, but now; now, in the sweating suffocation of nightmare, in paralysis of limbs, in the stammering of dislocated speech. In the name of civilisation these soldiers had been martyred, and it remained for civilisation to prove that their martyrdom wasn't a dirty swindle.
—SIEGFRIED SASSOON (QUOTED IN FUSSELL, 1983, p. 141)

People have always gathered in communities and organizations for aid in dealing with outside challenges. They seek close emotional relationships with others in order to help them anticipate, meet, and integrate difficult experiences. Emotional attachment is probably the primary protection against feelings of helplessness and meaninglessness; it is essential for biological survival in children, and without it, existential meaning is unthinkable in adults. For young children, the family is usually a very effective source of protection against traumatization, and most children are amazingly resilient as long as they have a caregiver who is emotionally and physically available (Werner, 1989; McFarlane, 1988). Mature people also rely on their families, colleagues, and friends to provide such a protective membrane. In recognition of this need for affiliation as a protection against trauma, it is widely accepted that the central issue in disaster management is the provision and restoration of social support (see Chapter 20, this volume).

Societies are in large part defined by their different norms regarding the mutual obligations between individuals and their surroundings; as a result, different societies foster different ways of coping with traumatizing experiences (see Chapter 17, this volume). Regardless of the relative value a society places on individualism or conformity, there seems to be a universal tendency for people under threat to form very close attachments to other people or communities. Freud (1926/1959) observed that the more terrifying the external threat, the stronger the allegiance to the group becomes; under extreme conditions, such as war, people may go so far as to sacrifice their own lives in order to assure survival of the group. Ernest Becker (1973) called the resulting deep sense of belonging "the taming of terror." In analogy to Freud's notion that trauma results in a rupture in the "membrane of the mind" (1919/1921), Lindy and Titchener (1983) have called the social support that surrounds victims "the trauma membrane."

When people's own resources are depleted, outside help needs to be mobilized to compensate for their helplessness (Hobfoll & deVries, 1995). During acute trauma, the social environment tends to respond with generosity; from tribal mourning ceremonies to Red Cross disaster relief, every society seems to have evolved social and religious structures that are geared to helping acutely distressed people until they can resume looking after themselves. External validation about the reality of a traumatic experience in a safe and supportive context is a vital aspect of preventing and treating posttraumatic stress. However, the creation of such a context for recovery can become very complicated when the psychological needs of victims and the needs of their social network conflict. When victims' helplessness persists (as in chronic posttraumatic stress disorder [PTSD]), or when the meaning of the trauma is secret, forbidden, or unacceptable (as in intrafamilial abuse or government-sanctioned violence), the trauma is unlikely to result in the mobilization of external resources, in restitution, or in the meting out of justice. Because of the lack of validation and support, traumatic memories are more likely to continue to prey on the victims' minds, and to be expressed as anger, withdrawal, or otherwise disrupted and disrupting behaviors.

RELIGION, COMMUNITY, AND TRAUMA

One core function of human societies is to provide their members with traditions, institutions, and value systems that can protect them against becoming overwhelmed by stressful experiences. Religion fulfills the critical function of providing a sense of purpose in the face of terrifying realities by placing suffering in a larger context and by affirming the commonality of suffering across generations, time, and space. Thus, religion can help people transcend their inbeddedness in their individual suffering. The principal feature that distinguishes one religion from another is the particular solution to the uncontrollability of life's experiences that each one offers. However, after having been traumatized, only a minority of victims seem to escape the notion that their pain, betrayal, and loss are meaningless. For many, this realization is one of the most painful lessons that the trauma brings; they often feel godforsaken and betrayed by their fellow human beings. Usually, suffering does not bring an increased sense of love and meaning; rather, it results in loneliness and disintegration of belief. Some traumatized people deal with their encounter with unpredictability and meaninglessness by converting to fundamentalist political or religious sects that have rigid codes of behavior, exclusionary criteria for belonging, and a designated group of outsiders who embody evil (see Chapter 17).

The very notion that PTSD occurs as a normal response to an abnormal condition would imply that, ordinarily, people can have control over their fate—a decidedly optimistic position. This belief that individuals can control their own destinies seems to be a relatively recent development. It is likely that the decline of religion is a function of a rise in the apparent predictability of life, which is accompanied by the hope that human beings can be in charge of their own future without divine assistance. Eastern religions, in particular, do not hold out the promise to their followers that they will be able to control their destiny; both Hinduism and Islam teach that life is entirely determined by fate and that one has to submit oneself to the gods' or Allah's will. Since no comparative scientific work has been done on the relative prevalence of PTSD in areas of the world where these religions have a large following, no information is available on how such religious beliefs shape people's responses to trauma.

THE NATURE OF TRAUMA: THE CRITICAL ISSUE OF MEANING

Victims of trauma often become subjects of passionate concern in those around them—concern that may have no direct connection to their actual well-being. Often voiceless about their innermost fears, and accustomed to life happening *to* them, victims of trauma are vulnerable to being used for a variety of political and social ends, both for good and ill; they can be nurtured and idealized, or just as easily spurned, stigmatized, and rejected. Solomon (1995) has described how, between 1947 and 1982, Israeli society moved from the latter to the former position in its attitude to Holocaust survivors, without ever resting in the middle of the continuum by treating them as fellow human beings who had been exposed to the unspeakable.

The personal meaning of traumatic experience for individuals is influenced by the social context in which it occurs. Victims and the significant people in their surroundings may have different and fluctuating assessments of both the reality of what has happened and of the extent of the victims' suffering. As a result, victims and bystanders may have strongly conflicting agendas to repair, create, forget, or take revenge. These conflicts between the victims' and the bystanders' assessment of the meaning of the trauma may set the stage for the trauma to be perpetuated in a larger social setting; soon the allocation of blame and responsibility, not the trauma itself, may become the central issue.

Traumas provoke emotional reactions in proportion to the degree of threat and horror accompanying them. One way of dealing with these intense emotions is to look for scapegoats who can be held responsible for the tragic event. Family members and other sources of social support can be so horrified at being reminded of the fact that they, too, can be struck by tragedies beyond their control that they start shunning the victims and blame them for what has happened—a phenomenon that has been called "the second injury" (Symonds, 1982). Many personal testimonies of trauma survivors indicate that not being supported by the people they counted on, and being blamed for bringing horrendous experiences upon themselves, have left deeper scars than the traumatic event itself (e.g., Lifton, 1983). Victims often feel the same way about themselves: They feel ashamed and disgusted by their failure to prevent what has happened. Thus, for many victims, a breach in their relationship to their expectations of themselves and of their culture becomes part of the traumatic experience.

Ironically, both the victims of PTSD, and the larger society that is asked to respond with compassion, forbearance, or financial sacrifices, have a stake in believing that the trauma is not really the cause of the victims' suffering. On the one hand, society becomes resentful about having its illusions of safety and predictability ruffled by people who remind them of how fragile security can be. On the other hand, many victims suffer from an impaired capacity to translate their intense emotions and perceptions related to the trauma into communicable language. Not being able to give a coherent account of the trauma to others, or even to themselves, without feeling traumatized all over again makes it difficult for them to articulate their needs (see Chapters 12 and 13, this volume). The combination of the wish of the bystanders not to be disturbed by the raw emotions of injured people, and the problems of victims in articulating what they feel and need, can make it extremely difficult for the victims to stay focused on working through the impact of the trauma. Because the victims cannot make clear-cut statements that convey the reality of what has happened, traumatic memories start leading a life of their own as disturbing symptoms (e.g., Langer, 1990), and the victims become patients.

When the memories of the trauma remain unprocessed, traumatized individuals tend to become like Pavlov's dogs: Subtle reminders become conditioned stimuli for the reexperiencing of frightening feelings and perceptions belonging to the past. In addition, actual injuries may leave a legacy of physical pain and suffering. If loved ones have been killed, grief adds to the trauma, so that victims are caught between wishing to avoid the memory of the horror and feeling that they need to be living memorials for the lost persons and world. After interpersonal violence, such as domestic abuse and rape, the sadism of perpetrators can radically disturb victims' sense of trust; even the prospect of emotional and physical intimacy may become a reminder of horror, shame, and fear. Many victims cope with their exquisite sensitivity by organizing their lives around not seeing, feeling, or participating in life on an emotional level. Many of them plunge into their work—the area of life in which they may feel least vulnerable. In the Grant Study, a 50-year study of Harvard men from the 1940s to the 1990s, the men who developed PTSD after World War II were much more likely to be listed in *Who's Who in America* than their nontraumatized peers (Lee, Vaillant, Torrey, & Elder, 1995). However, even professional success cannot compensate for the deeply held feeling of many victims that they no longer fit in, that they are aliens belonging to a lost world.

INDIVIDUAL VERSUS SOCIETAL RESPONSIBILITY

Society's reactions to traumatized people are rarely the results of objective and rational assessments. Rather, they are primarily the results of conservative impulses in the service of maintaining the belief that the world is essentially just, that "good" people are in charge of their lives, and that bad things only happen to "bad" people. Although people are capable of profound bursts of spontaneous generosity to victims of acute trauma, the continued presence of the victims as victims constitutes an insult to the belief (at least in the Western world) that human beings are essentially the masters of their fate. Victims are the members of society whose problems represent the memory of suffering, rage, and pain in a world that longs to forget.

Since the effects of trauma touch on the fundamental social issue of individual responsibility, it is very difficult to remain emotionally neutral when working with traumatized individuals. As Judith Herman (1992) put it,

> To study psychological trauma is to come face to face both with human vulnerability in the natural world and with the capacity for evil in human nature. To study psychological trauma means bearing witness to horrible events. When the traumatic events are of human design, those who bear witness are caught in the conflict between the victim and the perpetrator. It is morally impossible to remain neutral in this conflict. The bystander is forced to take sides. It is very tempting to take the side of the perpetrator. All the perpetrator asks is that the bystander do nothing. He appeals to the universal desire to see, hear and speak no evil. The victim, on the contrary, asks the bystander to share the burden or pain. The victim demands action,

engagement and remembering. After every atrocity one can expect to hear the same predictable apologies: it never happened, the victim lies, the victim exaggerates, the victim brought it on herself and in any case there is time to forget the past and move on. The more powerful the perpetrator, the greater is his prerogative to name and define reality and the more completely his arguments prevail. In the absence of strong political movements for human rights, the active process of bearing witness inevitably gives way to the active process of forgetting. Repression, dissociation and denial are phenomena of a social as well as individual consciousness. (p. 8)

The issue of responsibility, individual and shared, is at the very core of how a society defines itself. Will the inescapably traumatic events that befall its members become a shared moral and financial burden, or will victims be held responsible and left to fend for themselves? Do people have the right to expect support when their own resources are insufficient, or do they have to live with their suffering and not expect any particular compensation for their pain? Are people encouraged to attend to their pain (and learn from the past), or should they cultivate a "stiff upper lip" and refrain from reflecting on the meaning of their experience? Clearly, both individuals and societies that become too focused on the past lose the flexibility they need to respond to the future. Conversely, individuals and societies without coherent myths about having successfully transcended adversity lack the identity necessary to serve as a guide on how to structure responses to current challenges. Although traumatized individuals and societies may benefit from acknowledging and coming to terms with past trauma through shared rituals and days of remembrance, they too may become fixated on revenge or compensation, at the expense of endurance and individual initiative (see Chapter 17).

Robert Hughes (1993) has eloquently argued in *The Culture of Complaint* that trauma and victimization can become overinclusive explanations that prevent uncomfortable self-examination. This is true for both individuals and societies. A nation such as Kuwait, which was occupied by an aggressive neighbor, may exploit the trauma by attributing a host of social problems solely to the widespread upheaval, destruction, and torture that occurred. Failure to identify the many different factors that are responsible for changes in individual and social attitudes undermines the development of effective strategies to address the individual and collective adaptation to trauma.

The complexity of the issue of social support is illustrated by the finding that, after suffering from heart attacks, men with good social support and a good internal locus of control did much better than men who had neither, but that men with good social supports and a poor internal locus of control did worse than those with poor social support but a solid internal locus of control (Kobasa & Puccetti, 1982). This suggests that social support in the absence of an internal locus of control may in fact *impair* healing processes. Since trauma is known to decrease victims' internal locus of control (see Chapter 5, this volume), the critical question becomes this: What is the optimal amount of social support that will restore a sense of self-efficacy?

Thus, whereas research has shown that adequate social support is one important protector against the development of trauma-related disorders (see Chapters 8 and 20, this volume), Kobasa and Puccetti's work suggests that social support does not necessarily result in a better outcome than no social support at all. The efficacy of social support depends, a least in part, on the amount of comfort that individual victims derive from it and the extent to which it motivates them to take charge of their lives again. This issue is further complicated by the fact that, regardless of the level of support offered, the denial of the posttraumatic probems of victims carries the risk of perpetuating trauma-related behavior, such as violence against self and others, lack of attention to tasks at hand, and poor personal and occupational functioning.

Since the collapse of Communism, the issue of society's willingness and capacity to provide support to the disadvantaged has become the subject of intense public reassessment in the industrialized world. After a gradually increasing social commitment to shared responsibility since the end of World War II in both Europe and North America, the collapse of the Iron Curtain has inspired a reexamination of the distribution of society's resources, including their allocation to traumatized, ill, and otherwise disdvantaged individuals. After half a century of emphasis on promoting social security, social Darwinism, in its current form of economic rationalism, argues that competition and survival of the fittest constitute a superior organizing dynamic for society, and that deprivation will foster creative adaptations. This frame of reference proposes that the care of helpless people interferes actively with their taking responsibility for their lives. Although in this new world of social Darwinism victims no longer demand the commitment to rehabilitation and alleviation of their suffering, they continue to fulfill a useful function: The more their plight differs from our own, the more secure we can feel about the notion that bad things only happen to "bad" people, or to people who are somehow genetically impaired.

Alarmingly, the need to ignore the reality of trauma in people's lives also pervades medical school departments of psychiatry, where the response to increasing levels of traumatization in society has generally been to ignore it. As was the case during previous pandemics of violence in society, the study of trauma and of its impact on the development of psychopathology runs the danger of becoming marginalized again (see Chapter 3, this volume). Medical students and psychiatric residents learn exhaustively about relatively obscure illnesses such as Huntington's chorea and obsessive–compulsive disorder (OCD), which do not confront them with the problems related to abuse and violence, while trauma-related disorders receive scant attention. This neglect is illustrated by the following: In 1992, 2,936,000 children in the United States were reported to have been abused and/or neglected (National Victim Center, 1993), and a substantial proportion of these are likely to develop trauma-related psychiatric disorders (see Chapters 9 and 14, this volume). However, as of the beginning of 1996, there was precisely one published controlled psychopharmacological study of the treatment of PTSD in children in the entire world literature (Famularo, Kinscherff, & Fenton, 1988). By contrast, in the past decade there have been 13 controlled studies on the psychopharmacological treatment of children with OCD, and 36 on the treatment of children with attention-deficit/hyperactivity disorder (ADHD). This latter disorder is of particular interest, since it has a high degree of comorbidity with PTSD. For example, Putnam (1994) found that of a sample of sexually abused girls, 28% met diagnostic criteria for ADHD, compared with 4% of a nontraumatized control group. Yet in none of these 36 studies on children with ADHD did the investigators measure past histories of trauma, comorbidity with PTSD, or the effects of the pharmacological agent studied on trauma-related symptomatology.

THE REENACTMENT OF TRAUMA IN SOCIETY

Central to the role of victims of crimes, wars, and accidents in any given society are the demands that they place on the community's moral and financial resources. Contrary to general perceptions, few victims make shrill demands for compensation and special privileges. Many victims quietly acquiesce in their suffering; they are contained by their sense of shame and helplessness, as well as a need to maintain their self-respect and independence. Others noisily reenact their traumas by either retraumatizing themselves or traumatizing other human beings, both inside and outside their own families (see Chapters 1 and 9, this volume).

Most victims who are conscious of the effects of trauma on their lives preserve their self-protective instincts and are highly ambivalent about having people find out what has happened to them. For example, rape victims are usually aware that they run a great risk of not being believed, of being blamed, and of having their sexuality exposed and scrutinized. Publicly admitting the reality of domestic violence can be made difficult or impossible by shame about not being loved by one's spouse, about being unable to protect oneself and one's children, about failing to bring security and happiness to one's family, and about acknowledging one's physical and financial powerlessness. In domestic and in dating relationships, the lines between appropriate trust and carelessness or failure to protect oneself are particularly difficult to draw. In recent years, some feminist groups have sought to introduce stringent rules for dating relationships, which such critics as Camille Paglia (1994) consider "condescending paternalism about victim-oriented social welfare workers" (p. 208). She adds, "Feminism has got to look honestly at the animal savagery and lust in all of us and stop blaming men for the darkness of the human condition" (p. 136).

The question of where to place the locus of responsibiity for self-protection is at the heart of the passions that PTSD stirs up in social debates. Intimate violence may entail conspiracies of silence; true and false accusations; and failures to take responsibility for violent, provocative, and humiliating behavior. Fear of abandonment is a central element in domestic violence: Violent partners attempt to control their families by inspiring fear; attachment to an abuser may override the urge to escape; and expectations of not being able to take care of oneself, or of not being believed, may cause a victim to be unable to consider alternatives (van der Kolk, 1989; Dutton & Painter, 1993). Many battered women and abused children are brought to emergency rooms with tissue damage and broken bones, only to make up cover stories to protect their abusers—usually much to the relief of the medical personnel, who then may feel excused from having to become involved in "other people's messes." Disclosing being a victim (or a perpetrator) involves confronting the shame associated with the relationship. Acknowledgment of the violence and of its impact on one's life demands being able to consider giving up the relationship and going on without it. Given these confusing realities, it is understandable that in recent years many health insurers have tried to refuse to cover women who are victims of domestic violence (no such limitations have been proposed for perpetrators of domestic abuse).

If memories of child abuse, domestic violence, wars, and torture are not worked through, they tend to be expressed as irrational symptoms—behaviors that represent derivativations of unresolved aspects of the trauma. People who have lived for long periods of time in abusive environments may never have learned, or may have forgotten, the rules of civilized conduct. The confusion and helplessness of many victims are expressed in passivity and failure to take responsibility. Patterns of fear and dissociation may interfere with the capacity to articulate feelings and wishes. When traumatized individuals feel threatened, their attitudes are often marked by fear of abandonment, expressed in pathetic compliance with their abusers. Their passivity may make them unable to recognize the role that they play in the continuation of their abuse. This passivity and helplessness may alternate with outbursts of rage and resentment, in which they seem to be unaware of the effects of their emotional displays and threats on other people. Neither the passivity nor the intimidation leaves room for mutuality and responsiveness to other people's needs.

Since both victims and bystanders experience intense emotions when confronted with these behaviors, they are likely to lose sight of the fact that they are rooted in past trauma. Instead, both will construct complex rationales to justify their reactions: elaborate grievances, in the case of the victims, and diagnostic constructs that invariably come to have a pejorative meaning, in the case of the bystanders. These grievances and diagnoses are designed to return a sense of control to the parties involved; ironically, however, both are likely to perpetuate the trauma in the interpersonal realm, which is dichotomized in terms of dominance and submission. After the breakdown of a healthy balance between collaboration and self-protective reserve, the resulting polarities assure that one person or group will be seen as powerful and the other as helpless. The trauma will thus continue to be played out between helpless supplicants/victims/caregivers and predators/manipulators/oppressors. Calling victims "survivors" is a euphemism that denies the reality of these dichotomies of powerlessness.

THE BENEFITS AND PRICE OF PROTECTION

Trauma may act as a catalyst for social change: By giving voice to their own misery, many social critics, political leaders, and artists have been able to transform their trauma into a way of helping other people. For example, Germaine Greer (1989), in describing her father's PTSD after World War II, wrote:

> When [the medical officers] examined men exhibiting severe disturbances they almost invariably found that the root cause [lay] in pre-war experience, mostly "domestic": the sick men were not first-grade fighting material. . . . The military proposition is [that it is] not war which makes men sick, but that sick men can not fight wars. The authorities compounded their distress by accusing them of fear. They were actually too tired and dispirited to feel fear. (pp. 327–328)

Greer's childhood exposure to and struggle to come to grips with her father's suffering prepared her to describe the consequences of sexual domination (in its ugly manifestations of rape, incest, and domestic violence) in her adult work. Similarly, many resistance leaders of World War II became leaders who were dedicated to the unification of Europe during the next half century. Anthony Eden and Harold Macmillan, both of whom were veterans of the trenches of France, became the Conservative prime ministers who were committed to the establishment of social security in the United Kingdom. Thus, although first-hand experience with trauma leads to personal suffering, it can be sublimated into social or artistic action and thus can serve as a powerful agent for social change.

Failure to deal with the plight of victims can be disastrous for a society. The costs of the reenactment of trauma in society, in the form of child abuse, continued violence, and lack of productivity, are staggering. Failure to face the reality of trauma may have devastating political consequences as well. For example, in the aftermath of World War I, the inability to face its effects on the capacity of the veterans to function effectively in society, and the social intolerance of their "weakness," may have substantially contributed to the subsequent rise of Fascism and militarism (see Chapter 3). The impossible war reparations of the Treaty of Versailles, motivated by a lust for revenge by the Allies, humiliated an already humiliated Germany. The German nation, in turn, dealt mercilessly with its own war veterans, who were accused of being moral invalids. This cascade of humiliations of the powerless set the stage for the ultimate debasement of human rights under the Nazi regime, the extermination of the weak and the different, and the moral justification for the subjugation of "inferior" people—the rationale for the ensuing war.

After World War II, somehow, the people in power learned their lesson after the defeat of Nazi Germany and imperial Japan: The United States massively helped the defeated nations by means of the Marshall Plan, which formed the economic foundation of the next 50 years of relative world peace. At home, the same spirit of generosity spawned the GI Bill, which gave millions of veterans educations that promoted general economic well-being by creating a broad-based, well-educated middle class. At the same time, the new Veterans Administration began building facilities throughout the country to help combat veterans with their health needs. Interestingly, however, with all this thoughtful attention to the returning veteran, no attention was paid to the psychological scars of war, and traumatic neuroses rapidly disappeared from the official psychiatric nomenclature. In 1982 one of us (van der Kolk) did a survey of over 300 World War II veterans in a medical outpatient clinic of a Veterans Administration hospital, and found that 85% of the patients suffered from PTSD but that none had a psychiatric diagnosis noted in their charts.

In order to move beyond trauma, people, institutions, and societies need to take adaptive action. A problem-solving approach is essential for such action, and excessive introspection may interfere with rebuilding (see Chapter 5). However, not looking back may keep victimized individuals and groups from learning from experience. Lack of awareness of the meaning of one's actions sometimes makes it difficult to draw the line between restorative action and actions that recreate the trauma. This may be true on both an individual and on a societal level. An all-too-common example was provided by Pelcovitz et al. (1995), who found that a group of traumatized adolescents minimized the effects of their severe physical abuse on their lives, but that they habitually engaged in predatory or victimized relationships with their peers, without awareness of the consequences of their actions.

When dealing with traumatized individuals who (or communities that) deal with their feelings through action, professionals and policy makers need, on the one hand, to respect the natural desire to take action to overcome posttraumatic helplessness, and on the other, to help people find ways of communicating about the dangers of recreating their traumas in new social contexts. When taking action fails to prevent the return of the trauma in feelings, images, or social interactions, both individuals and communities need to acknowledge the reality of what has happened and the pain associated with it.

Confronting the past is a delicate enterprise that should occur only with trusted people or institutions, since there is always a serious risk that the exposure of hurt will not be met with a constructive response, and that a call for help will be turned into a blaming of the victim.

SOCIAL ISOLATION VERSUS INTEGRATION

Reason and objectivity are not the primary determinants of society's reactions to traumatized people. Rather, as noted earlier, society's reactions seem to be primarily conservative impulses in the service of maintaining the beliefs that the world is fundamentally just, that people can be in charge of their lives, and that bad things only happen to people who deserve them. Bearers of bad tidings are generally considered dangerous; thus, societies tend to be suspicious that victims will contaminate the social fabric, undermine self-reliance, consume social resources, and live off the strong. The weak are a liability, and, after an initial period of compassion, are vulnerable to being singled out as parasites and carriers of social malaise. Society can only make a commitment to victims if it accepts these two ideas: (1) that victims are not responsible for the fact that they were traumatized; and (2) that if victims are not helped to deal with the memories of their trauma, they will become violent and anxious people, unreliable and easily distracted workers, inattentive parents, and/or people who use drugs and alcohol to help them cope with unbearable feelings.

The issue of blame is extraordinarily complicated. Research has repeatedly demonstrated that once people are traumatized, they are liable to be traumatized again. This notion is strongly supported by Russell's (1986) research, as well as by that of Breslau, Davis, and Andreski (1995): Once traumatized, people often lose their hold on self-protection and are prone to put themselves in harm's way. The issue of revictimization has enormous consequences for social policy. Is it possible to create a society in which victims can be given their due and protected against further harm? Have the welfare states of social democratic northern Europe been effective in preventing cycles of violence? And if they have, has this occurred at the expense of fostering initiative in the most motivated individuals in society? In the United States, have Head Start and similar efforts prevented cycles of violence through early intervention, or have all these programs been failed experiments in social engineering? Is it better to invest in school programs, day care centers, and other forms of early intervention, or should society's resources be invested in larger police departments and in the building of jails for offenders, whose temporary removal from the gene pool might make the rest of society safer? Do these questions present legitimate dichotomies? The answers to these questions are well beyond the scope of this volume, but they are researchable questions. Whatever answers policy makers and the electorate come up with will have a major impact on the amount of trauma that members of any given society are confronted with, as well as on the fate of trauma's victims.

Clinical work has taught us that the ability to tolerate the plight of victims is, at least in part, a function of how well people have dealt with their own misfortunes. When they have confronted the reality of their own hurt and suffering, and accepted their own pain, this generally is translated into tolerance and sometimes even compassion for others. Conversely, as long as people deny the impact of their own personal trauma and pretend that it did not matter, that it was not so bad, or that excuses can be made for their abusers, they are likely to identify with the aggressors and treat others with the same harshness with which they treat the wounded parts of themselves. Identification with the aggressor makes it possible to bypass empathy for themselves and secondarily for others.

THE "FALSE MEMORY" DEBATE

Providing reparation is part of the recognition that someone has been hurt. This raises difficult questions in forensic and psychiatric settings, where victims invite bystanders to pay attention to the issue of blame. On the assumption that wrongful accusation is more socially dangerous than not providing recourse for victims, the legal system requires strict rules of evidence against accused perpetrators. The "false memory" debate goes to the very heart of the principles of social justice, with both sides claiming the moral high ground. Victims have become the (by and large voiceless) bystanders in this acrimonious debate about whether traumatic memories can be trusted as accurate. Advocates on both sides of the debate frequently draw analogies to the Salem witch trials to demonstrate the dangers of miscarriage of justice, of suggestibility, and of false accusations. With the increasing suspicion (and an absence of scientific evidence) that many of their traumatic memories are "implanted" by their therapists, victims are readily suspected of making false accusations, whereas perpetrators are given the benefit of the doubt and may escape appropriate punishment. In the current political climate, it is more acceptable to trust the recollections of parents with documented histories of alcoholism and blackouts than of sober men and women who seek treatment for their intrusive images of past horrors.

In recent years, a few people have taken their alleged abusers to court after having become aware of their memories of sexual abuse, and a handful of accused perpetrators have been convicted. If the media are to be believed, this is a problem of epidemic proportions, but scrutiny of the court records of the Commonwealth of Masachusetts would suggest that these court cases are extremely rare, compared with the actual incidence of childhood sexual abuse. For example, in 1993 the Department of Social Services in Massachusetts substantiated 2,149 cases of sexual abuse; about 400 men were in jail for sexual offenses against children, and 575 were out on probation. Between 1990 and 1994, a total of four cases were tried in Massachusetts in which adults took alleged abusers to court after recovering traumatic memories. One of these cases was a celebrated case of a priest who was convicted of sexually molesting 155 children.

The "false memory" movement claims that thousands of unsuspecting white middle-class women go to therapists who implant false memories of abuse in their minds. However, current research shows that (1) there is no evidence that traumatic memories can be simply implanted in people's minds; (2) retrieving memories of forgotten traumatic memories is as common in men as in women, and is not more common in people who are in psychotherapy as in those who are not; (3) that posttraumatic amnesia is not a function of social class; and (4) that the rate of total amnesia following a traumatic experience is three times as high for Hispanics and twice as high for African-Americans as it is for whites (Elliot & Briere, 1994). Most cases of sexual abuse probably go unreported and never come to the attention of either mental health professionals or the legal system. Child custody issues greatly complicate the issue of false accusation, since they provide a motive for making them: Schetky and Green (1988) estimate that as many as 25% of sexual abuse allegations in child custody cases are false.

Although the occurrence of delayed memories following just about every conceivable form of trauma has consistently been documented for well over a century (see Chapter 12), there are considerable complications regarding the accuracy of these retrieved memories. One contributing factor is that traumatic memories have a fragmentary sensory quality, and the narrative that victims construct to account for these imprints is a function of the developmental level at which the trauma occurred and is subject to social demands. As in a similar debate a century ago (see Chapter 3), the campaign about these issues has focused on the problems of uncovering repressed memories and the problems of suggestibility.

The "false memory" debate illustrates, on the one hand, that people who attempt to lift the veil of the secrets of domestic abuse can be retraumatized by being subjected to intense suspicions; and, on the other, that careful attention needs to be paid to preventing false accusations of abuse. After all, being accused of such a heinous crime itself constitutes a traumatic experience with immeasurable consequences. There has recently been an increasing public backlash about accusations of sexual abuse. Accused parents and an advisory board of experts have set up a highly effective advocacy organization called the False Memory Syndrome Foundation, which aims to discredit the accounts of adults who claim to have been sexually abused as children. This organization claims that there is an epidemic of false accusations created by psychotherapists, whom they call the "recovered memory movement." The basis of this organization's existence is the claim that there exists a "false memory syndrome" that is produced by inappropriate techniques used by therapists working with highly suggestible patients. To date, there is no scientific evidence for the existence of such a syndrome. However, there is no dispute about the fact that some psychotherapists tend to reduce most psychological problems in their patients to childhood histories of sexual abuse—just as there are numerous mental health professionals who ignore the relevance of childhood abuse in the genesis of psychiatric problems, and who dismiss the clinical importance of the vast research literature on its devastating effects on further personality development.

The issue of true and false accusations of sexual abuse is extremely emotive because of the enormous distress that these memories cause in victims, and the disruptions that accusations of abuse create both for people who are justifiably accused and for falsely accused parents. In reaction, the False Memory group has called for the passage of Consumer Mental Health Protection Act (CMHPA) in several states—legislation that would declare "memory retrieval therapy" a felony. This proposed legisation has pitted the accused parents against professional organizations such as the American Psychological Association, whose Council of Representatives concluded that "on closer inspection [the CMHPA] contain[s] many provisions that will actually harm consumers and curtail the availability of quality services," and that "while seeming to protect the consumer, [the CMHPA] actually creates a bureaucracy and unnecessary barriers that interfere with consumer access to mental health services" (Director of Legal and Regulatory Affairs, 1995).

Although psychotherapists have taken most of the heat in this debate, the legal process has become embroiled in it as the final social arbiter on these matters. The adversarial environment of the courtroom, which promotes accusation and counterclaims, is less than an ideal forum for the resolution for the questions at stake. The highly publicized court cases have further obscured the fact that the issue of "repressed memories" is only relevant to a relatively small proportion of sexual abuse cases (see Chapter 12). It would be most unfortunate if the legitimate concern with the predicament of the wrongfully accused were to obscure concern with the real damage caused by childhood abuse.

The "false memory" debate has further polarized opinions between "believers" and "skeptics" about the reality of the significance of traumatic stress; the clinical and scientific questions are increasingly being lost in the heat of the argument. Given the estimate by the U.S. Department of Justice that every year 250,000 children are sexually abused, perpetrators have a significant interest in sweeping the effects of abuse and molestation under the rug. Moreover, it is not necessarily only people who run child prostitution rings, pedophiles, rapists, and child and spouse abusers who have a vital interest in denying the reality of the impact of trauma. Powerful social institutions such as insurance companies and the armed forces, for whom enormous amounts of money are at stake for damage claims and insurance reimbursements, also benefit from downplaying the impact of trauma on people's lives. Unfortunately, the multifaceted interest in denying the reality of trauma is so powerful, the fear of being taken advantage of is so deep, and the human need to find specific individuals and organizations to blame for our ills is so pervasive that this debate is unlikely ever to be driven primarily by attention to the facts.

THE LEGACIES OF TRAUMA IN SOCIETY

As noted earlier, victims often find themselves trapped by their tendency to recreate their traumatic past. This compulsion to repeat is graphically illustrated by victims of child sexual abuse, whom Kluft (1991) has described as "sitting ducks" for further victimization. Many traumatized individuals organize their lives around a core conflict between a fear of revictimization and a need for external reassurance. These anxieties and demands can provoke angry, dismissive, or even outright sadistic responses in the professionals to whom victims turn for redress and protection. Their conveying an extraordinary sense of helplessness, or behaving with extreme aggression, is likely to result in their being victimized over and over again. For the professionals entrusted with the care of people who have been traumatized, the emotional tight rope between empathy, rage, and helplessness means that dealing with them can be extraordinarily draining. Professionals all too readily get caught in the roles of rescuers or persecutors, both of which are likely to result ultimately in a repetition of the trauma (see Chapter 9). Relationships with victims require therapists to have a continual awareness of their own subjective reactions and their need to defend themselves against the tidings conveyed by their traumatized fellow men and women who have plumbed the darkest depths of life.

Social institutions play an important role in defining reactions and attitudes to victims. For example, the legal system has an important symbolic and practical role in channeling aggressive impulses; the penal code in any given society represents the principal internal check against violence, victimization, and revenge. By taking permission for revenge out of the hands of individual citizens, it provides a system of controlled revenge and humiliation of perpetrators, and prevents the escalation of conflict within society. The suffering of victims needs to be contained in ways similar to the legal system's containment of violence and revenge. The challenge for any civilized society is to find ways both to contain the excesses of violence, suffering, and deprivation, and to provide an umbrella under which children can be raised without being brutalized, victims can get redress for their grievances, and people can grow old without becoming helpless.

Other social structures and customs besides the courts and the medical and social service systems fulfill critical functions in helping people make meaning out of their rage and humiliation. Days of remembrance and communal memorials, such as the Vietnam War Memorial in Washington, D.C., or Yad Vashem, the Holocaust Memorial in Jerusalem, provide times and places where people can come to transcend their helplessless and rage in commemoration. The social transformation of trauma is also embodied in individuals who have transcended rage and revenge in the face of suffering and oppression. Martin Luther King Jr. and Mahatma Gandhi are two contemporary examples of individuals who rose above their individual grief and suffering to address the suffering of all humanity.

The themes of revenge, justice, and meaning making have been central human concerns since ancient times. For example, about 2,500 years ago, the playwright Aeschylus (458 B.C./1977) made the issue of containment of post-traumatic rage and revenge in human communities the central theme in his great trilogy, the *Oresteia*, in which raw issues of revenge are ultimately transformed into issues of social justice. In the trilogy, Orestes, who is both a victim (of his mother's murder of his father) and a perpetrator (by virtue of his revenge killing of her), is able to still the haunting memories of these deeds by submitting himself to the rules of law—the rules made to channel and contain the raw forces of "man's inhumanity to man."

Submitting impulses for revenge to the arbitration of the rule of law, finding common symbols and memorials, establishing agencies responsible for social security, and honoring and identifying with people who are symbols of righteousness—all these issues present particular challenges to societies that have been marked by oppression and brutality. Citizens of countries recently freed from totalitarian rule, such as the countries of Eastern Europe and the former Soviet Union, need to find new ways of containing the effects of past trauma in a political environment of increasing freedom. In totalitarian societies, systematic brutalization of the population is the principal instrument of social control: The state succeeds in subjugating its citizens when they come to concentrate on containing their memories of terror, at the expense of being active participants in planning their lives. The Soviets are estimated to have killed between 20 and 60 million citizens. Gulag survivors and the relatives of those killed were forbidden to speak of their losses or to grieve. Children denounced their fathers, and women remarried without knowing the fates of their husbands in the Gulags (Remnick, 1993).

Various important questions emerge from these facts. How are the memories of brutalization and cruelty stored at a societal level? How does this affect people's capacity for loyalty, personal and social commitments, belief in individual sacrifices for the common good, belief in justice, willingness to delegate decision making to elected representatives, and belief in the meaning of laws and rules? Historically, shared trauma promotes the emergence of tightly knit organizations that encourage their followers to adopt a paranoid stance, in which "outsiders" are singled out as scapegoats who are responsible for their current plight. In a way, such primitive forms of social organization constitute the nucleus of a social structure that provides a communal sense of shared suffering. Unfortunately, the price for shared suffering often seems to be shared hatred and a commitment to taking revenge. In regard to the current political developments in formerly totalitarian countries, it will be fascinating to see whether the neo-Darwinist belief in the forces of the market, embodied in a commitment to the individual accumulation of wealth, can successfully substitute for the traditional transformation of past suffering into a drive to take revenge. It would be remarkable if the drive to accumulate capital could still the desire for revenge for past injuries.

The function of social denial of the past needs to be better understood. For example, was it a coincidence that shortly after Mikhail Gorbachev publicly revealed his own family's history of trauma under the Soviet regime, he was removed from power? It is a critical question whether public acknowledgment and validation of the personal suffering of traumatized individuals in places such as Rwanda, Bosnia, Lebanon, Cambodia, and the inner cities of the United States is a useful social process that can promote a shared sense of trust, empathy and personal responsibility. Can individuals and nations afford to face the awful truths about their past, as long as life's basic necessities have not been provided for? What does it mean that it took a defeated but powerfully restored Germany over 40 years to face up publicly to its traumatic past, while Japan, at least equally successful in its recovery, continues in its social denial over half a century after the end of World War II (Buruma, 1994)?

Somehow, it is possible for societies to make a transition from cycles of victimization and revenge. For example, during the late Middle Ages, the murder rate in European cities was even higher than in U.S. cities today. What are the processes that allow societies to reestablish a social contract, in which goverments are once again trusted to rule for the benefit of the ruled? Why did the rate of violence in London drop so dramatically between Dickens's time and the time after World War I? How did nations like Japan and Germany not come to reenact their war trauma on a societal level after World War II? The opportunities to project the blame of the traumatic past on the enemy during the Cold War, as exemplified by West Germany's pinning the legacy of Fascism on East Germany and vice versa, may well have facilitated their recovery. Did the official denial of the reality of the impact of World War II on these societies help in their incredible economic resurgence? What price was paid by suffering individuals for keeping silent about their pain? Can people abandon their personal sense of injury when they have a sense of being participants in a social contract? The focus of most nations' collective myths is on their struggle against oppression and on the sacrifices made by their martyrs. Do nations, in order to function effectively, need a shared history of trauma to forge a sense of national community that creates a sense of belonging and security in its citizens?

TRAUMA AND THE NEWS MEDIA

The news media play a pivotal role in the ways that societies deal with traumatized individuals. The media are the prime purveyors of traumatic news, and they determine whether victims are treated with compassion and understanding, or with scorn and neglect. For reasons that are far from clear, people always seem to have had a well-nigh insatiable appetite for tales of trauma, as long as they do not personally involve the listeners or demand compassion for the victims. However, when such demands are made, such as after major earthquakes and other natural disasters, there tends to be an outpouring of public support. With the advent of satellite technology, it has become possible to supplement an insufficient daily trauma quota in the local area with tales of horror from Sri Lanka, Rwanda, or Bosnia, which are piped right into people's living rooms in such a lifelike fashion that the television watchers could be spectators in the local sports arena. The function of this daily smorgasbord of stereotyped and insensitive images of accidents, crimes, and disasters has barely been explored, but it is sure to blunt concern and trivialize the suffering involved.

The media can have very positive effects on people's awareness and sensitivities as well. During the Vietnam War, television coverage provided a grotesque portrayal of the mutilation and horror of war that allowed the citizens of the United States to move beyond abstract principles of patriotism into facing the realities of the cruelties and suffering involved. These images did much to change U.S. public opinion about the war. Television coverage can just as easily create exciting and surreal images. For example, the use of "smart" laser-guided bombs in the Gulf War made combat look more like a computer game than like the intentional infliction of mass death. These pictures succeeded in inducing excitement and exhilaration, while ignoring the fear and horror experienced both by the pilots flying through antiaircraft defenses and, to an even greater extent, by the million unnamed Iraqi soldiers who were subjected to continuous and merciless bombardments.

These vicarious thrills provide facile depictions of reality. Most television images gloss over the immediate impact of trauma on its victims, and give no indication whatever of the long-term effects. Portrayal of the lasting effects of trauma demands a perseverance of interest that goes beyond most people's attention spans. By ignoring the real dimensions of personal suffering, these portrayals tend to create an acceptance of violence as a reasonable and inevitable method of resolving conflict. Clearly, creating awareness of the social cost of trauma and violence could help educate people to the realities of human violence, and could motivate politicians and their constituencies to develop sophisticated interventions to change these behaviors.

THE CLINICIAN: OBJECTIVE OBSERVER OR ADVOCATE?

Because of their immediate exposure to the suffering of real human beings, clinicians and researchers who work with traumatized children and adults cannot afford to gloss over their reality in the same way that the general population and the news media do. However, clinicians and researchers are not exempt from developing the same ambivalence and numbing that victims provoke in the general public. Although the primary task of researchers and clinicians is to understand and heal victims, their continuous confrontation with the brutal facts of life may make it very difficult for them to maintain a detached scientific attitude. Working with trauma confronts everyone with the essence of human suffering, with "man's inhumanity to man," and with the essential lack of purity of people's interactions with each other. Individuals, and even entire cultures, build up elaborate defenses in order to keep these stark realities out of conscious awareness.

The practices of medicine and psychology cannot be divorced from the cultural context in which they occur. Being confronted with so much suffering, members of the medical profession may be even more reluctant to acknowledge the effects of trauma on people's lives than professionals in other disciplines. Military psychiatry, of which large numbers of psychiatrists have been a part during and after the various wars of the 20th century, exemplifies some of the dilemmas that arise when physicians are confronted with traumatized individuals. In these settings, doctors need to deny their empathy for individual soldiers as part of their obligation to maintain the fighting strength of the military. Thus, military psychiatrists confront the impossible ethical dilemma of having to decide whether soldiers are fit for combat, and thus ready to lay down their lives. When faced with such moral dilemmas, issues of suffering are easily reduced to such simple diagnoses as "failure to take responsibility" or "cowardice"; for example, during World War I, a common designation for soldiers who failed to function in the face of horrendous exposure to death and mutilation used to be "moral invalids."

Even in peacetime, physicians have similar conflicts of interest—in their allegiance to the patients on the one hand, and to the hospitals, insurance companies, or other organizations that are required to finance the provision of succor and compensation on the other. There is generally a profound divergence between the victims' own experience and the way physicians and other health care providers (as well as lawyers and pension managers) understand their patients' trauma. Professionals cannot be expected to become political activists; yet how are they to respond when they are confronted with child abuse and domestic violence, and there are no agencies that can take over and no rules to govern their obligations? Undoubtedly, the fear of getting sucked into "other people's messes" forms the basis of the traditional failure by medicine in general, and by psychiatry in particular, to identify and vigorously address the consequences of child abuse. After all, physicians and psychologists are not trained to be social crusaders or to confront social illusions about family values and the dark side of human behavior. Would it be possible to continue to practice one's profession if one could not distance oneself from other people's suffering and protect oneself by stigmatizing and blaming the victims? If professionals are to provide effective intervention and treatment, these feelings and attitudes must somehow be dealt with. Unless the reality of trauma is acknowledged, and bystanders can somehow deal with their own revulsion at being confronted with these realities, effective treatment is impossible.

CONCLUSION

The impact of the suffering of victims on observers makes it difficult to maintain an objective stance about the effects of trauma. Yet, in order to fully comprehend the effects of trauma on people's psychological and biological makeup, and in order to find out what constitutes truly effective treatment, scientific methods need to be rigorously applied to transform subjective experience into empirical data. Although the scientific approach runs the risk of obscuring the personal experience of trauma, and of losing perspective on the suffering that is the real subject of investigation, rigorously observing the individual components of people's response to trauma should enable us to analyze the totality of the experience, and thus to plan effective interventions and treatment. Despite a century of episodic denial of the reality of the impact of trauma on people's minds and bodies (see Chapter 3), objective data may yet be able to make a positive contribution in shaping society's attitudes to victims. As Freud (who was not always faithful to his own dicta) noted, "the voice of reason may be small, but it is persistent."

The principal task entrusted by society to professionals is that of creating a sense of controllability and predictability, and thereby of protecting society against the full impact of the tragic aspects of existence. The creation of diagnostic categories provides a sense of order as a protection against the bizarre and irrational, but it does not necessarily provide better ways to alleviate suffering. Therapists who claim that treatment of trauma victims is easily accomplished with standard protocols run the danger of minimizing the profound personal, social, and biological disruption caused by trauma. In an attempt to maintain their own sense of mission in the face of frightening realities, some therapists may be vulnerable to overestimating the effectiveness of their therapeutic interventions in undoing the effects of devastation in their patients (see Chapter 18, this volume).

Medicine, psychiatry, and psychology must find a way of acknowledging human beings' primitive wish to dominate and remain in control, and to suppress contradictory evidence when self-interest (be it economical or sexual) is at stake. Professionals are placed in the unique position of witnessing the predatory nature of our species, whose members are capable of victimizing others, even their own closest relatives. The study of trauma inevitably confronts us with issues of morality and social values—a questioning that we often avoid by hiding behind a cloak of objectivity. In this regard, artists have traditionally fulfilled the function of holding up a mirror to humankind; they present the issues of trauma with a clarity that contrasts sharply with the traditional obfuscation of these issues in the field of mental health. Let us hope that careful attention to the scientific data as they emerge will help us face the realities of trauma and of their effects on the human community.

REFERENCES

Aeschylus (1977). *The Oresteia* (R. Fagles, Trans.). London. Penguin Books. (Original works performed ca. 458 B.C.)

Becker, E. (1973). *The denial of death.* New York: Free Press.

Caruth, C. (Ed.). (1995). *Trauma and memory.* Baltimore: Johns Hopkins University Press.

Breslau, N., Davis, G. C., & Andreski, P. (1995). Risk factors for PTSD related traumatic events: A prospective analysis. *American Journal of Psychiatry, 152,* 529–535.

Buruma, I. (1994). *The wages of guilt: Memories of war in Germany and Japan.* New York: Farrar Straus Giroux.

Director of Legal and Regulatory Affairs, American Psychological Association Practice Directorate. (1995, January). *Memorandum on Consumer Mental Health Protection Act to state psychological associations.* Washington, DC: American Psychological Association.

Dutton, D. G., & Painter, S. (1993). Emotional attachments in abusive relationships: A test of traumatic bonding theory. *Violence and Victims, 8*(2), 105–120.

Elliot, M., & Briere, J. (1995). Posttraumatic stress associated with delayed recall of sexual abuse: A general population study. *Journal of Traumatic Stress, 8,* 629–647.

Famularo, R., Kinscherff, R., & Fenton, T. (1988). Propranolol treatment for childhood posttraumatic stress disorder, acute type. *American Journal of Diseases of Children, 142,* 1244–1247.

Freud, S. (1921). Enleitung zu Zur Psychoanalyse der Kriegsneurosen (*Gesammelte werke,* 12, pp. 321–324). Introduction in E. Jones (Ed.), *Psychoanalysis and the war neuroses* (The International Psychoanalytic Library No. 2, pp. 1–4). London: International Psychoanalytic Press. (Original work published 1919)

Freud, S. (1959). Inhibitions, symptoms and anxiety. In J. Strachey (Ed. and Trans.), *The standard edition of the complete psychological works of Sigmund Freud* (Vol. 20, pp. 75–175). London: Hogarth Press. (Original work published 1926)

Fussell, P. (1983). *Siegfried Sassoon's long journey.* New York: Oxford University Press.

Greer, G. (1989). *Daddy, we hardly knew you.* London: Viking Penguin.

Herman, J. L. (1992). *Trauma and recovery.* New York: Basic Books.

Hobfoll, S. E., & deVries, M. W. (Eds.). (1995). *Extreme stress and communities: Impact and intervention.* Dordrecht, The Netherlands: Kluwer.

Hughes, R. (1993). *The culture of complaint.* New York: Oxford University Press.

Kluft, R. P. (1991). Multiple personality disorder. In A. Tasman & S. Goldfinger (Eds.), *Review of psychiatry* (pp. 375–384). Washington, DC: American Psychiatric Press.

Kobasa, S. C., & Puccetti, M. C. (1982). Personality and social resources in stress resistance. *Journal of Personality and Social Psychology, 45,* 839–850.

Langer, L. L. (1990). *Holocaust testimonies: The ruins of memory.* New Haven, CT: Yale University Press.

Lee, K. A., Vaillant, G. E., Torrey, W. C., & Elder, G. H. (1995). A 50-year prospective study of the psychological sequelae of World War II combat. *American Journal of Psychiatry, 152*(4), 516–522.

Lifton, R. (1983). *The broken connection.* New York: Basic Books.

Lindy, J. D., & Titchener, J. (1983). "Acts of God and man": Long term character change in survivors of disaster and the law. *Behavioral Science and the Law, 1,* 85–96.

McFarlane, A. C. (1988). Recent life events and psychiatric disorder in children: The interaction with preceding extreme adversity. *Journal of Clinical Psychiatry, 29*(5), 677–690.

National Victim Center (1993). *Crime and victimization in America: Statistical overview.* Arlington, VA: Author.

Paglia, C. (1994). *Vamps and tramps: New essays.* New York: Vintage Press.

Pelcovitz, D., Kaplan, S., Goldenberg, B., Mandel, F., Lehane, J., & Guarrera, J. (1995). Post-traumatic stress disorder in physically abused adolescents. *Journal of the American Academy of Child and Adolescent Psychiatry, 33*(3), 305–312.

Putnam, F. W. (1994). *Developmental pathways following sexual abuse.* Paper presented at the annual meeting of the Society for Adolescent Psychiatry, San Francisco.

Remnick, D. (1993). *Lenin's tomb: The last days of the Soviet Empire.* New York: Random House.

Russell, D. (1986). *The secret trauma.* New York: Basic Books.

Schetky, D. H., & Green, A. H. (1988). *Child sexual abuse.* New York: Brunner/Mazel.

Solomon, Z. (1995). From denial to recognition: Attitudes toward Holocaust survivors from World War II to the present. *Journal of Traumatic Stress, 8,* 215–228.

Symonds, M. (1982). Victim's response to terror: Understanding and treatment. In F. Ochberg & D. Soskis (Eds.), *Victims of terrorism* (pp. 95–103). Boulder, CO: Westview.

van der Kolk, B. A. (1989). The compulsion to repeat the trauma: Re-enactment, revictimization, and masochism. *Psychiatric Clinics of North America, 12*(2), 389–411.

Werner, E. E. (1989). High-risk children in young adulthood: A longitudinal study from birth to 32 years. *American Journal of Orthopsychiatry, 59,* 72–81.

CHAPTER 3

History of Trauma in Psychiatry

BESSEL A. VAN DER KOLK
LARS WEISAETH
ONNO VAN DER HART

> *All the famous moralists of olden days drew attention to the way in which certain events would leave indelible and distressing memories—memories to which the sufferer was continually returning, and by which he was tormented by day and by night.*
>
> —JANET (1919/1925, p. 589)

Awareness of the role of psychological trauma in the genesis of various psychiatric problems has waxed and waned throughout the history of psychiatry. People have always known that exposure to overwhelming terror can lead to troubling memories, arousal, and avoidance: This has been a central theme in literature, from the time of Homer (Alford, 1992; Shay, 1994) to today (Caruth, 1995). In contrast, psychiatry as a profession has had a very troubled relationship with the idea that reality can profoundly and permanently alter people's psychology and biology. Psychiatry itself has periodically suffered from marked amnesias in which well-established knowledge has been abruptly forgotten, and the psychological impact of overwhelming experiences has been ascribed to constitutional or intrapsychic factors alone. Mirroring the intrusions, confusion, and disbelief of victims whose lives are suddenly shattered by traumatic experiences, the psychiatric profession has gone through periods of fascination with trauma, followed by periods of stubborn disbelief about the relevance of patients' stories.

From the earliest involvement of psychiatry with traumatized patients, there have been vehement arguments about trauma's etiology. Is it organic or psychological? Is trauma the event itself or its subjective interpretation? Does the trauma itself cause the disorder, or do preexisting vulnerabilities cause it?

Are these patients malingering and suffer from moral weakness, or do they suffer from an involuntary disintegration of the capacity to take charge of their lives? The history of these arguments is summarized in this chapter, and the status of current knowledge is presented in the rest of this book.

TRAUMATIC STRESS: EMOTIONAL OR ORGANIC?

The conflict over whether trauma has organic or psychological origins, along with the dispute as to whether it represents malingering or genuine breakdown, was at the center of the earliest scientific discussions about its effects, which focused on whiplash injuries and "railroad spines." The English surgeon John Eric Erichsen (1866, 1886) ascribed the psychological problems of severely injured patients to organic causes, and warned against confusing these symptoms with those of hysteria—a condition that he and most of his contemporaries claimed only occurred in women. Not unlike their present-day counterparts, physicians in those days struggled with trying to understand body–mind relationships; physical signs of anxiety then, as now, were easily misdiagnosed as symptoms of organic illness. Erichsen's fellow surgeon Page (1885) disagreed, and proposed instead that the symptoms of "railroad spine" had psychological origins. He claimed that "many errors in diagnosis have been made because fright has not been considered of itself sufficient" (p. 29). The German neurologist Herman Oppenheim (1889), who was the first to use the term "traumatic neurosis," was an organicist; he proposed that functional problems are produced by subtle molecular changes in the central nervous system. The frequent occurrence of cardiovascular symptoms in traumatized persons, particularly in combat soldiers, started a long tradition of associating posttraumatic problems with "cardiac neuroses." This began with such names as "irritable heart" and "soldiers' heart" (Myers, 1870; Da Costa, 1871) and progressed to "disorderly action of the heart" or "neurocirculatory asthenia" during World War I (Merskey, 1991).

Ascribing an organic origin to traumatic neuroses was particularly important in combat soldiers. Such an attribution offered an honorable solution for all parties who might be compromised by people breaking down under stress: The soldier preserved his self-respect, the doctor did not have to diagnose personal failure or desertion, and military authorities did not have to explain psychological breakdowns in previously brave soldiers, or bother with such troublesome issues as cowardice, low unit morale, poor leadership, or the meaning of the war effort itself. But if trauma was an illness, how could it be defined? Charles Samuel Myers (1915), a British military psychiatrist, was the first to use the term "shell-shock" in the medical literature. However, since "shell-shock" could be found in soldiers who had never been directly exposed to gunfire, it gradually became clear that the causes were often purely emotional. Myers came to play an important role in rejecting a relationship between battle neuroses and such organic factors as "molecular commotion in the brain," and declared emotional disturbance alone to be enough of an explanation. He, like so many after him, emphasized the close resemblance of the war neuroses to hysteria (Myers, 1940). Moran (1945) described how, despite the acceptance of diagnosis of shell-shock, doctors found it extremely difficult to distinguish it from cowardice. More than 200 British soldiers were executed for cowardice during World War II; a notable fact is that only 11% of those who were condemned to death for desertion were actually executed.

Psychological explanations for traumatic neuroses were easier to pursue in civilian settings. The American neurologist James J. Putnam (1881) developed a theory based on Hughlings Jackson's notion of illness, in which psychic traumatization was considered a functional regression toward earlier, simple, reflexive, automated modes of functioning (Putnam, 1898; MacLeod, 1993). These notions were similar to those set forth by Pierre Janet at the Salpêtrière in Paris. In his doctoral thesis, Janet (1889) had documented the relationships between trauma and psychological automatisms. When Harvard Medical School inaugurated its new buildings in 1906, Putnam was instrumental in inviting Janet to Boston to lecture on these common interests; these lectures were later published in expanded form as *The Major Symptoms of Hysteria* (Janet, 1907/1920).

TRAUMA, SUGGESTIBILITY, AND SIMULATION

An association between psychological trauma and hysteria has been noted ever since psychiatry has tried to be a scientific discipline. As early as 1859, the French psychiatrist Briquet started to make the first connnections between the symptoms of "hysteria" (including somatization) and childhood histories of trauma. Of the 501 hysterical patients he described, Briquet reported specific traumatic origins as the cause of their illness in 381 (Crocq & DeVerbizier, 1989). Sexual abuse of children was well documented during the second half of the 19th century in France by researchers such as Tardieu (1878), a professor of forensic medicine. Almost as soon as the issue of sexual trauma in children was identified, the thorny issue of false memories was raised by people like Alfred Fournier, who described "*pseudologica phantastica*" in children who were thought to have falsely accused their parents of incest.

Similar problems arose when the first systematic explorations of the relationships between trauma and psychiatric illness were conducted at the Salpêtrière. The great neurologist Jean-Martin Charcot (1887) described how traumatically induced "*choc nerveux*" could put patients into a mental state similar to that induced by hypnosis. This so-called "hypnoid state" was believed to be a necessary condition of what Charcot called "hystero-traumatic autosuggestion." Thus, Charcot became the first to describe both the problems of suggestibility in these patients, and the fact that hysterical attacks are dissociative problems—the result of having endured unbearable experiences.

While Charcot inspired Janet to study the nature of dissociation and traumatic memories (Janet, 1887, 1889, 1894), two of Charcot's other pupils, Gilles de la Tourette and Joseph Babinski, focused their further research on hysterical suggestibility. When Babinski took over as head of the Salpêtrière in 1905, Charcot's notions about the traumatic origins of hysteria were rejected as worthless (Ellenberger, 1970). In their place, simulation and suggestibility became to be considered as the hallmarks of the now emphatically neurological disease entity "hysteria" (Babinski, 1901, 1909). This development set the stage for the overriding interest during World War I, among Babinski and his French students as well as among many German psychiatrists, in treating "simulation" rather than in alleviating the horror of patients' traumatic memories (Nonne, 1915; Babinski & Froment, 1918). For many French and German neurologists and psychiatrists, the treatment of war syndromes became a battle against simulation.

With the focus on simulation, the notion of "will" became the dominant issue. "War neurosis" ("war hysteria"), for many psychiatrists, was essentially a disease of the will, a *Willenskrankheit* (Fischer-Homberger, 1975). Hence, largely for political reasons, the medical diagnosis of posttraumatic stress in Germany during World War I and during subsequent decades was recast as a failure of the individual soldier's willpower (*Willenversagung, Willenshemmung, Willensperrung, Wille zur Krankheit*). As a result, treatment consisted of "causal will therapies": The patients' "desire for health" had to be stimulated and bolstered by physiological exercises. The treatment was so painful that many patients preferred front-line duty, and were thus considered "cured." Chapter 2 of this volume has noted that this way of conceptualizing people's reactions to terrifying experiences, and the acceptance of these forms of "treatment," may have contributed to the popularity of the Nazi party and thus to the origins of World War II.

VULNERABILITY, PREDISPOSITION, AND COMPENSATION

The issue of predisposition could be studied with more detachment in civilian settings, where national pride was not at stake, and compensation was less of a potentially massive economic issue. The Swiss psychiatrist Edouard Stierlin (1909, 1911), the first researcher in disaster psychiatry, published two works based on studies of earlier calamities: an earthquake in Messina, Italy, in 1907, and a mining disaster in 1906. Stierlin was the first to study nonclinical populations, which brought him face to face with the issue of vulnerability and resiliency. He agreed with his predecessors at the Salpêtrière that violent emotions are the most important etiological factors of "fright neuroses." He was concerned that physicians had little awareness that emotions can cause serious long-term psychoneurotic problems, and that laypeople tended to equate posttraumatic psychological problems with simulation.

Stierlin found that a substantial proportion of victims developed long-lasting posttraumatic stress symptoms. For example, after the Messina earthquake in 1907, which killed 70,000 of the town's inhabitants, 25% of the survivors suffered from sleep disturbances and nightmares. He made the important observation that traumatic neurosis is the only psychogenic symptom complex for which no psychopathological predisposition is required. He also suggested that the term "neurosis" was not a good descriptor, and took issue with Kraepelin (1899), who claimed in his famous textbook of psychiatry that the type of traumatic neurosis in which fear played the dominant etiological role was rare and "atypical."

In the period following World War I, the leading German psychiatrist Bonhoeffer (1926) and his colleagues founded a school of thought that regarded traumatic neurosis as a social illness that could only be cured by social remedies. However, these social cures did not consist of an amelioration of social conditions. Since Bonhoeffer concluded that practically all of his 142 cases of traumatic neurosis had hereditary predispositions, dealing with these patients' inherent weakness, rather than preventing and ameliorating their misery, became the critical issue. Bonhoeffer and his colleagues believed that the real cause of traumatic neurosis among their patients was the availability of compensation (*"Das Gesetz ist die Ursache der Unfallsneurosen"*—"The law is the cause of traumatic neuroses"). In other words, the disorder was caused by secondary gain. Traumatic neurosis was not an illness, but an artifact of the insurance system—a *Rentenneurose* (a compensation neurosis). This compensation neurosis was thought to occur primarily in predisposed individuals: Jaspers (1913) had previously proclaimed that patients with psychogenic disorders (including the traumatic neuroses) lacked premorbid personality problems and therefore had a good prognosis. This blind acceptance of psychiatric dogma meant that a poor outcome must be the result of premorbid vulnerabilities.

The *Reichversicherungs Ordnung* (RVO—The National Health Insurance Act) of 1926 cemented this position in Germany. Traumatic neurosis was not to be compensated. The philosophy behind this decision was that traumatic neurosis was incurable if and as long as patients were awarded pensions or other compensations. Only immediate shock reactions were accepted. If the victim's problems persisted, this was blamed on the interplay among predisposition, constitution, "degenerative inclination," and compensation. The social backdrop of this discussion was a time of economic chaos and social distress in Germany. The RVO lasted through the Nazi period and beyond. It was slightly modified in 1959, but today German compensation practices continue to be much more restrictive than those of most other countries (Venzlaff, 1975).

THE PSYCHOLOGICAL PROCESSING
OF TRAUMA: REALITY IMPRINT
VERSUS INTRAPSYCHIC ELABORATION

In retrospect, the issue of the traumatic origins of hysteria is probably the most important legacy of psychiatry in the last decades of the 19th century. As noted earlier, Charcot (1887) had first proposed at the Salpêtrière that the symptoms of his hysterical patients had their origins in histories of trauma. In his first four books, Pierre Janet described a total of 591 patients and reported a traumatic origin of their psychopathology in 257 (Crocq & Le Verbizier, 1989). Janet noted that hysterical patients were unable to attend to their internal processes as guides for adaptive action. In line with the prevailing thinking of his day (e.g., Bergson, 1896), he considered self-awareness to be the central issue in psychological health. He believed that an individual's being in touch with his or her personal past, combined with having accurate perceptions of current situations, determines whether the person is able to respond appropriately to stress. Janet coined the word "subconscious" to describe the collection of memories that form the mental schemes that guide a person's interaction with the environment (Janet, 1904; van der Kolk & van der Hart, 1989). In his view, appropriate categorization and integration of memories of past experience allow people to develop meaning schemes that prepare them to cope with subsequent challenges.

Janet proposed that when people experience "vehement emotions," their minds may become incapable of matching their frightening experiences with existing cognitive schemes. As a result, the memories of the experience cannot be integrated into personal awareness; instead, they are split off (dissociated) from consciousness and from voluntary control. Thus, the first comprehensive formulation of the effects of trauma on the mind was based on the notion that extreme emotional arousal results in failure to integrate traumatic memories. Janet stated that people are "unable to make the recital which we call narrative memory, and yet they remain confronted by [the] difficult situation"(Janet, 1919/1925, Vol. 1, p. 661). This results in "a phobia of memory" (p. 661), which prevents the integration ("synthesis") of traumatic events and splits these traumatic memories off from ordinary consciousness (Janet, 1909, p. 145). The memory traces of the trauma linger as unconscious "fixed ideas" that cannot be "liquidated" as long as they have not been translated into a personal narrative; instead, they continue to intrude as terrifying perceptions, obsessional preoccupations, and somatic reexperiences such as anxiety reactions (Janet, 1889, 1930).

Janet observed that his traumatized patients seemed to react to reminders of the trauma with responses that had been relevant to the original threat, but that currently had no adaptive value. Upon exposure to reminders, the somatosensory representations of the trauma predominated (Janet, 1889; see Chapter 12, this volume). He proposed that when patients fail to integrate the traumatic experience into the totality of their personal awareness, they become "attached" (Freud would later use the term "fixated") to the trauma: "Unable to integrate traumatic memories, they seem to have lost their capacity to assimilate new experiences as well. It is . . . as if their personality has definitely stopped at a certain point, and cannot enlarge any more by the addition or assimilation of new elements" (Janet, 1911, p. 532). Later, he noted that "all [traumatized] patients seem to have had the evolution of their lives checked; they are attached to an insurmountable obstacle" (Janet, 1919/1925, Vol. 1, p. 660). Janet proposed that the efforts to keep the fragmented traumatic memories out of conscious awareness eroded the psychological energy of these patients. This, in turn, interfered with their capacity to engage in focused and creative actions and to learn from experience. Unless the dissociated elements of the trauma were integrated into personal consciousness, the patients were likely to experience a slow decline in personal and occupational functioning (van der Kolk & van der Hart, 1989; see also Chapter 13, this volume).

Until psychoanalysis—the doctrine of intrapsychic conflict and repressed infantile sexuality—crowded out competing schools of thought, Janet's clinical observations were widely accepted as the correct formulations of the effects of trauma on the mind. William James, Jean Piaget, Henry Murray, Carl Jung, Charles Myers, William MacDougal, and such students of dissociation as Ernest Hilgard all acknowledged the influence of Janet's work on their understanding of mental processes. In accepting dissociation as the core pathogenic process that gives rise to posttraumatic stress, they all disagreed with the psychoanalytic notion that catharsis and abreaction are the treatments of choice. Instead, they emphasized the role of synthesis and integration (van der Hart & Brown, 1992). Despite Janet's large body of work and his profound influence both on his contemporaries and on the next generation of psychiatrists, his legacy was slowly forgotten. Janet's extensive work on trauma, memory, and the treatment of dissociative states was not integrated with contemporary knowledge of PTSD until the role of dissociation in the origins of PTSD was rediscovered in the 1980s (van der Kolk & van der Hart, 1989; van der Hart & Friedman, 1989; Putnam, 1989; Nemiah, 1989).

FREUD AND TRAUMA

When Sigmund Freud visited Charcot at the end of 1885, he adopted many of the ideas then current in the Salpêtrière, which he expressed and acknowledged in his early papers on hysteria (Breuer & Freud, 1893–1895/1955; Freud, 1896b/1962; see also MacMillan, 1980, 1991). In much that he wrote between 1892 and 1896, Freud followed the notion that the "subconscious" contains affectively charged events encoded in an altered state of consciousness. In "On the Psychical Mechanism of Hysterical Phenomena: A Lecture" (Freud, 1893/

1962), he wrote on the nature of hysterical attacks: "We must point out that we consider it essential for the explanation of hysterical phenomena to assume the presence of a dissociation—a splitting of the content of consciousness . . . the regular and essential content of a (recurrent) hysterical attack is the recurrence of a psychical state which the patient has experienced earlier" (p. 30). When Breuer and Freud expanded this work in "Studies on Hysteria," they acknowledged their debt to Janet and stated that "hysterics suffer mainly from reminiscences . . . the traumatic experience is constantly forcing itself upon the patient and this is proof of the strength of that experience: the patient is, as one might say, fixated on his trauma" (Breuer & Freud, 1893–1895/ 1955). Citing Janet, Breuer and Freud thought that something becomes traumatic because it is dissociated and remains outside conscious awareness. They called this state "hypnoid hysteria." As late as 1896, Freud proposed in "Heredity and the Aetiology of Neuroses" (Freud, 1896a/1962) that "a precocious experience of sexual relations . . . resulting from sexual abuse committed by another person . . . is the specific cause of hysteria . . . not merely (as Charcot had claimed), an agent provocateur" (p. 152).

In "The Aetiology of Hysteria," Freud (1896b/1962) began to develop the concept of "defense hysteria," in which he for the first time abandoned dissociation as the central pathogenic process related to trauma, thereby beginning to make his own original contributions by claiming that repressed instinctual wishes form the foundation of the neuroses. Freud later claimed that "I find . . . that there are no grounds whatever for presupposing the presence of such hypnoid states" (Freud, 1896a/1962, p. 195). Although during World War I he again became interested in the nature of traumatic neuroses, the relationship between actual childhood trauma and the development of psychopathology was henceforth ignored. In Freud's view, it is not the actual memories of childhood trauma that are split off from consciousness, but rather the unacceptable sexual and aggressive wishes of the child, which threaten the ego and motivate defenses against the conscious awareness of these wishes.

In "An Autobiographical Study" (1925/1959), Freud wrote:

> I believed these stories [of childhood sexual trauma] and consequently supposed that I had discovered the roots of the subsequent neurosis in these experiences of sexual seduction in childhood. If the reader feels inclined to shake his head at my credulity, I cannot altogether blame him. . . . I was at last obliged to recognize that these scenes of seduction had never taken place, and that they were only fantasies which my patients had made up. (p. 34)

Freud henceforth argued that the memory disturbances and reenactments seen in hysteria are not the results of a failure to integrate new data into existing meaning schemes, but stem from the active repression of conflict-laden sexual and aggressive ideas and impulses, centering around the Oedipal crisis at about age 5 (Freud, 1900/1953).

Although he tried, Freud never was able to reconcile his notions about repressed infantile sexuality with actual trauma: "Keeping up the seduction theory would mean to abandon the Oedipus complex, and with it the whole importance of phantasy life, conscious or unconscious phantasy" (Anna Freud, quoted by Masson, 1984, p. 113). Focusing on intrapsychic reality and subjective experience crowded out interest in external reality. Psychiatry as a discipline came to follow Freud in his explorations of how the normal human psyche functioned: Real-life trauma was ignored in favor of fantasy.

However, just as his early hysterical patients seemed incapable of getting rid of their traumatic memories, Freud kept coming back to the issue of "fixation on the trauma." World War I temporarily confronted the world, including Freud, with the inescapable reality of the effects of trauma on people's spirits. During this time, he revived Janet's notion of "vehement emotions" as being at the root of traumatic neuroses: He declared that the overwhelming intensity of the stressor, the absence of abreactive verbal or motoric channels, and the unpreparedness of the individual cause a failure of the stimulus barrier (*Reitschutz*). The organism is unable to deal with the excitement, flooding the mental apparatus, resulting in mental paralyses and intense affect storms (Freud, 1920/1955). In 1920 Freud testified in the case against Wagner-Jauregg, the leading Viennese psychiatrist and subsequent Nobel laureate, who was accused of torturing patients who suffered from war neuroses by applying brutal electrical treatments. Eissler's 1986 book on Freud's statements and Wagner-Jauregg's explanations during the inquest is most informative about the concepts of war neurosis at that time. Freud stated before the commission (1) that every neurosis has a purpose and (2) constitutes a flight into illness by subconscious intentions; he also believed (3) that at the end of the war the war neuroses would disappear. He was wrong on all three counts.

Rather than integrating his observations of the war neuroses with those of 20 years earlier, Freud responded by developing two separate models of "trauma" (Krystal, 1978). One was the "unbearable situation" model; the other was the "unacceptable impulse" model, in which symptoms may be produced through the mobilization of defense mechanisms. Freud proposed that the compulsion to repeat is a function of repression itself: ". . . we therefore concluded that the keeping away from consciousness is the main characteristic of hysterical repression" (1920/1955, p. 18). Because the memory is repressed, the patient "is obliged to repeat the repressed material as a contemporary experience, instead of . . . remembering it as something belonging to the past" (p. 18). In the "Introductory Lectures on Psycho-Analysis" (1916–1917/1963), Freud stated: "The traumatic neuroses give a clear indication that a fixation to the traumatic incident lies at their root. These patients regularly repeat the traumatic neuroses in their dreams, where . . . we find that the attack conforms to a complete transplanting of the patient into the traumatic situation. It is as if the patient has not finished with the traumatic situation" (p. 369).

In "Beyond the Pleasure Principle" (1920/1955), Freud was close to reintegrating his earliest observations with his later understanding of intrapsychic reality: "The symptomatic picture presented by traumatic neurosis approaches that of hysteria . . . but surpasses it as a rule in its strongly marked signs of subjective ailment as well as the evidence it gives of a far more comprehensive general enfeeblement and disturbances of mental capacities" (1920/1955, p. 12). He was struck by the fact that patients suffering from traumatic neuroses often experienced a lack of conscious preoccupation with the memories of their accidents. He postulated that "perhaps they are more concerned with NOT thinking of it" (p. 13), but he did not connect this observation with the notion of *"la belle indifférence"* in hysterics.

The acceptance of psychoanalytic theory resulted in a total absence of research on the effects of real traumatic events on children's lives. From 1895 until very recently, no studies were conducted on the effects of childhood sexual trauma. Although psychoanalysts, including Freud, tended to acknowledge sexual trauma as tragic and harmful (Freud, 1905/1953, 1916–1917/1963), the subject seems to have been too awful to seriously consider in civilized company. One notable exception was Sandor Ferenczi (1933/1955), who presented a paper entitled "The Confusion of Tongues between the Adult and the Child: The Language of Tenderness and the Language of Passion" to the Psychoanalytic Congress in 1929. In this presentation he talked about the helplessness of the child when confronted with an adult who uses the child's vulnerability and need for affection to gain sexual gratification. Ferenczi talked with more eloquence than any psychiatrist before him about the helplessness and terror experienced by children who are victims of interpersonal violence, and he introduced a critical concept: that the predominant defense available to children thus traumatized is "identification with the aggressor." The response of the psychoanalytic community seems to have been one of embarrassment, and the paper was not published in English until 1949, 17 years after Ferenczi's death (Masson, 1984).

THE BEGINNINGS OF INTEGRATION: ABRAM KARDINER

Although several psychiatrists tried to apply the lessons of World War I to prevention and early intervention in civilian settings, their influence on psychiatry was minor and did not result in institutional change (Merskey, 1991). One notable exception was Abram Kardiner, who began his career treating traumatized U.S. war veterans. Starting in 1923, after finishing his analysis with Freud, he first unsuccessfully tried to create a theory of war neuroses based upon the concepts of early psychoanalytic theory. From 1939 on, as World War II was breaking out, he reassessed the meaning of his entire body of careful clinical observations, which he published in *The Traumatic Neuroses of War* (Kardiner, 1941). Like the previous great pioneers of psychological trauma, Kardiner was a master of detailed descriptions of the complex and unusual symptoms of his patients, and a meticulous chronicler of the plethora of previous diagnoses these patients had received before a connection between the trauma and their current symptoms was made. These included hysteria, malingering, or epileptiform disorders. More than anyone else, Kardiner defined PTSD for the remainder of the 20th century.

Kardiner noted that sufferers from "traumatic neuroses" develop an enduring vigilance for and sensitivity to environmental threat, and stated that "the nucleus of the neurosis is a *physioneurosis*. This is present on the battlefield and during the entire process of organization; it outlives every intermediary accommodative device, and persists in the chronic forms. The traumatic syndrome is ever present and unchanged" (p. 95; emphasis Kardiner's). He described extreme physiological arousal in his patients, who suffered from sensitivity to temperature, pain, and sudden tactile stimuli: "These patients cannot stand being slapped on the back abruptly; they cannot tolerate a misstep or a stumble. From a physiologic point of view there exists a lowering of the threshold of stimulation, and from a psychological point of view a state of readiness for fright reactions" (p. 95). (See also Chapter 10, this volume.)

Aside from the physiological alterations, Kardiner noted that the "pathological traumatic syndrome" consists of an altered conception of the self in relation to the world, based on being fixated on the trauma and having an atypical dream life, with chronic irritability, startle reactions, and explosive aggressive reactions. The phobic elaborations on the trauma made his patients look as if they were suffering from long-standing neuroses. However, he believed that it was the result of the fact that "the ego dedicates itself to the specific job of ensuring the security of the organism, and of trying to protect itself against recollection of the trauma" (p. 184). Patients became "stuck" in the trauma, and frequently had what he called "the Sisyphus dream," in which "whatever activity [they engage in] is greeted with a certain stereotyped futility." This sense of futility often overtook them; they became withdrawn and detached, even when they had functioned well prior to combat. Over four decades later, Tichener (1986) would rediscover this phenomenon and label it "posttraumatic decline."

Kardiner acknowledged that it is often difficult to differentiate between hysterical and organic origins of symptoms, and he noted the variety of ways in which traumatic memories are stored. Describing many patients who developed unusual physical symptoms, he recognized that this may sometimes be an adaptive mode of "remembering," since medical complaints are both socially acceptable and financially compensated. However, he cautioned that such symptoms cannot be explained by secondary gain alone (van der Kolk, Herron, & Hostetler, 1994).

Central in Kardiner's thinking, as it had been for Janet and Freud, was this fact: "The subject acts as if the original traumatic situation were still in existence and engages in protective devices which failed on the original occasion. This means in effect that his conception of the outer world and his conception of himself have been permanently altered" (p. 82). Sometimes patients' fixation on the trauma would take the form of dissociative fugue states. For example, triggered by a sensory stimulus, a patient might lash out, employing language suggestive of his trying to defend himself during a military assault. Many patients, while riding the subway and especially upon entering a tunnel, had flashbacks to being in the trenches. In other cases, patients had panic attacks in response to stimuli reminiscent of the trauma, while failing to make a conscious connection between their emotional states and their prior traumatic experience.

Kardiner was aware of the healing power of the process of psychotherapy, but also of the dangers and difficulties of talking about traumas. One of the issues that all therapists of "traumatic neuroses" continue to grapple with is how and whether to help patients bring unconscious traumatic material into awareness. In one case study, Kardiner urged the patient to discuss his combat traumas, believing this to be the cause of his frequent and severe headaches and dissociative spells. However, the patient was not amenable to this:

> . . . he showed unusual strength and emphatically refused to enter into any discussion about [the trauma], although he denied that any discussion would be painful for him. In other words, the original trauma and all its secondary ramifications seemed to be entirely encapsulated and to have no apparent connection with the patient's other psychic spheres. The prognosis, therefore, appeared to be practically hopeless, since no bridge remained between the patient's conscious life and the activity of the trauma in unconsciousness. (cited in van der Kolk et al., 1994, p. 591)

WORLD WAR II AND ITS AFTERMATH

Although Kardiner's work was available for practical application when World War II broke out, most of the lessons of front-line psychiatry from World War I had been forgotten and needed to be rediscovered. Thus, initially, the same inadequate treatment procedures (including evacuation from the front) were practiced as during World War I, resulting in great cost to the individual soldier and in manpower loss for the military (Stouffer, 1949; Ahrenfeldt, 1958). However, the essential elements of front-line psychiatry—the principles of "proximity, immediacy, and expectancy"—were soon practiced at the front. For the first time, there was research on protective factors such as training, group cohesion, leadership, motivation, and morale (Belenky, 1987; Grinker & Spiegel, 1945).

In the United States, many of the best minds of that generation tried to apply Kardiner's lessons in the combat theater. Lawrence Kubie, Roy Grinker, Herbert Spiegel, John Spiegel, Walter Menninger, and Lawrence Kolb were just a few of the pioneers in U.S. psychiatry who were actively involved in the treatment of combat neuroses, both in the field and at home. They confirmed Kardiner's observations about the persistence of profound conditioned biological responses in traumatized patients. In response, they pioneered the use of somatic therapies. In the process of trying to find an effective cure, they rediscovered that patients "remembered" the somatosensory aspects of the traumatic experience in an altered state of consciousness. Following this observation, they reintroduced, for the first time in four decades, hypnosis and narcosynthesis to help patients "remember" and abreact the trauma. They also confirmed Janet's observation that abreaction without transformation and substitution did not help. Grinker and Spiegel (1945) noted that the lasting imprint left by traumatic memories on the psyche "is not like the writing on a slate that can be erased, leaving the slate like it was before. Combat leaves a lasting impression on men's minds, changing them as radically as any crucial experience through which they live" (p. 371). The U.S. Army pioneered the use of group stress debriefing (Shalev & Ursano, 1990).

As a result of their war experiences, psychiatrists such as Walter Menninger in the United States, and Bion and his British colleagues at the Tavistock Clinic, discovered the use of group psychotherapy and the therapeutic community (Main, 1989). Clearly, the group had become a focus for psychiatric interest. War, as well as disasters, made the mental health profession aware that under extreme conditions, the group rather than the individual is the basic unit of study and treatment (see Chapters 19, 20, and 25, this volume). Given the vast experience gained during the war, the dedication of the practitioners, and the solid collection of data on the combat neuroses, it is astounding how the memory of war trauma was again completely forgotten for the subsequent quarter-century. An interesting example is that Roy Grinker, who was the co-author of one of the two most important books to come out of World War II (Grinker & Spiegel, 1945) went on to become a pioneer in the study of borderline personality disorder (Grinker, Werble, & Drye, 1968) without seeming to make the obvious connection between these two areas of interest.

Studies of Concentration Camp Survivors

After World War II, an independent line of investigation emerged with the study of the long-term effects of trauma in survivors of the Holocaust and other war-related traumas. Studies by Eitinger and Strøm (Eitinger, 1964; Eitinger & Strøm, 1973) showed that in terms of prewar health, concentration camp survivors were a representative sample of their national populations. Their increased mortality, general somatic morbidity, and psychiatric morbidity were thoroughly documented (Venzlaff, 1966; Hocking, 1970; Bastiaans, 1970). These investigators coined the term "concentration camp syndrome," which included not only the symptoms currently listed under PTSD, but also enduring personality changes. Perhaps the most consistent finding from these studies, however, was the devastating effect of extreme and long-lasting stress on subsequent health. This was also shown in the so-called "war sailor syndrome" from the Allied Convoy Service (Askevold, 1976–1977) and in survivors of Japanese concentration camps (Archibald & Tuddenham, 1956). The studies of people who had undergone concentration camp experiences once again showed that extreme trauma had severe biological, psychological, social, and existential consequences, including a diminished capacity to cope with both psychological and biological stressors later in life.

Henry Krystal (1968, 1978, 1988), a psychoanalyst who studied the long-term outcome of massive traumatization in concentration camp victims, suggested that the core experience of being traumatized consists of "giving up" and accepting death and destruction as inevitable. Like Janet and Kardiner before him, but in the language of psychoanalysis, Krystal noted that the trauma response evolves from a state of hyperalert anxiety to a progressive blocking of emotions and behavioral inhibition. He noted that trauma leads to a "dedifferentiation of affects." Developmentally, children learn to interpret bodily states in terms of emotions that are indicators of personal significance, and that come to serve as guides for subsequent action; in contrast, the chronic hyperarousal of traumatized people leads to a loss of ability to grasp the personal meaning of bodily feelings. Traumatized patients come to experience emotional reactions merely as somatic states, without being able to interpret the meaning of what they are feeling. Unable to "know" what they feel, they become prone to undifferentiated affect storms and psychosomatic reactions, which are devoid of personal meaning and cannot lead to adaptive responses. According to Krystal, this development of "alexithymia" is central to the psychosomatic symptoms typical of chronically traumatized individuals.

Most of the studies carried out in the aftermath of World War II were conducted by investigators who could identify with the "unbearable situation"; the majority had been participants in the war or concentration camp survivors themselves (Helweg-Larsen et al., 1952; Eitinger, 1964; Krystal, 1968; Davidson, 1984; Klein, 1974; Des Pres, 1976). The physician who first described the "war sailor syndrome" had himself been a sailor on a torpedoed vessel (Egede-Nissen, 1978).

THE EMERGENCE OF PTSD AS A DIAGNOSTIC CATEGORY

In recent decades, much of the impetus for the development of an integrated understanding of the effects of trauma on social, psychological, and biological functions has continued to come from the participation of individuals who themselves were exposed to trauma, such as Vietnam veterans (e.g., Figley, 1978), and from people working with two hitherto entirely neglected traumatized populations: women and children. Amazingly, between 1895 and 1974, the study of trauma centered almost exclusively on its effects on white males. In 1974, Ann Burgess and Linda Holstrom at Boston City Hospital first described the "rape trauma syndrome," noting that the terrifying flashbacks and nightmares seen in these women resembled the traumatic neuroses of war. At about the same time, the Kempes (1978) started their work on battered children, and the first systematic research on trauma and family violence began to appear (Walker, 1979; Carmen [Hilberman], & Munson, 1978; Strauss, 1977; Gelles & Strauss, 1979). Although in 1980 the leading U.S. textbook of psychiatry still claimed that incest happened to fewer than one in a million women, and that its impact was not particularly damaging (Kaplan, Friedman, & Sadock, 1980), people like Judith Herman (1981) began to document the widespread sexual abuse of children and the devastation that it caused. Sarah Haley, one of the people most directly involved in the acceptance of PTSD as a diagnostic category in the *Diagnostic and Statistical Manual of Mental Disorders*, third edition (DSM-III), was both the daughter of a World War II veteran with severe "combat neurosis" and an incest victim herself. She wrote the first comprehensive paper on the problems with tolerating reports of atrocities in the therapeutic setting (Haley, 1974).

In 1970 two New York psychiatrists, Chaim Shatan and Robert J. Lifton, started "rap groups" with recently returned veterans belonging to Vietnam Veterans Against the War, in which they talked about their war experiences. These "rap sessions" rapidly spread around the country, and formed the nucleus for an informal network of professionals concerned about the lack of recognition of the effects of the war on these men's psychological health. They started to read Kardiner, the literature on Holocaust survivors, and the existing work on burn and accident victims (Andreasen, 1980). Based on this, they made a list of the 27 most common symptoms of "traumatic neuroses" reported in the literature. They compared these with over 700 clinical records of Vietnam veterans, from which they distilled what they thought were the most critical elements. Not by accident, since Kardiner's work had helped to guide this enterprise, the final classification system was very close to the one that Kardiner described in 1941. As the DSM-III process unfolded, there were numerous committee meetings and presentations at conventions of the American Psychiatric Association (APA), culminating in the inclusion of PTSD in the DSM-III (APA, 1980). All the different syndromes—the "rape trauma syndrome," the "battered woman syndrome," the "Vietnam veterans syndrome," and the "abused child syndrome"—were subsumed under this new diagnosis. However, all of these different syndromes originally had been described with considerable variations from the eventual definition of PTSD.

The DSM-III PTSD diagnosis was not a result of careful factor-analytic studies of the symptom picture of people suffering from "traumatic neuroses," but a compilation of symptoms that were arrived at on the basis of literature searches, scrutiny of clinical records, and a thoughtful political process. Only later was the relevance of PTSD as a diagnostic classification subjected to closer scrutiny, and both its advantages and limitations more fully explored (see Chapters 6 and 9, this volume). Scientific field trials were not conducted until the PTSD diagnosis was reconsidered for the DSM-IV (APA, 1994), and most of the results of those trials were tabled for further exploration (see Chapter 9).

As part of the DSM-III process, another group of researchers and clinical psychiatrists created a diagnostic system for dissociative disorders, without any known communication with the PTSD work group. Initially, there simply seems to have been no awareness of the relation between dissociation and trauma, and an entirely separate classification for the dissociative disorders was set up (Nemiah, 1980; see Chapter 13, this volume). Once these two subcommittees came to understand that they were essentially entrusted with creating diagnostic systems of overlapping phenomena, there were several attempts to merge both the subcommittees and the diagnostic categories. However, their unanimous recommendation to combine the two groups and to create a broader diagnostic system were tabled by both the DSM-III-R and the DSM-IV Task Forces (see Chapter 6).

In the United States in the mid-1970s, four authors made critical linkages between the trauma of war and the traumas of civilian life. Mardi Horowitz's (1978) *Stress Response Syndromes* built a model for effective psychotherapy of acute life-threatening experiences. Building on Erich Lindemann's (1944) observations after the fire at the Cocoanut Grove nightclub in Boston, Horowitz defined the biphasic responses to trauma—the alternating phases of intrusion and numbing (which we now know do not alternate, but coexist)—and presented a systematic dynamic psychotherapy for acute trauma. Lenore Terr (1979, 1983) introduced a developmental focus on the effects of trauma on psychological functioning when she started to publish her research on the children involved in a school bus kidnapping in Chowchilla, California. Henry Krystal's (1978) paper "Trauma and Affects" spelled out the effect of trauma on the capacity to verbalize inner experience, as well as the resulting somatization and impairment of symbolic functioning. Charles Figley (1978), a Vietnam combat veteran, edited the first significant book on Vietnam war trauma. Most of these publications appeared too late for inclusion in the DSM-III definition of PTSD, but the revised DSM-III-R definition (APA, 1987) incorporated much of this work. The history of the diagnostic classification systems is further discussed in Chapter 6 by Brett.

PROGRESS SINCE 1980

In this book we survey the explosion of scientific research on, and clinical understanding of, many aspects of human traumatization since 1980. This work reflects a rapidly evolving knowledge base and the discovery of often surprising new insights into the problems that vexed our predecessors. During this time, a great many basic and clinical researchers have devoted their professional lives to the study and treatment of psychological trauma. Presently there exists at least one journal exclusively devoted to the study of psychological trauma, the *Journal of Traumatic Stress*. Another, *Dissociation*, is devoted to specialized issues regarding that topic; a number of other peer-reviewed journals, including *Child Abuse and Neglect* and *Developmental Psychopathology*, focus exclusively on traumatized children. Starting in 1985, professional organizations focusing on the study of the effects of trauma on children and adults were founded in Europe, Australia, the United States, South Africa, and Israel. In the United States, the National Institute of Mental Health founded a Violence and Traumatic Stress branch. In the remainder of this chapter, we outline what we consider to be the most critical developments of recent years.

Epidemiology of PTSD

Some of the best psychiatric epidemiology research has been conducted in the area of PTSD. The National Vietnam Veterans Readjustment Study (Kulka et al., 1990) showed that 15.2% of male Vietnam theater veterans suffered from PTSD almost 20 years after the war; an additional 11.1% suffered from partial PTSD. In 1989, 960,000 Vietnam veterans had had full-blown PTSD at some time after leaving Vietnam. This illustrates both the pervasive occurrence of PTSD and the fact that not everyone who is exposed to potentially traumatic experiences develops the disorder. In an urban population followed by a health maintenance organization, Breslau, Davis, Andreski, and Peterson (1991) found that 9.3% of this group had a lifetime incidence of PTSD. These studies and many others (see Chapter 8, this volume) indicate that PTSD is, along with the mood disorders, among the most common of psychiatric illnesses.

Vulnerability and Course

While previous wartime studies of traumatized individuals had always been retrospective, a new generation of prospective disaster studies was started in the 1970s (Weisaeth, 1994; see Chapters 5, 8, and 20, this volume). In order for such systematic studies to be conducted, reliable and valid rating scales had to be developed (see Chapter 11). This improved technology has permitted the systematic scaling of the effects of different degrees of exposure, as well as the determination of quantitative dose–response relationships. Many different nontreatment-seeking traumatized populations have now been studied for vulnerability factors after having been exposed to similar stressors. The results indicate that vulnerability does play a significant role in the development, as well as in the long-term adjustment to living with the legacy of traumatic stress (see Chapter 15, this volume).

Developmental Impact of Trauma

Since 1980, a large number of studies have shown that in both children and adults, the security of the attachment bond is the primary defense against trauma-induced psychopathology (Finkelhor & Browne, 1984; McFarlane, 1987). Trauma interferes with children's capacity to regulate their arousal levels. This seems to be related to a wide spectrum of problems, from learning disabilities to aggression against self and others (see Chapters 9 and 14, this volume). The capacity to regulate internal states and behavioral responses to external stress defines both one's core concept of oneself and one's attitude toward one's surroundings. People who were traumatized as children have been shown to tend to act rather than to reflect, and abused children have a marked impairment in their capacity to describe affect states in words (Cicchetti & White, 1990). Since a sense of "self" is derived from the interactions between the child and his or her caregivers and is founded on the important relationships of early childhood, trauma during this period interferes with the development of ego identity and with the capacity to develop trusting and collaborative relationships (Cole & Putnam, 1992; Herman, 1992).

During the past decade, research has shown that vast numbers of psychiatric patients have trauma histories. For example, borderline personality disorder, dissociative disorders, and a variety of aggressive behaviors against self and others are usually associated with childhood histories of trauma (Herman, Perry, & van der Kolk, 1989). The link between childhood trauma and the behaviors and affect states of borderline patients clarifies many of Kernberg's astute clinical observations (Kernberg, 1978; van der Kolk et al., 1994). Further research indicates that the acknowledgment of the trauma in psychotherapy can have significant effects on outcome of these patients (Perry, Herman, van der Kolk, & Hoke, 1990).

The differential effects of trauma at different stages of human development have been put in sharp focus by such investigators as Dante Cicchetti (Cicchetti & Toth, 1994) and Frank Putnam (in press). It has become increasingly clear that PTSD is a diagnosis that is most appropriate for traumatized adults; children develop much more complex reactions that are not easily subsumed under that diagnosis (see Chapters 9 and 14). As a first step in the recognition of the differential effects of trauma at different stages of development, the DSM-IV (APA, 1994) includes a listing of "Associated Features and Disorders" for PTSD, which integrates disorders of affect regulation, dissociation, somatization, and permanent character changes. The classification system of the World Health Organization (1992), which is used in many countries outside the United States, contains broader categorizations and places a range of "reactions to severe stress and adjustment disorders" (F43) side by side with "dissociative disorders" (F44) and "somatoform disorders" (F45), under the rubric of "neurotic, stress-related and somatoform disorders." It also recognizes posttraumatic personality changes under "enduring personality changes [following catastrophic stress]" (F62).

Trauma's Effects on Both Soma and Psyche

Although the clinical descriptions of traumatized adults from 100 years ago tend to be as fresh as those of today, modern technology and advances in the neurosciences and in psychopharmacology have allowed contemporary trauma work to gain a deeper understanding of the biological underpinnings of the "traumatic neuroses." In this process, the Cartesian dualism that has dominated so much of the debate about trauma over the past century has virtually disappeared. Modern advances in the neurosciences no longer allow us to draw clear demarcations between "psychological" and "biological" processes. In the quest to understand the biological underpinnings of PTSD in humans, the vast literature on how animals respond to extreme stress has proven to be extremely helpful (van der Kolk, Greenberg, Boyd, & Krystal, 1985).

Lawrence Kolb, who as a young U.S. army psychiatrist had served in the Pacific theater and studied the effects of World War II on combat soldiers, returned to study "traumatic neuroses" after formally retiring from a long and very distinguished career in psychiatry. A student of Kardiner, he was the first to apply contemporary knowledge about the biology of information processing to PTSD (Kolb, 1987), coining the term "conditional emotional reaction" to describe the biological underpinnings of PTSD. He proposed that excessive stimulation of the central nervous system at the time of the trauma may result in permanent neuronal changes, which have negative effects on learning, habituation, and stimulus discrimination. Research during this past decade has convincingly shown that people with PTSD have a defect in the ability to evaluate intensive but irrelevant stimuli, and to mobilize appropriate levels of physiological arousal (see Chapter 10). Contemporary research shows that the failure to "get over" the trauma, and the tendency to replay the trauma over and over again in feelings, images, and actions, are mirrored biologically in the persistent appraisal of innocuous physiological stimuli as potential threats.

In recent years, researchers have been able to replicate in the laboratory what Janet and Kardiner first described in their clinical observations: that autonomic arousal can precipitate the experience of visual images and affect states associated with prior traumatic experiences. The injection of drugs such as lactate (Rainey et al., 1987) and yohimbine (Southwick et al., 1993), which stimulate autonomic arousal, may result in either panic attacks or flashbacks (exact reliving experiences) of earlier trauma in subjects with PTSD, but not in controls.

Various neurotransmitter functions have been studied in people with PTSD; abnormalities have now been demonstrated in catecholamines, endogenous opioids, corticosteroids, and serotonin. Also, the new brain imaging techniques are beginning to demonstrate the neuroanatomical correlates of PTSD symptomatology (see Chapter 10). This improved understanding of the psychobiology of trauma has been accompanied by the invention of effective pharmacological interventions to help people with PTSD become less hyperaroused and less fixated on the trauma (see Chapter 23).

Integration of Dissociative Disorders and PTSD

Although both Janet and Kardiner understood that dissociative processes were fundamental to the trauma experience, the authors of the DSM-III, unaware of this earlier work, failed to juxtapose these disorders in 1980. However, the 1980s saw a proliferation of studies on the dissociative disorders (see Chapter 13). One consistent finding has emerged: Dissociation at the moment of the trauma appears to be the single most important predictor for the establishment of chronic PTSD. This understanding is fundamental for realizing the differences between memories of traumatic events and memories of everyday experiences (see Chapter 12). The connection between childhood histories of severe trauma and the emergence of dissociative disorders has become increasingly clear. The most recent published study on the subject showed that 15% of psychiatric inpatients suffer from a dissociative disorder, almost invariably associated with childhood histories of sexual abuse (Saxe et al., 1993).

Treatment

Although much of the treatment of PTSD still rests on accumulated wisdom and clinical anecdotes, research has begun to use appropriate scientific methodology to assess various treatment approaches (Weisaeth & Eitinger, 1993). Some treatments have proven to be surprisingly disappointing, but others show much promise. Naturally, only systematic research on treatment efficacy can eventually guide good clinical practice. (See the chapters on treatment in Part VI of this book.)

CONCLUSIONS

Perhaps the most important lesson from the history of psychological trauma is the intimate connection between cultural, social, historical, and political conditions on the one hand, and the ways that people approach traumatic stress on the other (Fischer-Homberger, 1975). Traumatic neurosis seems to be an "episodic" illness, in which, for better or worse, psychiatric explanations and theories reflect the spirit of the age. History demonstrates that psychiatry is imbedded in social forces, possibly more so than any other branch of medicine. These cultural forces include the status of women and children, patriotic and financial consideration, legal processes, traditions about workers' compensation, and other economic and political processes.

Psychiatry's amnesia about the importance of psychic trauma has taken the strange form of a "repetition compulsion." Because of periodic denials about the reality of trauma's effects on the human soma and psyche, hard-earned knowledge has been repeatedly lost and subsequently rediscovered *de novo*. In some ways the attitudes of health care personnel have closely paralleled those of the public at large, though generally they have lagged behind. Whereas compassionate lay observers have always recognized that extreme life experiences can cause psychiatric illnesses, the medical profession has been capable of maintaining decades of denial about the reality of psychic trauma. Many pioneers in the area of PTSD have been sustained in their lonely pursuits by their own firsthand experiences with psychic trauma. This is true both for those who have studied war trauma and for investigators of domestic abuse and violence.

Throughout the last century, a few professional "outliers" have worked on lifting psychiatry's amnesia about the importance of psychic trauma. However, it has taken the massive traumas of war to break the denial temporarily. The most recent resurgence of awareness started in the 1970s. As could be expected during a period following massive denial, some enthusiasts came to inflate the concept of trauma, and found in it the overarching explanation for all psychic ills of humankind. Psychiatry is a field of fashions; dominant schools of thought, therapist ideology, and the charisma of particular clinicians have always had a powerful impact on developing untenable biases. Too often, these have led to acrimonious polarizations within the profession, at the expense of good patient care.

In psychiatry, each generation seems to have a need to formulate psychogical phenomena in a new language—to find a contemporary voice, in keeping with the political tenor of the times. This may not be so serious, as long as the true nature of the phenomena is understood and communicated. However, though this continual reinvention of the psychological wheel may make for interesting careers, it does not foster a solid accumulation of knowledge or the development of an effective treatment repertoire.

Is there yet a risk that the recognition of psychic trauma and its consequences will again be denied? A hundred years of research have shown that patients often cannot remember, and instead reenact their dramas in interpersonal misery. The professionals attending to these patients have had similar problems with remembering the past, and thrice in this century have drawn a blank over the hard-earned lessons. It is not likely that these amnesias and dissociations will be things of the past; they are likely to continue as long as we physicians and psychologists are faced with human breakdown in the face of overwhelming stress, which flies in the face of our inherent hubris of imagining ourselves as masters of our own fate, and as long as we need to hide from the intolerable reality of "man's inhumanity to man."

REFERENCES

Ahrenfeldt, R. H. (1958). *Psychiatry in the British army in the Second World War.* London: Routledge & Kegan Paul.

Alford, C. F. (1992). *The psychoanalytic theory of Greek tragedy.* New Haven, CT: Yale University Press.

American Psychiatric Association (APA). (1980). *Diagnostic and statistical manual of mental disorders* (3rd ed.). Washington, DC: Author.

American Psychiatric Association (APA). (1987). *Diagnostic and statistical manual of mental disorders* (3rd ed., rev.). Washington, DC: Author.

American Psychiatric Association (APA). (1994). *Diagnostic and statistical manual of mental disorders* (4th ed.) Washington, DC: Author.

Andreasen, N. C. (1980). Post-traumatic stress disorder. In H. I. Kaplan, A. M. Freedman, & B. J. Sadock (Eds.), *Comprehensive textbook of psychiatry* (Vol. 2, pp. 1517–1525). Baltimore: Williams & Wilkins.

Archibald, H., & Tuddenham, R. (1956). Persistent stress reaction after combat. *Archives of General Psychiatry, 12,* 475–481.

Askevold, F. (1976–1977). War sailor syndrome. *Psychotherapy and Psychosomatics, 27,* 133–138.

Babinski, J. (1901). Définition de l'hystérie. *Revue Neurologique, 9,* 1074–1080.

Babinski, J. (1909). Démembrement de l'hystérie traditionelle: Pithiatisme. *La Semaine Médicale, 59*(1), 3–8.

Babinski, J., & Froment, J. (1918). *Hystérie-pithiatisme et troubles nerveux d'ordre reflexe en neurologie de guerre.* Paris: Masson & Cie.

Bastiaans, J. (1970). Over de specificiteit en de behandeling van het KZ-syndroom [On the specifics and the treatment of the concentration camp syndrome]. *Nederlands Militair Geneeskunde Tijdschrift, 23,* 364–371.

Belenky, G. (Ed.). (1987). *Contemporary studies in combat psychiatry.* New York: Greenwood Press.

Bergson, H. (1896). *Matière et mémoire.* Paris: Alcan.

Bonhoeffer, M. (1926). Beurteilung, Begutachtung und Rechtsprechung bei den sogenannten Unfallsneurosen. *Deutsche Medizinische Wochenschrift, 52,* 179–182.

Breslau, N., Davis, G. C., Andreski, P., & Peterson, E. (1991). Traumatic events and posttraumatic stress disorder in an urban population of young adults. *Archives of General Psychiatry, 48,* 216–222.

Breuer, J., & Freud, S. (1955). Studies on hysteria. In J. Strachey (Ed. and Trans.), *The standard edition of the complete psychological works of Sigmund Freud* (Vol. 2, pp. 1–305). London: Hogarth Press. (Original work published 1893–1895)

Briquet, P. (1859). *Traité clinique et thérapeutique de l'hystérie* [*Clinical and therapeutic treatise on hysteria*]. Paris: Ballière.

Burgess, A. W., & Holstrom, L. (1974). Rape trauma syndrome. *American Journal of Psychiatry, 131,* 981–986.

Carmen [Hilberman], E., & Munson, M. (1978). Sixty battered women. *Victimology, 2,* 460–471.

Caruth, C. (Ed.). (1995). *Trauma and memory.* Baltimore: Johns Hopkins University Press.

Charcot, J. M. (1887). *Leçons sur les maladies du système nerveux faites à la Salpêtrière* [*Lessons on the illnesses of the nervous system held at the Salpêtrière*] (Vol. 3). Paris: Progrès Médical en A. Delahaye & E. Lecrosnie.

Cicchetti, D., & Toth, S. (Eds.). (1994). *Rochester Symposium on Developmental Psychopathology: Disorders and dysfunctions of the self.* Rochester, NY: University of Rochester Press.

Cicchetti, D., & White, J. (1990). Emotion and developmental psychopathology. In N. Stein, B. Leventhal, & T. Trebasso (Eds.), *Psychological and biological approaches to emotion* (pp. 359–382). Hillsdale, NJ: Erlbaum.

Cole, P., & Putnam, F. W. (1992). Effect of incest on self and social functioning: A developmental psychopathology perspective. *Journal of Consulting and Clinical Psychology*, *60*, 174–184.

Crocq, L., & De Verbizier, J. (1989). Le traumatisme psychologique dans l'oeuvre de Pierre Janet. *Annales Médico-Psychologiques*, *147*(9), 983–987.

Da Costa, J. M. (1871). On irritable heart: A clinical study of a form of functional cardiac disorder and its consequences. *American Journal of the Medical Sciences*, *61*, 17–52.

Davidson, S. (1984). Human reciprocity among the Jewish prisoners of the Nazi concentration camps. In *Proceedings of the Fourth Yad Vashem International Historical Conference* (pp. 555–572). Jerusalem: Yad Vashem.

Des Pres, T. (1976). *The survivor: An anatomy of life in the death camps.* New York: Oxford University Press.

Egede-Nissen, A. (1978). Krigsseilersyndromet [War sailor syndrome]. *Tidsskrift for Den Norske Lægeforening*, *98*, 469. (English summary)

Eissler, K. R. (1986). *Freud as an expert witness: The discussion of war neuroses between Freud and Wagner-Jauregg.* Madison, CT: International Universities Press.

Eitinger, L. (1964). *Concentration camp survivors in Norway and Israel.* Oslo: Universitetsforlaget.

Eitinger, L., & Strøm, A. (1973). *Mortality and morbidity after excessive stress: A follow-up investigation of Norwegian concentration camp survivors.* Oslo: Universitetsforlaget.

Ellenberger, H. F. (1970). *The discovery of the unconscious: The history and evolution of dynamic psychiatry.* New York: Basic Books.

Erichsen, J. E. (1866). *On railway and other injuries of the nervous system.* London: Walton & Moberly.

Erichsen, J. E. (1886). *On concussion of the spine, nervous shock and other obscure injuries to the nervous system in their clinical and medico-legal aspects.* New York: William Wood.

Ferenczi, S. (1955). The confusion of tongues between the adult and the child: The language of tenderness and the language of passion. In M. Balint (Ed.), *Final contributions to the problems and methods of psychoanalysis* (pp. 156–167). New York: Brunner/ Mazel. (Original work presented 1933)

Figley, C. (1978). *Stress disorders among Vietnam veterans: Theory, research and treatment implications.* New York: Brunner/Mazel.

Finkelhor, D., & Browne, A. (1984). The traumatic impact of child sexual abuse: A conceptualization. *American Journal of Orthopsychiatry*, *55*, 530–541.

Fischer-Homberger, E. (1975). *Die Traumatische Neurose, von somatischen zum sozialen Leiden.* Bern: Verlag Hans Huber.

Freud, S. (1953). The interpretation of dreams. In J. Strachey (Ed. and Trans.), *The standard edition of the complete psychological works of Sigmund Freud* (Vol. 4, pp. 1–338; Vol. 5, pp. 339–627). London: Hogarth Press. (Original work published 1900)

Freud, S. (1953). Three essays on the theory of sexuality. In J. Strachey (Ed. and Trans.), *The standard edition of the complete psychological works of Sigmund Freud* (Vol. 7, pp. 125–243). London: Hogarth Press. (Original work published 1905)

Freud S (1955). Beyond the pleasure principle. In J. Strachey (Ed. and Trans.), *The standard edition of the complete psychological works of Sigmund Freud* (Vol. 18, pp. 3–64). London: Hogarth Press. (Original work published 1920)

Freud, S. (1959). An autobiographical study. In J. Strachey (Ed. and Trans.), *The standard edition of the complete psychological works of Sigmund Freud* (Vol. 20, pp. 3–74). London: Hogarth Press. (Original work published 1925)

Freud, S. (1962). On the psychical mechanism of hysterical phenomena: A Lecture. In J. Strachey (Ed. and Trans.), *The standard edition of the complete psychological works of Sigmund Freud* (Vol. 3, pp. 25–39). London: Hogarth Press. (Original work published 1893)

Freud, S. (1962). Heredity and the aetiology of the neuroses. In J. Strachey (Ed. and Trans.), *The standard edition of the complete psychological works of Sigmund Freud* (Vol. 3, pp. 141–156). London: Hogarth Press. (Original work published 1896a)

Freud S. (1962). The aetiology of hysteria. In J. Strachey (Ed. and Trans.), *The standard edition of the complete psychological works of Sigmund Freud* (Vol. 3, pp. 189–221). London: Hogarth Press. (Original work published 1896b)

Freud, S. (1963). Introductory lectures on psycho-analysis. In J. Strachey (Ed. and Trans.), *The standard edition of the complete psychological works of Sigmund Freud* (Vol. 15, pp. 1–240; Vol. 16, pp. 241–496). London: Hogarth Press. (Original work published 1916–1917)

Gelles, R. J., & Strauss, M. A. (1979). Determinants of violence in the family: Toward a theoretical integration. In W. R. Burr, R. Hill, & F. I. Nye (Eds.), *Contemporary theories about the family.* New York: Free Press.

Grinker, R. R., & Spiegel, J. P. (1945). *Men under stress.* Philadelphia: Blakiston.

Grinker, R. R., Werble, B., & Drye, R. C. (1968). *The borderline syndrome: A behavioral study of ego functions.* New York: Basic Books.

Haley, S. (1974). When the patient reports atrocities. *Archives of General Psychiatry, 30,* 191–196.

Helweg-Larsen, P., Hoffmeyer, H., Kieler, J., Thaysen, J. H., Thygesen, P., & Wulff, M. H. (1952). Famine disease in German concentration camps: Complications and sequelae. *Acta Psychiatrica et Neurologica Scandinavica* (Suppl. 83), 1–460.

Herman, J. L. (1981). *Father–daughter incest.* Cambridge, MA: Harvard University Press.

Herman, J. L., Perry, J. C., & van der Kolk, B. A. (1989). Childhood trauma in borderline personality disorder. *American Journal of Psychiatry, 146,* 490–495.

Herman, J. L. (1992). *Trauma and recovery.* New York: Basic Books.

Hocking, F. (1970). Psychiatric aspects of extreme environmental stress. *Diseases of the Nervous System, 31,* 1278–1282.

Horowitz, M. J. (1978). *Stress response syndromes.* New York: Jason Aronson.

Janet, P. (1887). L'anesthésie systématisée et la dissociation des phénomènes psychologiques. *Revue Philosophique, 23*(1), 449–472.

Janet, P. (1889). *L'automatisme psychologique.* Paris: Alcan.

Janet, P. (1894). Histoire d'une idée fixe. *Revue Philosophique, 37,* 121–163.

Janet, P. (1904). L'amnésie et la dissociation des souvenirs par l'émotion. *Journal de Psychologie, 1,* 417–453.

Janet, P. (1909). *Les nervoses.* Paris: Flammarion.

Janet, P. (1911). *L'état mental des hystériques* (2nd ed.). Paris: Alcan.

Janet, P. (1920). *The major symptoms of hysteria.* New York: Hafner. (Original work published 1907)

Janet, P. (1925). *Psychological healing* (Vols. 1–2) (C. Paul & E. Paul, Trans.). New York: Macmillan. (Original work published 1919)

Janet, P. (1930). Autobiography. In C. A. Murchinson (Ed. and Trans.), *A history of psychology in autobiography* (Vol. 1). Worcester, MA: Clark University Press.

Jaspers, K. (1913). *Allgemeine Psychopathologie.* Berlin: Springer-Verlag.

Kaplan, H. I., Freedman, A. M., & Sadock, B. J. (Eds.). (1980). *Comprehensive textbook of psychiatry* (2 vols.). Baltimore: Williams & Wilkins.

Kardiner, A. (1941). *The traumatic neuroses of war.* New York: Hoeber.

Kempe, R. S., & Kempe, C. H. (1978). *Child abuse.* Cambridge, MA: Harvard University Press.

Kernberg, O. (1978). Borderline personality organization. *Journal of the American Psychoanalytic Association, 15,* 641–685.

Klein, H. (1974). Delayed affects and aftereffects of severe traumatization. *Israeli Annals of Psychiatry, 12,* 293–303.

Kolb, L. C. (1987). Neurophysiological hypothesis explaining posttraumatic stress disorder. *American Journal of Psychiatry, 144,* 989–995.

Kraepelin, E. (1899). *Psychiatrie* (6th ed.). Leipzig: Verlag von Johann Ambrosius Barth.

Krystal, H. (Ed.). (1968). *Massive psychic trauma.* New York: International Universities Press.

Krystal, H. (1978). Trauma and affects. *Psychoanalytic Study of the Child, 33,* 81–116.

Krystal, H. (1988). *Integration and self healing: Affect, trauma, and alexithymia.* Hillsdale, NJ: Analytic Press.

Kulka, R. A., Schlenger, W. E., Fairbank, J. A., Hough, R. L., Jordan, B. K., & Marmar, C. R. (1990). *Trauma and the Vietnam War generation: Report of findings from the National Vietnam Veterans' Readjustment Study.* New York: Brunner/Mazel.

Lindemann, E. (1944). Symptomatology and management of acute grief. *American Journal of Psychiatry, 101,* 141–148.

MacLeod, A. D. (1993). Putnam, Jackson and post-traumatic stress disorder. *Journal of Nervous and Mental Disease, 181*(11), 709–710.

MacMillan, M. (1980). *Freud evaluated: The completed arc.* Amsterdam: North-Holland.

MacMillan, M. (1991). Freud and Janet on organic and hysterical paralyses: A mystery solved? *International Review of Psychoanalysis, 17,* 189–203.

Main, T. (1989). *"The ailment" and other psychoanalytic essays.* London: Free Association Press.

Masson, J. (1984). *The assault on truth.* New York: Farrar, Straus & Giroux.

McFarlane, A. C. (1987). Posttraumatic phenomena in a longitudinal study of children following a natural disaster. *Journal of the American Academy of Child and Adolescent Psychiatry, 26,* 764–749.

Merskey, H. (1991). Shell-shock. In *150 years of British psychiatry 1841–1991* (pp. 245–267). London: Gaskell/The Royal College of Psychiatrists.

Moran, Lord. (1945). *Anatomy of courage.* London: Constable.

Myers, A. B. R. (1870). *On the aetiology and prevalence of disease of the heart among soldiers.* London: J. Churchill.

Myers, C. S. (1915). A contribution to the study of shell shock. *Lancet,* 316–320.

Myers, C. S. (1940). *Shell shock in France 1914–18.* Cambridge, England: Cambridge University Press.

Nemiah, J. C. (1980). Psychogenic amnesia, psychogenic fugue, and multiple personality. In H. I. Kaplan, A. M. Freedman, & B. J. Sadock (Eds.), *Comprehensive textbook of psychiatry* (Vol. 2, pp. 942–957). Baltimore: Williams & Wilkins.

Nemiah, J. C. (1989). Janet redivivus [Editorial]. *American Journal of Psychiatry, 146,* 1527–1529.

Nonne, M. (1915). Zur therapeutischen Verwendung der Hypnose bei Fêllen von Kriegshysterie. *Medizinische Klinik, 11*(51), 1391–1396.

Oppenheim, H. (1889). *Die traumatische Neurosen.* Berlin: Hirschwald.

Page, H. (1885). Injuries of the spine and spinal cord without apparent mechanical lesion. In M. R. Trimble (Ed.), *Posttraumatic neurosis: From railroad spine to whiplash* (p. 29). London: J. Churchill.

Perry, J. C., Herman, J. L., van der Kolk, B. A., & Hoke, L. A. (1990). Psychotherapy and psychological trauma in borderline personality disorder. *Psychiatric Annals, 20,* 33–43.

Putnam, F. W. (1989). Pierre Janet and modern views on dissociation. *Journal of Traumatic Stress, 2*(4), 413–430.

Putnam, F. W. (in press). *Child and adolescent dissociative disorders.* New York: Guilford Press.

Putnam, J. J. (1881). Recent investigations into patients of so called concussion of the spine. *Boston Medical and Surgical Journal, 109,* 217.

Putnam, J. J. (1898). On the etiology and pathogenesis of the posttraumatic psychoses and neuroses. *Journal of Nervous and Mental Disease, 25,* 769–799.

Rainey, J. M., Aleem, A., Ortiz, A., Yaragani, V., Pohl, R., & Berchow, R. (1987). Laboratory procedure for the inducement of flashbacks. *American Journal of Psychiatry, 144,* 1317–1319.

Saxe, G., van der Kolk, B. A., Hall, K., Schwartz, J., Chinman, G., Hall, M. D., Lieberg, G., & Berkowitz, R. (1993). Dissociative disorders in psychiatric inpatients. *American Journal of Psychiatry, 150*(7), 1037–1042.

Shalev, A., & Ursano, R. J. (1990). Group debriefing following exposure to traumatic stress. In J. E. Lundeberg, U. Otto, & B. Rybeck (Eds.), *War medical services* (pp. 192–207). Stockholm: Försvarets Forskningsanstalt.

Shay, J. (1994). *Achilles in Vietnam: Combat trauma and the undoing of character.* New York: Atheneum.

Southwick, S. M., Krystal, J. H., Morgan, C. A., Johnson, D., Nagy, L. M., Niculaou, A., Heninger, G. R., & Charney, D. S. (1993). Abnormal noradrenergic function in posttraumatic stress disorder. *Archives of General Psychiatry, 50,* 266–274.

Stierlin, E. (1909). *Über psychoneuropathische Folgezustände bei den Überlebenden der Katastrophe von Courrières am 10. Marz 1906* [*On the psychoneuropathic consequences among the survivors of the Courrierès catastrophe of 10 March 1906*]. Unpublished doctoral dissertation, University of Zürich.

Stierlin, E. (1911). Nervöse und psychische Störungen nach Katastrophen [Nervous and psychic disturbances after catastrophes]. *Deutsches Medizinische Wochenschrift, 37,* 2028–2035.

Stouffer, S. A. (1949). Studies in social psychology in World War II. In *The American soldier: Vol. 2. Combat and its aftermath.* Princeton, NJ: Princeton University Press.

Strauss, M. A. (1977). Sociological perspective on the prevention and treatment of wife-beating. In M. Roy (Ed.), *Battered women: A psychological study of domestic violence.* New York: Van Nostrand Reinhold.

Tardieu, A.-A. (1878). *Etude médicolégale sur les attentats aux moeurs* [A medico-legal study of assaults on decency]. Paris: Ballière.

Terr, L. C. (1979). Children of Chowchilla: A study of psychic trauma. *Psychoanalytic Study of the Child, 34,* 552–623.

Terr, L. C. (1983). Chowchilla revisited: The effects of psychic trauma four years after a school-bus kidnapping. *American Journal of Psychiatry, 140,* 1543–1550.

Tichener, J. L. (1986). Post-traumatic decline: A consequence of unresolved destructive drives. In C. Figley (Ed.), *Trauma and its wake* (Vol. 2, pp. 5–19). New York: Brunner/Mazel.

van der Hart, O., & Brown, P. (1992). Abreaction re-evaluated. *Dissociation, 5(4),* 127–140.

van der Hart, O., & Friedman, B. (1989). A reader's guide to Pierre Janet on dissociation: A neglected intellectual heritage. *Dissociation, 2(1),* 3–16.

van der Kolk, B. A., Greenberg, M. S., Boyd, H., & Krystal, J. H. (1985). Inescapable shock, neurotransmitters, and addiction to trauma: Toward a psychobiology of post-traumatic stress. *Biological Psychiatry, 20,* 314–325.

van der Kolk, B. A., Herron, N., & Hostetler, A. (1994). The history of trauma in psychiatry. *Psychiatric Clinics of North America, 17,* 583–600.

van der Kolk, B. A., & van der Hart, O. (1989). Pierre Janet and the breakdown of adaptation in psychological trauma. *American Journal of Psychiatry, 146,* 1530–1540.

Venzlaff, U. (1966). Das akute und das chronische Belastungssyndrom. *Medizinsche Welt, 17,* 369–376.

Venzlaff, U. (1975). Aktuelle Probleme der forensischen Psychiatrie. In K. P. Kisker, J. E. Meyer, C. Müller, & E. Strømgren (Eds.), *Psychiatrie der Gegenwart* (pp. 920–932). Bertin: Springer-Verlag.

Walker, L. (1979). *The battered women.* New York: Harper & Row.

Weisaeth, L. (1994). Psychological and psychiatric aspects of technological disasters. In R. J. Ursano, C. S. McCaugley, & C. Fullerton (Eds.), *Individual and commu-*

nity response to trauma and disaster: The structure of human chaos (pp. 72–102). Cambridge, England: Cambridge University Press.

Weisaeth, L., & Eitinger, L. (1993). Posttraumatic stress phenomena: Common themes across wars, disasters and traumatic events. In J. P. Wilson & B. Raphael (Eds.), *International handbook of traumatic stress syndromes* (pp. 69–77). New York: Plenum Press.

World Health Organization (1992). *The ICD-10 classification of mental and behavioral disorders: Clinical descriptions and guidelines.* Geneva: Author.

PART II

ACUTE REACTIONS

CHAPTER 4

Stress versus Traumatic Stress

From Acute Homeostatic Reactions to Chronic Psychopathology

ARIEH Y. SHALEV

> *The disease is due essentially to a disordered imagination,*
> *whereby the part of the brain chiefly affected is that part in*
> *which the images . . . are located. This is the inner part of*
> *the brain where the vital spirits constantly surge back and*
> *forth through the nerve fibers in which the impressions . . .*
> *are stored. Once the vital spirits have made a path for*
> *themselves and widened it they find it easier, as in sleep, to*
> *take the same path again and again.*
> —HOFFER (1678; QUOTED IN ROSEN, 1975, p. 342)

Within psychiatric nomenclature, there exist many terms that are now obsolete or difficult to justify. Salient examples are diagnoses that locate the origins of psychological problems in body organs (e.g., "hysteria," "hypochondria") or bodily humors (e.g., "melancholia"). Although the term "posttraumatic stress disorder" (PTSD) is a much newer diagnostic label, it is an equally problematic term, for a number of reasons. First, "traumatic stress" confounds two distinct constructs—"stress" and "mental traumatization." Second, the idea of "posttraumatic" fosters a retrospective definition of events as traumatic, based on their long-term pathogenic effects. Third, the inclusion within a single framework of common unfortunate incidents (e.g., road traffic accidents) and colossal atrocities (e.g., the Holocaust) creates an unbalanced foundation for an etiological theory of stress-related disorders.

Much of the research on PTSD has been based on widely held but as yet unproven assumptions. The first of these is that the initial response to the trauma, which eventually leads to PTSD, is a normal response to an abnormal event. Another assumption is that of continuity—namely, that the reaction that takes place immediately after a trauma continues in some way into the chronic PTSD. Lastly, it is often assumed that there is an analogy between traumatic stress and milder forms of stress. This chapter challenges these concepts, examining the available literature, and finally proposes a model that attempts to explain the perseverance of PTSD symptoms.

IS PTSD A NORMAL RESPONSE TO ABNORMAL CIRCUMSTANCES?

The belief that PTSD is a normal response to abnormal situations is itself based upon two other assumptions: (1) that the incident that causes the PTSD is "abnormal"; and (2) that all of the reactions seen are within the limits of a normal response to such a stressor, and in fact would be expected to be seen in the majority of people experiencing the trauma (American Psychiatric Association, 1980). This is not a new belief; it appeared early in the traumatic stress literature. It continues to appear in more recent texts, as in this example: "What was of survival value in, for example, the jungle of Vietnam—an activation of noradrenergic and the [corticotropin-releasing factor/hypothalamic–pituitary–adrenal] axis systems, the strong engraving of memory traces of the event, promotion of the startle response, and heightened attention and vigilance—may represent pathology when the veteran is sitting at the dinner table with family [members] 20 years after the war" (Bremner, Davis, Krystal, Southwick, & Charney, 1993). In this case, PTSD is conceptualized as a normal response that continues over an extended time period, beyond its usefulness. A similar hypothesis appears in the psychodynamic literature, in which PTSD is seen as incomplete mental processing—in other words, a normal response that is not properly finished (e.g., Horowitz , 1974, 1986; Horowitz, Wilner, & Alvarez, 1979; Marmar, Foy, Kagan, & Pynoos, 1993). Behavioral approaches are also based on this assumption: Symptoms are normal learned responses, and in PTSD these responses do not extinguish (e.g., Keane, Fairbank, Caddell, Zimering, & Bender, 1985).

The "normal response" hypothesis suggests that PTSD is, in essence, a failure to recover from mental traumatization. Implicitly, recovery is always possible, especially when the subject is empowered so that the "normal" recovery process may occur (Herman, 1993). However, the contention that trauma invariably results in psychopathology is not always borne out by quantitative data . This is seen in the fact that a large number of survivors of the most extreme traumatization in modern history, the Holocaust (e.g., Levav & Abramson, 1984; Eaton, Sigal, & Weinfeld, 1982), have somehow recovered and lived normally. Results of the National Vietnam Veterans Readjustment Study (Kulka et al., 1990) similarly show that only 15.2% of male Vietnam veterans suffer from prolonged PTSD. McFarlane (1984) has suggested that mental illness should never be considered the *expected* reaction to major life events such as disasters.

The alternative viewpoint—that PTSD is in fact an abnormal response—has not really been considered within the literature, and only recently have sufficient data accumulated from outcome studies to permit us to examine this concept in a more critical light. The first important aspect to have emerged is that PTSD symptomatology occurs after ordinary as well as extraordinary events. Recent studies have shown that traumatic events frequently happen to civilians during peacetime, as well as to soldiers and war victims, and that many survivors of such frequent events develop PTSD (Breslau & Davis, 1992). Clinical descriptions similarly show that PTSD may follow events of lesser magnitude, such as road traffic accidents (e.g., Mayou, Bryant, & Duthie, 1993), medical procedures (Shalev, Schreiber, Galai, & Melmed, 1993c) or myocardial infarcts (Kutz, Shabtai, Solomon, Neumann, & David, 1994). The fact that a chronically disabling disorder such as PTSD can result from such common events argues against the "normality" of the response. Following is a review of the extensive literature on the predictors of PTSD, which will deepen this discussion of the nature of the immediate response to trauma.

PREDICTORS OF PTSD

The immediate response to trauma is but one step in the chain of causality that eventually leads to PTSD. Hence its intensity predicts, at best, only part of the variance of the pathological outcome. In order to put the effects of the immediate response in perspective, Table 4.1 summarizes 38 studies of predictors of PTSD. These predictors relate to pretrauma vulnerability, magnitude of the stressor, preparedness for the event, quality of the immediate and short-term responses, and postevent "recovery" factors.

Pretrauma Vulnerability

Pretrauma vulnerability encompasses genetic and biological risk factors, as well as factors related to one's life course, rearing environment, mental health, and personality. Biological constitutional factors include family history of mental disorders (Davidson, Smith, & Kudler, 1989), gender (Breslau & Davis, 1992),

TABLE 4.1. Predictors of PTSD

Author	N/Population/Design/Instruments	Variable(s) predicted	Predictors
Abenhaim et al., 1992	254 survivors of terrorist attacks in France; survey	PTSD	+ Severity of injury # Sex, age
Basoglu et al., 1994	55 torture survivors and 55 controls (political activists without torture); case control; questionnaires, interviews	PTSD and PTSD symptoms	+ Torture # Preparedness; commitment; social supports
Bownes et al., 1991	51 rape victims; survey	PTSD	+ Rapes by strangers; use of physical force or weapons; injury
Breslau & Davis, 1987	69 Vietnam veterans (inpatients); survey	PTSD, panic disorder, major depression, mania	+ (PTSD): participation in atrocities; cumulative exposure to combat stressors # (Panic disorder and major depression): combat intensity and atrocities
Breslau & Davis, 1992	1,007 young urban adults; survey	Chronic PTSD	+ Family history of antisocial behavior; female gender
Breslau et al., 1991	1,007 young urban adults; survey	Exposure to trauma; PTSD	+ (Exposure): lower education; male gender; early conduct problems; extraversion; family history of psychiatric disorder + (PTSD): early separation from parents; neuroticism; preexisting anxiety or depression; family history of anxiety

Buydens-Branchey et al., 1990	84 Vietnam veterans; survey	PTSD	+ Combat intensity and duration; physical injury
Chemtob et al., 1990	57 Vietnam veterans (special forces); survey	PTSD symptoms	+ Poor preservice relationships; being wounded; friends MIA; guilt over death of a friend; lack of preparation to leave the unit; failure to discuss feelings on return
Clarke et al., 1993	69 Cambodian young refugees of the Pol Pot regime; survey, interviews	PTSD and depressive symptoms	+ (PTSD): war trauma; resettlement strain + (Depression): recent stressful events
Davidson et al., 1991	2,985 residents of Piedmont, North Carolina; epidemiological survey	PTSD	+ Job instability, family history of psychiatric illness; parental poverty; history of child abuse; parental separation prior to age 10
Feinstein & Dolan, 1991	48 civilian survivors of physical trauma; survey, questionnaires (GHQ)	PTSD; psychiatric morbidity	+ Distress postinjury # Severity of the stressor predicts initial distress but not 6-month morbidity
Foy et al., 1984	43 help-seeking Vietnam veterans; survey, MMPI profiles, self-reports	PTSD	+ Combat exposure; military adjustment; MMPI scores; anxiety # Preliminary adjustment

TABLE 4.1. (cont.)

Author	N/Population/Design/Instruments	Variable(s) predicted	Predictors
Gallers et al., 1988	60 Vietnam combat veterans (30 with PTSD and 30 without PTSD); case control; questionnaires	PTSD and PTSD symptoms	+ Traumatic violence; distress at having participated in such acts # Preliminary adjustment; drug and alcohol use
Gidycz & Koss, 1991	1,213 sexual assault victims; survey, questionnaires	Anxiety and depression	+ History of mental health problems; aggressiveness of assault; belief that people are not trustworthy; conservatism regarding sex
Goldberg et al., 1990	715 monozygotic twin pairs discordant for military service in southeast Asia	PTSD	+ Combat exposure (nine-fold increase in prevalence from noncombat to high combat exposure)
Green et al., 1990	200 Vietnam veterans; survey, interviews	PTSD	+ Intensity of the stressor; exposure to grotesque death; level of education; social support at homecoming
Green & Berlin, 1987	60 help-seeking Vietnam veterans; survey	PTSD	+ Combat intensity; current impact of previously experienced events, concurrent level of life stress # Social support during the first year of return from Vietnam; preservice psychosocial functioning

Study	Sample; method	Outcome	Findings
Kilpatrick et al., 1989	294 adult female crime victims; survey	Crime-related PTSD	+ (PTSD): Life threat during crime; physical injury; completed rape
Laufer et al., 1985	326 Vietnam combat veterans	PTSD and PTSD symptoms	+ Combat exposure; exposure to abusive violence and killing; subjective "experiential" coping
McCranie et al., 1992	57 Vietnam veterans with PTSD (inpatients); survey	PTSD symptoms and severity	+ Negative parenting behaviors predict PTSD symptom severity at lower levels of combat exposure
McFall et al., 1991	489 Vietnam veterans seeking help for drug abuse; survey	PTSD	+ Combat exposure; age at war zone duty; duration of war zone duty; physical injury
McFarlane, 1988	469 firefighters exposed to bushfire; prospective; follow-up, questionnaires	PTSD	+ Introversion, neuroticism; family history of psychiatric disorder # Trauma intensity; threat; loss
McFarlane, 1989	469 firefighters exposed to bushfire disaster; follow-up at 4, 11, and 29 months	Posttraumatic morbidity	+ Neuroticism, past history of treatment for a psychological disorder # Exposure, loss
Nader et al., 1990	100 elementary school children exposed to sniper shooting; follow-up at 14 months after event	Severity of posttraumatic stress reaction	+ Level of exposure; guilt; knowing the child who was killed
North & Smith, 1992	900 homeless men and women in St. Louis; survey, interviews (DIS)	PTSD	+ Childhood histories of abuse and family fighting # Psychiatric diagnoses

(cont.)

TABLE 4.1. (cont.)

Author	N/Population/Design/Instruments	Variable(s) predicted	Predictors
North et al., 1994	136 civilian survivors of mass shooting; survey 1 month after the event, interview (DIS)	PTSD	+ Predisaster psychiatric disorder (MDD) predicted PTSD in women but not men # Most PTSD subjects had no history of mental illness
Patterson et al., 1990	54 inpatients with major burn injury; weekly follow-up during and after admission	PTSD	+ Total body surface area burn; female sex; lack of responsibility for the injury
Perry et al., 1992	51 inpatients with burn injuries; follow-up at 1 week and 2 ($n = 51$), 6 ($n = 40$), and 12 ($n = 31$) months	PTSD	+ Subjective variables: emotional distress, perceived social support # Severity of burns
Resnick et al., 1992	295 female crime victims; survey	PTSD	+ High crime stress; significant interaction among crime stress level; precrime depression and PTSD
Schnurr et al., 1993	131 male Vietnam-era veterans; studied premilitary MMPI and current PTSD; interviews (SCID)	PTSD and PTSD symptoms	+ (PTSD symptoms): MMPI scales of hypochondriasis, psychopathy, masculinity–femininity, and paranoia + (PTSD): depression, hypomania, and social introversion
Shalev, 1992	15 injured survivors of a terrorist attack; prospective follow-up for 10 months	PTSD	# Symptoms of intrusion and denial recorded 1 week after the trauma

84

Study	Sample	Outcome measure	Findings
Smith et al., 1990	46 hotel employees who survived a jet plane crash; survey, interview 4–6 weeks after the event	PTSD, major depression GAD, alcohol abuse and dependence	+ Predisaster psychiatric histories predict postdisaster psychiatric disorders
Solkoff et al., 1986	100 Vietnam combat veterans (50 with PTSD and 50 without PTSD); case control; structured interview	PTSD	+ Combat experience; perceptions of homecoming # Childhood family history; preservice factors
Solomon, Avitzur, & Mikulincer, 1990	255 Israeli war veterans of the Lebanon war; follow-up at 1 and 2 years after the war, questionnaires	PTSD	+ Social support (++); life events; internal locus of control
Solomon et al., 1991	348 Israeli veterans of the Lebanon war with combat stress reaction; Miller Behavioral Style Scale	Trauma-related psychopathology	+ Blunting coping strategies
Speed et al., 1989	62 World War II POWs; survey, interviews	PTSD	+ Proportion body weight lost during captivity; experience of torture # Weak: family history of mental illness; preexisting psychopathology
Sutker et al., 1990	193 World War II and Korea POWs; survey	PTSD	+ Confinement; weight loss; lower socioeconomic status; greater hardship; lower military rank
Zaidi & Foy, 1994	20 Vietnam veterans (inpatients); survey	PTSD symptoms	+ History of physical abuse

Note. GHQ, General Health Questionnaire; MMPI, Minnesota Multiphasic Personality Inventory; DIS, Diagnostic Interview Schedule; SCID, Structured Clinical Interview for DSM-III-R; +, finding of a significant event on the outcome measure; #, finding of no significant effect on the outcome measure.

and possibly also heightened conditionability (Peri, Ben-Shachar, & Shalev, 1994) or neuroendocrine vulnerability factors (e.g., low cortisol response to stress; Yehuda et al., 1993). True et al. (1993) have shown that genetic factors account for 13% to 30% of the variance in likelihood for symptoms in the reexperiencing cluster, 30% to 34% for symptoms in the avoidance cluster, and 28% to 32% for symptoms in the arousal cluster. Foy, Resnick, Sipprelle, and Carroll (1987) found that a positive family history for psychiatric disorders (especially alcohol) predicted PTSD under conditions of low combat exposure, whereas combat trauma exposure, homecoming environment, and social support during the first 6 months after military discharge predicted PTSD under conditions of high combat exposure.

Personality traits, such as neuroticism, introversion, and prior mental disorders, also increase the risk for developing PTSD. Factors related to life events include early traumatization (e.g., childhood sexual and physical abuse) and exposure to similar trauma (e.g., repeated combat experience or rape experience). Negative parenting behavior, early separation from parents, parental poverty, and lower education independently predict both exposure (Breslau, Davis, Andreski, & Peterson, 1991) and PTSD following exposure (e.g., Green, Grace, Lindy, Gleser, & Leonard, 1990; Davidson, Hughes, Blazer, & George, 1991; McCranie, Hyer, Boudewyns, & Woods, 1992). The last four variables interact with one another and may represent different facets of a common socioeconomic factor.

Magnitude of the Stressor

The intensity of the traumatic event, expressed in terms of combat intensity and duration (Foy, Rueger, Sipprelle, & Carroll, 1984; Solkoff, Gray, & Keill, 1986; Breslau & Davis, 1987; Green & Berlin, 1987; Buydens-Branchey, Noumair, & Branchey, 1990; Goldberg, True, Eisen, & Henderson, 1990; McFall, Mackay, & Donovan, 1991), dangerousness of a rape incident (Kilpatrick et al., 1989; Bownes, O'Gorman, & Sayers, 1991), intensity of a torture experience (Basoglu et al., 1994; Speed, Engdahl, Schwartz, & Eberly, 1989), or extent of physical injury (e.g., Abenhaim, Dab, & Salmi, 1992), contributes significantly to the development of PTSD (for a review, see March, 1993). Green (1990) has proposed eight generic dimensions of traumatic stressors that "cut across different types of traumatic events": (1) threat to one's life and body integrity; (2) severe physical harm or injury; (3) receipt of intentional injury/harm; (4) exposure to the grotesque; (5) witnessing or learning of violence to loved ones; (6) learning of exposure to a noxious agent; and (7) causing death or severe harm to another. When genetic variance was controlled for, Goldberg et al. (1990) found a positive relationship between combat intensity and the incidence of PTSD.

Preparation for the Event

Studies have shown that adequate preparation for a stressful event, when such preparation is possible, protects individuals from the effect of stress (e.g., Chemtob et al., 1990). It reduces uncertainty, increases one's sense of control, and teaches automatic responses that are less readily eroded under stress. The psychological effect of preparation may even exceed the content of the training. Hytten (1989) analyzed the rescue maneuvers of helicopter pilots who, prior to having crashed into the North Sea, had received simulator escape training. It was found that effective rescue maneuvers during the actual crash differed from those rehearsed during training; yet the survivors perceived the training exercises as very helpful. The author interpreted these findings as suggesting that training was effective in generating positive response outcome expectancy, rather than in teaching a specific life-saving routine.

Immediate and Short-Term Responses

Individual responses during the impact phase of a stressor (recently referred to as "peritraumatic"; Marmar et al., 1994) have received increasing attention in the last few years. Peritraumatic responses include (1) observable behaviors or symptoms (e.g., conversion, agitation, stupor); (2) emotional or cognitive experiences (e.g., anxiety, panic, numbing, confusion); or (3) mental processes or functions (e.g., defenses). These three dimensions (i.e., symptoms, experiences, and mental functions) are often confounded. Dissociation, for example, is at one and the same time an observable behavior, an experience, and a form of defense against pain, distress, or humiliation.

A central point here is the extent to which particular peritraumatic reactions (e.g., dissociation, freezing/surrender, disorganization) specifically predict prolonged distress. Early authors (e.g., Grinker & Spiegel, 1945) felt that some people develop excessive responses under stress and that such responses are often transformed into prolonged disorders:

> Fear and anger in small doses are stimulating and alert the ego, increasing efficacy. But, when stimulated by repeated psychological trauma, the intensity of the emotion heightens until a point is reached at which the ego loses its effectiveness and may become altogether crippled. . . . The clinical description of the *neurotic reactions to severe combat stress* is thus a passing parade of every type of psychological and psychosomatic symptom, and of maladaptive behavior. In addition, one of the major characteristics of traits of neurotic reactions to battle is the manner in which symptoms alter with the laps of time. What begins as a severe anxiety reaction in the combat area may end up as a severe depression in the rear area or at home. (Grinker & Spiegel, 1945, pp. 82–83; emphasis added)

Grinker and Spiegel (1945, p. 84) also proposed a hierarchy of combat anxiety states:

> [In] mild anxiety states . . . the subjective and motor signs of anxiety are present but function is not yet interfered with. In moderate anxiety states the same symptoms may have progressed to the point where the flier makes mistakes in flying and now has his own incapacity to fear as well . . . *Severe anxiety states* [are characterized by] much regression of the ego, confusion in regard to the environment, mutism and stupor. (p. 84; emphasis added)

Horowitz (1986) similarly described an "acute catastrophic stress reaction," characterized by panic, cognitive disorganization, disorientation, dissociation, severe insomnia, and agitation.

Following Grinker and Spiegel (1945), Solomon (1993) described, in combat veterans of the 1982 Lebanon War, an initial "combat stress reaction" encompassing anxiety, psychomotor agitation, and depression. The symptoms of combat stress reaction were found to be nonspecific and unstable ("polymorphous and labile"), and no specific constellation was found to be predictive of PTSD.

Another hypothetical predictor is dissociation. A recent elaboration of Janet's concept of traumatic dissociation (van der Kolk & van der Hart, 1989), studies showing heightened dissociability in PTSD (Spiegel, Hunt, & Dondershine, 1988), and reports of frequent dissociative reactions during stressful events (Cardeña & Spiegel, 1993) jointly propound that dissociation may have a specific role in the pathogenesis of PTSD. Several studies have provided empirical support for the dissociation–PTSD relationship. Holen (1993) studied survivors of the North Sea oil rig disaster and showed that reported dissociation during the trauma was significantly associated with the outcome of the disaster. Carlson and Rosser-Hogan (1991) showed a relationship among trauma severity, dissociative symptoms, and posttraumatic stress in Cambodian refugees. Bremner et al. (1992) found that Vietnam veterans with PTSD reported having experienced higher levels of dissociative symptoms during combat, in comparison to veterans without PTSD. Koopman, Classen, and Spiegel (1994) found that dissociative symptoms reported by survivors of the Oakland/Berkeley, California, firestorm early after the event predicted PTSD symptoms 7 months later. Finally, Marmar et al. (1994) found that peritraumatic dissociation reported by Vietnam veterans predicted PTSD above and beyond the effects of combat exposure.

In a recent prospective study of 51 injured trauma survivors in Israel (Shalev, Peri, Caneti, & Schreiber, 1996), it was found that peritraumatic dissociation, as reported 1 week after the trauma on the Marmar et al. (1994) Peritraumatic Dissociative Experience Scale, explained 30% of the variance in PTSD symptoms at a 6-month follow-up, over and above the effects of gender, education, age, and event severity, as well as intrusion, avoidance anxiety, and depression following the event. Thirteen of the 51 subjects (25.4%) had developed PTSD at follow-up, and peritraumatic dissociation was also the strongest predictor of PTSD status 6 months after the event.

Chaotic or disorganized responses such as "freezing," "stupor," or "surrender," and the ensuing perception of events as uncontrollable and unpredictable, strongly affect long-term outcome (Foa & Rothbaum, 1989). According to Baum, Cohen, and Hall (1993), "one of the possible reasons for chronic stress following traumatic events is the disorganizing effect of loss of control and violation of expectations for regulating aspects of one's life" (p. 276).

Dimensions of coping during the event have also been studied as predictors of PTSD. Coping during combat has been defined as "any attempt to increase the gap between combat stress and subjective distress" (Shalev & Munitz, 1989, p. 173). Coping includes a broad range of cognitive and behavioral strategies, generally construed as "problem-focused," "emotion-focused," and "appraisal-related" (e.g., Haan, 1969; Lazarus & Folkman, 1984). Solomon, Avitzur, and Mikulincer (1990) and Solomon, Mikulincer, and Arad (1991) found a positive relationship between emotion-focused coping and blunting coping strategies on the one hand, and long-term psychiatric symptoms on the other hand. Problem-focused coping and monitoring coping strategies, however, moderated the detrimental effects of emotion-focused coping on mental health. By contrast, Spurrell and McFarlane (1993) found that all coping strategies were equally associated with the presence of PTSD.

These conflicting results may be attributable to the fact that *successful coping*, rather than any particular coping strategy, may ultimately moderate the effect of stress. Effective coping results in relief of personal distress, maintenance of a sense of personal worth, conservation of one's ability to form rewarding social contacts, and sustained capability to meet the requirements of the task (Pearlin & Schooler, 1978). In order to succeed, however, coping efforts must match the circumstances of the event and the resources of the individual. Hence, passive surrender, stoic acceptance, and cognitive reframing may be appropriate in situations where the stressor is uncontrollable, whereas acting directly on the stressor, seeking help, and other active coping strategies may be adaptive in other circumstances. In a study of survivors of a terrorist attack, we (Shalev et al., 1993b) described a wide variety of coping efforts during the impact phase of the stressor. These included actively rescuing other survivors, sharing important information with the rescuers, preserving one's dignity by covering one's body, or controlling the disclosure of information about the event to one's relatives. Even survivors who were severely injured seemed to have engaged in some mode of coping during and immediately after the event. The survivors described that successfully achieving their individual coping goals increased their sense of control and reduced their distress.

Posttrauma Responses

During the days and weeks that follow the impact phase of a trauma, subjects show a variety of responses, some of which have been associated with the later development of PTSD. Distress during the days that follow a trauma seems to be ubiquitous. However, the amount of subjective distress is correlated with the later development of PTSD (Laufer, Brett, & Gallops, 1985; Feinstein & Dolan, 1991; Perry, Difede, Musngi, Frances, & Jacobsberg, 1992).

Symptoms resembling those of PTSD are frequently observed during the early days that follow a trauma. Intrusive symptoms, in particular, seem to appear within 48 hours after the event in the majority of survivors (Shalev, 1992). Survivors differ, however, in the amounts of discomfort, arousal, and dissociation that accompany such early intrusive recall, and for some survivors these repeated memories are intolerable. Clinical observation suggests that many survivors are judging themselves and reevaluating their actions (or their failure to act) with particular intensity during that period. Theory suggests (e.g., Foa, Steketee, & Rothbaum, 1989) that these reevaluations may yield a non-specific and overgeneralized appraisal of the stressor and of one's resources, thereby leading to the formation of negative beliefs about oneself and others.

In this area, again, symptomatology is often confounded with underlying mental processes. That is, the amount or intensity of observable behavior, rather then the effect of such behavior, is being evaluated as a predictor. To borrow Piaget's terminology, peritraumatic stress responses involve mainly *adaptation* (i.e., responding to external demand by using resources and structures that are already available), whereas postexposure processes are, in essence, a matter of *assimilation* (i.e., changing internal structures in response to novelty). As a rule of thumb, therefore, I propose that clinicians involved in the treatment of recent trauma victims should evaluate the *effectiveness* of the intrusive phenomena as promoters of assimilation, rather than their peak intensity. In evaluating this effectiveness, they should note the extent to which engaging in illness behavior and expressing symptoms recruit help and support from others, increase communication ability, and do not interfere with physiological needs for sleep and nutrition. Such recommendation, however, has not received an empirical confirmation.

Early PTSD symptoms subside with time in many survivors. Foa and Rothbaum (1989) described PTSD symptoms in 94% of rape victims 1 week after the trauma, but only in 52.4% 2 months later and 47.1% 9 months later. Other studies (e.g., Saigh, 1988; Patterson, Carrigan, Questad, & Robinson, 1990) found that a larger proportion of survivors recovered from early PTSD symptoms.

The frequent occurrence of such symptoms during the few days that follow a trauma decreases their predictive value—particularly because of low specificity. Two studies, performed at the Center for Traumatic Stress at Hadassah University Hospital in Jerusalem, have assessed the capacity of such symptoms to predict PTSD (Shalev, Schreiber, & Galai, 1993b; Shalev et al., 1996). The first study found that symptoms of intrusion and avoidance, recorded immediately after the event, failed to predict PTSD, PTSD symptoms, or general psychiatric symptoms at follow-up. The second study, as described earlier, evaluated 51 civilian trauma survivors 1 week and 6 months after the trauma. Thirteen subjects (25.5%) met PTSD diagnostic criteria at the 6-month assessment. The PTSD subjects did not differ from those who did not develop PTSD in their initial report of event severity and trait anxiety. PTSD subjects reported higher levels of intrusion, avoidance, depression, and state anxiety in the week that followed the trauma. An initial Impact of Event Scale (IES) score of over 19 correctly classified 12 of 13 subjects who later developed PTSD (sensitivity of 92%). However, only 13 of the 38 subjects who did not develop PTSD had initial IES scores of 19 or less (specificity of 34%). Overall, 72.5% of the subjects (37 of the 51) had IES scores of over 19 during the first week after the trauma. Interestingly, symptoms of intrusion did not increase in PTSD subjects between the 1-week and the 6-month examinations (IES Intrusion subscale scores of 27.2 at 1 week and 28.6 at follow-up). These symptoms remained elevated in PTSD subjects, while decreasing in subjects who did not develop PTSD. Avoidance symptoms, in contrast, increased dramatically in PTSD subjects (from 5.5 to 19.4 on the IES Avoidance subscale), while remaining low in subjects who did not develop PTSD. Similar results were reported by Perry et al. (1992), who assessed the presence of psychiatric disorder in 43 adult inpatients at discharge from a regional burn center and 4 months later, and found that symptoms of avoidance and emotional numbing tended to emerge after discharge from the hospital. McFarlane (1992) similarly suggested that avoidance may be a defensive strategy to contain the distress generated by the reexperiencing of the disaster. The time of the first evaluation of PTSD symptoms strongly affects their predictive value: McFarlane (1992) studied 113 firefighters exposed to a natural disaster, and found that scores on the Intrusion subscale of the IES 4 months after the event strongly predicted PTSD at 29 and 42 months.

In summary, the work on predictors of PTSD presents a complex picture of the development of the disorder. Until recently, the variables examined reflected the underlying assumption that the response to trauma is always a normal one, and this has led to difficulties in differentiating between normal responses and the responses of those who later develop PTSD. More recently, studies have begun to look at excessive or specific responses to see whether these are better predictors of PTSD. For example, the work on dissociation appears to support this as a possible differentiating variable.

IS PTSD A STRESS DISORDER?

A second example of confusion related to the label "PTSD" is the controversy regarding the specificity of traumatic stress as opposed to nontraumatic stress. The definition of PTSD in the *Diagnostic and Statistical Manual of Mental Disorders*, third edition (DSM-III; American Psychiatric Association, 1980) resulted in attempts to delineate extreme catastrophic or traumatic stress. Traumatic stress has been intuitively associated with events such as wars, captivity, torture, disasters, and racial extermination. Furthermore, events that do not involve extreme stress can be perceived by some survivors as threatening and by others as challenging (Shalev, 1992). Indeed, no one has successfully distinguished traumatic from stressful events.

Historically, the field of traumatic stress has evolved independently from the preexisting domain of stress and coping. Despite attempts to articulate theoretical links between "stress" and "traumatic stress" research (e.g., Kahana, Kahana, Harel, & Rosner, 1988; Hobfoll, 1988; Baum, 1990; Baum et al., 1993), there has been very little interaction between the two fields. Indeed, the conjunction between the two is rather problematic.

Stress theory is one of the central paradigms of 20th-century psychology. Early stress researchers have shown that excessive demands on the organism, whether somatic or psychological, produce a typical sequence of physiological responses involving sympathetic activation and activation of the hypothalamic–pituitary–adrenal axis. These responses attempt to keep the effect of the stressor on the organism within viable homeostatic boundaries. They "buffer" the effects of external demands, so to speak, often defending vital functions (e.g., central temperature, supply of oxygen to the brain) at the expense of secondary functions (e.g., digestion, peripheral temperature). Stress responses follow a generic triphasic pattern: an acute response, a phase of resistance, and either recovery or exhaustion. Research on psychological stress has emphasized the pathogenic effects of controllability and predictability of the stressor, and the modulating effects of coping and appraisal. By analogy with the homeostatic physiological model, the psychological responses to stress have also been conceived of as regulatory mechanisms aimed to keep the mental responses within manageable boundaries.

The core of stress theory, therefore, consists of a homeostatic model of self-conservation and resource allocation in response to adversity (e.g., Cannon, 1932; Selye, 1956). Such responses usually occur under stress or in the immediate proximity of the stressor. The intermediate and long-term consequences of exposure, however, are beyond the scope of the model. In the classical example of the body's response to massive bleeding, Selye's (1956) model focuses on immediate coping responses, which adaptively attempt to reduce the effects of such bleeding on vital functions of the organism. It does not address the healing of the wound that has caused the bleeding to occur. Neither does it say anything about the recovery from eventual renal failure or brain damage, which may result from unsuccessful coping with the bleeding. Stress, however, becomes traumatic precisely when psychological damage analogous to this type of physical damage occurs—that is, damage to a hypothetical stimulus barrier (Freud, 1920/1955), to the "self" (Laufer, 1988), to one's cognitive assumptions (Janoff-Bulman 1985), to one's affect (Krystal, 1978), to neuronal mechanisms governing habituation and learning (Kolb, 1987), to one's memory network (Pitman, 1988), or to emotional learning pathways (LeDoux, Romanski, & Xagoraris, 1989).

It is, therefore, in the best tradition of stress theory that Lazarus and Folkman's (1984) seminal monograph *Stress, Appraisal and Coping*, which was published 4 years after the DSM-III definition of PTSD appeared, does not mention PTSD (or any other Axis I disorder) as a possible consequence of exposure to stress . These authors suggested that impaired social functioning, decreased morale, and poor somatic health are typical forms of negative outcome resulting from the failure to cope with stress. Lazarus and Folkman deliberately chose to study the effect of mild stressors.

Lindemann's (1944) "traumatic grief" and Horowitz's (1986) "stress response syndrome" are often cited as extensions of "classical" stress theory (e.g., Hobfoll, 1988, p. 6). These models, however, include a recovery or assimilation phase, which consists of a prolonged struggle with the results of exposure. Survivors often experience discomfort, distress, anxiety, and grief during this period. Confusingly, these reactions have been vaguely referred to as "stress" or "chronic stress." Baum (1990), for example, has defined stress as a "negative emotional experience accompanied by biochemical, physiological, and behavioral changes" (p. 654). Chronic stress, accordingly, is not limited to situations in which stressors persist for long periods of time. Responses may habituate before a stressor disappears, or may persist beyond the physical presence of the stressor. Theoretically, however, the use of the term "stress" for both acute and chronic responses is problematic. Recent neuroendocrinological studies show reduced cortisol levels in PTSD (as opposed to elevated cortisol during acute stress), thereby supporting the distinction between acute stress and the prolonged states of posttraumatic morbidity.

Stress research and the traumatic stress literature differ also in a number of methodological dimensions. Most of the research on traumatic stress has been focused on evaluating the relationship between a trauma and subsequent disorders, thereby evaluating the traumatogenic nature of events rather than their stressfulness. New psychometric instruments, such as the IES (Horowitz et al., 1979) and the Mississippi Scale for Combat-Related PTSD (Keane, Caddell, & Taylor, 1988), have been created in order to assess these specific consequences of trauma. These instruments differ considerably from those used by stress researchers.

The stress literature is mostly experimental, using exploratory designs and controlled conditions. The traumatic stress literature, in contrast, is mostly naturalistic, retrospective, and observational. Traumatic stress researchers tend to use categorical outcome measures (mainly measures of the development of a disorder). The stress literature, on the other hand, has almost no inherent categorical outcome meaures, although it may borrow such measures from other areas (e.g., in studying the relationship between stress and increased mortality rates from myocardial infarction, mortality becomes a categorical measure). The stress researcher, therefore, feels more comfortable with continuous measures (e.g., blood pressure, urinary epinephrine excretion) than with predefined syndromes.

Hobfoll (1988) has suggested a view that bridges the gap between "stress" and "traumatic stress"—namely, that massive stressors lead to a qualitatively different type of stress reaction, in which the primary concern is to conserve resources ("playing dead"). A similar view is held by Krystal (1978), who, within psychoanalytic theory, has suggested that psychic surrender and "freezing of affect" (and subsequent loss of affective modulation and alexithymia) are central features of a "traumatic" response to extreme adversity. Other descriptors of extreme responses to massive stressors are "dissociation" (e.g., Marmar et al., 1994; Speigel et al., 1988) and "disorganization" (McFarlane, 1984).

Metaphorically, the two opposing positions here involve homeostasis, adaptation, and "normality" on the one hand, and bifurcation, discontinuity, and psychopathology on the other. The belief that PTSD is a "stress" disorder, and is in some way an adaptive response to environmental changes, strongly supports one side of this argument.

CONCLUSION

Is PTSD a Biopsychosocial Trap?

Extreme stress produces a variety of long-term consequences, such as depression, phobias, and pathological grief. PTSD, however, involves a unique combination of hyperarousal, learned conditioning, shattered meaning propositions, and social avoidance. Such complexity is best accounted for by the co-occurrence of several pathogenic processes, including (1) a permanent alteration of neurobiological processes, resulting in hyperarousal and excessive stimulus discrimination; (2) the acquisition of conditioned fear responses to trauma-related stimuli; and (3) altered cognitive schemata and social apprehension, resulting from a profound dissonance between the traumatic experience and one's previous knowledge of the world. This combination, which may not exist in other stress-induced disorders, makes PTSD a "biopsychosocial trap," in which one level of impairment prevents self-regulatory healing mechanisms from occurring on other levels (Shalev & Rogel-Fuchs, 1993; Shalev, Galai, & Eth, 1993a). For example a neurophysiological impairment in down-regulation of arousal may prevent the spontaneous extinction of learned conditioning from occurring. Avoidance of internal cues reminiscent of the trauma (i.e., traumatic memories) may impair effective grief. Similarly, the mistrust and insecurity that may result from the traumatic experience may preclude protective social interactions between the survivor and others. The complex causation of PTSD, exemplified by the large variety of predictors outlined above, thus reflects the complexity of the disorder.

"Aging" of PTSD Symptoms

This chapter has outlined some of the conceptual problems that must be dealt with in order for the understanding of PTSD to be furthered. Specifically, the assumption that PTSD reflects an adaptive, normal response to an extraordinary event must be reevaluated in the light of recent work. Symptoms of PTSD seem to resemble those seen in survivors of trauma, immediately after the event, but over time, these symptoms may no longer represent reparative attempts. Instead, they may reflect permanent damage and change. Recurrent and intrusive recollections of the trauma may "age" with time, and come to represent an obsessively repetitive dysfunction of memory. Conditioned fear responses may similarly become indelible and inaccessible to desensitization. The resistance of PTSD to most treatment modalities likewise suggests that the disorder is most often immutable and resistant to change. Theory also predicts (Post, Weiss, & George, 1994) that neurobiological scars of psychic trauma create irreversible changes in the brain structure. PTSD symptoms, therefore, may reflect different underlying processes at different stages of the disorder. Future research should focus on the ways in which stress responses are indelibly transformed and become a permanently disabling disorder.

REFERENCES

Abenhaim, L., Dab, W., & Salmi, L. R. (1992). Study of civilian victims of terrorist attacks (France 1982–1987). *Journal of Clinical Epidemiology, 45,* 103–109.

American Psychiatric Association. (1980). *Diagnostic and statistical manual of mental disorders* (3rd ed.). Washington, DC: Author.

Basoglu, M., Paker, M., Paker, O., Ozmen, E., Marks, I., Incesu, C., Sahin, D., & Sarimurat, N. (1994). Psychological effects of torture: A comparison of tortured with nontortured political activists in Turkey. *American Journal of Psychiatry, 151,* 76–81.

Baum, A. (1990). Stress, intrusive imagery, and chronic distress. *Health Psychology, 9,* 653–675.

Baum, A., Cohen, L., & Hall, M. (1993). Control and intrusive memories as possible determinants of chronic stress. *Psychosomatic Medicine, 55,* 274–286.

Bownes, I. T., O'Gorman, E. C., & Sayers, A. (1991). Assault characteristics and posttraumatic stress disorder in rape victims. *Acta Psychiatrica Scandinavica, 83,* 27–30.

Bremner, J. D., Southwick, S., Brett, E., Fontana, A., Rosenheck, R., & Charney, D. S. (1992). Dissociation and posttraumatic stress disorder in Vietnam combat veterans. *American Journal of Psychiatry, 149,* 328–332.

Bremner, J. D., Davis, M., Southwick, S. M., Krystal, J. H., & Charney, D. S. (1993). Neurobiology of posttraumatic stress disorder. In *Annual review of psychiatry.* Washington, DC: American Psychiatric Press.

Breslau, N., & Davis, G. C. (1987). Posttraumatic stress disorder: The etiologic specificity of wartime stressors. *American Journal of Psychiatry, 144*(5), 578–583.

Breslau, N., & Davis, G. C. (1992). Posttraumatic stress disorder in an urban population of young adults: Risk factors for chronicity. *American Journal of Psychiatry, 149,* 671–675.

Breslau, N., Davis, G. C., Andreski, P., & Peterson, E. (1991). Traumatic events and posttraumatic stress disorder in an urban population of young adults. *Archives of General Psychiatry, 48,* 216–222.

Buydens-Branchey, L., Noumair, D., & Branchey, M. (1990). Duration and intensity of combat exposure and posttraumatic stress disorder in Vietnam veterans. *Journal of Nervous and Mental Disease, 178,* 582–587.

Cannon, W. B. (1932). *The wisdom of the body.* New York: Norton.

Cardeña, E., & Spiegel, D. (1993). Dissociative reactions to the San Francisco Bay Area earthquake of 1989. *American Journal of Psychiatry, 150,* 474–478.

Carlson, E. B., & Rosser-Hogan, R. (1991). Trauma experiences, posttraumatic stress, dissociation, and depression in Cambodian refugees. *American Journal of Psychiatry, 148,* 1548–1551.

Chemtob, C. M., Bauer, G. B., Neller, G., Hamada, R., Glisson, C., & Stevens, V. (1990). Post-traumatic stress disorder among Special Forces Vietnam veterans. *Military Medicine, 155,* 16–20.

Clarke, G., Sack, W. H., & Goff, B. (1993). Three forms of stress in Cambodian adolescent refugees. *Journal of Abnormal Child Psychology, 21,* 65–77.

Davidson, J. R. T., Hughes, D., Blazer, D. G., & George, L. K. (1991). Post-traumatic stress disorder in the community: An epidemiological study. *Psychological Medicine, 21,* 713–721.

Davidson, J. R. T., Smith, R., & Kudler, H. (1989). Familial psychiatric illness in chronic posttraumatic stress disorder. *Comprehensive Psychiatry, 30,* 339–345

Eaton, W. W., Sigal, J. J., & Weinfeld, M. (1982). Impairment in Holocaust survivors after 33 years: Data from an unbiased community sample. *American Journal of Psychiatry, 139,* 773–777.

Feinstein, A., & Dolan, R. (1991). Predictors of post-traumatic stress disorder following physical trauma: An examination of the stressor criterion. *Psychological Medicine, 21,* 85–91.

Foa, E. B., & Rothbaum, B. O. (1989). Behavioural psychotherapy for post-traumatic stress disorder. *International Review of Psychiatry, 1,* 219–226.

Foa, E. B., Steketee, G., & Rothbaum, B. O. (1989). Behavioral/cognitive conceptualization of post-traumatic stress disorder. *Behavior Therapy, 20,* 155–176.

Foy, D. W., Resnick, H. S., Sipprelle, R. C., & Carroll, E. M. (1987). Premilitary, military, and postmilitary factors in the development of combat-related posttraumatic stress disorder. *The Behavior Therapist, 10,* 3–9

Foy, D. W., Rueger D. B., Sipprelle, R. C., & Carroll, E. M. (1984). Etiology of post-traumatic stress disorder in Vietnam veterans: Analysis of premilitary, military, and combat exposure influences. *Journal of Consulting and Clinical Psychology, 52,* 79–87.

Freud, S. (1955). Beyond the pleasure principle. In J. Strachey (Ed. and Trans.), *The standard edition of the complete psychological works of Sigmund Freud* (Vol. 18, pp. 3–64). London: Hogarth Press. (Original work published 1920)

Gallers, J., Foy, D. W., Donahoe, C. P., Jr., & Goldfarb, J. (1988). Post traumatic stress disorder in Vietnam veterans: Effect of traumatic violence exposure and military adjustment. *Journal of Traumatic Stress, 1,* 181–192.

Gidycz, C. A., & Koss, M. P. (1991). Predictors of long-term sexual assault trauma among a national sample of victimized college women. *Violence Victims, 6,* 175–190.

Goldberg, J., True, W. R., Eisen, S. A., & Henderson, W. G. (1990). A twin study of the effects of the Vietnam War on post traumatic stress disorder. *Journal of the American Medical Association, 263,* 1227–1232.

Green, B. L. (1990). Defining trauma: Terminology and generic stressor dimensions. *Journal of Applied Social Psychology, 20,* 1632–1642.

Green, B. L., Grace, M. C., Lindy, J. D., Gleser, G. C., & Leonard, A. (1990). Risk factors for PTSD and other diagnoses in a general sample of Vietnam veterans. *American Journal of Psychiatry, 147,* 729–733.

Green, M. A., & Berlin, M. A. (1987). Five psychosocial variables related to the existence of post-traumatic stress disorder symptoms. *Journal of Clinical Psychology, 43*(6), 643–649.

Grinker, R. R., & Spiegel, J. P. (1945). *Men under stress.* Philadelphia: Blakiston.

Haan, N. (1969). A tripartite model of ego functioning: Value and clinical research application. *Journal of Nervous and Mental Disease, 148,* 14–30.

Hobfoll, S. E. (1988). *The ecology of stress.* New York: Hemisphere.

Holen, A. (1993). The North Sea oil rig disaster. In J. P. Wilson & B. Raphael (Eds.), *International handbook of traumatic stress syndromes* (pp. 471–478). New York: Plenum Press.

Herman, J. L. (1993). Sequelae of prolonged and repeated trauma: Evidence for a complex posttraumatic syndrome (DESNOS). In J. R. T. Davidson & E. B. Foa (Eds.), *Posttraumatic stress disorder: DSM-IV and beyond* (pp. 213–228). Washington, DC: American Psychiatric Press.

Horowitz, M. J. (1974). Stress response syndromes: Character style and dynamic psychotherapy. *Archives of General Psychiatry, 31,* 768–781.

Horowitz, M. J. (1986). Stress-response syndromes: A review of posttraumatic and adjustment disorders. *Hospital and Community Psychiatry, 37*(3), 241–249.

Horowitz, M. J., Wilner, N., & Alvarez, W. (1979). Impact of Event Scale: A measure of subjective stress. *Psychosomatic Medicine, 41,* 209–218.

Hytten K. (1989). Helicopter crash in water: Effects of simulator escape training. *Acta Psychiatrica Scandinavica, 80,* 73–78.

Janoff-Bulman, R. (1985). The aftermath of victimization: Rebuilding shattered assumptions. In C. R. Figley (Ed.), *Trauma and its wake: The study and treatment of post-traumatic stress disorder* (pp. 15–36). New York: Brunner/Mazel.

Kahana, E., Kahana, B., Harel, Z., & Rosner, T. (1988). Coping with extreme trauma. In J. P. Wilson, Z. Harel, & B. Kahana (Eds.), *Human adaptation to extreme stress from the Holocaust to Vietnam* (pp. 55–80). New York: Plenum Press.

Keane, T. M., Caddell, J. M., & Taylor, K. L. (1988). Mississippi Scale for Combat-Related Posttraumatic Stress Disorder: Three studies in reliability and validity. *Journal of Consulting and Clinical Psychology, 56,* 85–90.

Keane, T. M., Fairbank, J. A., Caddell, M. T., Zimering, R. T., & Bender, M. E. (1985). A behavioral approach to assessing and treating post-traumatic stress disorders in Vietnam veterans. In C. R. Figley (Ed.), *Trauma and its wake: The study and treatment of post-traumatic stress disorder* (pp. 257–294). New York: Brunner/Mazel.

Kilpatrick, D. G., Saunders, B. E., Amick-McMullan, A., Best, C. L., Veronen, L. J., & Resnick, H. S. (1989). Victim and crime factors associated with the development of crime-related post-traumatic stress disorder. *Behavior Therapy, 20,* 199–214.

Kolb, L. C. (1987). A neuropsychological hypothesis explaining posttraumatic stress disorders. *American Journal of Psychiatry, 144*(8), 989–995.

Koopman, C., Classen, C., & Spiegel, D. (1994). Predictors of posttraumatic stress symptoms among survivors of the Oakland/Berkeley, California, firestorm. *American Journal of Psychiatry, 151,* 888–894.

Krystal, H. (1978). Trauma and affect. *Psychoanalytic Study of the Child, 33,* 81–116.

Kulka, R. A., Schlenger, W. E., Fairbank, J. A., Hough, R. L., Jordan, B. K., Marmar, C. R., & Weiss, D. S. (1990). *Trauma and the Vietnam War generation: Report of Findings from the National Vietnam Veterans Readjustment Study.* New York: Brunner/Mazel.

Kutz, I., Shabtai, H., Solomon, Z., Neumann, M., & David, D. (1994). Post-traumatic stress disorder in myocardial infarction patients: Prevalence study. *Israel Journal of Psychiatry and Related Science, 31,* 48–56.

Laufer, R. S. (1988). The serial self: War trauma, identity and adult development. In J. P. Wilson, Z. Harel, & B. Kahana (Eds.), *Human adaptation to extreme stress from the Holocaust to Vietnam* (pp. 33–54). New York: Plenum Press.

Laufer, R. S., Brett, E., & Gallops, M. S. (1985). Dimensions of posttraumatic stress disorder among Vietnam veterans. *Journal of Nervous and Mental Disease, 173,* 538–545.

Lazarus, R. S., & Folkman, S. (1984). *Stress, appraisal and coping.* New York: Springer.

LeDoux, J. E., Romanski, L., & Xagoraris, A. (1989). Indelibility of subcortical emotional networks. *Journal of Cognitive Neuroscience, 1,* 238–243.

Levav, I., & Abramson, J. H. (1984). Emotional distress among concentration camps survivors: A community study in Jerusalem. *Psychological Medicine, 14,* 215–218.

Lindemann, E. (1944). Symptomatology and management of acute grief. *American Journal of Psychiatry, 101,* 141–148.

March, J. S. (1993). What constitutes a stressor? The Criterion A issue. In J. R. T. Davidson & E. B. Foa (Eds.), *Posttraumatic stress disorder: DSM-IV and beyond* (pp. 37–54). Washington, DC: American Psychiatric Press.

Marmar, C. R., Foy, D., Kagan, B., & Pynoos, R. S. (1993). An integrated approach for treatment of posttraumatic stress disorder. In J. M. Oldham, M. B. Riba, & A. Tasman (Eds.), *American Psychiatric Press review of psychiatry* (Vol. 12, pp. 239–271). Washington, DC: American Psychiatric Press.

Marmar, C. R., Weiss, D. S., Schlenger, W. E., Fairbank, J. A., Jordan, K., Kulka, R. A., & Hough, R. L. (1994). Peritraumatic dissociation and posttraumatic stress in male Vietnam theater veterans. *American Journal of Psychiatry, 151,* 902–907.

Mayou, R., Bryant, B., & Duthie, R. (1993). Psychiatric consequences of road traffic accidents. *British Medical Journal, 307,* 647–651.

McCranie, E. W., Hyer, L. A., Boudewyns, P. A., & Woods, M. G. (1992). Negative parenting behavior, combat exposure, and PTSD symptom severity: Test of a person–event interaction model. *Journal of Nervous and Mental Disease, 180,* 431–438.

McFall, M. E., Mackay, P. W., & Donovan, D. M. (1991). Combat-related PTSD and psychosocial adjustment problems among substance abusing veterans. *Journal of Nervous and Mental Disease, 179,* 33–38.

McFarlane, A. C. (1984). Life events, disasters and psychological distress. *Mental Health in Australia, 1*(13), 4–6.

McFarlane, A. C. (1988). The aetiology of post-traumatic stress disorders following a natural disaster. *British Journal of Psychiatry, 152,* 116–121.

McFarlane, A. C. (1989). The aetiology of post-traumatic morbidity: Predisposing, precipitating, and perpetuating factors. *British Journal of Psychiatry, 154,* 221–228.

McFarlane, A. C. (1992). Avoidance and intrusion in posttraumatic stress disorder. *Journal of Nervous and Mental Disease, 180,* 439–445.

Nader, K., Pynoos, R., Fairbanks, L., & Frederick, C. (1990). Children's PTSD reactions one year after a sniper attack at their school. *American Journal of Psychiatry, 147,* 1526–1530.

North, C. S., & Smith, E. M. (1992). Posttraumatic stress disorder among homeless men and women. *Hospital and Community Psychiatry, 43,* 1010–1016.

North, C. S., Smith, E. M., & Spitznagel, E. L. (1994). Posttraumatic stress disorder in survivors of a mass shooting. *American Journal of Psychiatry, 151,* 82–88.

Patterson, D. R., Carrigan, L., Questad, K. A., & Robinson, R. (1990). Post-traumatic stress disorder in hospitalized patients with burn injuries. *Journal of Burn Care Rehabilitation, 11,* 181–184.

Pearlin, L. I., & Schooler, C. (1978). The structure of coping. *Journal of Health and Social Behavior, 22,* 337–356.

Peri, T., Ben-Shachar, G., & Shalev, A. (1994, May). *Heightened conditionability in PTSD and panic disorder.* Paper presented at the 147th Annual Meeting of the American Psychiatric Association, Philadelphia.

Perry, S., Difede, J., Musngi, G., Frances, A. J., & Jacobsberg, L. (1992). Predictors of posttraumatic stress disorder after burn injury. *American Journal of Psychiatry, 149,* 931–935.

Pitman, R. K. (1988). Post-traumatic stress disorder, conditioning, and network theory. *Psychiatric Annals, 18*(3), 182–189.

Post, R. M., Weiss, S. R. B., & George, M. S. (1994, May). *Sensitization and kindling components of PTSD.* Paper presented at the 147th Annual Meeting of the American Psychiatric Association, Philadelphia.

Resnick, H. S., Kilpatrick, D. G., Best, C. L., & Kramer, T. L. (1992). Vulnerability–stress factors in development of posttraumatic stress disorder. *Journal of Nervous and Mental Disease, 180,* 424–430.

Rosen, G. (1975). Nostalgia: A forgotten psychological disorder. *Psychological Medicine, 5,* 344–347.

Saigh, P. A. (1988). Anxiety, depression, and assertion across alternating intervals of stress. *Journal of Abnormal Psychology, 97*(3), 338–341.

Schnurr, P. P., Friedman, M. J., & Rosenberg, S. D. (1993). Premilitary MMPI scores as predictors of combat-related PTSD symptoms. *American Journal of Psychiatry, 150,* 479–483.

Selye, H. (1956). *The stress of life.* New York: McGraw-Hill.

Shalev, A.Y. (1992). Posttraumatic stress disorder among injured survivors of a terrorist attack: Predictive value of early intrusion and avoidance symptoms. *Journal of Nervous and Mental Disease, 180,* 505–509.

Shalev, A. Y., Galai, T., & Eth, S. (1993a). "Levels of trauma": Multidimensional approach to the psychotherapy of PTSD. *Psychiatry, 56,* 166–177.

Shalev, A. Y., & Munitz, H. (1989). Combat stress reaction. In N. D. Ries & E. Dolev (Eds.), *Manual of disaster medicine* (pp. 169–182). Berlin: Springer-Verlag.

Shalev, A. Y., Peri, T., Caneti, L., & Schreiber, S. (1996). Predictors of PTSD in injured trauma survivors. *American Journal of Psychiatry, 53,* 219–224.

Shalev, A. Y., & Rogel-Fuchs, Y. (1993). Psychophysiology of the post-traumatic stress disorder: From sulfur fumes to behavioral genetics. *Psychosomatic Medicine, 55,* 413–423.

Shalev, A. Y., Schreiber, S., & Galai, T (1993b). Early psychiatric responses to traumatic injury. *Journal of Traumatic Stress, 6,* 441–450.

Shalev, A. Y., Schreiber, S., Galai, T., & Melmed, R. (1993c). Post traumatic stress disorder following medical events. *British Journal of Clinical Psychology, 32,* 352–357.

Smith, E. M., North, C. S., McCool, R. E., & Shea, J. M. (1990). Acute postdisaster psychiatric disorders: Identification of persons at risk. *American Journal of Psychiatry, 147*(2), 202–206.

Solkoff, N., Gray, P., & Keill, S. (1986). Which Vietnam veterans develop posttraumatic stress disorders? *Journal of Clinical Psychology, 42,* 687–698.

Solomon, Z. (1993). *Combat stress reaction.* New York: Plenum Press.

Solomon, Z., Avitzur, E., & Mikulincer, M. (1990). Coping styles and post-war psychopathology among Israeli soldiers. *Personality and Individual Differences, 11*(5), 451–456.

Solomon, Z., Mikulincer, M., & Arad, R. (1991). Monitoring and blunting: Implications for combat-related post-traumatic stress disorder. *Journal of Traumatic Stress, 4,* 209–221.

Speed, N., Engdahl, B., Schwartz, J., & Eberly, R. (1989). Posttraumatic stress disorder as a consequence of the POW experience. *Journal of Nervous and Mental Disease, 177,* 147–153.

Spiegel, D., Hunt, T., & Dondershine, H. E. (1988). Dissociation and hypnotizability in posttraumatic stress disorder. *American Journal of Psychiatry, 145,* 301–305.

Spurrell, M. T., & McFarlane, A. C. (1993). Post-traumatic stress disorder and coping after a natural disaster. *Social Psychiatry and Psychiatric Epidemiology, 28,* 194–200.

Sutker, P. B., Bugg, F., & Allain, A. N. J. (1990). Person and situation correlates of post-traumatic stress disorder among POW survivors. *Psychological Reports, 66,* 912–914.

True, W. R., Rice, J., Eisen, S. A., Heath, A. C., Goldberg, J., Lyons, M. J., & Nowak, J. (1993). A twin study of genetic and environmental contributions to liability for posttraumatic stress symptoms. *Archives of General Psychiatry, 50,* 257–264.

van der Kolk, B. A., & van der Hart, O. (1989). Pierre Janet and the breakdown of adaptation in psychological trauma. *American Journal of Psychiatry, 146,* 1530–1540.

Yehuda, R., Southwick, S. M., Krystal, J. H., Bremner, J. D., Charney, D. S., & Mason, J. W. (1993). Enhanced suppression of cortisol following dexamethasone administration in posttraumatic stress disorder. *American Journal of Psychiatry, 150,* 83–86.

Zaidi, L. Y., & Foy, D. W. (1994). Childhood abuse experience and combat related PTSD. *Journal of Traumatic Stress, 7,* 33–42.

Acute Posttraumatic Reactions in Soldiers and Civilians

ZAHAVA SOLOMON
NATHANIEL LAOR
ALEXANDER C. McFARLANE

Very few of the many studies on traumatic stress have focused on describing or investigating the cause of the range of immediate reactions. Wartime and disasters are obviously very difficult times to conduct research: Both subjects and researchers are inevitably preoccupied with their own survival, which demands attention to the external world rather than to the private world of suffering and recollection. In fact, the essence of an acute traumatic reaction is that it hampers this critical process of survival and adaptation. Abnormal behavior that interferes with survival is the characteristic that best defines acute traumatic reactions. This chapter focuses on the description of these states. Their long-term significance is also discussed, although the longitudinal course of such reactions is discussed by McFarlane in Chapter 8 of this volume.

In the area of war, there have been many descriptive reports of the nature of acute stress reactions to combat (Solomon et al., 1993). Apart from the Israeli studies (Solomon, 1993), Rachman's (1990) study of the Blitz in London, and Saigh's (1984) study of students in Beirut, very little systematic research has been done in this area. Studies of acute reactions to other traumatic events include studies of victims of terrorist bombings (Shalev, 1992), a factory explosion (Weisaeth, 1989a, 1989b), and motor vehicle accidents (Malt, Hoivik, & Blikra, 1993; Mayou, Bryant, & Duthie, 1993; Atchison & McFarlane, 1995); however, research of this type is rare and constitutes an area of critical interest as the acute patterns of reaction to trauma (e.g., dissociation) are thought to play a primary etiological role in vulnerability to and onset of posttraumatic stress disorder (PTSD). However, as discussed by Shalev in Chapter 4 of this volume, little is known about the nature of the reactions that lead to PTSD or about the range of acute responses to traumatic events.

This chapter examines the immediate psychological reactions to war stress in both soldiers and civilians, to exemplify the nature of acute reactions and their relationship to long-term outcome. To date, the study of other events has not specifically examined acute stress reactions in sufficient detail to allow the link between such reactions and PTSD to be discussed in a systematic manner. Despite the differences in type of the exposed populations (active combatants and passive civilians), the data on both of them appear to validate the new diagnosis of acute stress disorder (ASD) in the *Diagnostic and Statistical Manual of Mental Disorders*, fourth edition (DSM-IV; American Psychiatric Association [APA], 1994) and the *International Classification of Diseases*, 10th revision (ICD-10; World Health Organization [WHO], 1992).

The defintion of ASD is significantly different in these two classification systems. The DSM-IV definition places a major emphasis on the presence of an acute dissociative reaction in combination with phenomena of PTSD, which emerge at the time of exposure to the event. These criteria reflect the interest of U.S. psychiatry in the importance and role of acute dissociation as a critical component of long-term posttraumatic reactions (see Chapter 6, this volume), and incorporate observations about the role of dissociation in disasters (Koopman, Classen, & Spiegel, 1994) as well as in combat settings. In contrast, the ICD-10 definition is more reflective of the descriptions that have been accumulated from military psychiatry, and is perhaps more specific to combat. This definition focuses on the polymorphic nature of the symptoms, notes that anxiety and depression are important features, and indicates that the phenomenology can fluctuate rapidly.

These two sets of criteria will have an important impact on the investigation of the nature and prevalence of acute stress reactions, in the same way that the diagnostic criteria for PTSD in DSM-III (APA, 1980) provided a benchmark for the investigation of chronic traumatic reactions. In particular, they will provide a focus for investigating these critical questions: What particular features of acute stress reactions are particularly detrimental to long-term adaptation, and what is their relationship to the psychophysiology and biochemistry of the normal stress response?

COMBAT STRESS REACTION

Definition

In both World Wars, many astute clinical observations were made about the psychiatric casualties of battle, who eventually came to be termed sufferers from "combat stress reaction" (CSR). The treatment concepts of "proximity, immediacy, and expectancy" were developed in this setting to deal with the significant psychiatric toll of war. CSR remains a matter of major concern to medical services and field commanders in war because of its impact on the fighting capacity of a force and the need for casualty facilities at the front. For example, in the 1982 Lebanon War, CSR casualties constituted 23% of all Israeli casualties (Solomon, 1993)—a figure very similar to that for the U.S. forces in World War II. CSR is the most studied type of acute stress reaction because of its practical significance.

CSR is a labile, polymorphic disorder, characterized by high variability and rapid changes in manifestation (Solomon, 1993). Among its prevalent somatic and affective manifestations are restlessness, irritability, psychomotor retardation, apathy, psychological withdrawal, sympathetic activity, startle reactions, anxiety and depression, constriction of affect, confusion, abdominal pains, nausea and vomiting, aggressive and hostile behaviors, paranoid reactions, and ill-concealed earfulness (Bar-On, Solomon, Noy, & Nardi, 1986; Bartemeier, 1946; Grinker, 1945; Solomon, 1993). These symptoms are universal and have been observed among combatants of different wars, at different times, and from different cultures (Bar-On et al., 1986).

CSR's polymorphic and labile nature makes it difficult to construct clear diagnostic criteria; most armies thus use a functional gauge, in which the defining criterion for CSR is that the soldier ceases to function militarily and acts in a manner that may endanger himself and/or his fellow combatants (Kormos, 1978). The use of such a functional definition is problematic. The identification of CSR is generally based on the judgment of nonprofessionals— the afflicted soldier himself[1] or his comrades or field commanders—who have little if any clinical knowledge. It is made under conditions of extreme stress and the life threats of battle, which are not necessarily conducive to a clear perception of abnormal changes, either in one's own behaviors or in those of others. Moreover, the loose behavioral criterion is relative; it depends on the "identification threshold" of those making the judgment—that is, on the level of psychopathology that either the individual or the unit can tolerate without labeling the soldier a CSR casualty (Moses & Cohen, 1984). This level is determined by the suffering that the individual can bear, by the judgment of

[1]For the sake of simplicity, masculine pronouns are used in this chapter to refer to the individual soldier, even though women have recently begun to play front-line roles in the armies of some nations.

either the individual himself or those in his environment of what constitutes a normal or acceptable reaction to battle stress, by the ability of the unit to serve as a holding environment, and by such factors as unit morale and motivation. It thus tends to vary from situation to situation, as suggested by the disparities in the proportion of identified CSR casualties in different wars. The relativity and subjectivity of the identification threshold may have detrimental consequences. A high identification threshold may result in a soldier's not getting the immediate care that has been shown to mitigate later emotional disturbances (Solomon & Benbenishty, 1986). A low identification threshold may result in labeling normal reactions to stress as psychopathology.

Taxonomy

The remoteness of the loose functional definition of CSR from its clinical picture has led to a number of attempts on the part of mental health professionals to formulate an orderly taxonomy. Some attempts were based on dominant manifestations (Cavenar & Nash, 1976; Grinker, 1945); others were based on the severity of symptoms (Bartemeier, 1946) or prognosis (Bailey, Williams, Komora, Salmon, & Fenton, 1929). All, however, relied on clinical impressions and lacked any quantitative component. During the Lebanon War, a team from the Israeli Defense Forces Medical Corps's Mental Health Department constructed a taxonomy based on an empirical approach (Yitzhaki, Solomon, & Kotler, 1991). Using 100 clinical records made on or near the front, they compiled a list of all the CSR manifestations. Analysis of the data yielded two major findings. First, it confirmed the labile and polymorphic nature of CSR as observed by others (McGrath & Brooker, 1985): 48% of the cases were polymorphic, and 11% were labile. Second, it emphasized the predominance of anxiety and depression in those cases that were not polymorphic. Anxiety states characterized 13% of the sample, and depression 9%. Moreover, in the polymorphic cases anxiety was the most prevalent symptom, followed by depression. The most prevalent change in the labile cases was from anxiety to depression; usually anxiety was the first manifestation of the CSR, and depression the last.

A study of 104 subjects in the first year after the war documented the sequence of events leading to the soldiers' breakdowns, along with how they felt and acted before, during, and after (Solomon, Mikulincer, & Benbenishty, 1989; Solomon, 1993). Several manifestations were particularly widespread: Acute anxiety was cited in over 48% of the cases, fear of death in about 26%, and crying in about 21%. Psychic numbing was reported in about 18% of the cases, and a feeling of total vulnerability in about 17%.

In order to identify CSR patterns, a factor analysis was performed. Six main factors were derived, together accounting for about 62% of the variance:

1. Distancing (20% of the total variance) included reports of psychic numbing, fantasies of running, and thoughts about civilian life. All of these were means by which the soldiers tried to block the intrusion of unbearably threatening battlefield stimuli and/or to distance themselves mentally and emotionally from the fighting (see also Beebe & Apple, 1951; Shontz, 1975).

2. Anxiety (11% of the total variance) included reports of paralyzing anxiety, fear of death, and thoughts of death. Its association with insomnia suggests that the problems casualties had in falling and staying asleep were caused by their fears.

3. Fatigue and guilt about poor performance in combat (9% of the total variance) were reported together. The guilt seems to have been largely over the breakdown per se, and over the casualties' inability to function effectively as combatants—a reaction not unlike survival guilt (Lifton, 1968).

4. Loneliness and vulnerability (8% of the total variance) also occurred together. The loneliness of the casualties may have resulted from their being away from their homes and families; from being new in a unit; from the loss of friends and buddies in combat; and from the recognition that, however one lives, in death one is alone. The feeling of vulnerability arose from the reality that the soldiers had few means of effectively countering or evading the dangers to which they are exposed (Maier & Seligman, 1976; Silver & Wortman, 1980). The two emotions were related, in that the battlefield deaths that brought on feelings of loneliness did more than anything else, on a psychological level, to bring home to the surviving soldiers their diminished chances of survival.

5. Loss of self-control (7% of the total variance) covered weeping, screaming, and a range of impulsive behaviors, as well as somatic reactions such as vomiting, wetting, and diarrhea. All these behaviors are indicative of the inability of casualties' to control their responses to the threat of injury and death.

6. Disorientation (6.5% of the total variance) included difficulty in concentrating, focusing thoughts, and making mental associations. In extreme cases, the soldiers might not know where they were, what unit they were in, or what time or day of the week it was. Disorientation, too, has been noted in previous wars and is usually brief (Bartemeier, 1946; Cavenar & Nash, 1976; Grinker, 1945).

This taxonomy of CSR is not unlike earlier classifications; the similarity suggests the universality of the pattern of response, regardless of the culture or the war being studied. The factors isolated appeared in Grinker's (1945) and Cavenar and Nash's (1976) taxonomies under different names. For example, the loneliness and vulnerability cited in the present taxonomy correspond to what Grinker (1945) called the passive–dependent type of reaction; loss of self-control overlaps with their psychosomatic and hostile–aggressive types. Although Grinker (1945) did not define anxiety as a separate type, he regarded it as the core of all CSR.

Some of the major manifestations of CSR are not limited to CSR casualties. Fear, anxiety, and a sense of vulnerability are prevalent emotions in threatening situations, and are certainly to be expected in war. In fact, these emotions may be adaptive in highly threatening environments by augmenting alertness or caution (Eberly, Harkness, & Engdahl, 1991). In CSR, however, fear becomes intense enough to impair the soldier's judgment, paralyze his limbs, make him lose consciousness, or cause him to engage in counterphobic activities that lead to unnecessary risk taking. The psychic numbing becomes so pervasive that it blocks not only pain, horror, and grief, but also the perceptions needed to make realistic judgments. And the fatigue, depression, and withdrawal become so intense that they impair effective action.

Long-Term Sequelae

With the end of a war, the pathogenic effects of combat stress may abate in some cases; in others, profound, prolonged, and varied psychological sequelae may ensue. Titchener and Ross (1974) have likened trauma to the flooding of a piece of land. When the flood water covers the earth, one cannot foresee its consequences. Sometimes, when the water recedes and the land reemerges, the preflood order reappears, reinforcing the notion that the damage can be quickly corrected. On other occasions, however, the flood leaves behind long-lasting damage. Similarly, following a traumatic event, when the stressor recedes, the injured person sometimes recovers quickly and the emotional trauma becomes a transitory life episode; at other times, the trauma causes impairment that is most difficult to remedy.

Posttraumatic Stress Disorder

The most common and conspicuous long-term sequela of combat stress is PTSD. A decline in PTSD rates was observed among the Yom Kippur War veterans, with higher recovery rates found among controls than among CSR casualties: 37% of CSR casualties who reported having suffered from PTSD in the past, still suffered from the syndrome at the time of the study, in comparison to 23% of the control group (Solomon & Kleinhauz, in press). Not all CSR casualties suffer from long-term maladjustment, however. The findings also show a substantial pattern of recovery over time. Following an acute reaction, some individuals may regain their equilibrium and cope well. Although for many soldiers CSR marks the beginning of long-term chronic distress which puts them at high risk for subsequent stress, for other soldiers CSR may be a transient episode. The link between CSR and PTSD may result from several sources. First, it may reflect the stressfulness of the trauma. Intense traumatic events may induce both immediate CSR and long-term PTSD. This relationship may also reflect the vulnerability of the individual: A more vulnerable individual may suffer more severe CSR and more severe PTSD. Finally, the positive relation may reflect the fact that PTSD generally involves ruminations about one's reactions during the trauma. Individuals who exhibit CSR remain preoccupied with their breakdowns, which in turn can exacerbate posttraumatic reactions.

Other Long-Term Disturbances

CSR soldiers experience a wide range of distress and non-PTSD psychiatric symptoms (Solomon, 1989, 1993); this again indicates that PTSD is only one of a range of posttraumatic adaptations. Combat stress may also have long-lasting effects on the social aspects of a veteran's life (DeFasio, Rustin, & Diamond, 1975; Figley, 1978). CSR casualties of the Lebanon War reported more problems in work performance, family functioning, sexual functioning, and various aspects of social functioning than did controls (Solomon, 1993). The difficulties in most of these areas did not abate with time. Only problems in family functioning were reported by fewer soldiers 3 years after the war than at the end of the first year (Solomon, 1994). Finally, a higher percentage of CSR casualties than of controls reported higher rates of somatic complaints and behaviors potentially detrimental to their health (Solomon, 1988; Solomon & Mikulincer, 1987; Solomon, Mikulincer, & Kotler, 1987). In general, the CSR casualties reported poorer health than the controls (Solomon, 1994).

ACUTE CIVILIAN REACTIONS TO WAR

The acute reactions of Israeli civilians during the Gulf War conflict and in the months prior to this war, when the threat of chemical attack hung over Israelis' heads, are the best-studied civilian reactions. These studies highlight that undifferentiated fear should not be forgotten as a primary determinant of behavior in attempts to create more complex classification systems for acute stress reactions. In the end, weapons of mass destruction were not used in the Gulf War; however, 18 conventional missile attacks all caused destruction of property, bodily injury, and some loss of life. Bleich, Dycian, Koslovsly, Solomon, and Weiner (1992) examined the 1,059 war-related hospital emergency room admissions. Of these, only 22% were direct casualties injured either by the missiles or by flying debris; the other 78% were indirect casualties, that is, "injuries" stemmed from fear when the air raid alerts were sounded. Of these, 11 persons died—7 from suffocation caused by faulty use of the gas masks, and 4 from heart attacks. That is, more people died from fear than from actual exposure to the missiles.

Evidently, under certain circumstances fear may be not only distressing, but fatal. A quarter of all emergency hospital admissions at this time suffered physical injuries while rushing to safety at the sound of the warning siren; others needlessly injected themselves with atropine (the nerve gas antidote that was distributed to all residents of Israel prior to the outbreak of the war). Over half the admissions (554, 51% in all) came with symptoms of acute psychological distress. Most of the admissions for acute distress or for self-injected atropine came right after the first missile attack; this points to progressive habituation to the threat, and perhaps to a quick learning process. Any strategy for dealing with the acute impact of disasters or war must take account of the critical role that the emotional determinants of behavior play in the survival of the individual and the society (McFarlane, 1995). Warning information must be presented in forms that take into account the effects of fear and denial on people's ability to digest information.

Solomon et al. (1993) investigated the impact of serious damage or destruction of houses by missiles in two stages: the first a week after the missile strikes, the second a year later. Most evacuees initially showed a very high level of nonspecific distress. What was most striking, however, was the very high level of PTSD symptomatology found. A full 80% of those assessed with the PTSD Inventory displayed a constellation of symptoms consistent with DSM-III-R criteria for the disorder (APA, 1987). This finding was similar to the very high levels of distress found among rape victims in the immediate aftermath of their trauma (Foa, Riggs, & Gershuny, 1995). Although a formal diagnosis of PTSD cannot be considered so soon after a traumatic event (according to the DSM-IV, a 1-month minimum duration of symptoms is required), the finding does indicate that the vast majority of people respond to traumatic events with a level of stress and a constellation of symptoms that would be deemed pathological if they persisted. It suggests that even if the symptoms may abate with time, the acute stress reaction constellation is almost universal.

One year later, a follow-up assessment showed that although trauma-related symptomatology declined somewhat, it was more persistent than in other similar studies (Karlehagen et al., 1993; Shalev, 1992): The PTSD rates fell from 80% to under 60%. Similarly, intrusion responses also declined only modestly. Moreover, the decline in intrusion was matched by an increase of avoidance. This later emergence of avoidance has also been observed in other groups of victims (e.g., Shalev, 1992), which raises some questions about the validity of the inclusion of these avoidance phenomena in the DSM-IV criteria for ASD. Among road accident victims, Mayou et al. (1993) found a subgroup of victims for whom this avoidance dominated the clinical picture, so that they had the features of a specific phobia about travel, with insufficient intrusive phenomena for these to contribute to the diagnosis.

CURRENT CONCEPTS OF ACUTE STRESS DISORDER

The empirical findings reviewed here and elsewhere (see Koopman, Classen, Cardeña, & Spiegel, 1995) support the definition of ASD as a separate independent clinical entity. Until recently, the trauma literature paid only limited attention to immediate reactions to stress. The recent inclusion of the diagnosis in the DSM-IV (APA, 1994) is a major contribution that will stimulate further research and result in increased knowledge of this disorder.

According to the DSM-IV formulation (APA, 1994), trauma survivors suffering from dissociative, intrusive, avoidance, anxiety, and hyperarousal symptoms of at least 2 days' duration are diagnosed as suffering from ASD. These symptoms must also markedly interfere with social or occupational functioning, or prevent an individual from pursuing some necessary task. Until the recent formulation of ASD in the DSM-IV, this diagnosis was mainly functional rather than clinical, as noted above in the case of CSR. Several reasons contributed to the adoption of a functional definition, among them the concept that the distinction between normative and pathological reaction to stress during adversity is a highly complex matter. Acute stress reactions were often perceived as short, transient crisis reactions. Moreover, labeling stress reactions as pathological was, and is, perceived by many professionals to be an impediment to recovery.

The DSM-IV (APA, 1994) formulation also recognizes the significance of functional impairment in ASD. The implicit concept that underpins the disorder is the distinguishing of "normal" from "abnormal" on the dimension of adaptability. One should recall that under traumatic circumstances, some of the symptoms listed in the DSM-IV may serve an adaptive purpose. For example, a degree of anxiety on the battlefield seems to be useful in promoting a soldier's survival. The factors distinguishing dysfunctional from functional anxiety are therefore its intensity and the extent to which it interferes with functioning.

The clinical picture of immediate response to stress that we have presented in this chapter also validates the new diagnostic entity. Specifically, immediately following their traumatic exposure to missile attack, civilian survivors reported elevated levels of intrusive, avoidance, hyperarousal, and anxiety symptoms. Similarly, studies examining the clinical picture of CSR among combatants also indicate that anxiety, dissociation, loss of control, disorientation, loneliness, guilt, and a sense of vulnerability are prominent parts of this disorder.

At the same time, two important criticisms should be mentioned. The first is the time frame defined in the DSM-IV. The manual states that ASD may last from a minimum of 2 days to a maximum of 4 weeks. However, research and clinical experience in Israel indicate that episodes of dissociation, anxiety, numbing, and an impaired sense of control that last over a period of 2 days following exposure to traumatic threat may be within the range of normal. The studies reviewed above, especially those of the civilian population in the Gulf War, indicate that a period of confusion and trauma can be followed by accommodation and organization in a large proportion of the population exposed to intense stress. It thus seems that the DSM-IV criteria may result in an overdiagnosis of transient reactions that will spontaneously abate with time. On the other hand, this problem emphasizes the need to consider the value of a categorical system of description in this situation, compared with a dimensional one, which may have more utility in describing the range of reactions.

Another important issue concerns the labile and polymorphic nature of the acute stress reaction, which has been consistently documented in the military psychiatric literature on CSR over decades. Naturally, a standardized set of diagnostic criteria cannot always capture the elusive nature of ASD. In fact, the labile and polymorphic qualities of the disorder make the adequacy of the diagnostic criteria questionable. However, the costs and benefits of the rigidity of standardized criteria should always be taken into account. In this regard, the flexibility of the ICD-10 criteria (WHO, 1992) may make them more clinically useful than the DSM-IV criteria.

It should not be forgotten that in most disasters and accidents involving civilians there is little need for such classification because it is very rare for specific interventions to be needed in this setting or for individuals' behavior to demand containment (McFarlane, 1995). Most accident and disaster populations will be provided with psychological first aid and debriefing, regardless of whether they have ASD or whether they are distressed. It is in the military setting where these diagnostic judgments take on genuine importance, because the critical issue is how to deal with a soldier who is unable to fight. Is he a coward, or is he sick? The German army did not recognize CSR in World War II. The moral imperative of this issue is reflected in the following statement about the way CSR was dealt with in World War I:

> A man was shot for cowardice. The volley failed to kill. The officer-in-charge lost his nerve, turned to the assistant provost marshal and said, "Do your own bloody work, I cannot." We understand that the sequel was that he was arrested. Officially, this butchery has to be applauded, but I have changed my ideas. There are no two ways. A man either can or cannot stand up to his environment. With some, the limit for breaking is reached sooner. The human frame can only stand so much. Surely, when a man becomes afflicted, it is more a case for the medicals than the APM. How easy for the generals living in luxury, well back in their chateau, to enforce the death penalty and with the stroke of a pen sign some poor wretch's death warrant—maybe of some poor, half-witted farm yokel, who once came forward of his own free will without being fetched. It makes one sick. (Evans, quoted in Winter, 1978, p. 140)

To conclude, the inclusion of this new diagnostic entity in the DSM-IV represents important progress. It focuses the attention of professionals on a fairly neglected area. As with every diagnostic criterion, its improvement is dependent on systematic research and clinical work. Its formulation will stimulate more research, which should increase our knowledge of this disorder and the range of normal and abnormal reactions to trauma.

REFERENCES

American Psychiatric Association (APA). (1980). *Diagnostic and statistical manual of mental disorders* (3rd ed.) Washington, DC: Author.

American Psychiatric Association (APA). (1987). *Diagnostic and statistical manual of mental disorders* (3rd ed., rev.). Washington, DC: Author.

American Psychiatric Association (APA). (1994). *Diagnostic and statistical manual of mental disorders* (4th ed.). Washington, DC: Author.

Atchison, M., & McFarlane, A. C. (1995). *Acute responses to trauma*. Manuscript submitted for publication.

Bailey, P., Williams, F. E., Kormora, P. O., Salmon, T. W., & Fenton, N. (1929). *The medical department of the United States Army in the World War: Vol. 10. Neuropsychiatry*. Washington, DC: U.S. Government Printing Office.

Bar-On, R., Solomon, Z., Noy, S., & Nardi, C. (1986). The clinical picture of combat stress reactions in the 1982 war in Lebanon: Cross-war comparisons. In N. A. Milgram (Ed.), *Stress and coping in time of war: Generalizations from the Israeli experience* (pp. 103–109). New York: Brunner/Mazel.

Bartemeier, L. H. (1946). Combat exhaustion. *Journal of Nervous and Mental Disease, 104*, 359–425.

Beebe, G. W., & Apple, J. W. (1951). *Variation in psychological tolerance to ground combat in World War II* (Final Report). Washington, DC: National Academy of Sciences, National Research Council, Division of Medical Sciences.

Bleich, A., Dycian, A., Koslovsky, M., Solomon, Z., & Weiner, M. (1992). Psychiatric implications of missile attacks on civilian population. *Journal of the American Medical Association, 268*, 613–615.

Cavenar, J. O., & Nash, J. L. (1976). The effects of combat on the normal personality: War neurosis in Vietnam returnees. *Comprehensive Psychiatry, 17*, 647–653.

DeFasio, V. J., Rustin, S. X., & Diamond, A. (1975). Symptom development in Vietnam era veterans. *American Journal of Orthopsychiatry, 45*, 158–163.

Eberly, R. E., Harkness, A. R., & Engdahl, B. E. (1991). An adaptational view of trauma response as illustrated by the prisoner of war experience. *Journal of Traumatic Stress, 4*, 363–380.

Figley, C. R. (1978). Psychosocial adjustment among Vietnam veterans: An overview of the research. In C. R. Figley (Ed.), *Stress disorders among Vietnam veterans* (pp. 57–70). New York: Brunner/Mazel.

Foa, E. B., Riggs, D. S., & Gershuny, B. S. (1995). Arousal, numbing and intrusion: Symptom structure of PTSD following assault. *American Journal of Psychiatry, 152*, 116–120.

Grinker, K. P. (1945). Psychiatric disorders in combat crews overseas and in returnees. *Medical Clinics of North America, 29*, 729–739.

Karlehagen, S., Malt, U., Hoff, H., Tibell, E., Herrstromer, U., & Hildingson, K. (1993). The effect of major railway accidents on the psychological health of train drivers: II. A longitudinal study of the one-year outcome after the accident. *Journal of Psychosomatic Research, 37,* 807–817.

Koopman, C., Classen, C., Cardeña, E., & Spiegel, D. (1995). When disaster strikes, acute stress disorder may follow. *Journal of Traumatic Stress, 8,* 29–46.

Koopman, C., Classen, C., & Spiegel, D. (1994). Predictors of posttraumatic stress symptoms among survivors of the Oakland/Berkeley, California, firestorm. *American Journal of Psychiatry, 151,* 888–894.

Kormos, H. R. (1978). The nature of combat stress. In C. R. Figley (Ed.), *Stress disorders among Vietnam veterans* (pp. 3–22). New York: Brunner/Mazel.

Lifton, R. J. (1968). *Death in life: The survivors of Hiroshima.* New York: Random House.

Maier, S. F., & Seligman, M. E. P. (1976). Learned helplessness: Theory and evidence. *Journal of Experimental Psychology, 105,* 3–46.

Malt, U. F., Hoivik, B., & Blikra, G. (1993). Psychosocial consequences of road accidents. *European Psychiatry, 8,* 227–228.

Mayou, R., Bryant, B., & Duthie, R. (1993). Psychiatric consequences of road traffic accidents. *British Medical Journal, 307,* 647–651.

McFarlane, A. C. (1995). Stress and disaster. In S. E. Hobfa & M. W. deVries (Eds.), *Extreme stress and communities* (pp. 247–267). Dordrecht, The Netherlands: Kluwer.

McGrath, T. R., & Brooker, A. E. (1985). Combat stress reaction: A concept in evolution. *Military Medicine, 150,* 186–190.

Moses, R., & Cohen, I. (1984). Understanding and treatment of combat neurosis: The Israeli experience. In H. J. Schwartz (Ed.), *Psychotherapy of the combat veteran* (pp. 269–303). New York: Spectrum.

Rachman, S. (1990). *Fear and courage.* New York: Freeman.

Saigh, P. (1984). Pre- and postinvasion anxiety in Lebanon. *Behavior Therapy, 15,* 185–190.

Shalev, A. Y. (1992). Posttraumatic stress disorder among injured survivors of a terrorist attack: Predictive value of early intrusion and avoidance symptoms. *Journal of Nervous and Mental Disease, 180,* 505–509.

Shontz, F. C. (1975). *The psychological aspects of physical illness and disability.* New York: Macmillan.

Silver, R. L., & Wortman, C. B. (1980). Coping with undesirable events. In J. Garber & M. E. Seligman (Eds.), *Human helplessness: Theory and application* (pp. 279–340). New York: Academic Press.

Solomon, Z. (1988). Somatic complaints, stress reaction and post-traumatic stress disorder: A 3-year follow-up study. *Behavioral Medicine, 14,* 179–186.

Solomon, Z. (1989). Characteristic psychiatric symptomatology in PTSD veterans: A three year follow-up. *Psychological Medicine, 19,* 927–936.

Solomon, Z. (1993). *Combat stress reaction: The enduring toll of war.* New York: Plenum Press.

Solomon, Z. (1994). *The psychological aftermath of combat stress reaction: An 18-year follow-up.* Technical report, Israeli Ministry of Defense.

Solomon, Z., & Benbenishty, R. (1986). The role of proximity, immediacy, and expectancy in frontline treatment of combat stress reaction among Israelis in the Lebanon War. *American Journal of Psychiatry, 143,* 613–617.

Solomon, Z., & Kleinhauz, M. (in press). War induced psychic trauma: An 18 year follow-up of Israeli veterans. *American Journal of Orthopsychiatry.*

Solomon, Z., Laor, N., Weiler, D., Muller, U. F., Hadar, O., Waysman, M., Koslowsky, M., Ben-Yakar, M., & Bleich, A. (1993). The psychological impact of the Gulf War: A study of acute stress in Israeli evacuees. *Archives of General Psychiatry, 50,* 320–321.

Solomon, Z., & Mikulincer, M. (1987). Combat stress reaction, post-traumatic stress disorder and somatic complaints among Israeli soldiers. *Journal of Psychosomatic Research, 31,* 131–137.

Solomon, Z., Mikulincer, M., & Bebenishty, R. (1989). Combat stress reaction: Clinical manifestations and correlates. *Military Psychology, 1,* 35–47.

Solomon, Z., Mikulincer, M., & Kotler, M. (1987). A two year follow-up of somatic complaints among Israeli combat stress reaction casualties. *Journal of Psychosomatic Research, 31,* 463–469.

Tichener, J. L., & Ross, W. O. (1974). Acute and chronic stress as determinants of behavior, character and neurosis. In S. Arieti & E. B. Brody (Eds.), *American handbook of psychiatry: Adult clinical psychiatry* (pp. 47–70). New York: Basic Books.

Weisaeth, L. (1989a). The stressors and the post-traumatic stress syndrome after an industrial disaster. *Acta Psychiatrica Scandinavica, 80,* 25–37.

Weisaeth, L. (1989b). A study of behavioural responses to an industrial disaster. *Acta Psychiatrica Scandinavica, 80*(Suppl. 355), 13–24.

Winter, D. (1978). *Death's men.* London: Allen Lane.

World Health Organization (WHO). (1992). *International classification of diseases* (10th revision). Geneva: Author.

Yitzhaki, T., Solomon, Z., & Kotler, M. (1991). The clinical picture of the immediate combat stress reaction (CSR) in the Lebanon War. *Military Medicine, 156,* 193–197.

PART III

ADAPTATIONS TO TRAUMA

CHAPTER 6

The Classification of Posttraumatic Stress Disorder

ELIZABETH A. BRETT

The question of how posttraumatic stress disorder (PTSD) should be classified was raised in the deliberations prior to publication of the *Diagnostic and Statistical Manual of Mental Disorders*, fourth edition (DSM-IV; American Psychiatric Association [APA], 1994). Although the DSM-IV Advisory Subcommittee on PTSD voted unanimously to place PTSD in a new stress response category (Brett, 1993), the DSM-IV Task Force did not support this position, and PTSD remains classified as an anxiety disorder (as it has been since DSM-III). The classification of PTSD was controversial in the revision of DSM-III as well. Subcommittee members debated heatedly whether PTSD should be located within the anxiety or the dissociative disorders (Brett, Spitzer, & Williams, 1988). The consideration of classification in both instances was driven by the necessity to reach a decision for the new edition of the diagnostic manual. Although this exigency focused discussion, it also narrowed it. In this chapter, the freedom from the need to endorse a concrete proposal allows a broader consideration of the issues involved.

The chapter reviews the history of the placement of PTSD and its predecessors within the international and American diagnostic nosologies. The question of how PTSD should be classified is replaced by the more fruitful consideration of the ways in which thinking of PTSD as a particular type of disorder illuminates and extends our understanding of the syndrome or limits and constrains it.

A HISTORICAL REVIEW
OF CLASSIFICATIONS OF PTSD

Let us look at the evolution of diagnoses for traumatic stress reactions. War has always been a stimulus to the description and study of trauma. Experience with psychiatric casualties in World War II led to a profound reformulation of the existing concepts for mental disorder. At "the beginning of World War II, American psychiatry, civilian and military, was using a system of naming developed primarily for the needs and case loads of public mental hospitals. . . . Military psychiatrists, induction station psychiatrists, and Veterans Administration psychiatrists found themselves operating within the limits of a nomenclature specifically not designed for 90% of the cases handled" (APA, 1952, p. vi). The kinds of cases for which the previous classification had no terms included minor personality disturbances, psychosomatic reactions, neurotic symptoms, and reactions to combat stress.

During and immediately following the war, the American Armed Forces and the Veterans Administration each developed new diagnostic classsifications. In 1948, when the World Health Organization (WHO) decided to include mental disorders in the sixth revision of the *International Statistical Classification of Diseases, Injuries, and Causes of Death* (ICD-6), they were organized on the basis of the Armed Forces' categories. In 1952, when the APA revised its nosology dating from 1933, it did so on the basis of psychiatry's experience with the Armed Forces, Veterans Administration, and ICD-6 systems (APA, 1952, 1993). Thus both the international and American classifications were formulated by psychiatrists who had extensive experience with posttraumatic pathology.

How did the experience with soldiers and civilians in World War II affect diagnoses? The Armed Forces and the Veterans Administration defined traumatic reactions as short-lived responses in essentially normal individuals. Transient situational syndromes were acute reactions to overwhelming stress occurring in individuals with no premorbid or concurrent psychopathology. This perspective was carried through in both the international and American classifications.

In ICD-6 (see Table 6.1), PTSD prototypes were called "acute situational maladjustments." DSM-I labeled them "transient situational personality disturbance." DSM-II (APA, 1968) was based on the mental disorders section of ICD-8 (WHO, 1969), and both used the same term, "transient situational disturbance." There were no changes in mental disorders in ICD-7. ICD-9 (WHO, 1977) employed the compatible but more specific designation "acute reaction to stress."

ICD-10 (WHO, 1992) and DSM-III (APA, 1980) presented significantly different conceptions of posttraumatic reactions (see Table 6.2). The most important change was, and is, that stress disorders are no longer restricted to

TABLE 6.1. Comparison of International and American Diagnoses for Traumatic Stress, 1948 to 1977

International	American
ICD-6 (1948)	DSM-I (1952)
Acute situational maladjustment	Transient situational personality disturbance
	Gross stress reaction
	Adult situational reaction
	Adjustment reaction of:
	Infancy
	Childhood
	Adolescence
	Late life
ICD-8 (1968)	DSM-II (1968)
Transient situational disturbance	Adjustment reaction of:
	Infancy
	Childhood
	Adolescence
	Adult life
	Late life
ICD-9 (1977)	
Acute reaction to stress:	
With predominant disturbance of emotions	
With predominant disturbance of consciousness	
With predominant psychomotor disturbance	
Other mixed	

acute responses in healthy individuals. Traumatic stress can cause chronic reactions, and responses to traumatic stress can occur with previous and simultaneous conditions. A second significant change was that the new diagnosis, PTSD, was placed in the anxiety disorders section of DSM-III. The conceptualization of PTSD as an anxiety disorder is thus a relatively recent American phenomenon. International and American classifications of anxiety have also come to differ over the inclusiveness of the group of anxiety disorders. The American approach encompasses obsessive–compulsive disorder (OCD) as well as PTSD, regarding the anxiety in each as a core phenomenon. Europeans, on the other hand, regard anxiety as a common and nonspecific feature of many disorders, and locate OCD and PTSD on the basis of other features (Jablensky, 1993).

Several other characteristics of the DSM and ICD systems are worth noting. ICD-10 has more variety in the diagnoses for traumatic reactions, with the inclusion of enduring personality changes after catastrophic experience. In the

TABLE 6.2. Comparison of International and American Diagnoses for Traumatic Stress, 1980 to 1994

International	American
ICD-10 (1992)	DSM-III, DSM-III-R (1980,1987)
Acute stress reaction	Post-traumatic stress disorder
Posttraumatic stress disorder	DSM-IV (1994)
Enduring personality changes	Acute stress disorder
after catastrophic experience	Posttraumatic stress disorder

American manuals from DSM-I to DSM-II, there was a dilution in the concept of traumatic disorders. DSM-I contained "gross stress reaction," which was to be recorded as a response to military or civilian catastrophe. DSM-II eliminated gross stress reaction; all that remained were "adjustment reactions," syndromes that are not differentiated on the basis of the nature or severity of the stress response. The authors of DSM-II pointed out that the adjustment disorder diagnosis allowed for reactions of psychotic proportions, whereas the DSM-I category did not. Nevertheless, the combining of adjustment and stress disorders represented a simultaneous loss of differentiation.

Specificity about reactions to trauma reappeared in DSM-III. This was the result of psychiatric evaluation and treatment of Vietnam veterans (Spitzer, personal communication, March 1994). Like World War II, the Vietnam War stimulated the study of trauma. It is not difficult to see that closeness to large populations of traumatized individuals enhances the ability to describe and retain descriptions of traumatic stress, and that distance from such populations diminishes this ability. The waxing and waning of knowledge about trauma has often been noted in reviews of the field (Brett & Ostroff, 1985; Herman, 1992; Horowitz, 1986; Trimble, 1985).

This fluctuation is even more apparent when one looks at the history behind the diagnostic criteria for PTSD. The criteria were based on Abram Kardiner's formulation of traumatic neurosis, derived from his treatment of World War I veterans. Kardiner built on Freud's observations concerning the alternating repetitions and defensive processes so characteristic of traumatic neurosis. He added the idea that the traumatic event has a direct physiological impact on the individual; he also emphasized that the traumatic event initiates a neurotic reaction that is not accounted for by premorbid factors. In anticipation of World War II, Kardiner (1941) published a book about his observations. Following the war, he added new case material from World War II in a second edition of the book, but he did not change his conceptualization and description of traumatic neurosis (Kardiner & Spiegel, 1947).

In the introduction to his first book, Kardiner noted that his work with World War I veterans had not influenced views of peacetime trauma, which, he asserted, has the same structure as the wartime version. Kardiner's views were rediscovered during and following World War II, but it was not until the third rediscovery of his work in the preparation for DSM-III that a fuller recognition of his contribution was possible—that both his description of the symptoms and the generic nature of the syndrome could be appreciated.

PTSD AS AN ANXIETY DISORDER

DSM-III and its successors have taken posttraumatic reactions out of an adjustment and stress category and placed them in the anxiety disorders. Barlow makes the most comprehensive and persuasive argument for considering PTSD an anxiety disorder (Barlow, 1988; Jones & Barlow, 1990). This argument rests on noting "the presence of the fundamental components of anxiety in behavioral, cognitive and physiological response systems" in PTSD (Jones & Barlow, 1990, p. 308). Barlow applies his model of the development and consolidation of anxiety disorders to PTSD, and then uses the similarity of panic disorder and PTSD to further demonstrate the utility of considering PTSD an anxiety disorder.

According to Barlow, when individuals with both biological and psychological vulnerability experience stressful life events, they develop beliefs that these stressful events are unpredictable and uncontrollable. The environmental triggers may either be (1) events that cause stress or (2) "alarms," events that cause intense fear or panic. If the individuals do not possess adequate coping skills or social support, they will become fearful about the repetition of the stress; this creates a cycle of chronic overarousal and "anxious apprehension." It is this preoccupation with and anticipation of future stress that is at the core of the disorder. Hypervigilance, attention narrowing, and distortions in the processing of information are features of anxious apprehension.

Barlow's model of panic disorder is based on the recognition that panic may occur in reaction to either realistic or irrational dangers. If an individual becomes anxious about the recurrence of panic, a cycle of anxious apprehension and of secondary conditioning to cues associated with the panic creates the self-perpetuating feedback loop necessary for the development and maintenance of the panic disorder. Panic disorder and PTSD are distinguished in this model on the basis of the realistic versus unrealistic nature of the original stressful events. For PTSD patients, the original dangers are realistic. From a symptomatological perspective, Barlow finds panic disorder and PTSD similar in the presence of intrusive thoughts about the stressful event or alarm, efforts to avoid the disturbing material, hypervigilance, and heightened arousal.

Barlow's is a strong argument. In essence, he asserts that although PTSD and other anxiety disorders may look as if they differ on the basis of the nature and role of the stressor, they are similar in that the cycle of anxious apprehension is what creates the disorder. This is Barlow's response to the contention that PTSD should be classified as a stress disorder on the basis of etiology. He argues that since so many people exposed to traumatic stressors do not develop PTSD, an explanation that accounts for how some and not others develop the disorder is necessary.

How does considering PTSD an anxiety disorder extend our understanding of the disorder? A number of models of PTSD have borrowed heavily from concepts used for anxiety disorders (Foa, Steketee, & Rothbaum, 1989; Chemtob, Roitblat, Hamada, Carlson, & Twentyman, 1988; Keane, Zimering, & Caddell, 1985; Litz & Keane, 1989). The same has happened with lines of research (Rainey et al., 1987; Southwick et al., 1993) and approaches to treatment (Fairbank & Keane, 1982; Fairbank & Brown, 1987; Saigh, 1987; Resick, Jordan, Girelli, Hulter, & Marhoefeo-Dvorak, 1988; Foa, Rothbaum, Riggs, & Murdock, 1991).

Jones and Barlow (1990) review research on PTSD and conclude that it supports the similarity between PTSD and the anxiety disorders in the following areas: genetic vulnerability, psychological predisposition, pathophysiology, symptomatology, and response to treatment. In contrast, four other reviews conclude that PTSD is best thought of as a stress disorder, not an anxiety disorder (Brett, 1993; see particularly Davidson & Foa, 1991; Davidson & Fairbank, 1993; and Pittman, 1993). The authors of these reviews, it should be acknowledged, were all members of the DSM-IV Advisory Subcommitttee on PTSD. At this point, research in this area is preliminary and suggestive, and can be interpreted from a variety of points of view. It has not yet provided definitive answers.

Three fundamental objections can be made to the anxiety disorder perspective:

1. The questions of whether the arousal in PTSD is anxiety and whether PTSD has the same pathophysiology as the other anxiety disorders remain unanswered. Pittman (1993) argues trenchantly that the arousal in PTSD is not simply anxiety and does not share the same physiological pathways. This issue awaits further clarification.

2. Although Barlow's description of PTSD as an anxiety disorder shows some goodness of fit with the clinical features of the disorder, one can argue that the recurrent and overlapping phases of reexperiencing and numbing are much closer phenomenologically to processes of mourning and bereavement. In fact, Horowitz has frequently emphasized this similarity, and his recommendation for the creation of a stress response category in DSM-IV includes normal and pathological bereavement (Horowitz, Weiss & Marmar, 1987).

3. The distinctive and unique posttraumatic aspects of the disorder that have to do with memory are not focused on or further differentiated in as much detail as they might be. Barlow's perspective is most useful in considering the features and processes generic to a variety of disorders. Although it accounts for some aspects of reexperiencing and avoidance, it does not provide new avenues for illuminating and distinguishing the processes of encoding traumatic memories, with their fragmentation, dissociation, and diverse forms of repetition and avoidance. We do not have new approaches to considering the formal properties of memories that range from indistinct to vivid and lifelike, illusory, and hallucinatory. One of the chief attractions of the study of the dissociative disorders to PTSD investigators is that the field of dissociation is focused on the further explication of just these features of the posttraumatic experience.

PTSD AS A DISSOCIATIVE DISORDER

One of the most salient features of the literature on dissociation is the richness of the descriptions of posttraumatic symptomatology. Spiegel and Cardeña (1991), in their article on the dissociative disorders for DSM-IV, discuss derealization, depersonalization, dazed states, disorientation, out-of-body experiences, and amnesias; reexperiencing phenomena, including reenactments, intrusive images, and flashbacks; and alterations in body image, time passage, and visual and auditory perceptions, including illusory and hallucinatory experiences. It is significant that the new DSM-IV diagnosis of acute stress disorder was proposed by the Advisory Subcommittee on Dissociative Disorders. The elaboration of the posttraumatic and dissociative symptom criteria for the new diagnosis follows naturally from this descriptive orientation. The attentiveness to posttraumatic reactions is further demonstrated in the recognition that the diagnoses of dissociative amnesia and dissociative fugue frequently occur after traumatic stressors. Spiegel and Cardeña mention that both often have been reported as responses to combat.

The focus on the distinctive characteristics of PTSD, and the sponsoring of acute stress disorder, are particularly salient in the context of the history of posttraumatic diagnoses. As I have mentioned in the review of classifications of PTSD, distance from experience with traumatized populations can lead to a dilution of posttraumatic diagnoses and their homogenization with other disorders. This was seen, for example, in the loss of gross stress reaction in DSM-II; after this, adjustment disorders became the only way to diagnose traumatic syndromes. One of the dangers of a perspective derived from the anxiety disorders is that the communalities with nonposttraumatic disorders are emphasized and the differences receive less attention. The advantage of the perspective derived from the dissociative disorders is that reactions to traumatic stressors and alterations in memory are central foci and therefore less easily ignored or forgotten.

In the last few years, the dissociation literature has stimulated a significant amount of research on PTSD, dissociation, and memory. This work is just beginning to be reported (see Chapter 13, this volume), but it is expected that the findings of these investigations will provide valuable information and insights.

There are two objections to considering PTSD a dissociative disorder as opposed to considering it a posttraumatic disorder. First, as Spiegel and Cardeña (1991) point out, there is confusion about the precise meaning of "dissociation." The difficulties in definition are that different terms are used to describe the same phenomena in some cases (e.g., "dissociation" and "repression" are used in various traditions to describe the same defensive maneuver) and that a single term is used to describe different phenomena in other instances (e.g., "dissociation" is used to refer to a broad spectrum of defensive processes) (Braun, 1992). At this stage of inquiry, it is most useful to distinguish both similarities and differences, without losing sight of either. The second objection to considering PTSD a dissociative as opposed to a posttraumatic disorder is that although there is overlap in symptoms between acute stress disorder and PTSD on the one hand and the dissociative disorders on the other, there are also significant differences in pathology.

THE ADVANTAGES AND DISADVANTAGES OF CURRENT APPROACHES TO DIAGNOSIS

The description of PTSD in 1980 was part of the new atheoretical, phenomenologically based approach to diagnosis introduced in DSM-III and used since then in its successors. The specification of the symptom criteria fostered the appreciation of the generic features of posttraumatic syndromes, which spurred the creation of the field of traumatic stress studies. Clinicians working with many different traumatized populations began to use a common language. Research investigators developed reliable and valid measures of PTSD, and research expanded dramatically.

There have been disadvantages to the DSM's diagnostic approach, however. There are several ways in which this conceptualization may narrow options:

1. The focus on one posttraumatic syndrome can hinder exploration of alternate forms or variations of the disorder. A clear example of this is the controversy over the inclusion of "disorders of extreme stress not otherwise specified" (DESNOS), sometimes called "complex PTSD," in DSM-IV. The decision for DSM-IV (APA, 1994) was not to include DESNOS. By contrast,

the ICD-10 (WHO, 1992) does include personality changes after traumatic experience.

2. The restriction of the diagnostic criteria to essential features (i.e., only those symptoms necessary for making the diagnosis) leaves out many characteristics of the disorder which have clinical and treatment relevance. Despite the DSM's cautionary statements about this (APA, 1987), the criteria are often used by clinicians as if they were complete descriptions of mental disorders. Research from the DSM-IV field trials confirmed the existence and frequency of DESNOS (most often in conjunction with PTSD) and its relation to variables such as age of onset, severity, and type of stressor (van der Kolk, Roth, Pelcovitz, & Mandel, 1993). The restriction of the diagnosis to its most essential features can result in two types of clinical errors: Either a clinician may miss the PTSD diagnosis because associated features are most prominent, or the associated features may be overlooked because of the presence of the PTSD. Blank (1994) has written a useful guide for the clinician evaluating posttraumatic responses, in which he repeatedly emphasizes the variety of reactions to trauma.

3. The cross-sectional nature of diagnosis can impede effforts to conceptualize the course of stress disorders as they evolve over years in an individual's life. The extreme complexity and subtlety of posttraumatic responses have been noted since Kardiner's (1941) postulation of a two-stage response to trauma. In Kardiner's description, the first stage is the core traumatic neurosis (what we now call PTSD). The second stage can have any diagnostic manifestation and is the personality's adaptation to and reorganization in the face of its compromised functioning caused by the traumatic neurosis. In a review of the recent research findings concerning the course of PTSD, Blank (1993) documents the intricacy of the long-term effects of trauma. This includes PTSD and its variants; dissociative disorders; brief reactive psychosis and other disorders precipitated directly by a traumatic stressor; comorbid diagnoses with either a primary or secondary relation to the stressor; and issues such as delayed, intermittent, or recurrrent forms of the disorder. The danger of premature closure lies in losing this complexity.

SUMMARY

The historical review of diagnosis since World War II indicates the vulnerabilty of knowledge about trauma to erosion. It is sobering to contemplate the amount of time that elapsed between Kardiner's observations of World War I veterans and the incorporations of his insights into the DSM-III criteria. There are two principal areas in which information has been lost: the uniqueness and the variety of traumatic responses. Although perspectives from the anxiety and dissociative disorders have stimulated theory and research in traumatic stress studies, the primary tasks for the field remain just those that are vulnerable—namely, continuing to specify the unique features of traumatic stress responses, as well as the variety of forms they may take.

REFERENCES

American Psychiatric Association (APA). (1952). *Diagnostic and statistical manual of mental disorders* (1st ed.). Washington, DC: Author.
American Psychiatric Association (APA). (1968). *Diagnostic and statistical manual of mental disorders* (2nd ed.). Washington, DC: Author.
American Psychiatric Association (APA). (1980). *Diagnostic and statistical manual of mental disorders* (3rd ed.). Washington, DC: Author.
American Psychiatric Association (APA). (1987). *Diagnostic and statistical manual of mental disorders* (3rd ed., rev.). Washington, DC: Author.
American Psychiatric Association (APA). (1993). *DSM-IV draft criteria.* Washington, DC: Author.
American Psychiatric Association (APA). (1994). *Diagnostic and statistical manual of mental disorders* (4th ed.). Washington, DC: Author.
Barlow, D. H. (1988). *Anxiety and its disorders: The nature and treatment of anxiety and panic.* New York: Guilford Press.
Blank, A. S. (1993). The longitudinal course of posttraumatic stress disorder. In J. R. T. Davidson & E. B. Foa (Eds.), *Posttraumatic stress disorder: DSM-IV and beyond* (pp. 3–22). Washington, DC: American Psychiatric Press.
Blank, A. S. (1994). Clinical detection, diagnosis, and differential diagnosis of posttraumatic stress disorder. *Psychiatric Clinics of North America, 17*(2), 351–384.
Braun, B. G. (1993). Multiple personality disorder and posttraumatic stress disorder: Similarities and differences. In J. P. Wilson & B. Raphael (Eds.), *International handbook of traumatic stress syndromes* (pp. 35–47). New York: Plenum Press.
Brett, E. A. (1993). Classifications of posttraumatic stress disorder in DSM-IV: Anxiety disorder, dissociative disorder or stress disorder? In J. R. T. Davidson & E. B. Foa (Eds.), *Posttraumatic stress disorder: DSM-IV and beyond* (pp. 191–204). Washington, DC: American Psychiatric Press.
Brett, E. A., & Ostroff, R. (1985). Imagery and post-traumatic stress disorder: An overview. *American Journal of Psychiatry, 142,* 417–424.
Brett, E. A., Spitzer, R. L., & Williams, J. B. W. (1988). DSM-III-R criteria for posttraumatic stress disorder. *American Journal of Psychiatry, 145,* 1232–1236.
Chemtob, C., Roitblat, G. C., Hamada, R. S., Carlson, J. G., & Twentyman, C. T. (1988). A cognitive action theory of post-traumatic stress disorder. *Journal of Anxiety Disorders, 2,* 253–275.
Davidson, J. R. T., & Foa, E. B. (1991). Diagnostic issues in posttraumatic stress disorder: Considerations for the DSM-IV. *Journal of Abnormal Psychology, 100*(3), 346–355.
Davidson, J. R. T., & Fairbank, J. A. (1993). The epidemiology of posttraumatic stress disorder. In J. R. T. Davidson & E. B. Foa (Eds.), *Posttraumatic stress disorder: DSM-IV and beyond* (pp. 147–169). Washington, DC: American Psychiatric Press.

Fairbank, J. A., & Brown, T. A. (1987). Current behavioral approaches to the treatment of posttraumatic stress disorder. *The Behavior Therapist, 10,* 57–64.

Fairbank, J. A., & Keane, T. M. (1982). Flooding for combat-related stress disorders: Assessment of anxiety reduction across traumatic memories. *Behavior Therapy, 13,* 499–510.

Foa, E. B., Rothbaum, B. O., Riggs, D. S., & Murdock, T. B. (1991). Treatment of posttraumatic stress disorder in rape victims: A comparison between cognitive-behavioral procedures and counselling. *Journal of Consulting and Clinical Psychology, 59,* 715–723.

Foa, E. B., Steketee, G., & Rothbaum, B. O. (1989). Behavioral/cognitive conceptualizations of post-traumatic stress disorder. *Behavior Therapy, 20,* 155–176.

Herman, J. L. (1992). *Trauma and recovery*. New York: Basic Books.

Horowitz, M. J. (1986). *Stress response syndromes* (2nd ed.). Northvale, NJ: Jason Aronson.

Horowitz, M. J., Weiss, D. S., & Marmar, C. (1987). Diagnosis of posttraumatic stress disorder. *Journal of Nervous and Mental Disease, 175*(5), 267–268.

Jablensky, A. (1993). Concepts and classification of anxiety. *Torture, 1,* 36–40.

Jones, J. C., & Barlow, D. H. (1990). The etiology of posttraumatic stress disorder. *Clinical Psychology Review, 10,* 299–328.

Kardiner, A. (1941). *The traumatic neuroses of war.* New York: Hoeber.

Kardiner, A., & Spiegel, H. (1947). *War stress and neurotic illness.* New York: Hoeber.

Keane, T. M., Zimering, R. T., & Caddell, J. M. (1985), A behavioral formulation of post-traumatic stress disorder in Vietnam veterans. *The Behavior Therapist, 8,* 9–12.

Litz, B. T., & Keane, T. M. (1989). Information processing in anxiety disorders: Application to the understanding of post-traumatic stress disorder. *Clinical Psychology Review, 9,* 243–257.

Pittman, R. K. (1993). Biological findings in posttraumatic stress disorder: Implications for DSM-IV classification. In J. R. T. Davidson & E. B. Foa (Eds.), *Posttraumatic stress disorder: DSM-IV and beyond* (pp. 173–189). Washington, DC: American Psychiatric Press.

Rainey, J. M., Aleem, A., Ortiz, A., Yeragani, V., Pohl, R., & Berehou, R. (1987). A laboratory procedure for the induction of flashbacks. *American Journal of Psychiatry, 144,* 1317–1319.

Resick, P. A., Jordan, C. G., Girelli, A. A., Hulter, C. K., & Marhoefeo-Dvorak, S. (1988). A comparative victim study of behavioral-group therapy for sexual assault victims. *Behavior Therapy, 19,* 385–401.

Saigh, P. A. (1987). *In vitro* flooding of childhood posttraumatic stress disorders: A systematic replication. *Professional School Psychology, 2,* 133–144.

Southwick, S. M., Krystal, J. H., Morgan, C. A., Johnson, D., Nagy, L. M., Nicolauo, A., Heninger, G. R., & Charney, D. S. (1993). Abnormal noradrenergic function in posttraumatic stress disorder. *Archives of General Psychiatry, 50,* 266–274.

Spiegel, D., & Cardeña, E. (1991). Disintegrated experience: The dissociative disorders revisited. *Journal of Abnormal Psychology, 100*(3), 366–378.

Trimble, M. (1985). Posttraumatic stress disorders: History of a concept. In C. R. Figley (Ed.), *Trauma and its wake* (pp. 5–14). New York: Brunner/Mazel.

van der Kolk, B. A., Roth, S., Pelcovitz, D., & Mandel, F. (1993). *Complex PTSD: Results of the PTSD field trials for DSM-IV.* Washington, DC: American Psychiatric Association.

World Health Organization (WHO). (1948). *Manual of the international statistical classification of diseases, injuries, and causes of death* (6th revision). Geneva: Author.

World Health Organization (WHO). (1969). *Manual of the international statistical classification of diseases, injuries, and causes of death* (8th revision). Geneva: Author.

World Health Organization (WHO). (1977). *Manual of the international statistical classification of diseases, injuries, and causes of death* (9th revision). Geneva: Author.

World Health Organization (WHO). (1992). *ICD-10: International statistical classification of diseases and related health problems* (10th revision). Geneva: Author.

CHAPTER 7

The Nature of Traumatic Stressors and the Epidemiology of Posttraumatic Reactions

ALEXANDER C. McFARLANE
GIOVANNI DE GIROLAMO

History is always an ambiguous affair. Facts are hard to establish, and capable of being given many meanings. Reality is built on our own prejudices, gullibility, and ignorance, as well as on knowledge and analysis.
— SALMAN RUSHDIE (1981, pp. 99–100)

The role of the stressor in posttraumatic stress disorder (PTSD) raises a series of central issues about causation, treatment, and prevention. The stressor criterion as defined by the fourth edition of the *Diagnostic and Statistical Manual of Mental Disorders* (DSM-IV); American Psychiatric Association [APA], 1994) is somewhat simplified, thereby avoiding some serious questions. The early work on traumatic stress suggested that there were specific syndromes caused by specific types of trauma, such as the "concentration camp syndrome," the "rape trauma syndrome," or the "battered wife syndrome" (Herman, 1992). This tradition continues in many books in the traumatic stress field, which focus on the effects of a single type of traumatic event, such as disasters or torture. However, the notion behind PTSD is that there is a generalized reaction pattern to traumatic events, which is predetermined by the limited range of affective, cognitive, and behavioral responses that humans can have to overwhelming stress (Andreasen & Wasek, 1980). The currently accepted view, which is supported by a variety of systematic studies, is that the similarities of responses far outweigh the differences (Blank, 1993). This is an important issue, because it emphasizes the necessity of paying attention to the role of both biological and psychological adaptational processes as determinants of the posttraumatic response pattern.

In research on the effects of trauma, the time has arrived to consider the differences between different groups of trauma victims. For example, the demands of coping with repeated combat will be very different from being involved in a motor vehicle accident, which may last for a second and in which the victim has no control over the situation. Child abuse also tends to continue over a period of time, but in this circumstance the child has to cope with being in a dependent relationship with the abusive parent. The developmental stage of the child may also alter how he or she understands the trauma, and will influence the nature of possible psychological and behavioral responses (see Chapter 9, this volume). Child abuse and related traumas therefore have a much greater potential to disrupt stable relationships, and the development of appropriate ways of expressing affection and tolerating intense emotion, than a circumscribed traumatic event. Therefore, the time has come to reopen the question as to whether there exist subtypes of PTSD that are determined by the nature of the stressors.

After a brief background description of the fitful course of interest in traumatic stress and stressors over the years, this chapter first describes the dimensions that should be considered when describing the nature of traumatic events; second, it discusses the problems of constructing an objective picture of the impact of a traumatic event and the complexity of this task; and, third, it discusses the epidemiology of the effects of different types of traumatic events. The nature of the stressor is a central issue in traumatic stress studies, as is the role of the stressor as the primary etiological factor in determining the typical pattern of symptoms. At first glance, one would imagine that traumatic events such as disasters are truly independent events (i.e., events where the experience is not caused or modified by a victim). However, on closer examination the question is more complicated, as the intensity of exposure and survival behaviors can be critically determined by the victims. Therefore, the outcome following a stressful event may reflect a victim's capacity for adaptive behavior (Gibbs, 1989). The intensity of traumatic experience hence may reflect individuals' resilience and vulnerability. Epidemiology provides invaluable information about the range of traumatic responses and the characteristics of different traumas that appear to be particularly damaging (de Girolamo & McFarlane, in press).

BACKGROUND: THE RECOGNITION
OF TRAUMATIC STRESS AND STRESSORS

The interest in traumatic neurosis emerged out of the recognition that some events have a peculiar psychological toxicity (see Chapter 3, this volume). One of the characteristics of these events is their capacity to create fear and an intense sense of threat. Traumatic stressors are events that violate our existing ways of making sense of our reactions, structuring our perceptions of other people's behavior, and creating a framework for interacting with the world at large. In part, this is determined by our ability to anticipate, protect, and know ourselves. In the novel *Salem's Lot*, Stephen King (1975) describes this process. This passage conveys how meaning protects us and allows us to function in the face of threat and danger:

> She had always consciously or unconsciously formed fear into an equation: fear = unknown. And to solve the equation, one simply reduced the problem to simple algebraic terms, thus: unknown = creaky board (or whatever), creaky board = nothing to be afraid of. . . . But until now she had not believed that some fears were larger than comprehension, apocalyptic and nearly paralyzing. This equation was insoluble. The act of moving forward at all became heroism. . . . (King, 1975, p. 293)

The impact of these traumatic experiences is uniquely destabilizing to one's consciousness, as we can see in Lothar-Gunther Buchheim's description of enduring a depth charge attack on a German U-boat beneath the mid-Atlantic Ocean. This passage illustrates the complex process of the formation of a traumatic memory, which can become multitextured in the attempt to integrate the present according to the past:

> Three crashing sledgehammer blows spin me around. Half stunned, I hear a dull roar. What is it? Fear claws at my heart: that roaring! Finally I identify it: it's water pouring back into the vacuum created in the sea by the explosion. . . . I have a feeling that I've lived all this somewhere before. Images shift about in my mind, jostling, overlaying one another, merging into new combinations. My immediate impressions seem to be being transmitted by a complicated circuit to my brain centre, from which they re-emerged into my consciousness as memories. (quoted in Richler, 1994, p. 418)

Stressors such as this demand more than adaptation and coping. They necessitate a confrontation of the threat of helplessness, death, and mutilation—"induction into the ranks of the Undead" (King, 1975, p. 303).

A second element of these experiences is the way that they cannot be left behind in the past, and the resultant way that they come to haunt the individual's life in the present. This results in part from the need to try to construct a meaning network, in order to solve the equation of the fear and uncertainty that are provoked. Siegfried Sassoon described this process in his account of his journey back to England from the front in World War I after he had been injured:

> Next afternoon a train conveyed me to the Base Hospital. My memories of that journey are rather strange and terrible, for it carried a cargo of men in whose minds the horrors they had escaped from were still vitalized and violent ... every bandaged man was accompanied by his battle experience. Although many of them talked lightly and even facetiously about it, there was an aggregation of enormities in the atmosphere of that train. ... The Front Line was behind us; but it could lay its hand on our hearts, though its bludgeoning reality diminished with every mile. It was as if we were pursued by the Arras battle, which had now become a huge and horrible idea. We might be boastful or sagely reconstructive about our experience, in accordance with our different characters. But our minds were still out of breath and our inmost thoughts in disorderly retreat from the bellowing darkness and men dying out in shell-holes under the desolation of returning daylight. We were the survivors; few among us would ever tell the truth to our friends and relations in England. We were carrying in our heads which belonged to us alone, and to those we had left behind us in the battle. (quoted in Fussell, 1983, p. 120)

The failure to differentiate the quality of such events as these, even from other major life stressors such as the death of a spouse, has meant that the importance of the link between trauma and psychological disorder has been underestimated in much of the life events literature.

Traumatic stressors can be divided into different types. First, there are time-limited events such as an aircraft accident or a rape, which are characterized by the unpreparedness of the victim and the high intensity. By contrast, sequential stressors can have a cumulative effect; these stressors are particularly relevent for emergency service workers such as police. Finally, there are stressors characterized by long-lasting exposure to danger, which can evoke uncertainty and helplessness; such stressors include combat involving multiple exposures and repeated intrafamilial abuse affecting attachment bonds and disrupting a basic inner sense of security.

The first type of trauma to provoke systematic interest was traumatic neurosis following accidents that were subject to compensation claims. The author of an 1890 review article about medicine stated that the status of traumatic neuroses could be settled "if those terms (railway spine, railway brain, compensation neurosis) as well as the words 'concussion' and 'hysteria' were dropped" (Seguin, 1890, p. N-1). However, as soon as traumatic neuroses were recognized, the genuineness of this type of distress was questioned; many authors contended that this was simply a result of malingering (see Trimble, 1981). Malingering remains a catchword in medico-legal/forensic circles, in which the reality of these traumas is continually questioned (Appelbaum et al., 1993).

The same problem occurred when psychiatry first recognized the importance of sexual abuse in the etiology of hysteria in the closing decades of the 19th century. The initial wave of enthusiastic interest was followed by the claim that the trauma was the product of children's sexual fantasies (Brown, 1961). The prejudice that arose against such patients because of their "suggestibility" rapidly provoked a dismissal of their suffering and traumatization (see Chapter 3).

The massive slaughter and carnage of a generation of men in World War I were more difficult to deny; nevertheless, various strategies were used to minimize the significance of the suffering of these soldiers. In the immediate setting of battles, combat stress reactions were dismissed as consequences of cowardice. Attempts at organic explanations (e.g., the hypothesis that the vibration of exploding shells could cause microscopic neuronal damage) were another method of denying that the horror of battle was a sufficient cause to explain the psychological toxicity of combat. This would have meant that the officers had a responsibility for the psychological well-being of their troops, and would have increased the cost of war. Subsequently, the issues of compensation and pension entitlements were again seen as the causes of chronic combat-related traumatic neurosis. Such prejudice meant that many of the lessons of World War I were forgotten in the first years of World War II. What was striking was the lack of continuity in any systematic research or clinical concern. This is reflected in Kardiner and Spiegel's (1947) historic monograph about the effects of combat in World War II.

Following the war, DSM-I (APA, 1952) was published and only included the category "gross stress reaction." This implied that acute symptomatic distress following extreme trauma warranted a specific diagnostic category, whereas more prolonged disorders were conceptualized as being anxiety or depressive neuroses. In light of current knowledge, this raises more questions about the nature of psychiatric practice prior to 1980 than it does about the validity of PTSD. For example, Finkel (1976) when writing about the situation in World War II, indicated that 90% of patients at that time could not be classified adequately by existing diagnostic categories. Brill (1967) similarly indicated that many of the symptoms of combat veterans were inconsistent with the traditional neuroses. These are but a few of the many examples of the inadeqacy of previous diagnostic systems to describe the effects of traumatic stress, which implies a failure to acknowledge the specific quality of extreme trauma.

However, the exposure of many young psychiatrists and other future mental health professionals to combat led to changes in the way that clinicians thought about the effects of stress and trauma. Their interest was an important factor in the development of social psychiatry in the 1960s and 1970s, which investigated the role of adversity as a cause of psychiatric illness. Concerned clinicians began to systematically document the severe disruption that could occur in victims' lives after rape, disaster, burn injury, and violent crime. Survivors of the brutality and torture of the Nazi concentration camps, such as Eitinger (1980), began to describe the psychological scars they had endured. Initially, each investigator wrote about the psychiatric problems related to his or her particular experience. Each stressor was seen to produce a specific syndrome, and the occurrence of such events was believed to be rare. This state of confusion was reflected in some of the life events literature, where the distinction between traumatic experiences and other types of life events was sometimes neglected or its importance minimized. This is perhaps one of the reasons why the importance of traumatic events as a cause of psychological symptoms has not been fully recognized.

THE NATURE AND RANGE OF TRAUMATIC STRESSORS

Interestingly, there has been a general reluctance to acknowledge just how frequent traumatic experiences, and the resulting haunted preoccupation with them, are in people's lives. When PTSD was first defined in DSM-III (APA, 1980), the original stressor criterion characterized traumatic events as being outside the range of usual human experience. However, when the prevalence of such events is systematically examined, it is apparent that trauma is surprisingly commonplace. The first epidemiological study of PTSD found that it was a relatively rare disorder, with a prevalence of 1% (Helzer, Robins, & McEvoy, 1987). In succeeding years, studies using more sophisticated methodology have demonstrated an alarming prevalence of traumatic events, which suggests that the original definition of these experiences as being outside the province of most people's lives was erroneous.

In recent years, there have been attempts to better characterize the prevalence of experiences that might cause PTSD, as well as the relative risk of PTSD's arising after different types of traumatic events (Norris, 1992; Kessler, Sonnega, Bromeft, & Nelson, in press). Correspondingly, the definition of the events that can lead to PTSD has been changed, with DSM-IV (APA, 1994) proposing that such events should involve actual death or physical injury, or threat to the bodily integrity of oneself or other people. The *International Classification of Diseases*, 10th revision (ICD-10; World Health Organization, 1992), describes these events as exceptionally threatening or catastrophic and likely to cause distress to almost everyone.

The study of the epidemiology of PTSD has become a field of growing interest for researchers and clinicians, and has provided a substantial justification for the proliferating interest in the disorder. The scientific investigation of these issues has done much to counter the many influences that have mitigated against acceptance of the significance and prevalence of traumatic experiences.

There is little doubt that many people experience the threat and distress of these events without being disabled or developing long-term psychological symptoms. Kessler et al. (in press), as part of the National Comorbidity Survey, have used an epidemiological sample of 8,098 persons to examine the current and lifetime prevalence of PTSD in the U.S. population. They found that the most common causes of PTSD in men were combat and witnessing death or severe injury, whereas rape and sexual molestation were the most common in women. Among the male sample, 60.3% had experienced a trauma that met the DSM-IV stressor criterion and 17% a trauma that produced intrusive recollections but was not covered by the stressor criterion, whereas 50.3% of women had experienced a stressor that fulfilled the criterion. There were significant sex differences in the types of events experienced. For example, 25% of the men had had an accident, in contrast to 13.8% of the women; 9.2% of the women had been raped, in contrast to 0.7% of the men. The capacity of these events to produce PTSD in victims varied significantly, ranging from 48.4% of female rape victims to 10.7% of men witnessing death or serious injury.

Norris (1992), in a study of 1,000 adults in the southern United States, found that 69% of the sample had experienced a traumatic stressor in their lives, and that this included 21% in the past year alone. Although this was not a strictly random sample, Norris found that the most common trauma was tragic death, with sexual assault again leading to the highest rates of PTSD and motor vehicle accidents presenting the most adverse combination of frequency and impact. In both these studies, age, race, and sex had important effects on exposure to trauma. For example, Norris (1992) found that black men had the highest rates of exposure and young people had the highest rates of PTSD. Kessler et al. (in press) found that women's risk of developing PTSD following a trauma was twice as high as men's; they also found that there was no age effect in women, because PTSD at an early age has increased in recent cohorts of women.

Perhaps the prevalence of disasters best demonstrates that traumatic events are not confined to small pockets of society. Between 1967 and 1991, disasters around the world killed 7 million people and affected 3 billion (International Federation of Red Cross and Red Crescent Societies, 1993). Norris (1992) found that in the previous year, 2.4% of households in the southern United States were subjected to disaster or damage, with a lifetime exposure to disaster of 13%. This report highlights the differential impact of disasters in Third World countries. In the period 1967–1991, an average of 117 million people living in developing countries were affected by disasters each year, as compared to about 700,000 in developed countries (a striking ratio of 166:1!). War represents the most ancient and the most important form of human-made violence in terms of the magnitude of its effects. Since World War II, there have been 127 wars and 21.8 million confirmed war-related deaths (Zwi, 1991). The Red Cross estimates a total twice as high, or about 40 million people killed in wars and conflicts since World War II (International Federation . . . , 1993). Like those of natural disaster, the consequences of wars have worsenened over time, and there is also a striking geographical imbalance: All but 2 of the 127 wars have taken place in developing countries. War and political violence cause not only direct psychosocial health problems in the exposed populations, but additional trauma in the refugees who attempt to flee the fighting. Overall, the number of refugees and internally displaced persons has increased from 30 million in 1990 to more than 43 million in 1993 (Toole & Waldham, 1993).

Thus, exposure to these events is surprisingly widespread, indicating the relatively commonplace nature of traumatic threat. The available epidemiological studies suggest social and cultural dissociation about the prevalence of trauma and its impact. The ability of mental health professionals to dismiss the significance of these experiences in the past, as noted both above and in Chapter 3, is an issue that highlights the power of prevailing paradigms to influence observation and models of etiology. These are events that are so severe that they are likely to cause distress in almost everyone, although only a minority of those exposed develop PTSD. Defining these traumas from a psychological perspective depends on understanding how these events challenge people's capacity to adapt and survive.

Any classification of trauma needs to consider this question: What are the dimensions that modify the nature of the meaning and the distress provoked? For example, it is a commonly held opinion that technological and human-made disasters are likely to be more traumatic than natural disasters, as they provoke a greater sense of being the deliberate victim of one's fellow human beings (Smith & North, 1993). The trauma of rape, torture, and interpersonal assaults may have a greater capacity to disrupt an individual's psychological assumptions than such events as hurricanes and floods. On the other hand, a recent meta-analysis of the relationship between disasters and subsequent psychopathology (Rubonis & Bickman, 1991) came to the opposite conclusion—namely, that natural disasters resulted in greater rates of disorder. Therefore, an investigation of the severity of impact of traumatic events and the range of responses must involve an examination of the nature and intensity of the traumatic event.

THE PROBLEMS OF CHARACTERIZING THE NATURE OF TRAUMA

Central to the experience of traumatic stress are the dimensions of helplessness, powerlessness, and threat to one's life. Trauma attacks the individual's sense of self and predictability of the world. Oddly enough, there has been little discussion of the determinants of these dimensions of trauma, or of whether they had such importance at other times in history. Western society, in its current historical context, places far greater emphasis on the rights of the individual than on the value of obedience to the broader dictums of one's culture. Cultural values may influence how an unpredictable event will challenge an individual's sense of identity, as well as determining the quality of the sense of violation associated with such traumas as rape. It is imperative that these issues be investigated among various types of traumatic events and various subcultures. This is particularly important in developing countries, where the experience of natural disasters, war, and violence, combined with individuals' cultural values, may affect psychosocial responses and adaptations to trauma.

Despite the systematic methodology involved in constructing DSM-IV, many issues remain unresolved. For example, although the role of the stressor was examined in the field trials for DSM-IV (Kilpatrick et al., 1993), this revision has not confronted a number of core issues—perhaps understandably, given how controversial they are. The authority of the DSM has encouraged an acceptance of its conclusions with relatively little debate. A more vigorous discourse would have been better for the development of the traumatic stress field. For example, the DSM-IV field trials examined the role of the stressor within specific populations who had experienced a limited range of traumatic experiences. In addition, the trials were confined to the cultural environment of the United States. The importance of property loss as a determinant of PTSD in disaster populations is not reflected in the new Criterion A, because the field trial largely addressed the consequences of violence. In fact, the evidence for natural disasters would suggest that property loss is a better predictor of long-term psychopathology than is the intensity of exposure.

DSM-IV also modified the definition of the stressor by specifying that the person's response must involve fear, helplessness, or horror. This modification was made to indicate the importance of subjective perception and appraisal in response to the event (Davidson, 1994). However, such definitions are inevitably arbitrary. This one was in part designed to limit the use of PTSD in forensic proceedings, instead of being based on objectively defined parameters.

A further problem with the stressor criterion is its implication that a different causal relationship exists between PTSD and environmental factors than between other psychiatric disorders and such factors. It suggests that individual vulnerability plays a less important role in precipitating PTSD than in bringing about other psychiatric disorders. Yet studies of the prevalence of comorbidity provide a series of conceptual challenges to the specificity of the relation between PTSD and traumatic stress (McFarlane & Papay, 1992). Most systematic studies have found that the majority of victims of trauma develop a range of disorders, such as major depressive disorder, panic disorder, and generalized anxiety disorder, in addition to PTSD. This means that trauma does not have a unique association with the constellation of symptoms in PTSD and may be equally able to precipitate a range of other symptomatic outcomes. This is an issue that argues against the specificity of the effects of traumatic stress and needs to be considered by any biological or psychological etiological model of the effects of trauma.

Moreover, different types of traumas may have different consequences. Acute, circumscribed traumas may create a particular risk of uncomplicated PTSD, whereas cumulative stressors may lead to the recruitment of other psychiatric disorders (e.g., depression and panic disorder). Chronic and unpredictable stress may be more likely to create a series of enduring personality changes and disrupt the individual's basic sense of trust in relationships and confidence in the future (see Chapter 9, this volume). Thus issues such as the event's controllability, the individual's preparedness, and the extent of warning, as well as the severity and duration of the actual event, are all critical.

It is usually assumed that the critical factor in the psychological sequelae of traumatic events is the nature of the acute psychological reaction that the victims endure (see Chapter 4, this volume). However, in many instances the physical effects of the trauma are also important. At one extreme, World War II concentration camp survivors endured a range of stresses, including starvation, repeated physical assault, disease, and gross social deprivation. The experience of the victims of torture may include many of these same elements. A child who is sexually abused is likely also to have been emotionally neglected and physically abused. The physical injuries of trauma victims and even the treatment experience can create uncertainties and suffering equal to the immediate terror and threat of the event itself. This is perhaps best epitomized by burn patients, many of whom say that the pain and distress of treatment are so unendurable that they often wish they had been left to die. In general, many studies have found a close association between being wounded or suffering from severe physical exhaustion (e.g., severe malnutrition among prisoners of war) and the occurrence of PTSD (de Girolamo & McFarlane, in press).

The utility of PTSD as a psychopathological construct has created pressure to widen the definition of the stresses that qualify for the diagnosis. The challenge is that the typical symptoms can follow even apparently trivial stresses in some individuals, because of the particular meaning of the experience. Solomon and Canino (1990) showed that some common stressful events were related more closely to PTSD symptoms than were more extraordinary events. The argument against the inclusion of such events is that individual vulnerabilities are more important etiological factors than the objective nature of the experience. Many have argued that giving "victim" status to persons experiencing these lesser events is an abuse of this status. Such critics hold that defining these lesser events as "stressors" promotes a culture that externalizes the causes of personal distress, in contrast to a culture of individual responsibility. This issue was examined in the National Comorbidity Survey. The prevalence rates of PTSD were only increased by 30% when the stressor criterion was relaxed to include any stressful event that produced intrusive recollections (Kessler et al., in press).

A final challenge to the current definition of the stressor criterion is the issue of whether psychiatric disorders themselves can lead to secondary PTSD (McGorry et al., 1991; Shaner & Eth, 1989, 1991). Several studies have now demonstrated that patients who have been psychotic can develop a series of symptoms identical to PTSD in response to the experience of the illness. Thus, the experience of a psychological disorder can itself create the same sense of powerlessness and threat of disintegration that confront the victims of traumatic stress. As many as 50% of patients who have been acutely psychotic will develop a PTSD-type syndrome in response to their disorder (Shaw & McFarlane, 1995). For example, such patients may have a paranoid delusion that someone is trying to kill them, and this may have the same sense of reality to these individuals as an actual assault. Psychotic individuals are also confronted with the perception of their psychological disintegration and the associated terror. Why should not this experience be recognized as triggering the same disorder as an external life experience? As William Styron wrote about the experience of depression:

> In depression . . . faith in deliverance, in ultimate restoration, is absent. The pain is unrelenting, and what makes the condition intolerable is the foreknowledge that no remedy will come—not in a day, an hour, a month, or a minute. If there is mild relief, one knows that it is only temporary; more pain will follow. It is hopelessness even more than pain that crushes the soul. (1991, p. 62)

This description is an eloquent elaboration of the subjective experience required by the DSM-IV stressor criterion. This is an intriguing issue that remains to be debated.

THE EPIDEMIOLOGY OF POSTTRAUMATIC RESPONSES

Epidemiology, the study of the distribution and determinants of disorders in populations (Last, 1983), is a particularly important discipline in understanding the etiology of PTSD, because it provides a methodology for investigating the relative contribution of exposure and individual vulnerability. Such information can only be obtained from studies that examine either entire populations exposed to a particular trauma or representative samples (de Girolamo & McFarlane, in press). The role of the intensity of exposure is demonstrated by increasing prevalence rates with increasing intensity of exposure. In contrast, the role of vulnerability is highlighted by determining the distinguishing characteristics of individuals who do and do not develop PTSD after similar levels of exposure. These epidemiological investigations are also valuable in the design of treatment services after large-scale traumatic events, because they provide prevalence estimates that help define the size of the affected populations. Studies conducted a significant period after the trauma also provide essential information about the chronicity of symptoms and disability, which is a critical issue in arguing the case for service provision and prevention in the immediate aftermath of traumatic events. Issues of methodology are therefore critical in interpretation (de Girolamo & McFarlane, in press).

Studying treatment-seeking populations and other unrepresentative samples provides information that answers a different set of questions. The extent to which PTSD defines and characterizes the pattern of psychological symptoms in those seeking treatment is valuable information in understanding the specificity of the trauma response and the nature of the treatment required. However, a number of problems arise in attempts to extrapolate from these studies, because a variety of factors influence treatment seeking apart from having PTSD; a study by Brom, Kleber, and Hofman (1993) suggests that PTSD sufferers may account for only 10% of a traumatized population.

Although many studies (starting with studies on war-related disorders) have been carried out in the past to investigate the frequency of different types of events and their consequences for human behavior, the findings are hardly comparable because of the use of different concepts, competing diagnostic systems, assessment methodologies, and selective and nonrepresentative samples. Only the identification of operationally defined PTSD diagnostic criteria and the refinement of assessment methodologies have made it possible to carefully investigate the epidemiology of PTSD. In addition, within traumatized populations there will be significant variations in the levels of exposure and the intensity of threat experienced. Therefore, the prevalence of PTSD found in any study of a disaster will be partially determined by the level of exposure that is required before a subject can be included, given that studies of populations with high levels of exposure are likely to have higher prevalence estimates. Similarly, studies of clinical populations are likely to yield higher prevalence rates.

Prevalence of PTSD in General Population Samples

The first epidemiological study of PTSD was part of the Epidemiologic Catchment Area (ECA) study and was carried out in St. Louis. A lifetime PTSD rate of 0.5% among men and 1.3% among women was found. However, substantially more people were found to have experienced some symptoms after a trauma (15% among men and 16% among women) (Helzer et al., 1987). The rate of comorbidity with other psychiatric disorders (e.g., obsessive–

compulsive disorder, dysthymia, and bipolar disorder) was also high. At the St. Louis site, additional data were collected as part of the second wave of the same survey (Cottler, Compton, Mager, Spitznagel, & Janca, 1992), with an overall rate of PTSD of 1.35% being identified. This part of the study specifically examined the association between PTSD and substance use. Cocaine/ opiate users reported three times the number of traumatic events.

At the Duke University ECA site, lifetime and 6-month PTSD prevalence rates of 1.30% and 0.44%, respectively, were found (Davidson, Hughes, Blazer, & George, 1991). PTSD sufferers reported significantly more job instability, family history of psychiatric illness, parental poverty, experiences of child abuse, and separation or divorce of parents prior to the age of 10. PTSD was also associated with greater psychiatric comorbidity (e.g., somatization disorders, schizophrenia, and panic disorder). Interestingly, similar PTSD lifetime rates, on the order of 1.5%, have been found in two studies that employed control groups randomly selected from the general population (Kulka et al., 1990; Shore, Vollmer, & Tatum, 1989).

A fourth survey was carried out in a random sample of 1,007 young adults (aged 21–30 years) from a large health maintenance organization in Detroit, 39% of whom had been exposed to a traumatic event (Breslau, Davis, Andreski, & Peterson, 1991). PTSD was found in 23.6% of those exposed, yielding an overall lifetime prevalence rate of 9.2%. In this group, the prevalence of PTSD was preceded only by that of phobia, major depression, and alcohol and drug dependence. In the National Comorbidity Survey of 8,098 subjects, Kessler et al. (in press) found a lifetime prevalence of 6.5% and a 30-day prevalence of 2.8%. This study indicated the chronicity of symptoms in a significant minority, with little remission after 6 years—a finding similar to that of the 50-year follow-up study of Lee, Vaillant, Torrey, and Elder (1995). As noted earlier, Kessler et al. found that following exposure, women had twice the risk of developing PTSD; they also found that those with PTSD were at increased risk for other psychiatric disorders, especially anxiety and affective disorders. Resnick, Kilpatrick, Dansky, Saunders, & Best (1993) in a national U.S. survey of women, found that 12.3% of respondents (17.9% of those exposed) had a lifetime history of PTSD.

Lindal and Stefansson (1993) have reported the lifetime prevalence rates of anxiety disorders, including PTSD, in a cohort consisting of one-half of those born in the year 1931 ($n = 862$) and living in Iceland. Whereas the overall prevalence of anxiety disorders was 44%, the lifetime prevalence of PTSD was 0.6%; however, the disorder was found only in females (1.2%), and had a mean age of onset of 39 years. This low prevalence rate may reflect something of the lifestyle in that nation. Similarly, low prevalence rates of 0.6% were found in a sample of 7,229 in a community mental health survey in Hong Kong (Chen et al., 1993).

Prevalence of PTSD Following Specific Traumas

Epidemiological studies have examined the survivors of a range of different traumatic events, and generalizations are difficult to make for the reasons described earlier. A total of 15 studies assessed the prevalence of PTSD among victims of natural and technological disasters; of these, nine were carried out in the United States and the remaining six in other countries, including three developing countries (Colombia, Fiji, and Mexico). The rates vary significantly according to the sample and the type of disaster (see de Girolamo & McFarlane, in press). For example, Shore et al. (1989) examined the impact of the Mount St. Helens volcanic eruption and compared the exposed population with a control group. The lifetime prevalence in the Mount St. Helens group was 3.6%, compared to 2.6% in the controls. In contrast, McFarlane (1988) studied a representative sample of 469 volunteer firefighters exposed to a severe natural disaster in Australia. This study found a rate of 16% of PTSD, and fewer than half of the sufferers had gone into remission at 42 months (McFarlane, 1992). The Buffalo Creek disaster (a dam break and a subsequent flood), which occurred in 1972, is one of the best-studied disasters. Green, Lindy, Grace, and Leonard (1992) have found a 59% PTSD lifetime rate among the victims; 25% still met PTSD diagnostic criteria at the 14-year follow-up assessment.

A relatively large number of studies ($n = 35$) have been carried out among samples of war veterans (de Girolamo & McFarlane, in press). Twenty-five have been conducted in the United States and 20 of these either focused exclusively on Vietnam veterans or included such veterans. Sample size and composition, study setting, assessment methods, prevalence period (point, period, or lifetime), and inclusion of a comparison group are remarkably different among the various studies. These differences are reflected in a marked variation in prevalence rates, ranging between a low of 2% (current prevalence) in the Centers for Disease Control (1988) Vietnam Experience study, and a high of over 70% found in five studies. The National Vietnam Veterans Readjustment Study (NVVRS) is probably the most in-depth investigation (Kulka et al., 1990); it found that 15% of all male veterans who were involved in active war operations had current cases of PTSD, and that an additional 11% suffered from partial PTSD.

Another study evaluated the influence of military service during the Vietnam era on the occurrence of PTSD among a sample of over 2,000 male–male monozygotic veteran twin pairs (Goldberg, True, Eisen, & Henderson, 1990). A prevalence of PTSD of almost 17% was found in twins who served in Southeast Asia, compared with 5% in cotwins who did not. There was a ninefold increase in the rate of PTSD among twins who experienced high levels of combat, compared to those who did not serve in Vietnam. Changing the threshold for the definition of exposure to combat results in changes in reported prevalence rates, as demonstrated by the study by Snow, Stellman, Stellman, and

Sommer (1988). Among those in this study exposed to a median level of combat, the rate of PTSD was 28%; among those exposed to the highest level, the rate was 65%.

Eleven studies have been carried out among former prisoners of war and other types of prisoners, generally imprisoned for political reasons (Basoglu et al., 1994; Bauer, Priebe, Haring, & Adamczak, 1993; Beal, 1995; Burges-Watson, 1993; Crocq, Hein, Duval, & Macher, 1991; Eberly & Engdahl, 1991; Kluznik, Speed, Van Valkenburg, & McGraw, 1986; Kuch & Cox, 1992; Mellman, Randolph, Brawman-Mintzer, Flores, & Milanes, 1992; Speed, Engdahl, Schwartz, & Eberly, 1988; Sutker, Allain, & Winstead, 1993). Among these, six have been conducted in the United States, and one each in Germany, Turkey, Australia, France, and Canada. In all these studies, the PTSD rate was quite substantial, with the prevalence rate in six studies being equal to or higher than 50%, and three studies showing prevalence rates of 70% or more.

Five studies have focused on victims of terrorist attacks (Abenhaim, Dab, & Salmi, 1992; Bell, Kee, Loughrey, & Roddy, 1988; Curran et al., 1990; Shalev, 1992; Weisaeth, 1993), while one has assessed the PTSD rate among residents of Lockerbie, Scotland, who claimed compensation after the aircraft disaster there caused by a terrorist bomb explosion (Brooks & McKinlay, 1992). The rate of PTSD found has been substantial, exceeding 20% of the subjects studied, and in two cases being higher than 40% (Curran et al., 1990; Weisaeth, 1993).

Nine of the 12 studies that have assessed the rate of PTSD among samples of refugees have been carried out in the United States among samples of resettled refugees, mostly Southeast Asians (Carlson & Rosser-Hogan, 1991; Cervantes, Salgado de Snyder, & Padilla, 1989; Hauff & Vaglum, 1993; Hinton et al., 1993; Kinzie, Sack, Angell, Manson, & Rath, 1986; Kinzie et al., 1990; Kroll et al., 1989; Mollica, Wyshak, & Lavelle, 1987; Mollica et al., 1993; Moore & Boehnlein, 1991; Ramsay, Gorst-Unsworth, & Turner, 1993; Summerfield & Toser, 1991). Six of these studies have found a PTSD rate equal to or higher than 50%, demonstrating that refugees who seek treatment and have usually faced very difficult circumstances (including torture, starvation, witnessing killings, etc.) represent a highly traumatized population. They display a substantial rate not only of PTSD, but of other psychiatric disorders.

A number of studies ($n = 21$) have assessed the prevalence rate of PTSD among victims of different types of violence (de Girolamo & McFarlane, in press). The rate of PTSD was substantial in most investigations; only in three studies was the PTSD prevalence rate lower than 25% of the victims. The degree of life threat and the extent of physical injury were generally correlated with both the occurrence and the severity of PTSD.

Finally, 34 studies have investigated the prevalence of PTSD in a variety of samples of at-risk subjects (de Girolamo & McFarlane, in press). They include, for the most part, medical patients hospitalized or treated for different reasons (e.g., patients hospitalized because of major burns or injuries resulting from traffic or other accidents, or suffering from pain). Across these studies the rates of PTSD vary, depending on a number of factors related to the type, severity, length, and consequences of the stressor and to the psychiatric status of the subjects prior to the traumatic event. In particular, substantial rates of PTSD have been found among psychiatric patients specifically evaluated on measures of PTSD symptomatology, as well as among burn patients.

Thus, PTSD is a predictable consequence of traumatic events; however, specific prevalence rates are determined by a range of issues, such as the intensity of exposure, the prevalence of risk factors in the population, and the recruitment rates of different studies. Many methodological issues need to be addressed before these questions can be investigated more precisely.

PROBLEMS IN THE MEASUREMENT OF TRAUMATIC EXPOSURE

The measurement of the severity of life events and the associated distress has proved a vexing issue (Paykel, 1978). The many problems associated with measurement of life events have in part been responsible for the decrease in research activity over the last decade in this area. Against this background, it is perhaps surprising that few of the lessons from the life events literature have been considered in the traumatic stress literature.

First, scales are needed to quantify the severity of stress associated with a range of experiences in different populations, in order to overcome the problem of "effort after meaning" (Andrews & Tennant, 1978). In other words, people who have experienced particular types of adversity that have led to the onset of symptoms are likely to rank such adversity as being more distressing and demanding greater degrees of change than people who have not become ill but have experienced these events. This tendency to exaggerate the importance of an event arises from people's attempts to search their environment for an attributable cause of their distress. Moreover, in the development of scales such as the Schedule for Life Events, an important part of the process has been to compare a variety of different populations and the extent to which there are similarities and differences in their ranking of life events (Finlay-Jones, 1981). In the traumatic stress area, there has been little attempt to develop scaled measures of traumatic stress and to compare ratings on these measures made by different groups unexposed to the trauma. Furthermore, no attempt has been made to look at social and cultural influences affecting the perception of trauma. For example, trained personnel may perceive certain traumatic experiences as being much less distressing than those without training may perceive them. In addition, certain cultural and religious expectations about fate may similarly modify the perception of individual traumatic events.

Other assumptions about the construction of trauma scales have gone largely unexamined. Life events scales have assumed that there is an additive effect among individual events (Brown & Harris, 1978). The logic and rationale for using additive scales in the study of traumatic experiences have not been established. Another major problem demonstrated in the life events literature is the low test–retest reliability of most scales (Paykel, 1983). Even over relatively short periods of time, a great deal of variability of recall exists. There is some suggestion that the retrospective assessment of the severity of traumatic events inevitably biases the finding toward demonstrating the importance of the stressor. Part of the phenomenology of PTSD is the powerful imprinting of memories; however, the normal process of adaptation involves forgetting. It is easy to see how unaffected groups will tend to forget or minimize the severity of the traumatic stress if this is assessed some time after the event (McFarlane, 1989).

The issue of test–retest reliability in traumatic settings is particularly important in the area of disaster research, because of the natural process of forgetting involved in adaptation. Thus, the very process of remembering is likely to differ between those who have PTSD and those who do not; thus, retrospective recall of the traumatic event may naturally bias the data toward the finding of high levels of exposure in the PTSD group. The importance of avoidance as a mechanism of adaptation is also an important issue. A number of studies (Kinzie et al., 1990; Kolb, 1989) have demonstrated how avoidance may lead to a complete denial of the trauma. Clinical practice would also suggest that the trauma history taken is dependent in part upon the method of examination.

The impact of extremely traumatic events on the victims' behavior and mental state during such events may also be an important issue affecting the validity of measures of exposure. Dissociation is a common response during traumatic events, and this could lead to the potential underreporting and misperception of various aspects of the trauma. It is important that objective measures of events be used to validate individuals' recall, if at all possible. Although major traumatic events are clearly independent events in the sense that they have not been caused by the victims, the victims' mental state may have important effects on their behavior and consequent danger. People who panic or who respond in other maladaptive ways may effectively increase their apparent exposure. Thus, exposure can be a confounded measure of individuals' mental state at the time and the severity of the trauma. Furthermore, Breslau, Davis, and Andreski (1995) demonstrated that PTSD-related traumatic events are not completely random phenomena; they are related in part to personality and lifestyle issues.

In contrast to the effort put into the development of valid and reliable measures of adverse life events, surprisingly little attention has been given to the issue in the area of traumatic stress. Furthermore, the impact of social and cultural issues on people's recall has not been explored; for example, as noted earlier, the relative importance of property loss versus personal loss in different cultural settings needs to be examined. One of the only populations to rate the stressfulness of the items on the Holmes and Rahe (1967) scale in a significantly different way was a group of earthquake victims; surprisingly, they rated the severity of the impact of major losses lower than populations unaffected by disaster did (Janney, Masuda, & Holmes, 1977). This suggests that traumatized groups may have a different perspective on their experience than populations who have not confronted that particular event may have. This has the potential to create significant errors when investigators are trying to judge the severity of traumatic stressors and to determine which events are markedly distressing to most people.

Finally, there has been little systematic examination of the different dimensions of a traumatic experience and their interrelationship. Green (1993) has suggested eight generic dimensions of trauma that need to be taken into account. In attempts to grade exposure, the relative importance of a range of variables has not been considered. Figure 7.1 lists a series of components of a traumatic experience. These include the actual impingement of the event on the individual (e.g., injury), as well as the events the person saw. These issues will be influenced by the person's mental state (e.g., did he or she panic or dissociate?) and by the person's perception of the risks and capacity to act adaptively. On the one hand, there will be objective measures of exposure, such as seeing death and injury or actually being injured. Similarly, the duration of exposure and awareness of destruction and loss are objective issues. In contrast, matters that may be equally important in determining the degree of traumatization include the perceptions that one survived the experience through freak circumstances or was kept safe by chance, and that one had no control over the circumstances or one's behavior. The relative importance of these subjective components has increasingly been demonstrated to be the important issue in determining subsequent symptomatology (Feinstein & Dolman, 1991).

How to measure these variables and combine them into scales requires examination. Figure 7.1 implies a gradation of experience, with increasing distress and threat occurring with increasing intensity of exposure. There has been little systematic validation of the interrelationship of these phenomena or of whether it is appropriate to construct composite scales. The extent to which such a scale can be legitimately transferred from one population to another has also not been examined; this is an important issue, because subjective experiences may be quite variable within different cultural and social groups.

Therefore, the development of scales to quantify the severity of an individual's traumatic exposure is a complex and difficult issue. Whether mean-

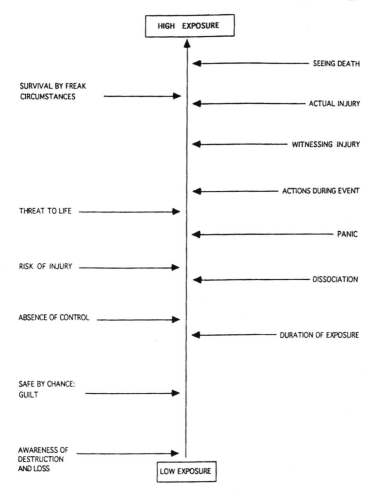

Figure 7.1. A hypothetical hierarchy of elements of a traumatic experience.

ingful scales can be developed that combine a range of very different experiences needs careful theoretical and methodological examination. For example, in a disaster situation, how does one compare the differential effects of coming close to being killed oneself and losing one's house? If one has also lost a relative, does this make the exposure and the impact twice or three times as bad? There has been little systematic examination of these and other assumptions and issues involved in constructing a valid quantitative representation of the experience of trauma.

CONCLUSION

"Stress" has been the great catchword of many health professionals as an explanatory model for psychological symptoms. Thus far, however, the traumatic stress field has failed to provide the insights and predictive ability that life events research first promised. The increasing refinement of our understanding of the nature of traumatic stress suggests that such events appear to have particular significance and a unique relationship with a range of psychiatric disorders, not just PTSD.

The high incidence of these experiences is a surprise to many, given the denial of mental health professionals in the past. However, no trauma is so severe that almost everyone exposed to the experience develops PTSD (Kessler et al., in press; Yehuda & McFarlane, 1995). There is also a large variability across events in producing PTSD, and it is very difficult to categorize those events that are traumatic and those that are not (Solomon & Canino, 1990). The issue is whether all people who develop intrusive recollections of any event are allowed to be diagnosed as having PTSD, if their symptoms are of sufficient severity. Logically, this would appear to be the way to go, as it would allow the investigation of the effects of these events and the relationship between the aspects of traumatic experience and individual vulnerability (Kessler et al., in press; Solomon & Canino, 1990).

One of the critical issues to which epidemiological research can contribute in the future is the relationship between PTSD and the comorbid disorders. Although various disorders predispose individuals to PTSD, both because of increased risk of exposure to trauma and increased risk of disorder following exposure, the boundaries between mood disorders and anxiety disorders are of primary interest. Longitudinal studies of traumatized populations will allow investigation of this question with a variety of sophisticated statistical techniques. Ultimately, this will clarify the unique aspects of traumatic adaptation, as opposed to nonspecific psychiatric morbidity, which will exist in any general population sample exposed to a trauma such as a disaster. We know from most epidemiological studies that between 20% and 29% of the population has suffered from a psychiatric disorder in the past year. The question is this: How does the PTSD thst arises in these people who are at greater risk differ from PTSD in those who have no past history of a psychological disorder?

Finally, there also needs to be a fine-grained analysis of the effects of different types of stressful events and the extent to which the type of event influences aspects of the symptoms. Now that the traumatic stress field has a more secure future, this will allow a more sophisticated analysis of the debate as to whether there are any trauma-specific syndromes. The more enduring impact of trauma on personality is an issue that requires similar scrutiny.

REFERENCES

Abenhaim, L., Dab, W., & Salmi, L. R. (1992). Study of civilian victims of terrorist attacks, France (1982–1987). *Journal of Clinical Epidemiology, 45*, 103–109.

American Psychiatric Association (APA). (1952). *Diagnostic and statistical manual of mental disorders* (1st ed.). Washington, DC: Author.

American Psychiatric Association (APA). (1980). *Diagnostic and statistical manual of mental disorders* (3rd ed.). Washington, DC: Author.

American Psychiatric Association (APA). (1994). *Diagnostic and statistical manual of mental disorders* (4th ed.). Washington, DC: Author.

Andreasen, N. C., & Wasek, P. (1980). Adjustment disorders in adolescents and adults. *Archives of General Psychiatry, 37*(10), 1166–1170.

Andrews, G., & Tennant, C (1978). Being upset and becoming ill: An appraisal of the relationship between life events and physical illness. *Medical Journal of Australia, 134*, 324–327

Appelbaum, P. S., Jick, R. Z., Grisso, T., Givelber, D., Silver, E., & Steadman, H. J. (1993). Use of posttraumatic stress disorder to support an insanity defense. *American Journal of Psychiatry, 150*(2), 229–234.

Basoglu, M., Paker, M., Paker, O., Ozmen, E., Marks, I., Incesu, C., Sahin, D., & Sarimurat, N. (1994). Psychological effects of torture: A comparison of tortured with nontortured political activists in Turkey. *American Journal of Psychiatry, 151*(1), 76–81.

Bauer, M., Priebe, S., Haring, B., & Adamczak, K. (1993). Long-term sequelae of political imprisonment in East Germany. *Journal of Nervous and Mental Disease, 181*, 257–262.

Beal, A. L. (1995). Posttraumatic stress disorder in prisoner of war and combat veterans of the Dieppe raid: A 50 year follow-up. *Canadian Journal of Psychiatry, 40*, 177–184.

Bell, P., Kee, M., Loughrey, G. C., & Roddy, R. J. (1988). Post-traumatic stress in Northern Ireland. *Acta Psychiatrica Scandinavica, 77*(2), 166–169.

Blank, A. S. (1993). The longitudinal course of posttraumatic stress disorder. In J. R. T. Davidson & E. B. Foa (Eds.), *Posttraumatic stress disorder: DSM-IV and beyond* (pp. 3–22). Washington, DC: American Psychiatric Press.

Breslau, N., Davis, G. C., & Andreski, P. (1995). Risk factors for PTSD related traumatic events: A prospective analysis. *American Journal of Psychiatry, 152*, 529–535.

Breslau, N., Davis, G. C., Andreski, P., & Peterson, E. (1991). Traumatic events and posttraumatic stress disorder in an urban population of young adults. *Archives of General Psychiatry, 48*, 216–222.

Brill, N. Q. (1967). Gross stress reactions: II. Traumatic war neuroses. In A. M. Freedman & H. L. Kaplan (Eds.), *Comprehensive textbook of psychiatry* (1st ed., pp. 1031–1035). Baltimore: Williams & Wilkins.

Brom, D., Kleber, R. J., & Hofman, M. C. (1993). Victims of traffic accidents: Incidence and prevention of post-traumatic stress disorder. *Journal of Clinical Psychology, 49*(2), 131–140.

Brooks, N., & McKinlay, W. (1992). Mental health consequences of the Lockerbie disaster. *Journal of Traumatic Stress, 5*, 527–543.

Brown, G. W., & Harris, T. O. (1978). *Social origins of depression.* London: Tavistock.

Brown, J. A. C. (1961). *Freud and the post-Freudians.* Ringwood, Australia: Penguin Books.

Burges-Watson, I. P. (1993). Post-traumatic stress disorder in Australian prisoners of the Japanese: A clinical study. *Australian and New Zealand Journal of Psychiatry, 27,* 20–29.

Carlson, E. B., & Rosser-Hogan, R. (1991). Trauma experiences, posttraumatic stress, dissociation, and depression in Cambodian refugees. *American Journal of Psychiatry, 148*(11), 1548–1551.

Centers for Disease Control. (1988). Health status of Vietnam veterans: I. Psychosocial characteristics. *Journal of the American Medical Association, 259,* 2701–2707.

Cervantes, R. C., Salgado de Snyder, N. V., & Padilla, A. M. (1989). Posttraumatic stress in immigrants from Central America and Mexico. *Hospital and Community Psychiatry, 40*(6), 615–619.

Chen, C., Wong, J., Lee, N., Chan, H., Mun-Wan, C. H., Tak-Fai Lau, J., & Fung, M. (1993). The Shatin community mental health survey in Hong Kong: II. Major findings. *Archives of General Psychiatry, 50*(2), 125–133.

Cottler, L. B., Compton, W. M., Mager, D., Spitznagel, E. L., & Janca, A. (1992). Post-traumatic stress disorder among substance users from the general population. *American Journal of Psychiatry, 149,* 664–670.

Crocq, M. A., Hein, K. D., Duval, F., & Macher, J. P. (1991). Severity of the prisoner of war experience and post traumatic stress disorder. *European Psychiatry, 6,* 39–45.

Curran, P. S., Bell, P., Murray, A., Loughrey, G., Roddy, R., & Rocke, L. G. (1990). Psychological consequences of the Enniskillen bombing. *British Journal of Psychiatry, 156,* 479–482.

Davidson, J. R. T. (1994). Issues in the diagnosis of PTSD. In R. S. Pynoos (Ed.), *PTSD: A clinical review* (pp. 1–15). Lutherville, MD: Sidran Press.

Davidson, J. R. T., Hughes, D., Blazer, D. G., & George, L. K. (1991). Post-traumatic stress disorder in the community: An epidemiological study. *Psychological Medicine, 21,* 713–721.

de Girolamo, G., & McFarlane, A. C. (in press). Epidemiology of posttraumatic stress disorders among victims of intentional violence: A review of the literature. *APA Review.*

Eberly, R. E., & Engdahl, B. E. (1991). Prevalence of somatic and psychiatric disorders among former prisoners of war. *Hospital and Community Psychiatry, 42*(8), 807–813.

Eitinger, L. (1980). The concentration camp syndrome and its late sequelae. In J. E. Dimsdale (Eds.), *Victims, survivors and perpetrators* (pp. 127–162). New York: Hemisphere.

Feinstein, A., & Dolan, R. (1991). Predictors of posttraumatic stress disorder following physical trauma: An examination of the stressor criterion. *Psychological Medicine, 21*(1), 85–91.

Finkel, N. J. (1976). *Mental illness and health: Its legacy, tensions and changes.* New York: Plenum Press.

Finlay-Jones, R. (1981). Types of stressful life events and the onset of anxiety and depression disorders. *Psychological Medicine, 11*(5), 803–815.

Fussell, P. (1983). *Siegfried Sassoon's long journey.* New York: Oxford University Press.

Gibbs, M. S. (1989). Factors in the victim that mediate between disaster and psychopathology: A review. *Journal of Traumatic Stress, 2,* 489–514.

Goldberg, J., True, W. R., Eisen, S. A., & Henderson, W. G. (1990). A twin study of the effects of the Vietnam War on posttraumatic stress disorder. *Journal of the American Medical Association, 263*(9), 1227–1232.

Green, B. L. (1993). Identifying survivors at risk: Trauma and stressors across events. In J. P. Wilson & B. Raphael (Eds.), *International handbook of traumatic stress syndromes* (pp. 135–144). New York: Plenum Press.

Green, B. L., Lindy, J. D., Grace, M. C., & Leonard, A. C. (1992). Chronic posttraumatic stress disorder and diagnostic comorbidity in a disaster sample. *Journal of Nervous and Mental Disease, 180,* 70–766.

Hauff, E., & Vaglum, P. (1993). Vietnamese boat refugees: The influence of war and flight traumatization on mental health on arrival in the country of resettlement. *Acta Psychiatrica Scandinavica, 88*(3), 162–168.

Helzer, J. E., Robins, L. N., & McEvoy, L. (1987). Post-traumatic stress disorder in the general population: Findings of the Epidemiologic Catchment Area survey. *New England Journal of Medicine, 317*(26), 1630–1634.

Herman, J. (1992). Complex PTSD: A syndrome in survivors of prolonged and repeated trauma. *Journal of Traumatic Stress, 5,* 377–391.

Hinton, W. L., Chen, Y. C. J., Du, N., Tran, C. G., Lu, F. G., Miranda, J., & Faust, S. (1993). DSM-III-R disorders in Vietnamese refugees: Prevalence and correlates. *Journal of Nervous and Mental Disease, 181,* 113–122.

Holmes, T. H., & Rahe, R. H. (1967). The Social Readjustment Rating Scale. *Journal of Psychosomatic Research, 11,* 213–218.

International Federation of Red Cross and Red Crescent Societies. (1993). *World disaster report, 1993.* Dordrecht, The Netherlands: Martinus Nijhoff.

Janney, J. G., Masuda, M., & Holmes, T. H. (1977). Impact of a natural catastrophe on life events. *Journal of Human Stress, 3*(2), 22–23, 26–34.

Kardiner, A., & Spiegel, H. (1947). War stress and neurotic illness. New York: Hoeber.

Kessler, R., Sonnega, A., Bromet, E., & Nelson, C. B. (in press). Posttraumatic stress disorder in the National Comorbidity Survey. *Archives of General Psychiatry.*

Kilpatrick, D. G., Resnick, H. S., Freedy, J. R., Pelcovitz, D., Roth, S., & van der Kolk, B. A. (1993). *Report of the findings from the DSM-IV PTSD field trial: Emphasis on Criterion A and overall PTSD diagnosis.* Washington, DC: American Psychiatric Association.

King, S. (1975). *Salem's lot.* London: Hodder & Stoughton.

Kinzie, J. D., Boehnlein, J. K., Leung, P. K., Moore, L. J., Riley, C., & Smith, D. (1990). The prevalence of posttraumatic stress disorder and its clinical significance among Southeast Asian refugees. *American Journal of Psychiatry, 147*(7), 913–917.

Kinzie, J. D., Sack, W. H., Angell, R. H., Manson, S. M., & Rath, B. (1986). The psychiatric effects of massive trauma on Cambodian children: I. The children. *Journal of the American Academy of Child Psychiatry, 25*(3), 370–376.

Kluznik, J. C., Speed, N., Van Valkenburg, C., & Magraw, R. (1986). Forty-year followup of United States prisoners of war. *American Journal of Psychiatry, 143,* 1443–1446.

Kolb, L. C. (1989). Chronic post-traumatic stress disorder: Implications of recent epidemiological and neuropsychological studies. *Psychological Medicine, 19*(4), 821–824.

Kroll, J., Habenicht, M., Mackenzie, T., Yang, M., Chan, S., Vang, T., Nguyen, T., Ly,

M., Phommasouvanh, B., Nguyen, H., Vang, Y., Souvannasoth, L., & Cabugao, R. (1989). Depression and posttraumatic stress disorder in Southeast Asian refugees. *American Journal of Psychiatry, 146*(12), 1592–1597.

Kuch, K., & Cox, B. J. (1992). Symptoms of PTSD in 124 survivors of the Holocaust. *American Journal of Psychiatry, 149*(3), 337–340.

Kulka, R. A., Schlenger, W. E., Fairbank, J. A., Hough, R. L., Jordan, B. K., Marmar, C. R., & Weiss, D. S. (1990). *Trauma and the Vietnam War generation: Report of findings from the National Vietnam Veterans Readjustment Study.* New York: Brunner/Mazel.

Last, J. M. (1983). *A dictionary of epidemiology.* New York: Oxford University Press.

Lee, K. A., Vaillant, G. E., Torrey, W. C., & Elder, G. H. (1995). A 50-year prospective study of the psychological sequelae of World War II combat. *American Journal of Psychiatry, 152*(4), 516–522.

Lindal, E., & Stefansson, J. G. (1993). The lifetime prevalence of anxiety disorder in Iceland as estimated by the US National Institute of Mental Health Diagnostic Interview Schedule. *Acta Psychiatrica Scandinavica, 88,* 29–34.

McFarlane, A. C. (1988). The phenomenology of posttraumatic stress disorders following a natural disaster. *Journal of Nervous and Mental Disease, 176*(1), 22–29.

McFarlane, A. C. (1989). The aetiology of post-traumatic morbidity: Predisposing, precipitating and perpetuating factors. *British Journal of Psychiatry, 154,* 221–228.

McFarlane, A. C. (1992). Avoidance and intrusion in posttraumatic stress disorder. *Journal of Nervous and Mental Disease, 180*(7), 439–445.

McFarlane, A. C., & Papay, P. (1992). Multiple diagnoses in posttraumatic stress disorder in the victims of a natural disaster. *Journal of Nervous and Mental Disease, 180*(8), 498–504.

McGorry, P. D., Chanen, A., McCarthy, E., Van Riel, R., McKenzie, D., & Singh, B. S. (1991). Posttraumatic stress disorder following recent-onset psychosis: An unrecognized postpsychotic syndrome. *Journal of Nervous and Mental Disease, 179*(5), 253–258.

Mellman, T. A., Randolph, C. A., Brawman-Mintzer, O., Flores, L. P., & Milanes, F. J. (1992). Phenomenology and course of psychiatric disorders associated with combat-related posttraumatic stress disorder. *American Journal of Psychiatry, 149*(11), 1568–1574.

Mollica, R. F., Donelan, K., Tor, S., Lavelle, J., Elias, C., Frankel, M., & Blendon, R. J. (1993). The effect of trauma and confinement on functional health and mental health status of Cambodians living in Thailand–Cambodia border camps. *Journal of the American Medical Association, 270,* 581–586.

Mollica, R. F., Wyshak, G., & Lavelle, J. (1987). The psychosocial impact of war trauma and torture on Southeast Asian refugees. *American Journal of Psychiatry, 144*(12), 1567–1572.

Moore, L. J., & Boehnlein, J. K. (1991). Posttraumatic stress disorder, depression, and somatic symptoms in U.S. Mien patients. *Journal of Nervous and Mental Disease, 179*(12), 728–733.

Norris, F. H. (1992). Epidemiology of trauma: Frequency and impact of different potentially traumatic events on different demographic groups. *Journal of Consulting and Clinical Psychology, 60*(3), 409–418.

Paykel, E. S. (1978). Contribution of life events to causation of psychiatric illness. *Psychological Medicine, 8*(2), 245–253.

Paykel, E. S. (1983). Methodological aspects of life events research. *Journal of Psychosomatic Research, 27*(5), 341–352.

Ramsay, R., Gorst-Unsworth, C., & Turner, S. (1993). Psychiatric morbidity in survivors of organised state violence including torture: A retrospective series. *British Journal of Psychiatry, 162,* 55–59.

Resnick, H. S., Kilpatrick, D. G., Dansky, B. S., Saunders, B. E., & Best, C. L. (1993). Prevalence of civilian trauma and posttraumatic stress disorder in a representative national sample of women. *Journal of Consulting and Clinical Psychology, 61*(6), 984–991.

Richler, M. (1994). *Writers on World War II.* New York: Knopf.

Rubonis, A., & Bickman, L. (1991). Psychological impairment in the wake of disaster: The disaster–psychopathology relationship. *Psychological Bulletin, 109,* 384–399.

Rushdie, S. (1981). *Midnight's children.* London: Cape.

Seguin, E. C. (1890). Traumatic neuroses. In C. E. Sajous (Ed.), *Annual of universal medical sciences* (pp. N-1–N-8). Philadelphia: F. A. Davis.

Shalev, A. Y. (1992). Posttraumatic stress disorder among injured survivors of a terrorist attack: Predictive value of early intrusion and avoidance symptoms. *Journal of Nervous and Mental Disease, 180,* 505–509.

Shaner, A., & Eth, S. (1989). Can schizophrenia cause posttraumatic stress disorder? *American Journal of Psychotherapy, 43*(4), 588–597.

Shaner, A., & Eth, S. (1991). Postpsychosis posttraumatic stress disorder. *Journal of Nervous and Mental Disease, 179*(10), 640.

Shaw, K., & McFarlane, A. C. (1995). *Posttraumatic stress disorder following psychosis.* Manuscript in preparation.

Shore, J. H., Vollmer, W. M., & Tatum, E. L. (1989). Community patterns of posttraumatic stress disorders. *Journal of Nervous and Mental Disease, 177*(11), 681–685.

Smith, E. M., & North, C. S. (1993). Posttraumatic stress disorder in natural disasters and technological accidents. In J. P. Wilson & B. Raphael (Eds.), *International handbook of traumatic stress syndromes* (pp. 405–419). New York: Plenum Press.

Snow, B. R., Stellman, J. M., Stellman, S. D., & Sommer, J. F. (1988). Post-traumatic stress disorder among American Legionnaires in relation to combat experience in Vietnam: Associated and contributing factors. *Environmental Research, 47,* 175–192.

Solomon, S. D., & Canino, G. J. (1990). Appropriateness of DSM-III-R criteria for posttraumatic stress disorder. *Comprehensive Psychiatry, 31*(3), 227–237.

Speed, N., Engdahl, B., Schwartz, J., & Eberly, R. (1989). Posttraumatic stress disorder as a consequence of the POW experience. *Journal of Nervous and Mental Disease, 177*(3), 147–153.

Styron, W. (1991). *Darkness visible: A memoir of madness.* London: Jonathon Cape.

Summerfield, D., & Toser, L. (1991). Low intensity war and mental trauma in Nicaragua: A study in a rural community. *Medicine and War, 7,* 84–99.

Sutker, P. B., Allain, A. N., & Winstead, D. K. (1993). Psychopathology and psychiatric diagnoses of World War II Pacific theater prisoner of war survivors and combat veterans. *American Journal of Psychiatry, 150*(2), 240–245.

Toole, M. J., & Waldham, R. J. (1993). Prevention of excess mortality in refugee and displaced populations in developing countries. *Journal of the American Medical Association, 263*, 3296–3302.

Trimble, M. R. (1981). *Posttraumatic neurosis: From railway spine to whiplash.* New York: Wiley.

Weisaeth, L. (1993). Torture of a Norwegian ship's crew: Stress reactions, coping, and psychiatric aftereffects. In J. P. Wilson & B. Raphael (Eds.), *International handbook of traumatic stress syndromes* (pp. 743–750). New York: Plenum Press.

World Health Organization. (1992). *International classification of diseases* (10th revision). Geneva: Author.

Yehuda, R., & McFarlane, A. C. (1995). The conflict between current knowledge about PTSD and its original conceptual basis. *American Journal of Psychiatry, 152*, 1705–1713.

Zwi, A. B. (1991). Militarianism, militarization, health and the Third World. *Medicine and War, 7*, 262–268.

CHAPTER 8

Resilience, Vulnerability, and the Course of Posttraumatic Reactions

ALEXANDER C. McFARLANE
RACHEL YEHUDA

If posttraumatic stress disorder (PTSD) is caused by an external traumatic event, why do only some trauma survivors develop this condition? This question is important, because it challenges the conceptual origins of PTSD as a syndrome that occurs in normal individuals as a direct consequence of trauma exposure. Those who have argued against the existence of specific posttraumatic syndromes have hypothesized that in the absence of vulnerability, individuals exposed to traumatic events should not develop this psychiatric disorder. On the other side, proponents of the original idea of PTSD as a condition that occurs as a direct result of trauma have argued that individual differences in resilience are responsible for the lower prevalence of PTSD than of trauma. The issue of vulnerability versus resilience continues to be highly charged among clinicians, because it directly affects how trauma survivors must be viewed and treated. The complex social dynamics that drive this debate have been discussed in Chapter 2 of this volume. This chapter reviews the evidence for vulnerability and resilience, by discussing factors other than the nature of exposure to the traumatic events that contribute to the development of PTSD and to the failure of symptoms to resolve.

One of the greatest difficulties in examining issues of vulnerability versus resilience is that the data base for the field of traumatic stress has been derived from retrospective studies. The extent to which the subjects of these studies are representative of the population of trauma survivors who would have been available prospectively is simply unknown. Although there have been recent attempts to examine trauma survivors prospectively, such studies are difficult to do for a variety of reasons, not least of which is the randomness with which trauma occurs in individuals. Nonetheless, it is helpful to elucidate the concrete issues that can be discussed in the context of exploring vulnerability versus resilience, and to evaluate the extent to which data have been provided by outcome studies. The types of studies that have primarily contributed to our understanding of the consequences of trauma have been prospective epidemiological studies of the longitudinal course of PTSD. Studies that have provided ancillary information are those that have attempted to characterize the psychological and neurobiological characteristics differentiating those who develop PTSD from those who demonstrate positive adaptations.

CONCEPTUAL FRAMEWORK

The longitudinal course of PTSD needs to be understood as a process (see Figure 8.1). This process has a series of stages. First, whereas exposure to many traumatic events is random (e.g., people cannot predict when an earthquake is going to occur), exposure to other traumas, such as being the victim of an assault or an auto accident(Breslau, Davis, & Andreski, 1995), may be determined by the individual to at least some extent. The way people behave during a disaster may also have an important impact on their survival; their prior experience of traumas and their training will play a role in their ability to maximize their chance of survival. Equally, a person's immediate emotional reaction at the time of the trauma will influence the capacity to respond to the threat in an adaptive way. For example, a dissociative response or a panic reaction is likely to put the individual at particular risk. The person's state of mind in the midst of the traumatic experience will also have a profound impact on the way the memory of the trauma is laid down and subsequently processed.

PTSD does not develop in the immediate aftermath of a traumatic event. Rather, this disorder emerges out of the pattern of the acute distress triggered by the event (see Chapter 5, this volume). To be distressed is a normal reaction to the horror, helplessness, and fear that are the critical elements of a traumatic experience. The typical pattern for even the most catastrophic experiences, however, is resolution of symptoms and not the development of PTSD (see Chapter 7, this volume). Only a minority of the victims will go on to develop PTSD, and with the passage of time the symptoms will resolve in approximately two-thirds of these (Kessler, Sonnega, Bromet, & Nelson, in press). Therefore, chronic PTSD many years after the triggering event may have some different determinants from what people suffer in the first 6 months after exposure to the trauma. The most chronic forms of PTSD represent the failure of healing and modulation of the acute traumatic response.

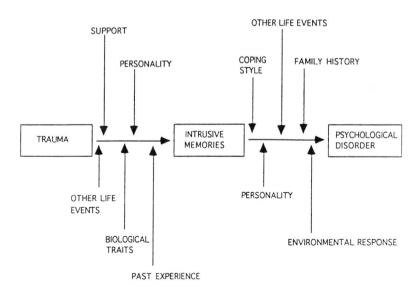

Figure 8.1 Etiological factors influencing the transition from distress to disorder following trauma.

The factors that influence the transition from health to disorder and back to recovery are of critical interest in understanding the longitudinal course of PTSD. The nature of this process is central to understanding the psychopathological consequences of trauma. This process can be divided into three stages: the acute stress response, the chronic response to the traumatic event, and finally the individual's adaptation to having to endure the chronic symptomatic state of PTSD. The acute process is described in Chapter 4. In the chronic forms of the disorder, the associated disability and handicap are more responses to the distress and disruption caused by the symptoms of the disorder than they are primary reactions to the experience of the traumatic event. The ability to tolerate suffering is therefore a critical determinant of long-term adaptation.

The individual's response at each step of this process will be influenced by a complex matrix of biological, social, temperamental, and experiential issues. For example, the neurobiology of an individual's stress response, the capacity for self-modulation, the ability to tolerate the fear and threat that trauma involves, and the ability to cope with any losses will be some of the factors influencing the individual's ultimate outcome. Some characteristics increase the probability of a pathological outcome. These are "vulnerability" factors; they are generally neither necessary nor sufficient to explain the onset of a disorder or predict its course, but rather place the individual at risk of a negative outcome. One example of a risk factor is having a family history of psychiatric illness (Breslau & Davis, 1992; McFarlane, 1992). On the other hand, some characteristics protect the individual or favor a path to recovery. These "resilience" factors may minimize the intensity of the individual's acute distress or allow the more rapid modulation of an abnormal reaction. One example is a person's ability to recruit his or her social network in the aftermath of a traumatic experience. Vulnerability and resilience factors may operate at any part of the process of the stress response—that is, at the time of the event, in the immediate aftermath, or in the longer term. A particular factor may be important at one point in the course of the disorder but not at another.

The longer PTSD lasts, the less important the role of the traumatic exposure becomes in explaining the underlying symptoms. Subsequent adversity, the demoralization of chronic hyperarousal, and the progressive disruption of the individual's underlying neurobiology play an increasing role in understanding the nature and course of chronic symptoms (see Chapter 1).

Research on the longitudinal course of PTSD is summarized below as a background to the discussion of the role of vulnerability and resilience factors. This chapter should be read in conjunction with Chapter 7, which emphasizes that only a minority of people exposed to traumatic events develop PTSD. The factors that influence the acute reactions to trauma are also examined in Chapters 4, 5, and 13.

THE LONGITUDINAL COURSE OF PTSD

The early clinical literature about traumatic neurosis emphasized the chronic course of the disorder and the progressive social decline caused in its more severe forms (Archibald & Tuddenham, 1956). Kardiner (1941), whose pioneering work with World War I veterans had a major impact on our current formulation of PTSD, wrote that the disorder was characterized by "deterioration . . . not dissimilar to that in schizophrenia. . . .The diminution of interest and intelligence is due to the continuous shrinkage of the field of affective functioning and the gratifications derived therefrom" (p. 249). Questions arise as to whether this is the typical outcome, what is the range of other adaptations, and whether these are modified by the nature of the stressor.

The differential effects of different traumatic events are discussed in Chapter 7. Breslau, Davis, Andreski, and Peterson (1991) suggested that the type of traumatic experience may have a major impact on the long-term course of PTSD. Somewhat surprisingly, brief and circumscribed traumas such as accidents may have more enduring effects than combat (Norris, 1992). However, the small numbers and limited range of traumas documented in these two studies limit the capacity to generalize from their findings.

The Effects of War

Epidemiological studies demonstrate that PTSD tends to be the exception rather than the rule after war. The National Vietnam Veterans Readjustment

Study (NVVRS) found that 19 years after combat exposure, 15% of veterans still suffered from PTSD (Kulka et al., 1990). The relationship between the acute effects of combat and long-term outcome has been investigated most thoroughly in veterans of the 1982 Lebanon War (see Chapter 5). This research found that soldiers who became acutely distressed at the time of combat had a much higher risk of PTSD, and that this emerged from combat stress reactions. On the other hand, the rates of PTSD among those who coped at the time of the combat were significantly lower.

This research also provided valuable insights into the pattern of PTSD symptom emergence. This pattern was similar in soldiers who did and did not have a combat stress reaction, suggesting that it is relatively independent of the acute pattern of response. Intrusive symptoms were also found to have low diagnostic specificity, compared to the combination of intrusive and avoidance symptoms. In addition, the prominence of intrusive symptoms decreased over a 2-year period while the avoidance increased (Blank, 1993). The relationship between the acute and chronic reactions to other types of traumatic events has not been so systematically investigated, because it is uncommon for people to present for treatment in the immediate aftermath of disasters and accidents.

A number of studies in progress are examining the impact of war both on the civilian population in general and on specific groups of war victims, such as in Kuwait. These will provide a unique body of prospective data about the effects of a large-scale traumatic event. Retrospective research examined these issues in 824 Dutch resistance fighters (Hovens, Falger, Op den Velde, DeGroen, & Van Duijn, 1994) and found that five decades later 27% of men and 20% of women were currently experiencing PTSD. However, although a directly comparable population sample was not available, the differences between this group and population norms on measures of anxiety and depression raise an ongoing question that has not been thoroughly addressed in any study to date.

The Effects of Disasters and Accidents

The longitudinal study of disaster and accident victims suggests a similar picture: Delayed PTSD is uncommon, and the typical course of PTSD is to begin in the immediate aftermath of the trauma and to continue. A study of 469 firefighters who were intensely exposed to a major fire disaster in the Australian bush (McFarlane & Papay, 1992) found that in the majority with a chronic course, the symptoms fluctuated significantly with the passage of time. This picture does not emerge from most retrospective studies. Delayed onset of PTSD was rare, and some who reported such a pattern of symptoms failed to recall their acute posttraumatic symptoms. In this group, only 15% had PTSD in the absence of an anxiety disorder or major depression, indicating that PTSD is only one of a number of psychiatric disorders that arise in such settings.

Forty-two months after the disaster, the symptoms remained in 56% of those who had PTSD immediately after the disaster. However, when the subjects were followed up 8 years after the disaster, only 4% continued to attract a diagnosis of PTSD. At this stage, 60% still had significant intrusive symptoms, and symptoms of disordered arousal were as common as at 42 months; failure to reach the diagnostic threshold for avoidance and estrangement represented the main reason why these subjects did not qualify for a diagnosis of PTSD. The *intensity* of intrusive symptoms decreased significantly over time, particularly in the first 2 years after the disaster; intrusive symptoms were also less specific to PTSD than were avoidance and disordered arousal. At 8 years, the disordered arousal was the most prominent clinical feature, suggesting that anxiety and depressive symptoms were the most prominent residual symptoms of the disorder. By contrast, among a clinical population that was followed after the same disaster, there tended to be a much greater stability of intrusive and avoidance symptoms. This comparison suggests that quite different pictures can emerge from community and clinical samples studied after the same event. It may be the case that there are different longitudinal courses of PTSD, depending on the initial severity. In the most severe forms, the symptoms may be relatively stable with the passage of time; with the less intense forms, the specific trauma-related symptoms of intrusion and avoidance may decrease, while the disordered affect and arousal may remain.

The variable impact of different traumatic experience on the symptomatic outcome is suggested when these data are compared with those from a recent study of 188 motor accident victims who were assessed soon after the accident and followed for up to 1 year (Mayou, Bryant, & Duthie, 1993). Eighteen percent were found to have an acute distress syndrome, characterized by anxiety and depression together with "horrific" intrusive memories of the accident. Only 15% of these 31 victims did not have persistent psychiatric complications at the end of 1 year, with 13 having a specific phobia of travel, 13 having a mood disorder or an anxiety disorder besides specific phobia, and 9 having PTSD. This suggests that in this setting, even when the initial reaction has the typical features of an acute traumatic reaction, PTSD accounts for only a minority of the psychopathological outcomes. These findings also indicate the enduring nature of the distress in those who develop acute traumatic reactions. Finally, they indicate that horrific memories are not ubiquitously associated with PTSD: One-third complained of these in the immediate aftermath of their accidents, whereas only 7% had PTSD at 1 year.

The longest follow-up of PTSD sufferers to date was conducted after the 1972 Buffalo Creek Dam collapse in the United States, which caused a devastating flood. Grace, Green, Lindy, and Leonard (1993) conducted a 14-year follow-up of 121 victims of this flood (32% of the original 381 victims participating in the study). This rate of participation highlights one of the central problems of conducting long-term follow-ups of trauma victims, and we therefore examine it in more detail. With regard to stressor experiences, bereavement levels were significantly higher for those who refused to participate in the follow-up than for those who did. This would suggest that most follow-up studies may have a bias in the sampling toward those who had less traumatic experiences. This is not surprising, given that people with extremely traumatic experiences may decline participation, in order to avoid reexposure to memories of the traumatic event.

The main goal of the investigation was to define specific aspects of individuals' stressor experiences and to examine the degree to which those experiences predicted long-term psychological impairment. The prevalence rate of PTSD decreased from 44% in 1974 to 28% in 1986. The symptoms in this population fluctuated with the passage of time, and this explained the emergence of what otherwise might have been conceived of as delayed-onset cases. In addition, the severity of the symptoms in the PTSD sufferers was found to decrease with the passage of time. The recovery environment may have played a role in the maintenance of symptom levels, as the flood had become a historical marker that made it hard for residents to put memories behind them.

Prospective and Controlled Studies

A unique body of data relating to these issues comes from a study of 2,092 monozygotic twin pairs who served in the U.S. military during the Vietnam era (Goldberg, True, Eisen, Henderson, 1990), which found a ninefold increase in the rates of PTSD in the combat-exposed twin group. These data provide an unusual opportunity to compare the relative importance of the longitudinal role of the traumatic experience with that of genetic predisposition in determining the different elements of PTSD. The effects of combat were strongest for avoidance of reminders of the trauma (odds ratio = 13.4) and intrusive painful memories (odds ratio = 12.6), and weakest for the symptoms of insomnia (odds ratio = 1.8) and disturbed concentration (odds ratio = 2.3), in the group who had high levels of combat. Thus, intense levels of combat only caused a moderate increase in the prevalence of the symptoms of arousal, the majority being accounted for by the background prevalence of symptoms (47% of the combat-exposed had insomnia, compared with 37% in the unexposed). In this way, trauma may make only a minor contribution to the disordered arousal associated with the diagnosis of PTSD, whereas the experience of trauma may be the major determinant of the reexperiencing phenomena.

Although other studies are of interest, they did not specifically assess the subjects for PTSD. Alexander (1993) conducted a unique longitudinal study of police involved in retrieving bodies after the Piper Alpha oil rig disaster. Most of the officers were free from psychiatric morbidity, and this appeared to be a robust finding, because predisaster baseline data were available on these men. Of particular note was the lack of signs of acute distress at 3 months in this group. However, it is difficult to generalize from these findings because of the possible protective role of training and support in this group. The health data base kept on Norwegian citizens provided a longitudinal record of the effects of the Alexander Kielland oil rig disaster, in which 123 men were killed (Holen, 1991). The 73 survivors were compared with the insurance records of 89 oil rig workers not exposed to the disaster. Predisaster data showed no differences between the populations. Increased rates of both psychiatric and physical disorders were observed for the survivors after the disaster, and this proved to be a persistent effect throughout the 8-year follow-up. The contrast was greatest for the psychiatric diagnoses, where the rates were 12.3 per 100 and 1.5 per 100 for the exposed and control populations, respectively. Norris and Murrell (1988) examined the longitudinal effects of a flood and found that predisaster symptoms were the predominant determinants of distress in this population.

Two cohorts of the Epidemiologic Catchment Area study were subsequently subjected to disasters; these provided a unique opportunity for prospective longitudinal effects to be studied. First, the Times Beach area was found to have been built on a dioxin dump, and floods also occurred in the region. Following this combined disaster, the exposed population had greater symptoms of depression, somatization, phobia, generalized anxiety, PTSD, and alcohol abuse. However, when the symptoms existing prior to the disaster were taken into account, the differences were less dramatic, with only those for depression and PTSD being significant. In contrast to the symptoms of PTSD, where the symptoms occurred *de novo*, the depressive symptoms were a recurrence of previous symptoms. Many of these symptoms had resolved within a year of the disaster. Second, the Puerto Rico cohort experienced a hurricane that involved loss of life and property, and similar findings were obtained (Solomon & Canino, 1990).

Thus, the longitudinal effects of trauma are complex. They include the initiation of new symptoms (particularly those of PTSD), but also the emergence of symptoms (e.g., of depression and anxiety) that represent both the onset of new symptoms and the reactivation of prior affective distress and hyperarousal. However, the trauma may serve to further increase the probability that these symptoms will become autonomous. PTSD is a syndrome that appears to have a variable course, and this course appears to be affected by the nature of the precipitating event, the characteristics of the traumatized individual, and the nature of the recovery environment.

RANGE OF THE LONG-TERM EFFECTS OF TRAUMA

As currently conceptualized, the definition of PTSD is insufficient to describe the full range of the effects of trauma (see Chapter 9, this volume). This range not only has important theoretical implications, but is often forgotten in the planning of treatment services for traumatized populations.

Comorbid Disorders

The current tendency to focus exclusively on the trauma may prevent the adequate assessment and treatment of comorbid disorders such as depression and substance abuse. Recently, the range of specific trauma-related disorders has received more attention, as has the nonspecific role of trauma as a trigger for a range of psychiatric disorders. There is a consistent finding across a variety of traumatic events that PTSD is only one of a number of psychiatric disorders that can occur in such settings. In fact, in the majority of cases even in community samples, PTSD is usually accompanied by another disorder (e.g., major depression, an anxiety disorder, or substance abuse) (Kulka et al., 1990; McFarlane & Papay, 1992).

Such findings call into question the longitudinal relationship between the experience of traumatic events and these other disorders. Interestingly, some victims of trauma do not develop PTSD but do develop other disorders, such as depression. On the other hand, while PTSD goes into remission, other disorders may become active. In populations of general psychiatric patients, the role of trauma in these patients' problems is easily underestimated, because of the apparent dominance of other disorders that are not obviously linked with a traumatic precipitant.

The relationship between traumatic stressors and general vulnerability to psychiatric disorder may vary significantly among different populations. For example, the Grant Study, which has followed the health of a group of sophomores recruited at Harvard University until the age of 65, found that the occurrence of PTSD was unrelated to the variables that predicted poor psychological health on a range of other parameters (Lee, Vaillant, Torrey, & Elder, 1995). This contrasts with the findings of other studies, which have not examined such an elite population. For example, Schnurr, Friedman, and Rosenberg (1993) found that Minnesota Multiphasic Personality Inventory scores prior to combat predicted subsequent PTSD. The National Comorbidity Survey (Kessler et al., in press) and Breslau and Davis (1992) have shown the role of prior disorders and family history as predictors of PTSD.

There has been surprisingly little research examining the extent to which trauma plays a role in the onset and maintenance of general psychiatric patients' various disorders. However, several investigations have now looked at the prevalence of child abuse in clinical samples and found prevalence rates on the order of 18–60% (Saxe et al., 1993). Davidson and Smith (1990) and McFarlane (1994) have also found that in general patient samples the lifetime rates of PTSD are significantly underestimated.

Multiple Forms of PTSD

In any attempt to understand the longitudinal consequences of trauma, it is important that information be derived from a range of victim groups, because the outcomes of different types of traumas may vary substantially. For example, clinical experience suggests that the long-term consequences of child abuse are very different from those of a natural disaster or other circumscribed trauma in adult life (Herman, 1992). Victims of childhood abuse are more likely to have amnesias of the trauma and a range of dissociative symptoms (Saxe et al., 1993).

Blank (1993) has highlighted that the longitudinal course of PTSD has multiple variations—namely, acute, delayed, chronic, intermittent, residual, and reactivated patterns. Longitudinal studies like the NVVRS (Kulka et al., 1990) and the Grant Study suggest a need to define a posttraumatic syndrome in which the full PTSD criteria are not met. An issue that has not been explored in depth is whether there are significant variations in the presentations of PTSD over time, such as interpersonal dysfunction's becoming more prominent with the passage of time. The impact of trauma on personality is specifically addressed by van der Kolk in Chapter 9. This is a critical question, particularly among people who were subjected to prolonged and recurrent trauma in childhood.

Impact on Beliefs and Attitudes

Trauma can also have a series of longitudinal consequences other than the onset of psychological disorders. The experience of such events can modify an individual's vulnerability to subsequent traumatic events, even in the absence of a symptomatic response. In particular, the meaning of a threat or traumatic loss can lead to a major shift in an individual's internal perceptual sensitivities (van der Kolk, 1989). Equally, such experiences can become powerful sources of motivation for some individuals, indicating that trauma can have positive effects on those who survive the ordeal; it need not necessarily result in an enduring sense of demoralization or of having been damaged. The role of the memory of traumatic experiences as a source of motivation and a determinant of human behavior is an issue that is one of the major preoccupations of literature and art. This is an indication of how the impact of such experiences on values and beliefs has important implications for both individuals and society. The accommodation to the possibility of loss and threat of danger plays a central role in shaping many social attitudes and responses.

Impact on Physical Health

The impact of trauma on physical health is a neglected topic. The question arises as to whether any specific pattern of associated physical symptoms arises as part of the traumatic stress response. Historically, PTSD was described by a series of names that focused on the physical accompaniments, such as "soldiers' heart" and "railway spine" (see Chapter 3, this volume). The controversy about the effects of herbicides on the physical health of Vietnam veterans similarly highlights how even in more recent times, the physical symptoms associated with PTSD can be the primary concern of traumatized populations.

Although a number of studies have noted an increased reporting of physical symptoms in persons with PTSD, the reasons for this association are unclear (McFarlane, Atchison, Rafalowicz, & Papay, 1994); a number of possible explanations exist. First, physical symptoms may be an integral part of the constellation of symptoms that constitutes PTSD. If so, PTSD would be similar in this respect to panic disorder or major depression, in which specific physical symptoms either are physical concomitants of the disorder (e.g., shortness of breath or palpitations in panic disorder, and sleeplessness or weight loss in depression) or occur via somatization (e.g., pain syndromes in depression). In these disorders, physical symptoms are often the focus of patients' distress and the main cause for consultation with professionals.

Second, the physical symptoms may be directly caused by the stressor responsible for the development of PTSD. In many instances, the stressors are life-threatening events such as accidents or combat, which cause physical injury to many of those exposed. Benedict and Kolb (1986) describe a sample of war veterans with undiagnosed PTSD attending a pain clinic. In all these patients, pain was localized to the site of a former injury. In this situation, the development of PTSD may influence the presentation of the symptoms rather than their onset.

Third, physical symptoms may be a nonspecific response to exposure to a traumatic experience, independent of the development of PTSD. Investigation of this question has important practical consequences for the assessment of patients who have been exposed to traumatic events in which they may have been injured—particularly when the symptoms become the subject of litigation, because their cause is often disputed. The presence of physical symptoms in the absence of an obvious cause should raise the possibility of undetected PTSD.

The majority of studies examining the relationship between physical symptoms and trauma have had war veterans as subjects. For example, Solomon and Mikulincer (1987), reporting on somatic complaints among Israeli soldiers 1 year after their combat experience in the 1982 Lebanon War, found an increase in self-reporting of physical symptoms among soldiers with acute or chronic psychological reactions. The existence of physical symptoms was also related to the use of new medication, alcohol consumption, cigarette use, and PTSD. Shalev, Bleich, and Ursano (1990) compared Lebanon War veterans with chronic PTSD to matched combat veterans without PTSD. The PTSD group reported higher rates of cardiovascular, neurological, gastrointestinal, audiological, and pain symptoms. This raises the possibility either that the physical symptoms are related to a psychological process, or that there are differences in the way PTSD sufferers report symptoms generally.

Many variables in combat veterans make extrapolation to civilian populations difficult, including bias in the initial selection for military service, the nature of the stressors of military life and combat, the nature of injuries sustained in combat, and the effect of pension entitlement schemes. Escobar, Canino, Rubio-Stipee, and Bravo (1992) reported on the development of new physical symptoms 1 year after a natural disaster in Puerto Rico. Victims of the disaster were more likely to report new gastrointestinal or pseudoneurological symptoms than persons not exposed to the disaster. Although these symptoms may have been indicators of psychopathology, no correlation was made with the presence of psychiatric illness.

The Grant Study has examined the impact of combat (Lee et al., 1995). Subjects in this study were selected for their physical and psychological health and high levels of achievement at Harvard University. Although 72 had a high level of combat exposure, only 1 retrospectively satisfied the diagnostic criteria for PTSD in 1946, with another 4 having a PTSD-like syndrome. (Of these five, two committed suicide, one became withdrawn and dropped out of the study, and another was murdered.) This suggests that PTSD is the exception among a group of highly competent and resourceful individuals. However, combat exposure predicted early death, independent of PTSD: 56% of the men who had experienced heavy combat were dead or chronically ill by the age of 65 (Lee et al., 1995). The length of follow-up in this study makes the results especially noteworthy, as these long-term effects of trauma may only emerge in old age, when the risk of physical illness is increased.

Similarly, the mortality of World War II concentration camp victims was much higher than in control populations and was most marked in the youngest age groups. The death rate was highest among those in the death camps. The duration of imprisonment had no influence upon the mortality, perhaps because survival reflected a positive selection factor. The initial deaths were due to infectious diseases, whereas in the later period coronary arterial disease, lung cancer, and violent death were especially common (Eitinger & Strom, 1973). Similar long-term health effects were observed among the merchant seamen who sailed the convoys in the North Atlantic in World War II (Askevold, 1980).

Behavioral and Interpersonal Disability and Handicap

The impact of trauma on the behavioral and interpersonal functioning of victims has also undergone little investigation. This is surprising, as one of the popular prejudices that emerged both in the 1880s in relation to "railway spine" and also in the aftermath of World War I was the notion that the cause of traumatic neurosis was the payment of compensation. This led the Germans to pay no compensation for trauma-related disorders in the aftermath of the war, and to develop punitive attitudes toward sufferers from combat stress reactions in World War II. There have now been four studies that have examined the impact of compensation on the outcome of PTSD (see Chapter 16, this volume). First, a study on victims of the Buffalo Creek disaster (Grace et al., 1993) compared a group who went through a litigation process with those who accepted an uncontested payment and found few differences in outcome. Mayou et al. (1993) found that being involved in compensation did not affect the outcome of motor accident victims—a similar finding to that after the Pan American Flight 103 crash over Lockerbie, Scotland (Brooks & McKinlay, 1992). Litigation also did not affect the outcome of the victims of the 1983 Australian Ash Wednesday disaster, although they felt very traumatized by the litigation process (McFarlane, in press-b). Thus, although trauma can have dramatic effects on the ability to perform in a variety of social roles, this variation cannot be substantially attributed to the payment of financial compensation. However, defining the optimal system for paying compensation and maximizing victims' motivation to play a useful social role are matters of critical concern.

It is important to distinguish the severity of individuals' symptoms from their ability to perform a range of social roles. For example, in the Grant Study, one of the men who was most troubled by traumatic memories of war became president of the United States—John F. Kennedy. As noted above, some people can have positive adaptations to trauma, using their experience as a source of motivation. For others, work becomes a method of distraction and of keeping the past at bay. Although their careers may be very successful, this success may be achieved at the expense of their family and interpersonal relationships. Still others become crippled by the intrusiveness of the past and their inability to focus on the present.

These social consequences have perhaps been best addressed in studies of concentration camp victim survivors (Eitinger & Strom, 1973). They had less stable working lives than controls, with more frequent changes in jobs, domiciles, and occupations. There were transitions to less qualified and well-paid work in 25% of the survivors, in contrast to 4% of the controls. The ex-prisoners from the lower socioeconomic classes seemed to be less able to compensate for their failing health than the more professional and skilled groups. Weisaeth's (1989) study demonstrated that the absences from work and problems with occupational functioning were accounted for not only by PTSD symptoms, but also a variety of psychosomatic complaints, conversion complaints, and vegetative symptoms.

The NVVRS (Kulka et al., 1990) examined the impact of Vietnam service in great detail and indicated that, as a group, veterans were disadvantaged in a variety of educational and social domains. This could not be accounted for simply by the payment of pension entitlements for PTSD, as a significant percentage of those entitled chose not to receive pensions. However, this issue has also been investigated among the 50,000 Australian Vietnam veterans who were not found to be occupationally disadvantaged (O'Toole, personal communication). This highlights how cultural issues and the available social roles may also play a central part in determining the impact of PTSD on the levels of disability and handicap.

The relationship between symptom improvement and function has been examined in a group of Israeli war veterans (Solomon, 1989). No change in high levels of social and interpersonal dysfunction were found in a longitudinal follow-up. This suggests that these consequences may be more resistant to remission than the intrusive phenomena. The potential for the social dislocation that can be caused by this disorder was demonstrated by North and Smith (1992), who found that PTSD was one of the most common psychiatric disorders among the homeless and that their disorder preceded rather than being caused by their homelessness.

Another aspect of the behavioral consequences of trauma was shown in a study of Australian female prisoners, which demonstrated that PTSD and a history of abuse were almost ubiquitous in these women, and that these factors contributed significantly to their criminal histories (Raeside, Shaw, & McFarlane, 1995). The investigation of the trauma history of attenders at a drug rehabilitation clinic also found a strong association between PTSD and the existence of drug abuse in 59% of cases (Fullilove et al., 1993). Thus, in its more malignant form, PTSD leads to a severe social decline that is associated with the most dysfunctional social groups. A comparison of PTSD patients to patients with other anxiety disorders showed that the PTSD group had a worse outcome on a range of dimensions of functioning (Warshaw et al., 1993). In this longitudinal study in a clinical setting, PTSD was found to have severe effects on quality of life in virtually all domains. The PTSD patients also had high levels of depression, suicide attempts and gestures, and alcohol abuse.

Given the enormous costs of financial compensation for the effects of traumatic stress, and the fact that the amount of compensation is often determined by the severity of the associated disability, it is an extreme paradox that this area has been so little investigated. It is also a critical issue for treatment, as we should not assume that the interventions that improve patients' symptoms of intrusion and hyperarousal will automatically modify their ability to work or function within families. At this point, we do not even know which of the posttraumatic symptoms is the most disabling. The role that personality and attitudes play in influencing these adaptations is of critical interest. For example, it is probable that individuals who have a stoical attitude are more likely to put their symptomatic distress to one side and maintain their usual levels of functioning, despite their suffering.

Another matter that has not been investigated is the question of returning people to work in jobs where they have been traumatized (e.g., emergency service workers, or bank employees who have been involved in a holdup). Does the return to work have a negative long-term impact on their adjustment, although they maintain their social role? Does this lead to the development of the use of dissociative defenses? At what point is such a return to the traumatizing environment against an individual's interests? Equally, *not* to make return to work a goal of rehabilitation can be very detrimental to an individual's sense of mastery and self-competence.

Modified Vulnerability to
Disordered Affect and Arousal

Some of the concepts developed in the literature about the outcome of the treatment of depression (Kupfer, 1993) can be usefully applied to the description of the longitudinal course of PTSD (McFarlane, in press-a). The issue then arises as to how to distinguish between remission of a disorder and recovery from it. This is an important concept, because the term "recovery" defines the end of an illness episode and presumes that a further episode is a recurrence of the disorder rather than a relapse of the current one. In medico-legal circles, where the prognosis of PTSD and its long-term outcome are of particular importance, there is an assumption that once the symptoms of PTSD have resolved, the disorder does not recur. This is based on the idea that PTSD is an adaptational response to an event (Yehuda & McFarlane, 1995)—a response that begins with an acute stress reaction, then follows a predictable course, and eventually resolves without sequelae. However, emerging evidence suggests that this is not the case. In particular, Solomon, Garb, Bleich, and Grupper (1987a) described 35 soldiers who had several exposures to combat and multiple episodes of PTSD. There was support for the concept of reactivation of the original PTSD in some soldiers, whereas in others the second episode may have been substantially independent of the first.

Both clinical and biological data suggest that in a significant number of individuals PTSD causes significant psychological and neurobiological changes, which endure even after the disorder remits. These may include a permanent modification of the individual's vulnerability to a range of psychiatric disorders, which may or may not be triggered by subsequent adverse life experience. Mellman, Randolph, Brawman-Mintzer, Flores, & Milanes, (1992) have suggested that the comorbid disorders triggered in relation to PTSD, particularly panic disorder, major depressive disorder, and phobias, become increasingly autonomous in their pattern of recurrence. This propensity of the concurrent disorder to have a recurrent course may in fact be one of the critical long-term consequences of trauma (McFarlane & Papay, 1992). A further issue is whether the constellation of symptoms in PTSD changes with the passage of time. For example, the interpersonal estrangement and emotional detachment may come to dominate the picture as the intrusive memories become less dominant. This may have important implications for treatment, as the effectiveness of different strategies may change according to the stage of the disorder (McFarlane, 1994).

The model of kindling in affective disorders has been developed from the clinical observation that life events play an important initiating role in the first episodes of an affective disorder, but that their importance progressively decreases as the neurobiology of the disorder becomes autonomous (Post, 1992). This model implies that there is a "biological memory" of the preceding episodes of the illness, and that the individual's current vulnerability to affective disorder is a consequence of this progressive sensitivity to affective de-stabilization. The observation that the symptoms of PTSD are maintained and triggered by day-to-day adverse life experiences, and that this process is a stronger determinant of current levels of symptomatic distress than the original trauma, suggests that a modification of the individual's stress responsiveness may be an important aspect of the dysregulation that is central to the psychobiology of PTSD (van der Kolk, Greenberg, Boyd, & Krystal, 1985; McFarlane, 1989; Koopman, Classen, & Spiegel, 1994). The work of Resnick and associates (cited in Yehuda, Resnick, Kahana, & Giller, 1993a), who found altered cortisol responsiveness in women who had been raped on a second occasion, indicates how the course of PTSD needs to take account of the similar transformations of stress responsiveness that are thought to be operating in affective disorders.

Therefore, research on the longitudinal course of PTSD and other post-traumatic states needs to consider the possibility that even if the symptoms of the immediate disorder remit, permanent changes may remain in the individual's vulnerability to disordered affect and arousal. The underlying neurobiology may be similar to that found in affective disorders, and van der Kolk et al. (1985) have proposed that kindling is a useful model to explain the changes in PTSD. Yehuda and Antelman (1993) have also suggested that a model of sensitization can explain the abnormalities of cortisol responsiveness in this disorder.

VULNERABILITY AND RESILIENCE: POSSIBLE FACTORS AND PROCESSES

How Do Vulnerability Factors Modify the Response to Stress?

It is necessary to be precise about what vulnerability does predict. Critical to this issue is the question of how individuals who are exposed to a traumatic event but do not develop a psychiatric disorder differ from those who develop PTSD. In particular, are there specific symptoms that differentiate people who survive a traumatic experience without being disabled from those who become severely symptomatic? Epidemiological studies of populations in the immediate aftermath of a trauma, and even studies of concentration camp survivors 50 years after the Holocaust, have found that many of the victims have intrusive memories of the trauma and some avoidance phenomena but do not have PTSD. Therefore, it is highly probable that different factors contribute to the different subsets of symptoms. It may be the case that the predictors of disordered arousal are the vulnerability factors that best distinguish those with PTSD.

Epidemiological studies are especially important in understanding etiology, as discussed in Chapter 7, because they allow comparisons of PTSD sufferers to individuals who have been exposed to the trauma but have not developed the disorder. In particular, PTSD cannot be explained entirely by the emergence of traumatic memories and the associated cognitive and biological processes, as these traumatic memories are present in many of those without PTSD. Thus the biology of memory is not a sufficient model to explain the characteristics differentiating those with PTSD from those who do not remain distressed following the trauma, although it is a critical intermediary process to the emergence of symptoms of disordered arousal.

The many studies of normal stress reactions may also be less relevant than is often assumed, as they do not deal with the variability of response that is critical to pathological outcomes. This is particularly the case in the light of the finding of hypocortisolemia and supersuppression on the dexamethasone suppression test (Yehuda et al., 1993b). These findings demonstrate that the biology of PTSD is not the biology of the "normal" acute stress response. This is a critical issue, because models of animal stress are often used to develop hypotheses about the etiology of PTSD; in reality, these paradigms may not be applicable. Similarly, many of the studies that are used to discuss the role of memory in PTSD refer to the investigation of memories of situations and experiences that are far from traumatic (see Chapter 12). Therefore, any model of predisposition or vulnerability should aim to explain the emergence of the features of PTSD that differentiate it from the normal stress response. The study by Resnick et al. (cited in Yehuda et al., 1993a) is of particular interest in this regard, as it demonstrated that women who had been previously raped tended to have a lower acute cortisol response to a subsequent rape than women who were raped for the first time. This pattern of reaction was associated with an increased risk of PTSD, which indicates that the normal stress response (with a characteristic major surge in cortisol) may protect against the development of PTSD.

Thus the concept of vulnerability is more complicated than it first appears. Kardiner (1941) suggested that the role of vulnerability factors in the development of acute symptoms differs from their role in regard to the chronic outcomes. The natural course of acute distress may be to dissipate—a finding highlighted by Weisaeth's (1989) follow-up study of a factory explosion. Chronic PTSD was associated with preexisting vulnerabilities, complicating life events, and low motivation; high trauma exposure was necessary, but not sufficient, to explain the emergence of chronic symptoms. Therefore, predisposition and lowered resilience may be more important in preventing the resolution and amelioration of the acute distress than in determining its occurence.

Hence, vulnerability can influence a series of different steps in the emergence of chronic PTSD, and the process can be modified in either a positive or a negative way at each step. First, the ability to tolerate traumatic events such as combat, rape, or assault is often assumed to be the critical determinant for the onset of chronic PTSD. This particularly prejudicial view accounts for much of the stigma connected with PTSD. It erroneously assumes that fear is the cause of PTSD, rather than the sense of threat and horror that becomes imbedded in the memory of an individual who may have coped well at the time of the trauma. The paradox is that there is no direct link between an individual's bravery and the existence of PTSD. For example, in World War I, men who developed shell-shock were as likely to be decorated as other soldiers, and officers with PTSD were overrepresented among those receiving decorations (Miller, 1940).

Second, the individual's behavior during the traumatic event and the development of acute stress-related symptoms at the time of the trauma or in the immediate aftermath are also considered to be central prerequisites of PTSD (see Chapter 9). The determinants of these acute patterns of stress response are therefore of primary interest in understanding vulnerability and resilience. Although it is true that soldiers with combat stress reactions are more likely to develop PTSD, PTSD is not an inevitable consequence (see Solomon et al., Chapter 5). Many individuals who develop PTSD after combat have not had an acute stress reaction. This is also true of other traumatic events: People who have been able to respond and manage in the face of the immediate trauma and suffering later succumb to the disorder. Therefore, the link between the acute response and PTSD is not a simple one-to-one relationship. The pattern of acute response, as discussed in Chapter 7, can be critically determined by the nature and predictability of the trauma. Thus, a range of acute stress reactions may need to be considered in relation to resilience. Furthermore, they may directly lead to PTSD, and hence it is necessary to consider the determinants of chronic posttraumatic states as a separate issue.

The Role of Vulnerability in the Initial Posttraumatic Period

Whether an individual's arousal normalizes once an acute traumatic reaction has been triggered is a critical process in the long-term adaptation to an event. The modulation of an individual's acute arousal is modified by a range of vulnerability factors. In the initial days after a traumatic event, distressing and intrusive recollections of the traumatic experience are universal and indicate an ongoing process of normal reappraisal. In this process, various representations of the trauma are entertained, and an attempt is made to integrate these with existing psychological schemata. This replaying of these memories allows the development of novel meaning constructs that are not part of the individual's inner world (see Chapter 7).

The emergence of an enduring exaggerated startle response, hypervigilance, increased irritability, sleep disturbance, and disturbed memory and concentration is what differentiates the victims who go on to develop PTSD (Weisaeth, 1989; McFarlane, 1992). This hyperarousal arises as a consequence of the constant replaying of the traumatic memories. The evidence for this relationship comes from epidemiological data (McFarlane, 1992; Creamer, Burgess, & Pattison, 1992) and provides the basis for a neural network model for the neurobiological changes that are central to PTSD (Galletly, Clark, & McFarlane, in press). Weisaeth (1989) indicated that failure of insomnia, anxiety, and general agitation to subside in the first weeks was a major predictor of PTSD. These observations may allow us to begin to define high-risk individuals, taking note of the fact that severity of exposure and extent of losses alone are not good predictors. The factors that facilitate or prevent the onset and maintenance of this pattern of hyperarousal are critical to understanding the role of vulnerability factors in the onset of PTSD.

What happens in the immediate aftermath of the trauma is critical. Often the reality of many aspects of a trauma only becomes apparent after a few days. For example, the significance of physical injuries may take some time to become apparent, and the extent of both the destruction of property and the number of deaths may only become clear at the end of extensive rescue and containment efforts. The ultimate meaning of the experience will be constructed from its impact on a variety of domains. These perceptions are influenced by previous life experiences, habitual coping skills, and general arousability (Freedy, Resnick, & Kilpatrick, 1992). The ability to mobilize appropriate relationships and support is another critical issue at this stage of the process of adaptation.

The progression from a state of distress to more severe symptoms is influenced by a range of other vulnerabilities, including a past or family history of psychiatric illness, neuroticism as a personality trait, a range of social mediators, and other life events or traumas occurring after the disaster (Kessler et al., in press; Breslau & Davis, 1992; McFarlane, 1989). It is important to emphasize once again that the development of chronic symptoms is the exception rather than the rule. Exposure to extreme stress can produce personal growth and lead to increased self-respect. Many people go through a process of reassessing their values and priorities. In any consideration of the long-term outcome and the interplay with an individual's resilience and vulnerability, the range of posttraumatic outcomes needs to be kept in mind. At this stage, the emotional state and propensity to experience anxiety of people with prior psychological problems may lead to difficulty in regaining homeostasis. For example, they may experience difficulty in negotiating social support because their own resources are inadequate, or they may have problems with finding or coming to terms with the personal meaning of the experience.

Several studies have now shown that the relationship between intrusive cognitions and arousal is less apparent in the immediate aftermath of the trauma (Shalev, 1992), and that avoidance symptoms only emerge over time (Solomon, Weisenberg, Schwarzwald, & Mikulincer, 1987b). Rapidly, over a period of several weeks, the typical constellation of PTSD begins to be manifested. At this early stage, the intensity of intrusions is probably not a good measure of their psychopathological significance; it is unclear at which stage traumatic memories develop the typically fixed and irreconcilable quality with the associated sense of retraumatization often experienced in PTSD. The inflexible quality of these traumatic memories represents a failure to resolve the issue of meaning (see Chapter 12). A corollary of this question is the nature of the process that leads to the onset of the avoidance phenomena. One view is that they represent a defense modulating the emotions associated with the intense traumatic cognitions, and thus are an integral part of the immediate trauma response (Janet, 1889; Lindemann, 1944; Horowitz, 1986). However, Shalev (1992) found in a study of terrorist attack victims that avoidance was not proportional to intrusions in the immediate post attack period. It appeared that avoidance only emerged after an individual was unable to work through these phenomena. These findings are in part supported by other work (Solomon et al., 1987b; McFarlane, 1992), which has suggested (1) that intrusions are common to many who have experienced traumatic events and not specific to PTSD; and (2) that avoidance is a phenomenon that emerges during the months after the trauma and is characteristic of having developed the disorder, rather than of having been exposed to a potentially traumatic stressor.

Very few prospective accounts have systematically examined survivors in the immediate aftermath and examined the relationship between immediate reactions and subsequent emergence of PTSD. Such studies are likely to provide critical evidence about the range of acute stress responses and their relationship to PTSD and the other psychiatric disorders that emerge in the setting of trauma. A systematic study of train drivers involved in railway accidents (Malt et al., 1993) found that whereas more than half reported moderate to high levels of intrusive memories in the immediate aftermath, fewer than one-third reported symptoms of acute psychophysiological arousal. Avoidance was uncommon. The correlations between the various measures increased progressively at 1 month and 1 year, suggesting that the relationships among these phenomena change with the passage of time.

The suggestion that initial levels of intrusion and avoidance do not predict the onset of PTSD points to the role of some other process, such as the destabilization of an individual's normal pattern of arousal, which will have a feedback effect on the processing of thoughts and feelings (Shalev, 1992). Thus the focus on a cognitive processing model, which underpins the current conceptualization of PTSD, may have hampered the investigation of what differentiates adaptive from maladaptive responses to trauma. As such, it may have diverted attention away from the impact of trauma on personality (see Chapter 9).

Resilience at the Time of the Trauma

The nature of the trauma and the strategies used to cope with it may vary substantially among different types of traumatic events. For example, in a motor vehicle accident the trauma probably has a very brief duration, and its ability to affect an individual eventual outcome may be minimal. The emotional reaction will be immediate fear, with little chance for anticipatory anxiety. In contrast, victims of repeated sexual abuse may have some opportunity to anticipate and develop strategies to cope with the trauma. Therefore, the issue of resilience at the time of the trauma is more of a concern with prolonged or recurrent traumas in which victims are required to contain their fear and arousal. However, with accident victims who sustain significant injuries, it is increasingly apparent that the experience of the rescue and acute treatment are as important predictors of the posttraumatic outcome as the trauma itself.

A second issue relates to an individual's emotional reaction at the time of the trauma. This point is discussed at length in this book (see Chapters 7 and 13), but it should suffice to say that people who dissociate at the time of the trauma are more vulnerable to posttraumatic reactions. However, it is important to emphasize that many individuals who develop PTSD do not dissociate at the time of the trauma. Dissociation also demonstrates the complexity of the determinants of vulnerability. The probability and severity of a dissociative response at the time of the trauma will be influenced by the duration and intensity of the exposure, as well as by the individual's personality, prior history of traumatization, and behavior triggered by the dissociation. Thus, the issue of resilience relates both to the behavior and the mental state of the individual at the time of the trauma.

The role of training in preventing PTSD is discussed by Ursano, Grieger, and McCarroll in Chapter 19. The emotional impact of a traumatic event can be substantially modified by preparation and training. The sense of helplessness is lessened as the individual gains an understanding of the behaviors that will aid in survival. Furthermore, the intensity of the exposure and the reality of the danger may be modified by the use of learned adaptive behaviors during the emergency, whether these are methods of resisting and managing being tortured, or ways of averting the dangers of assault or rape in particular settings. Training and leadership are obviously critical issues in the military and emergency services.

Adaptations to Chronic Symptoms

Once symptoms have emerged, the individual's capacity to cope with them is critical. As it stands, the coping behavior documented in PTSD sufferers tells us more about how they cope with the distress of their symptoms than how they coped with the trauma itself. Lazarus and Folkman (1984) have suggested that coping is largely determined by the meaning that people give to their experiences. According to this view, personal meaning is derived from the evaluation of how much one is harmed, threatened, and challenged by an experience, and by the evaluation of one's percieved options for mitigating the effects of the event. Thus, it is important to consider resilience and vulnerability in terms of both individuals' responses to the trauma and their capacity to cope with their reactions. To date, this issue has received surprisingly little research attention.

The distress of a psychological disorder can create the same sense of powerlessness and the same threat of disintegration that confront the victims of trauma. The comparative intensity of the distress caused by the experience of the trauma and that caused by the experience of symptoms is described by a British orthopedic registrar who was a veteran of the Falklands War and subsequently developed PTSD (Hughes, 1990). Hughes describes his experience in a graphic manner:

> For no obvious reason I had suddenly been overwhelmed by a crescendo of blind unreasoning fear, defying all logic and insight . . . nothing that General Galtieri's men had generated compared with the terrors that may own mind invented that night. Having looked death full in the eye on a windswept isthmus outside Goose Green and again, but two weeks later, on a barren hillside called Wireless Ridge, I think I can honestly say I no longer feared death or the things real and imagined that usually become the objects of phobias. I was afraid that night of the only thing that could still frighten me, myself. I was terrified of losing my control. (1990, p. 1476)

Several studies have demonstrated that patients who have been psychotic can develop symptoms identical to PTSD in response to their illness (McGorry et al., 1991; Shaner & Eth, 1989, 1991). Such findings lead one to question the effect that the experience of chronic PTSD itself has on the course of the disorder. In contrast to the actual trauma, which is a circumscribed experience, the symptoms of PTSD (e.g., the intense flashbacks and nightmares) can seem endless. The sufferer has to cope with the constant and unpredictable recurrence of the memory of the trauma, with little anticipation of relief. Thus, although the realistic danger of the trauma is long gone, continuing feelings of threat and fear are the emotional reality. These intrusions take away any sense of security or safety of retreat in the privacy of one's mind, and result in repeated traumatization. This is what leads to the disorder we call PTSD. Thus, in those who develop the disorder, the internal sense of threat and loss of control may present a new dimension of trauma. The attributes and appraisals of the individual that allow him or her to tolerate and modulate this distress are the critical determinants of the long-term outcome of the person's suffering.

Many of the problems seen in people who suffer from PTSD are actually the consequences of the secondary effects of the disorder, which include appraisal of the experience as it unfolds. The presence of nightmares and the sleep disturbance mean that even the safety of withdrawal into unconsciousness is lost. The irritability, emotional numbing, and anhedonia mean that the relationships that are critical to the individual's sense of identity and belonging may also be threatened and undermined by the PTSD sufferer's pattern of response to his or her symptoms. The very attachments that can provide a powerful motivation for survival in the face of extreme threat can themselves be threatened by these secondary responses. The disturbances of attention and concentration mean that the person is no longer able to interact with his or her current environment with the same sense of involvement. Even simple activities such as reading, participating in a conversation, and watching television demand greater effort. It is this sense of being damaged, rather than the immediate horror of the trauma, that many victims describe as the worst aspect of their ordeal in the long term.

CONCLUSION

From his more general review of longitudinal research into PTSD, Blank (1993) concluded that it is dangerous to generalize about the course of PTSD, as there appears to be significant variation among individuals, traumatic events, and the contexts in which events occur. Ultimately, answers to the many questions that still exist will only emerge with sophisticated prospective studies that investigate the interaction between the effects of traumatic events and the other vulnerability factors that influence the onset and course of psychiatric disorders in other settings. The important issue to emphasize is that both the type of outcomes and the enduring effects of trauma vary widely. The critical question yet to be answered is whether treatments that lead to a decrease in symptoms alter the long-term consequences of trauma. Of paramount importance is the need to demonstrate the effectiveness of preventive interventions, because the chronic effects of trauma have important implications for public health.

REFERENCES

Alexander, D. A. (1993). Stress among police body handlers: A long-term follow-up. *British Journal of Psychiatry, 163*, 806–808.

Archibald, H., & Tuddenham, R. (1956). Persistent stress reaction after combat: A twenty year follow up. *Archives of General Psychiatry, 12*, 475–481.

Askevold, F. (1980). The war sailor syndrome. *Danish Medical Bulletin, 77*, 220–223.

Benedict, R. A., & Kolb, L. C. (1986). Preliminary findings on chronic pain and posttraumatic stress disorder. *American Journal of Psychology, 143*, 908–910.

Blank, A. S. (1993). The longitudinal course of posttraumatic stress disorder. In J. R. T. Davidson & E. B. Foa (Eds.), *Posttraumatic stress disorder: DSM-IV and beyond* (pp. 3–22). Washington, DC: American Psychiatric Press,.

Breslau, N., & Davis, G. C. (1992). Posttraumatic stress disorder in an urban population of young adults: Risk factors for chronicity. *American Journal of Psychiatry, 149*(5), 671–675.

Breslau, N., Davis, G. C., & Andreski, P. (1995). Risk factors for PTSD related traumatic events: A prospective analysis. *American Journal of Psychiatry, 152*, 529–535.

Breslau, N., Davis, G. C., Andreski, P., & Peterson, E. (1991). Traumatic events and posttraumatic stress disorder in an urban population of young adults. *Archives of General Psychiatry, 48*, 216–222.

Brooks, N., & McKinlay, W. (1992). Mental health consequences of the Lockerbie disaster. *Journal of Traumatic Stress, 5*, 527–543.

Creamer, M., Burgess, P., & Pattison, P. (1992). Reaction to trauma: A cognitive processing model. *Journal of Abnormal Psychology, 101*, 452–459.

Davidson, J., & Smith, R. (1990). Traumatic experiences in psychiatric outpatients. *Journal of Traumatic Stress, 3*(3), 459–475.

Eitinger, L., & Strom, A. (1973). *Mortality and morbidity after excessive stress: A follow-up investigation of Norwegian concentration camp survivors.* New York: Humanities Press.

Escobar, J. I., Canino, G., Rubio-Stipee, M., & Bravo, M. (1992). Somatic symptoms after natural disasters: A prospective study. *American Journal of Psychiatry, 149*, 965–967.

Freedy, J. R., Resnick, H. S., & Kilpatrick, D.G. (1992). Conceptual framework for evaluating disaster impact: Implications for clinical intervention. In L. S. Austin (Eds.), *Clinical response to trauma in the community* (pp. 3–23). Washington, DC: American Psychiatric Press.

Fullilove, M. T., Fullilove, R. E., Smith, M., Michael, C., Panzer, P. G. & Wallace, R. (1993). Violence, trauma and post-traumatic stress disorder among women drug users. *Journal of Traumatic Stress, 6*, 533–543.

Galletly, C. A., Clark, C. R. & McFarlane, A. C. (in press). Artificial neural networks: A prospective tool for the analysis of psychiatric disorders. *Journal of Psychiatry and Neuroscience.*

Goldberg, J., True, W. R., Eisen, S. A., & Henderson, W. G. (1990). A twin study of the effects of the Vietnam War on posttraumatic stress disorder. *Journal of the American Medical Association, 263*(9), 1227–1232.

Grace, M. C., Green, B. L., Lindy, J. D., & Leonard, A. C. (1993). The Buffalo Creek disaster: A 14-year follow-up. In J. P. Wilson & B. Raphael (Eds.), *International handbook of traumatic stress syndromes* (pp. 441–449). New York: Plenum Press.

Herman, J. (1992). *Trauma and recovery.* New York: Basic Books.

Holen, A. (1991). A longitudinal study of the occurrence and persistence of posttraumatic health problems in disaster survivors. *Stress Medicine, 7*, 11–17.

Horowitz, M. J. (1986). Stress-response syndromes: A review of posttraumatic and adjustment disorders. *Hospital and Community Psychiatry, 37*(3), 241–249.

Hovens, J. E., Falger, P. R. J., Op den Velde, W., De Groen, J. H. M., & Van Duijn, H. (1994). Posttraumatic stress disorder in male and female Dutch resistance veterans of World War II in relation to trait anxiety and depression. *Psychological Reports, 74*, 275–285.

Hughes, S. (1990). Inside madness. *British Medical Journal, 301*, 1476–1478.

Janet, P. (1889). *L'automatisme psychologique.* Paris: Alcan.

Kardiner, A. (1941). *The traumatic neuroses of war.* New York: Hoeber.

Kessler, R., Sonnega, A., Bromet, E., & Nelson, C. B. (in press). Posttraumatic stress disorder in the National Comorbidity Survey.

Koopman, C., Classen, C. & Spiegel, D. (1994). Predictors of posttraumatic stress symptoms among survivors of the Oakland/Berkeley, California, firestorm. *American Journal of Psychiatry, 151*(6), 888–894.

Kulka, R. A., Schlenger, W. E., Fairbank, J. A., Hough, R. L., Jordan, B. K., Marmar, C. R., & Weiss, D. S. (1990). *Trauma and the Vietnam War generation: Report of findings from the National Vietnam Veterans Readjustment Study.* New York: Brunner/Mazel.

Kupfer, D. J. (1993). Management of recurrent depression. *Journal of Clinical Psychiatry, 54*(Suppl.), 29–33.

Lazarus, R. S., & Folkman, S. (1984). *Stress, appraisal and coping.* New York: Springer.

Lindemann, E. (1944). Symptomatology and management of acute grief. *American Journal of Psychiatry, 101,* 141–148.

Lee, K. A., Vaillant, G. E., Torrey, W. C., & Elder, G. H. (1995). A 50-year prospective study of the psychological sequelae of World War II combat. *American Journal of Psychiatry, 152*(4), 516–522.

Malt, U., Karlehagen, S., Hoff, H., Herrstromer, U., Hildingson, K., Tibell, E., & Leymann, H. (1993). The effect of major railway accidents on the psychological health of train drivers: I. Acute psychological responses to accident. *Journal of Psychosomatic Research, 37*(8), 793–805.

Mayou, R., Bryant, B., & Duthie, R. (1993). Psychiatric consequences of road traffic accidents. *British Medical Journal, 307,* 647–651.

McFarlane, A. C. (1988). The longitudinal course of posttraumatic morbidity: The range of outcomes and their predictors. *Journal of Nervous and Mental Disease, 176,* 30–39.

McFarlane, A. C. (1989). The aetiology of post-traumatic morbidity: Predisposing, precipitating and perpetuating factors. *British Journal of Psychiatry, 154,* 221–228.

McFarlane, A. C. (1992). Avoidance and intrusion in posttraumatic stress disorder. *Journal of Nervous and Mental Disease, 180*(7), 439–445.

McFarlane, A. C. (1994). Individual psychotherapy for posttraumatic stress disorder. *Psychiatric Clinics of North America, 17,* 393–408.

McFarlane, A. C. (in press-a). The longitudinal course of trauma. In E. Giller & L. Weisaeth (Ed.), *Baillière's clinical psychiatry: Posttraumatic stress disorder.* London: Ballière.

McFarlane, A. C. (in press-b). Attitudes to victims: Issues for medicine, the law & society. In C. Sumner, M. Israel, M. O'Conner, & R. Sarre (Eds.), *International victimology: Selected papers from the 8th International symposium on victimology.* Canberra: Australian Institute of Criminology.

McFarlane, A. C., Atchison, M., Rafalowicz, E., & Papay, P. (1994). Physical symptoms in post-traumatic stress disorder. *Journal of Psychosomatic Research, 38*(7), 715–726.

McFarlane, A. C., & Papay, P. (1992). Multiple diagnoses in posttraumatic stress disorder in the victims of a natural disaster. *Journal of Nervous and Mental Disease, 180*(8), 498–504.

McGorry, P. D., Chanen, A., McCarthy, E., Van Riel, R., McKenzie, D., & Singh, B. S. (1991). Posttraumatic stress disorder following recent-onset psychosis: An unrecognized postpsychotic syndrome. *Journal of Nervous and Mental Disease, 179*(5), 253–258.

Mellman, T. A., Randolph, C. A., Brawman-Mintzer, O., Flores, L. P., & Milanes, F. J. (1992). Phenomenology and course of psychiatric disorders associated with combat-related posttraumatic stress disorder. *American Journal of Psychiatry, 149*(11), 1568–1574.

Miller, E. (1940). *Neuroses in war.* London: Macmillan.

Norris, F. H. (1992). Epidemiology of trauma: frequency and impact of different potentially traumatic events on different demographic groups. *Journal of Consulting and Clinical Psychology, 60*(3), 409–418.

Norris, F. H., & Murrell, S. A. (1988). Prior experience as a moderator of disaster impact on anxiety symptoms in older adults. *American Journal of Community Psychology, 16*(5), 665–683.

North, C. S., & Smith, E. M. (1992). Posttraumatic stress disorder among homeless men and women. *Hospital and Community Psychiatry, 43*(10), 1010–1016.

Post, R. M. (1992). Transduction of psychosocial stress into the neurobiology of recurrent affective disorder. *American Journal of Psychiatry, 149*(8), 999–1010.

Raeside, C. W. J., Shaw, J. J., & McFarlane, A. C. (1995) *Posttraumatic stress disorder (PTSD) in perpetrators of violent crime.* Manuscript submitted for publication.

Saxe, G. N., van der Kolk, B. A., Berkowitz, R., Chinman, G., Hall, K., Lieberg, G. & Schwartz, J. (1993). Dissociative disorders in psychiatric inpatients. *American Journal of Psychiatry, 150*(7), 1037–1042.

Schnurr, P. P., Friedman, M. J., & Rosenberg, S. D. (1993). Premilitary MMPI scores as predictors of combat-related PTSD symptoms. *American Journal of Psychiatry, 150,* 479–483.

Shalev, A. Y. (1992). Posttraumatic stress disorder among injured survivors of a terrorist attack: Predictive value of early intrusion and avoidance symptoms. *Journal of Nervous and Mental Disease, 180,* 505–509.

Shalev, A. Y., Bleich, A., & Ursano, R. J. (1990). Posttraumatic stress disorder: Somatic comorbidity and effort in tolerance. *Psychosomatics, 31*(2), 197–203.

Shaner, A., & Eth, S. (1989). Can schizophrenia cause posttraumatic stress disorder? *American Journal of Psychotherapy, 43*(4), 588–597.

Shaner, A., & Eth, S. (1991). Postpsychosis posttraumatic stress disorder. *Journal of Nervous and Mental Disease, 179*(10), 640.

Solomon, S. D., & Canino, G. J. (1990). Appropriateness of DSM-III-R criteria for posttraumatic stress disorder. *Comprehensive Psychiatry, 31*(3), 227–237.

Solomon, Z. (1989). PTSD and social functioning: A three year prospective study. *Social Psychiatry and Psychiatric Epidemiology, 24,* 127–133.

Solomon, Z., Garb, R., Bleich, A., & Grupper, D. (1987a). Reactivation of combat-related posttraumatic stress disorder. *American Journal of Psychiatry, 144*(1), 51–55.

Solomon, Z., & Mikulincer, M. (1987). Combat stress reaction, posttraumatic stress disorder and somatic complaints among Israeli soldiers. *Journal of Psychosomatic Research, 31,* 131–137.

Solomon, Z., Weisenberg, M. Schwarzwald, J., & Mikulincer, M. (1987b). Post traumatic stress disorder amongst front line soldiers with combat stress reactions: The 1982 Israeli experience. *American Journal of Psychiatry, 144,* 448–454.

van der Kolk, B. A. (1989). The compulsion to repeat the trauma: Re-enactment, revictimization and masochism. *Psychiatric Clinics of North America, 12*(2), 389–411.

van der Kolk, B. A., Greenberg, M., Boyd, H., & Krystal, J. (1985). Inescapable shock, neurotransmitters, and addiction to trauma: Toward a psychobiology of posttraumatic stress. *Biological Psychiatry, 20*(3), 314–325.

Warshaw, M. G., Fierman, E., Pratt, L., Hunt, M., Yonkers, K. A., Maisson, A. D., & Keller, M. B. (1993). Quality of life and dissociation in anxiety disorder patients with histories of trauma or PTSD. *American Journal of Psychiatry, 150*(10), 1512–1516.

Weisaeth, L. (1989). A study of behavioural responses to an industrial disaster. *Acta Psychiatrica Scandinavica, 80*(Suppl. 355), 13–24.

Yehuda, R., & Antelman, S. M. (1993). Criteria for rationally evaluating animal models of posttraumatic stress disorder. *Biological Psychiatry, 33*, 479–486.

Yehuda R., & McFarlane, A. C. (1995). The conflict between current knowledge about PTSD and its original conceptual basis. *American Journal of Psychiatry, 152*, 1705–1713.

Yehuda, R., Resnick, H., Kahana, B., & Giller, E. L. (1993a). Long-lasting hormonal alterations to extreme stress in humans: Normative or maladaptive? *Psychosomatic Medicine, 55*, 287–297.

Yehuda, R., Southwick, S.M., Krystal, J. H., Bremner, D., Charney, D. S., & Mason, J. W. (1993b). Enhanced suppression of cortisol following dexamethasone administration in posttraumatic stress disorder. *American Journal of Psychiatry, 150*(1), 83–86.

CHAPTER 9

The Complexity of Adaptation to Trauma

Self-Regulation, Stimulus Discrimination, and Characterological Development

BESSEL A. VAN DER KOLK

. . . traumatized people are frequently misdiagnosed and mistreated in the mental health system. Because of the number and complexity of their symptoms, their treatment is often fragmented and incomplete. Because of their characteristic difficulties with close relationships, they are vulnerable to become re-victimized by caregivers. They may become engaged in ongoing, destructive interactions, in which the medical . . . system replicates the behavior of the abusive family.
—HERMAN (1992a, p. 123)

In the early 1970's, when psychiatry rediscovered the impact of trauma on soma and psyche, only a sparse literature on "traumatic neuroses" was available to guide the creation of a diagnostic construct for posttraumatic stress disorder (PTSD). The small group of clinicians who helped establish the diagnosis of PTSD in the third edition of the *Diagnostic and Statistical Manual of Mental Disorders* (DSM-III; American Psychiatric Association, 1980) relied on new clinical discoveries and on a very limited literature on traumatized adults—such as combat veterans (e.g., Kardiner, 1941), burn victims (Andreasen, Norris, & Hartford, 1971), and Holocaust survivors (Krystal, 1968)—to help them define PTSD. The committee eventually adopted a set of diagnostic criteria that was largely based on Abram Kardiner's 1941 descriptions in *The Traumatic Neuroses of War*. Subsequently, a vast research literature has confirmed the relevance of PTSD as a diagnostic construct. However, at the same time, studies of various traumatized populations have shown that the syndrome of intrusions, avoidance, and hyperarousal does not begin to capture the complexity of long-term adaptations to traumatic life experiences, particularly in children and in adults who were traumatized as children. These long-term adaptations vary a great deal according to the developmental level of the victim at the time of the trauma, the victim's personal relationship to the agent responsible for the trauma, temperamental predispositions, gender, cultural context, and other variables that we have tried to address in this book (Herman, 1992b; see Chapters 1, 4, 5, 7, 10, 13, and 14, this volume).

Exposure to extreme stress affects people at many levels of functioning: somatic, emotional, cognitive, behavioral, and characterological (e.g., van der Kolk, 1988; Kroll, Habenicht, & McKenzie, 1989; Cole & Putnam, 1992; Herman, 1992b; van der Kolk et al., 1993). For example, childhood trauma sets the stage for a variety of psychiatric disorders, such as borderline personality disorder (BPD; Herman, Perry, & van der Kolk, 1989; Ogata et al., 1989), somatization disorder (e.g., Saxe et al., 1994), dissociative disorders (e.g., Ross et al., 1990; Saxe et al., 1993; Kluft, 1991; Putnam, 1989), self-mutilation (van der Kolk, Perry, & Herman, 1991), eating disorders (Herzog, Staley, Carmody, Robbins, & van der Kolk, 1993), and substance abuse (Abueg & Fairbank, 1992). Naive one-to-one notions about the causal relationships between trauma and these disorders would oversimplify the very complex interrelationships among specific traumas, secondary adversities, environmental chaos and neglect, nature of preexisting and subsequent attachment patterns, temperament, special competencies, and other contributions to the genesis of these problems. However, if clinicians fail to pay attention to the contribution of past trauma to the current problems in patients with these diagnoses, they may fail to see that they seem to organize much of their lives around repetitive pattens of reliving and warding off traumatic memories, reminders, and affects. Whether clinicians accept the fundamental reality of past trauma in the lives of many of their patients will determine whether they understand their communications as psychotic distortions of reality or as derivations of inner experience. Therapists' attitudes toward these symptoms—whether they are viewed as bizarre behaviors that need to be abolished, or as misguided attempts at self-regulation—will critially determine approaches to treatment. If these patients' tales of past trauma are irrelevant or concocted, it is madness to join them in their delusions. On the other hand, if clinicians deny the essential truth of their patients' experiences, they can only aggravate feelings of rage and helplessness by invalidating the realities of their patients' lives.

Since the creation of the diagnosis of PTSD, it has become clear that the long-term effects of trauma are numerous and complicated (see Table 9.1). Intrapsychic, relational, and social factors are not the only issues that contribute to the long-term adjustment to trauma; the biological consequences of traumatization have a different impact at different stages of development as well. Although both adults and children may respond to a traumatic event with generalized hyperarousal, attentional difficulties, problems in stimulus discrimination, inability to self-regulate, and dissociative processes, these problems have very different effects on young children than they do on mature adults. For example, Pitman (1995) showed that people who developed PTSD secondary to child abuse had more profound physiological dysregulation in response to nontraumatic stimuli than did people who developed PTSD as adults. In addition, interpersonal traumas are likely to have more profound effects than impersonal ones. For example, a survivor of a hurricane may develop conditioned emotional responses to certain noises and weather conditions; by contrast, people who have been physically and sexually molested as children may develop a host of distrustful, fearful, and dissociative responses to a range of stimuli associated with intimacy, aggression, and the negotiation of trust.

After a brief discussion of the role of secure attachments in protecting individuals against being traumatized, this chapter then describes (1) how trauma leads to a variety of problems with the regulation of affective states, such as anger, anxiety, and sexuality; (2) how affect dysregulation makes

TABLE 9.1. Long-Term Effects of Trauma

Generalized hyperarousal and difficulty in modulating arousal
    Aggression against self and others
    Inability to modulate sexual impulses
    Problems with social attachments—excessive dependence or isolation

Alterations in neurobiological processes involved in stimulus discrimination
    Problems with attention and concentration
    Dissociation
    Somatization

Conditioned fear responses to trauma-related stimuli

Shattered meaning propositions
    Loss of trust, hope, and sense of agency
    Loss of "thought as experimental action"

Social avoidance
    Loss of meaningful attachments
    Lack of participation in preparing for future

people vulnerable to engage in a variety of pathological attempts at self-regulation, such as self-mutilation, eating disorders, and substance abuse; (3) how extreme arousal is accompanied by (a) dissociation and (b) the loss of capacity to put feelings into words (alexithymia and somatization); and (4) how failure to establish a sense of safety and security leads to characterological adaptations that include problems with self-efficacy, shame, and self-hatred, as well as problems in working through interpersonal conflicts. Such problems are expressed either in excessive dependence or in its counterpart— social isolation, lack of trust, and a failure to establish mutually satisfying relationships. The chapter concludes with a brief description of the deliberations concerning the definition of complex trauma in DSM-IV and ICD-10, as well as of treatment implications.

SECURE ATTACHMENTS AS A DEFENSE AGAINST TRAUMA

All people mature and thrive in a social context that has profound effects on how they cope with life's stresses. Particularly early in life, the social context plays a critical role in buffering an individual against stressful situations, and in building the psychological and biological capacities to deal with further stresses. The primary function of parents can be thought of as helping children modulate their arousal by attuned and well-timed provision of playing, feeding, comforting, touching, looking, cleaning, and resting—in short, by teaching them skills that will gradually help them modulate their own arousal. Secure attachment bonds serve as primary defenses against trauma-induced psychopathology in both children and adults (Finkelhor & Browne, 1984). In children who have been exposed to severe stressors, the quality of the parental bond is probably the single most important determinant of long-term damage (McFarlane, 1988).

As people mature, the safety of parent–child interplay gradually extends itself to include a combination of skills to regulate emotional arousal and to derive comfort from social supports. Coping with stress entails such factors as being able to mobilize one's skills to take care of oneself, knowing how to access social support, and being able to rely on protection from outside when one's own resources are inadequate. Our own studies (van der Kolk & Fisler, 1994) have shown that traumatized adults with childhood histories of severe neglect have a particularly poor long-term prognosis, compared with traumatized individuals who had more secure attachment bonds as children. Consistent external support appears to be a necessary condition for most children to learn to comfort and soothe themselves, and later to derive comfort from the presence of others.

AFFECT DYSREGULATION
IN TRAUMATIZED INDIVIDUALS

The Development of Affect
Regulation/Dysregulation

As noted above, caregivers play a critical role in modulating children's physiological arousal by providing a balance between soothing and stimulation; this balance, in turn, regulates normal play and exploratory activity. Stern (1983) calls this "affect attunement" between caregivers and infants. When very young children are removed from their primary caregivers (usually their mothers), they go through an initial period of behavioral agitation, accompanied by increases in heart rate and body temperature, followed by depression. During this time, they suffer from sleep problems (an increase in arousal and time spent awake) and show a decrease in autonomic activity (Reite, Seiler, & Short, 1978). Upon reunion with their mothers, children may continue to show behavioral changes; the caregivers' response during this time seems to play a critical role in modulating the long-term effects of separation (Field & Reite, 1984).

Whereas adequate caregivers maintain an optimal level of physiological arousal, unresponsive or abusive parents may promote chronic hyperarousal, which may have enduring effects on the ability to modulate strong emotions. Recent research has shown that as many as 80% of abused infants and children have disorganized/disoriented attachment patterns, including unpredictable alterations of approach and avoidance toward their mothers, as well as other conflict behaviors (e.g., prolonged freezing, stilling, or slowed "underwater" movements) (Lyons-Ruth, 1991). Thus, early attunement combines with temperamental predispositions to "set" the capacity to regulate future arousal; limitations in this capacity are likely to play a major role in long-term vulnerability to psychopathological problems after exposure to potentially traumatizing experiences.

As children mature, they gradually become less vulnerable to overstimulation and learn to tolerate higher levels of excitement. Over time, their need for physical proximity to their primary caregivers to maintain comfort decreases, and children start spending more time playing with their peers and with their fathers (Field, 1985). Secure children learn how to take care of themselves effectively as long as the environment is more or less predictable; simultaneously, they learn how to get help when they are distressed. In contrast, avoidant children learn how to organize their behavior effectively under ordinary conditions, but they remain unable to communicate or interpret emotional signals. In other words, they know how to handle cognition, but not affect (Crittenden, 1994).

Cole and Putnam (1992) have proposed that people's core concepts of themselves are defined to a substantial degree by their capacity to regulate their internal states and by their behavioral responses to external stress. The lack of development, or loss, of self-regulatory processes in abused children leads to problems with self-definition: (1) disturbances of the sense of self, such as a sense of separateness, loss of autobiographical memories, and disturbances of body image; (2) poorly modulated affect and impulse control, including aggression against self and others; and (3) insecurity in relationships, such as distrust, suspiciousness, lack of intimacy, and isolation . Abused children have trouble functioning in social settings; they tend either to draw attention to themselves or to withdraw from social interactions. Thus, they tend to display either angry, threatening, fearless, acting-out behavior or meek, submissive, fearful, incompetent behavior. Problems in articulating cause and effect make it hard for them to appreciate their own contributions to their problems and set the stage for paranoid attributions.

Manifestations of the Absence of Self-Regulation

The lack or loss of self-regulation is possibly the most far-reaching effect of psychological trauma in both children and adults. The DSM-IV field trials for PTSD clearly demonstrated that the younger the age at which the trauma occurred, and the longer its duration, the more likely people were to have long-term problems with the regulation of anger, anxiety, and sexual impulses (van der Kolk, Roth, Pelcovitz, & Mandel, 1993). Pitman, Orr, and Shalev (1993) have pointed out that in PTSD, hyperarousal goes well beyond simple conditioning. The fact that the stimuli that precipitate emergency responses are not conditioned enough and that many triggers not directly related to the traumatic experience may precipitate extreme reactions is merely the beginning of the problem. Loss/lack of self-regulation may be expressed in many different ways: as a loss of ability to focus on appropriate stimuli; as attentional problems; as an inability to inhibit action when aroused (loss of impulse control); or as uncontrollable feelings of rage, anger, or sadness. The results of a study by McFarlane, Weber, and Clark (1993) of event-related potentials in people with PTSD illustrate these various effects (see Chapter 10, this volume, for details).

In Chapter 10, I discuss how people with PTSD have at least two different abnormal levels of psychophysiological responses to their environment: (1) conditioned responses to specific reminders of the trauma, and (2) generalized hyperarousal to intense but intrinsically neutral stimuli. The first level involves heightened physiological arousal to sounds, images, and thoughts related to specific traumatic incidents. One way of measuring whether treatment has been effective is to see whether traumatized people are less physiologically aroused when they are reexposed to reminders of the trauma (Keane & Kaloupek, 1982). However, Shalev and Rogel-Fuchs (1993) have shown that desensitization to specific trauma-related mental images does not affect the overall physiological sensitivity of people with PTSD; they continue to have difficulty evaluating sensory stimuli and to mobilize excessive levels of physiological arousal to meet ordinary demands. The inability of people with PTSD to properly integrate memories of the trauma, and their tendency to get mired in revisiting the past over and over again, are mirrored physiologically in the continuing misinterpretation of innocuous stimuli as potential threats.

Problems with attention and simulus discrimination may account for the high comorbidity between PTSD and attention-deficit/hyperactivity disorder (ADHD) in traumatized children, such as sexually abused girls (Putnam, 1995). Problems with stimulus discrimination can also help explain the recurrent observation that, when aroused, traumatized people tend to lose the capacity to utilize their feelings as guides for assessing the available information and taking appropriate action; instead, emotional arousal comes to precipitate fight-or-flight reactions (Krystal, 1978; van der Kolk & Ducey, 1989). Thus, they often go immediately from stimulus to response, without making the necessary psychological assessment of the meaning of what is going on.

Traumatized patients experience current stressors with an intensity of emotion that belongs to the past, and that has little value in the present. Unaware of the traumatic antecedents, they tend to experience their own affect storms, as well as emotional reactions from others, as retraumatizing. Thus, the feelings that belong to the trauma are continually reexperienced on an interpersonal level; these patients lead traumatizing and traumatized lives. In an apparent attempt to compensate for their hyperarousal, traumatized people tend to "shut down." On a behavioral level, they do this by avoiding stimuli reminiscent of the trauma; on a psychobiological level, they do this through emotional numbing, which may extend to both trauma-related and everyday experience (Litz & Keane, 1989). Thus, people with chronic PTSD tend to suffer from numbing of responsiveness to the environment, which gets in the way of taking pleasure in ordinary events. This anhedonia is punctuated by intermittent excessive responses to traumatic reminders.

SELF-DESTRUCTIVE BEHAVIORS AS ATTEMPTS AT SELF-REGULATION

Traumatized people employ a variety of methods to regain control over their problems with affect regulation. Often these efforts are self-destuctive and bizarre; they range from self-mutilation to unusual sexual practices, and from bingeing and purging to drug and alcohol abuse (van der Kolk & Fisler, 1994; Briere & Runtz, 1988; Hall, Tice, Beresford, Wooley, & Hall, 1989; Palmer, Oppenheimer, Dignon, Chaloner, & Howells, 1990; van der Kolk et al., 1991; Browne & Finkelhor, 1986).

Self-Mutilation

Research has amply demonstrated that self-mutilation is a common reaction to social isolation and fear, both in humans and in nonhuman primates. For example, isolated young rhesus monkeys engage in self-biting, head slapping, and head banging (Kraemer, 1985). Green (1978) found that 41% of his sample of abused children engaged in head banging, self-biting, self-burning, and self-cutting. In a study of the traumatic antecedents of BPD, we found a highly significant relationship between childhood sexual abuse and various forms of self-harm later in life, particularly self-cutting and self-starving (van der Kolk et al., 1991). Clinical studies consistently report childhood his-tories of physical or sexual abuse, or repeated surgery, in self-mutilators (Favazza, 1987; Lacey & Evans, 1986; Bowlby, 1984; van der Kolk, 1987). Simpson and Porter (1981) concluded that "self-destructive activities were not primarily related to conflict, guilt, and superego pressure, but to more primitive behavior patterns originating in painful encounters with hostile caretakers during the first years of life" (p. 430).

Dissociation is a frequent concomitant of self-injury. Many of these patients report feeling numb and "dead" prior to harming themselves (Pattison & Kahan, 1983; Demitrack, Putnam, Brewerton, Brandt, & Gold, 1990). They often claim not to experience pain during self-injury, and report a sense of relief afterwards (Roy, 1985). Episodes of self-mutilation often follow feelings of disappointment or abandonment (Gardner & Cowdry, 1985; Stone, 1987; Leibenluft, Gardner, & Cowdry, 1987; Favazza, 1989; Simpson & Porter, 1981). The experience of dissociation itself may account for the urge to cut: The subjective sense of deadness and disconnection from others, which originally may have helped these individuals to cope with extreme distress, is also quite a dysphoric experience. Many people who habitually engage in deliberate self-harm report that self-mutilation makes them feel better and restores a feeling of being alive. In an unpublished study, I collaborated with eight self-mutilators, and measured their pain responses at times when they felt an extreme urge to cut themselves. During these times, six out of these eight subjects did not register pain in response to any painful stimulus that could be applied within ethical limits. Intravenous injection of naltrexone abolished the analgesia, but the subjects claimed that this did not provide as much relief as cutting or burning themselves did. This study suggested to me that these patients had develped a conditioned analgesic response to an environmental stressor, which made them feel numb. The fact that they were able to physically experience pain after a naltrexone injection suggested that this analgesia and numbing were mediated by endogenous opioids. Cutting, according to these patients, gave them relief and made them feel alive. I do not know what neurochemical agent may be released at the moment of cutting that may provide the sort of relief reported by these patients.

In a study of childhood antecedents of self-destructive behavior in psychiatric outpatients (van der Kolk et al., 1991), we found that the age at which their abuse and/or neglect had occurred played an important role in both the severity of their self-destructive behavior and the form it took: The earlier the abuse, the more self-directed the aggression. Abuse during early childhood and latency was strongly correlated with suicide attempts, self-mutilation, and other self-injurious behavior. In contrast, abuse in adolescence was significantly associated only with anorexia nervosa and with increased risk taking. In this prospective study we followed our subjects for an average of 4 years, measuring continued self-destructive behavior during this period. Histories of sexual abuse, in particular, predicted continued suicide attempts, self-mutilation, and other self-destructive acts. Severity of neglect scores predicted continued suicide attempts, self-mutilation, and other self-destructive behaviors. During this period, the subjects with the most severe separation and neglect histories were the most self-destructive. We concluded that childhood abuse contributes heavily to the initiation of self-destructive behavior, but that the lack of secure attachments maintains it. Those subjects who had sustained prolonged separations from their primary caregivers, and those who could not remember feeling special or loved by anyone as children, were least able to utilize interpersonal resources to control their self-destructive behavior during the course of the study.

Suicide attempts, self-cutting, and other self-injurious behaviors may serve different functions in regulating affective states. They may be active attempts to kill, injure, or quiet menacing hallucinations; they may also be ways to manage unbearable affects by altering interpersonal conditions as well as the biological homeostasis (Bowlby, 1984; van der Kolk, 1987; Field, 1985).

Eating Disorders

The relationships between eating disorders and childhood trauma is a controversional one. Histories of childhood trauma (and in particular of sexual abuse) keep showing up in studies of clinical populations with eating disorders, with rates ranging from 7% (Lacey, 1990) to 69% (Folsom, Krahn, Canum, Gold, & Silk, 1989). In nonclinical population samples, eating disorders are not consistently associated with histories of childhood trauma (Pope & Hudson, 1993). However, in a large epidemiological study of the high school population of Minnesota, Hernandez and DiClemente (1992) found that sexually abused girls were at a greater risk for developing eating disorders. In our BPD study (van der Kolk et al., 1991), we found that bulimia nervosa was not related to childhood abuse and neglect, whereas abuse in adolescence was related to anorexia nervosa. In a recent preliminary study of women with anorexia nervosa, bulimia nervosa, or both conditions, Herzog et al. (1993) found that severity of childhood sexual abuse was correlated with the duration and severity of eating disorders in all three groups. The relatively high frequencies of dissociation, self-mutilation, and inconsistent family rules reported by the eating-disordered subjects with childhood sexual abuse parallel the dissociative phenomena, self-destructive behaviors, and patterns of parental care commonly reported among patients with BPD (Herman et al., 1989; Sanders & Giolas, 1991). However, the precise relationship between childhood abuse and eating disorders remains to be defined. It is possible that unsupportive early environments, in which children's needs are left unattended, both make children vulnerable to sexual abuse and leave them to their own devices in attempts to regulate dysphoric affective states, which may come to include abnormal eating patterns.

Substance Abuse

Studies of populations with substance abuse consistently report childhood histories of abuse and neglect in much higher proportions than are found in the general population (e.g., Hernandez & DiClemente, 1992; Abueg & Fairbank, 1992; Lisak, 1993). In traumatized adults, high rates of alcohol and drug abuse have been reported as well (Keane & Wolfe, 1990; Kulka et al., 1990). Khantzian (1985) has proposed a self-medication theory of substance abuse, in which he suggests that drugs of abuse are selected according to their specific psychotropic effects. For example, heroin has powerful effects on muting feelings of rage and aggression, whereas cocaine has significant antidepressant action. Alcohol is probably the oldest medication for the treatment of posttraumatic stress, and may well be an effective short-term medication for sleep disturbances, nightmares, and other intrusive PTSD symptoms (Keane, Gerardi, Lyons, & Wolfe, 1988; Jellinek & Williams, 1987). Although alcohol may effectively dampen PTSD symptomatology, cessation of drinking may cause a rebound effect, in which people again experience sleep loss, nightmares, and other traumatic intrusions (Abueg & Fairbank, 1992). It is likely that substance abuse treatment of traumatized individuals can be more effective if the issue of recurrent posttraumatic problems during withdrawal is vigorously addressed. Self-help groups such as Alcoholics Anonymous seem to have grasped this issue intuitively, and, with extraordinary insight, seem to have incorporated effective posttraumatic treatment in their Twelve Steps.

DISSOCIATION

Many traumatized children, and adults who were traumatized as children, have noted that when they are under stress they can make themselves "disappear." That is, they can watch what is going on from a distance while having the sense that what is occurring is not really happening to them, but to someone else. In

Chapter 13, van der Hart, Marmar, and I discuss the central role of dissociation in the etiology and maintenance of PTSD. Recent research has rediscovered Janet's finding that dissociation is an integral aspect of PTSD (van der Kolk & van der Hart, 1989; Marmar et al., 1994; van der Kolk et al., in press). When people develop a split between the "observing self" and the "experiencing self," they report having the feeling of leaving their bodies and observing what happens to them from a distance (Gelinas, 1983; Noyes & Kletti, 1977; van der Hart, Steele, Boon, & Brown, 1993). During a traumatic experience, dissociation allows a person to observe the event as a spectator, to experience no, or only limited, pain or distress; and to be protected from awareness of the full impact of what has happened.

When children are repeatedly exposed to extreme stress, they develop what van der Hart (van der Hart, van der Kolk, & Boon, 1996) has called "tertiary dissociation": Elements of the traumatic experience may be organized by a separate state of mind, which may only come into play when that particular element of the traumatic experience is activated. Very complex forms of such secondary dissociations can be found in dissociative identity disorder (formerly called multiple personality disorder), which has also been described as a complex form of PTSD with origins in severe childhood traumatization (Kluft, 1991).The capacity to dissociate allows many of these patients to develop domains of competence that can make them quite sucessful in some areas of life, while dissociated aspects of the self contain the memories related to the trauma, usually leaving devastating traces in the capacity to negotiate issues related to intimacy and aggression. Dissociation can be an effective way to continue functioning while the trauma is going on, but if it continues to be utilized after the acute trauma has passed, it comes to interfere with everyday functioning. While providing protective detachment from overwhelming affects, it also results in a subjective sense of "deadness" and a sense of disconnection from others (see Chapter 13, this volume).

Adults who suffer from a dissociative disorder are also likely to suffer from nightmares and flashbacks, to have psychosomatic problems, to make suicide attempts,and to engage in self-mutilation and substance abuse. When Saxe et al. (1993, 1994) administered the Dissociative Experiences Scale (DES; Bernstein & Putnam, 1986) to 111 consecutive state hospital admissions, they found that 15% had very high scores. All of these patients reported histories of sexual abuse; 86% had histories of physical abuse; and 79% reported witnessing domestic violence. Of the high-scoring group, 100% also met diagnostic criteria for PTSD, 71% for BPD, and 64% for somatization disorder. Another study of patients with high DES scores found very high correlations with familial loss in childhood and with both intrafamilial and extrafamilial sexual abuse (Irwin, 1994). Unfortunately, almost none of these patients had been diagnosed as having a dissociative disorder or PTSD. Recent research increasingly supports the notion that making the appropriate diagnoses in these chronically traumatized patients has dramatic beneficial effect on their long-term prognosis (Ross, 1995).

Containing aspects of the traumatic exerience in a separate ego state can be understood as an exaggeration and fixation of normal developmental processes. School-age children are at a developmental level where they have learned object constancy. This is a stage of development in which they know that things are not necessarily what they appear. Children at that age take pleasure in trying on different roles; they spend endless hours trying out what it feels like to take on different identities (e.g., taking the roles of different television characters, or playing cowboys and Indians). When children live under conditions of extraordinary stress, some can utilize this capacity to disappear into the identities of different characters to escape their fate. However, young children only habitually come to utilize alternative identities to escape unbearable situations when their caregivers are unable or unwilling to do what caregivers usually do to help children change their internal states from agitated and dysphoric to calm and contented (e.g., stroking, rocking, verbalizing, and singing). This occurs not only in the context of intrafamilial violence and neglect, but also when children have to undergo repeated medical or surgical procedures. In recent years, Frank Putnam's (1995) prospective study of the development of sexually abused girls has shown that the expressions of such pathological dissociation include amnesias, rapid shifts in behavior, visual hallu- cinations, "spacing out," and "lying."

ALEXITHYMIA AND SOMATIZATION: LOSS OF WORDS AND SYMBOLS TO COMMUNICATE WITH SELF AND OTHERS

Henry Krystal (1978) was the first to suggest that trauma results in a "de-differentiation of affect"—that is, a loss of ability to identify specific emotions to serve as a guide for taking appropriate actions. He noted that this inability to create semantic constructs to identify somatic states is related to the development of psychosomatic reactions and to aggression against self and others. Our recent positron emission tomography (PET) scan study of people with PTSD (Rauch et al., in press) showed that when people with PTSD are exposed to stimuli reminiscent of their trauma, there is an increase in perfusion of the areas in the right hemisphere associated with emotional states and autonomic arousal. Moreover, there is a simultaneous decrease in oxygen utilization in Broca's area—the region in the left inferior frontal cortex responsible for generating words to attach to internal experience. These findings may account for the observation that trauma may lead to "speechless terror," which in some individuals interferes with the ability to put feelings into words, leaving emotions to be mutely expressed by dysfunction of the body. Recent studies (e.g., Harber

& Pennebaker, 1992) have documented that verbalization of traumatic experiences decreases psychosomatic symptoms.

Problems in the development of the utilization of words and symbols to identify feelings can start very early. Cicchetti and colleagues (Cicchetti & Beeghly, 1987; Cicchetti & White, 1990) have shown that maltreated toddlers use fewer words to describe how they feel and have more problems with attributing causality than do secure children of the same age. Secure children spend more time describing physiological states, such as hunger, thirst, and states of consciousness, and speak more often about negative emotions, such as hate, disgust, and anger. Not knowing how and what one feels may contribute to the impaired impulse control seen in abused children (Fish-Murray, Koby, & van der Kolk, 1987); having problems putting feelings into words and formulating flexible response strategies may make people likely to act on their feelings. Anticipating our recent PET scan findings, Cicchetti and White (1990) hypothesized that "the special difficulties that abused toddlers have expressing feelings in words may not be simply a reflection of psychological intimidation but rather a manifestation of neuroanatomical and neuro-physiological changes secondary to abusive or neglectful treatment" (p. 369).

People have been aware of a close association between trauma and somatization since the dawn of contemporary psychiatry. When Briquet (1859) published the first empirical investigation of hysteria, he concluded that hysteria seems to be associated with having a history of exposure to extreme stress. Briquet's descriptions of hysteria form the basis of the present-day diagnosis of somatization disorder (Mai & Mersky, 1980). Amnesia is one criterion for somatization disorder. Many studies describe histories of childhood sexual and/ or physical abuse in conjunction with dissociative processes in patients with somatoform disorders (Goodwin, Cheeves, & Connel, 1990; Loewenstein, 1990; Saxe et al., 1994; Spiegel, 1988a, 1988b; Terr, 1988). Studies since 1980 have repeatedly shown a close association between somatization and dissociation (e.g., Pribor, Yutzy, Dean, & Wetzel, 1993; Coons, Bowman, & Milstein, 1988; Putnam, Loewenstein, Silberman, & Post, 1984; Putnam et al., 1986; Ross, Heber, Norton, & Andreason, 1989; Loewenstein, 1990; Gorss, Doerr, Caldirola, Guzinski, & Ripley, 1980; Walker, Katon, Neraas, Jemelka, & Massoth, 1992; Saxe et al., 1994) and between somatization and PTSD (e.g., Walker et al., 1992; Saxe et al., 1994; McFarlane, Atchinson, Rafalowicz, & Papay, 1994) In one of the studies conducted in conjunction with the DSM-IV field trials for somatization disorder (Pribor et al., 1993), over 90% of 100 women with somatization disorder reported some type of abuse, and 80% reported being sexually abused as either children or adults. Somatization, dissociation, and abuse were significantly associated: The total number of somatization symptoms was directly proportional to the DES score.

In both the DSM-IV field trials for PTSD (van der Kolk et al., 1993) and our study of patients with dissociative disorders (Saxe et al., 1994), we came to the surprising conclusion that somatization rarely occurred in the absence of severe histories of trauma. In our study, 64% of patients with dissociative disorders also met criteria for somatization disorder (Saxe et al., 1994). Problems caused by reliance on action instead of symbolic representation are also common in traumatized adolescents: In the DSM-IV field trials for PTSD (Pelcovitz et al., in press) the abused adolescents were so out of touch with their feelings that they denied that their abuse had any impact on their lives. However, a high proportion were involved in abusive relationships with peers, or were engaged in high-risk behaviors and drug taking. Many of the girls had become pregnant at an early age.

Maybe these are the sorts of behaviors that fall within what Freud once called "the compulsion to repeat." Freud (1920/1955) pointed out that people who do not remember highly charged emotional events are at risk of repeating those unintegrated experiences both in the therapeutic relationship and in their current lives. He thought that when a memory is repressed, a patient "is obliged to repeat the repressed material as a contemporary experience, instead of . . . remembering it as something belonging to the past" (p. 18).

Prone to action, and deficient in words, these patients can often express their internal states more articulately in physical movements or in pictures than in words. Utilizing drawings and psychodrama may help them develop a language that is essential for effective communication and for the symbolic transformation that can occur in psychotherapy. Group psychotherapy may also be effective in providing them both with (inter)action and with borrowed words to express emotional states.

TRAUMA AND CHARACTER DEVELOPMENT

The combination of chronic dissociation, physical problems for which no medical cause can be found, and a lack of adequate self-regulatory processes is likely to have profound effects on personality development. These may include disturbances of the sense of oneself, such as a sense of separateness and disturbances of body image; a view of oneself as helpless, damaged, and ineffective; and difficulties with trust, intimacy, and self-assertion (van der Kolk, 1987; Herman, 1992a, 1992b; van der Kolk & Fisler, 1994; Cole & Putnam, 1992). Naturally, these processes have different impacts at different stages of personality development. Social support is an important factor in determining how the personality is shaped by problems of affect regulation. For example, we (Herman et al., 1989) found that most subjects who were diagnosed as suffering from BPD were first traumatized before the age of 7 within their own families, and suffered from substantial degrees of neglect as well.

What is striking about the impact of trauma on character is that, regardless of preexisting vulnerabilities, a previously well-functioning traumatized adult can experience an overall sharp deteriorization in his or her functioning (Tichener, 1986; Kardiner, 1941). Posttraumatic decline following adult trauma has been repeatedly documented in the World War II literature (e.g., Archibald & Tuddenham, 1956). Kardiner (1941) wrote that traumatic neurosis included "a deterioration that is not dissimilar to that in schizophrenia. . . . The diminution of interest and intelligence is due to the continuous shrinkage of the field of effective functioning and the gratifications derived therefrom" (p. 249). Kardiner noted that, once traumatized, a person "acts as if the original traumatic situation were still in existence and engages in protective devices which failed on the original occasion. This means in effect that this conception of the outer world and his conception of himself have been permanently altered" (p. 82).

The Internalization of the Trauma

On a cognitive level, people's life experiences shape the assumptions that determine the perceptions they select for day-to-day attention. These schemes then serve as road maps for subsequent actions and expectations (van der Kolk & Ducey, 1989; Pearlman & Saakvitne, 1995). Janoff-Bulman (1992) has spoken of the shattered assumptions in traumatized adults, while others (Cole & Putnam, 1992; Herman, 1992a, 1992b) have spelled out in great detail and with much clarity how trauma affects the development of character and concepts of the self.

Trauma-based internal schemes come to occupy a place in the traumatized person's views of himself or herself and the world (see Chapter 13). Often parallel schemes coexist, and these are activated in a state-dependent manner: High levels of competence and interpersonal sensitivity often exist side by side with self-hatred, lack of self-care, and interpersonal cruelty. Many people who were traumatized in their own families have great difficulty taking care of their own basic needs for hygiene, rest, and protection, even as they are exquisitely responsive to other people's needs. Many repeat their family patterns in interpersonal relationships, in which they may alternate between playing the role of victim and that of persecutor, often justifying their behavior by their feelings of betrayal and helplessness. The use of projective identification—attributing to others one's own most despised attributes, without consciously acknowledging the existence of those characteristics in oneself—has been thoroughly described by Kernberg (1975).

Impairment of Basic Trust

Trauma at any age, but particularly trauma that is inflicted by caregivers, generally has a profound effect on the capacity to trust (Burgess, Hartman, & McCormick, 1987; Nadelson, Notman, Zackson, & Gornick, 1982; Oates, 1984; Terr, 1983; Briere, 1988; Mezey & King, 1989; Pynoos et al., 1987). After traumatic events, perceptions of relationships tend to become filtered through those experiences. In our BPD study, most traumatized patients were clinging and dependent on the one hand, but socially isolated without mutually rewarding relationships on the other (Herman et al., 1989). Many had retreated into social isolation after years of frantic searches for rescuers. Having a history of helplessness with people in power, they tended to cast most subsequent relationships in terms of dominance and submission. When they were in a position of power, they often inspired fear and loathing; when they were in a subordinate position, they often felt helpless, behaved submissively, did not stand up for themselves, and tended to engage in idealization (and/or devaluation) at the expense of being able to experience their own competence. Clearly, treatment cannot address past trauma unless its reenactment in current relationships is vigorously taken up as well. Treatment often starts with prolonged negotiations centering around the issues of trust, power, and safety. Often little is accomplished until a major conflict arises and is negotiated successfully.

Lack of a Sense of Responsibility

One critical issue related to fixation at the developmental level of the trauma is the lack of capacity to attribute responsibility properly. Young children, by virtue of their cognitive level of development, attribute everything that happens to their own actions or their own magical thinking. However, trauma-related self-blame, guilt, and shame are not confined to traumatized children; those feelings are also found in more mature people, and may reflect a general loss of internal locus of control (Ferenczi, 1932/1955; Kluft, 1990; Ogata et al., 1989; Piaget, 1962; Paris & Zweig-Frank, 1992; Perry, Herman, van der Kolk, & Hoke, 1990; Rutter & Hersov, 1985; Sullivan, 1940). The DSM-IV field trials for PTSD confirmed that many traumatized people (particularly those who had been first traumatized as children) suffered from a profound sense of responsibility not only for their own abuse, but for subsequent problems over which they had no control. They are like preoperational children in that their lack of conservation and object constancy seemed to make it impossible for them to see that they were not the center of the universe; they often continued to have great difficulty in seeing various people's contributions to interpersonal problems.

Negative Effects on Identity

Traumatized people often fail to maintain a personal sense of significance, competence, and inner worth. If they have been victims of interpersonal abuse, they often identify with the aggressor and express hate for people who remind them of their own helplessness. Identifying with the aggressor seems to help them deal with their anxiety. Many of these patients have learned to behave competently and responsibly early in life, and continue to act that way as adults. Simultaneously, they tend to perceive themselves as being unlovable, despicable, and weak. Traumatized patients are frequently triggered by current sensory and affective stimuli into a reliving of feelings and memories of their past trauma. Being so easily propelled into feeling aroused, anxious, freightened, and dissociated, they cannot count on themselves to have a stable presence in the world, and to react consistently to their environment. This inner sense of hatefulness and unpredictability will generally be expressed in social isolation and avoidance of intimate relationships. These patients often experience their competence as part of a "cover story" with which they "fake" their way through life.

Impact on Play and Relationships with Others

One of the principal tasks of childhood is to learn to negotiate collaborative relationships with other human beings. Many studies of traumatized children have established that they often have serious problems in their capacity to play (Terr, 1988; Pynoos & Nader, 1988). After exposure to trauma, children tend either to be excessively shy and withdrawn, or to bully and frighten other children (Cicchetti & White, 1990). Their inability to regulate their arousal, to articulate their feelings in words, or to attend to appropriate stimuli, and the ease with which they are triggered to reexperience feelings and sensations related to the trauma, make it difficult for them to be attuned to their environments. The functions of childhood play are to enable children to try out different roles and different outcomes; to learn to appreciate how others experience the world; and to gain mastery over dreaded feelings, people, and situations. When play is curtailed, the capacity to integrate the positive and negative is aborted: Good and bad, power and helplessness, affection and anger continue to be experienced as separate ego states. This promotes the likelihood of continuing the characteristic way of coping with fear—by dissociating, thereby consciously disavowing and not personally "owning" the reality of the situation. The overall result is that many traumatized children miss a critical developmental stage in which issues of competition, intimacy, and play are being negotiated. Without these skills, adult life tends to be bleak and devoid of meaning. One of our studies (van der Kolk et al., 1991) indicated that the capacity to derive comfort from the presence of another human being was eventually a more powerful predictor than the trauma history itself of whether patients improved and were able to give up chronically self-destructive activities.

Excessive Interpersonal Sensitivity

After exposure to interpersonal abuse, people learn to watch their fellow human beings like hawks. Many people who were traumatized by their own caregivers develop an uncanny ability to read the needs and feelings of people who may have power over them. This may well alternate with episodes of extraordinary failure to understand other people's motives. Early exposure to abusive and unpredictable parents makes many children exquisitely aware of other people's needs—a capacity that they can subsequently utilize for self-protection. Unfortunately, such exquisite interpersonal sensitivity often lacks a feeling of personal satisfaction, as it is a mere replication of a survival skill acquired in childhood, and not accompanied by a sense of trust, belonging, and intimacy.

The Compulsion to Repeat the Trauma

Many traumatized people become involved in social situations that bear a striking similarity to the context in which they were first traumatized. An example from a classic movie is the title role in *The Pawnbroker*, played by Rod Steiger. People engaged in these behavioral reenactments are rarely consciously aware that they are repeating earlier life experiences. Freud (1896/1962) thought that the aim of such repetitions is to gain mastery, but clinical experience shows that this rarely happens; instead, repetition causes further suffering for the victims or for other people in their surroundings. Children seem more likely than adults to engage in compulsive behavioral repetition accompanied by a lack of conscious awareness of the trauma (Bowlby, 1984). In behavioral reenactments of the trauma, a person may play the role of victim, victimizer, or both.

Victimizing Others

Numerous studies of family violence have found a direct relationship between the severity of childhood abuse and later endencies to victimize others (Burgess et al., 1987; Green, 1983; Pynoos & Nader, 1988; Widom, 1987; Mezey & King, 1989; Burgess, Hartman, McClausland, & Powers, 1984; Groth, 1979; Lewis et al., 1988; Lewis, Lovely, Yeager, & Della Femina, 1989; Werner, 1989). Reenactment of one's own victimization seems to be a major cause of the cycle of violence (Widom, 1987). Numerous studies have shown that criminals often have histories of physical and/or sexual abuse (e.g., Burgess et al., 1987). In a prospective study of 34 sexually molested boys, Burgess et al. (1987) found that many began to engage in drug abuse, juvenile delinquency, and criminal behavior within a few years of the start of their abuse. Lewis et al. (1988, 1989) have extensively studied the association between childhood abuse and subsequent victimization of others. As an example, they found in one study (Lewis et al., 1988) that of the 14 juveniles condemned to death for murder in the United States in 1987, 12 had been brutally physically abused, and 5 had been sodomized by relatives.

Revictimization

Once people have been traumatized, they are vulnerable to being victimized on future occasions (Hilberman, 1980; Mezey & Taylor, 1988; Mezey & King, 1989; Groth, 1979; Russell, 1986). Rape victims are more likely to be raped again, and women who were physically or sexually abused as children are more likely to be abused as adults. Victims of child sexual abuse are at high risk of becoming prostitutes (Field, 1985; Finkelhor & Browne, 1984). Diane Russell (1986), in a careful study on the effects of incest on the life of women, found that few women made a conscious connection between their childhood victimization and their drug abuse, prostitution, and suicide attempts. Whereas 38% of a random sample of women reported incidents of rape or attempted rape after age 14, 68% of those with a childhood history of incest did. Twice as many women with a history of incest as women without such a history reported physical violence in their marriages (27%), and more than twice as many (53%) reported unwanted sexual advances by an unrelated authority figure, such as a teacher, clergyman, or therapist. Victims of father–daughter incest were four times more likely than nonvictims to report being asked to pose for pornography.

Increased Attachment in the Face of Danger

Writers and psychiatrists have long noted that people who are brutalized sometimes form very close attachments to their tormentors. Well-known examples in the United States include Patricia Hearst and Hedda Nussbaum. It is well understood that people in general, and children in particular, seek increased protection when they are frightened (van der Kolk, 1989). Most cultures have rituals designed to provide such increased care when members of those cultures have been traumatized. When nobody else is available, people may turn towards the sources of their fear for comfort: Both adults and children tend to develop strong emotional ties with people who intermittently harass, beat, and threaten them (Dutton & Painter, 1981; Herman, 1992a). This phenomenon was initially described as the "Stockholm syndrome." Hostages have put up bail for their captors and expressed wishes to marry them or have sexual relations with them (Dutton & Painter, 1981); abused children often cling to their parents and resist being removed from the home (Dutton & Painter, 1981; Kempe & Kempe, 1978); battered spouses may form intense attachments to their tormentors (Walker, 1979). Central components of these increased attachment bonds in response to threat include captivity, a lack of permeability, and absence of outside support (van der Kolk, 1989; Herman, 1992a).

People who were abused as children (many of whom learned to blame themselves early for the violence around them) are particularly likely to become partners in abusive relationships later, as suggested above. With their tendency to cast relationships in terms of power and dominance, these patients tend either to require total control over the relationship, or, when accepting a submissive position, to operate from the assumption that love, dedication, and exemplary behavior will enable them to avoid repeating the past (Frieze, 1983; Krugman, 1987; Walker, 1979). When the inevitable disagreements and power struggles that are part of any relationship cannot be managed with either total control or perfect submission, people with abuse histories tend to be unable to articulate their wishes, to fail to understand the other person's point of view, and to be unable to compromise. Having had little experience with nonviolent resolution of differences, partners in such relationships often alternate between an expectation of perfect behavior leading to perfect harmony, and a state of helplessness in which all verbal communication seems futile. A return to earlier coping mechanisms, such as self-blame, numbing (by means of emotional withdrawal or substance abuse), and physical violence, sets the stage for a repetition of the childhood trauma and "return of the repressed" (Ainsworth, 1967; Freud, 1939/1964; Frieze, 1983).

Trauma and the Development of Borderline Personality Disorder

In the mid-1980s, Judith Herman and I started a collaboration with Christopher Perry to study the relationship between childhood trauma and the development of BPD. On the basis of our work with incest victims and with Vietnam veterans, we proposed (Herman & van der Kolk, 1987) that trauma, especially prolonged trauma at the hands of people on whom one depends for nurturance and security, will significantly shape one's ways of organizing one's internal schemes and ways of coping with external reality. We theorized that the characteristic splitting of the self and others into "all-good" and "all-bad" portions represents a developmental arrest—a continued fragmentation of the self and a fixation on earlier modes of organizing experience. We proposed that self-mutilation, which is often experienced by therapists as a display of masochism or as a manipulative gesture (van der Kolk et al., 1991), may in fact be a way of regulating the psychological and biological equilibrium when ordinary ways of self-regulation have been disturbed by early trauma (Herman & van der Kolk, 1987). In this framework, psychotic episodes in borderline patients can be understood much like the flashbacks seen in Vietnam veterans: as intrusive recollections of traumatic memories that were not integrated into the individual's personal narrative, and instead were stored on a somatosensory level (see Chapter 10, this volume). This idea first introduced the issue of dissociation into our work; subsequent research in BPD has found dissociation to be highly correlated both with the degree of BPD psychopathology and with severity of childhood trauma (Kluft, 1990; Putnam, 1989).

Our study (Herman & van der Kolk, 1987) showed that many psychiatric patients had histories of trauma, but that the BPD patients stood out by having the most severe abuse histories: More than half of all BPD patients had histories of severe physical or sexual abuse starting before the age of 6. Trauma in patients with other diagnoses usually started much later, near puberty. Of our subjects who met diagnostic criteria for BPD, 13% did not report childhood histories of trauma; half of this 13% were amnesic for most of their childhoods, making their reports unreliable. However, a small proportion of our BPD patients did actually seem not to have a trauma history. Those subjects tended to report having been shy and frightened as children. Our explanation was that BPD is a function of having been chronically terrified during one's early development. For children who are being abused, for those who are pathologically shy, for those who have a chronic illness, or for those who experience frequent separations, the world can be a terrifying place. Exquisitely sensitive children may interpret normative growth experiences as terrifying. However, our study suggested that shyness and biological vulnerability are not the predominant factors leading people to develop BPD; the superimposition of childhood terror upon adult situations is most likely to be the key.

In our study we also found high correlations between having been sexually abused, particularly early in life, and self-mutilation and suicide attempts. We found a less significant relationship between anorexia nervosa and childhood sexual abuse. The younger patients were when they were abused and neglected, the more likely they were to engage in self-mutilation and other self-destructive acts; the abuse was engraved on both psychological and biological levels. In the long range, the patients with the most severe neglect histories were the ones who benefited least from psychotherapy. Since we did our study, several other investigations have found similar incidences of histories of physical and sexual abuse in BPD patients (e.g., Ogata et al., 1989; Zanarini, Gunderson, Marino, Schwartz, & Frankenburg, 1989).

COMPLEX TRAUMA AND THE DSM-IV

Aware of much of the research literature cited in this chapter, the committee charged with defining PTSD for the DSM-IV (American Psychiatric Association [APA], 1994) made an attempt to incorporate some of these findings into a more comprehensive definition of PTSD. The committee distilled various core symptoms out of the vast research literature as tentative criteria for "disorders of extreme stress not otherwise specified" (DESNOS), and clustered these symptoms into five main categories (Pelcovitz et al., in press; Herman 1992a, 1992b). These are listed in Table 9.2.

The DSM-IV field trials found that people who had been traumatized at an early age tended to have problems in all of these categories; these apparently disparate problems tended to occur together in the same individuals (van der Kolk et al., 1993, in press; Pelcovitz et al., in press). Trauma affected a whole range of core psychological functions: regulation of feelings; thinking clearly about what had happened in the past and was currently happening; ways in which feelings are expressed by the body; and people's views of themselves, strangers, and intimates. The older the victims were, and the shorter the duration of the trauma, the more likely they were to develop only the core PTSD symptoms; the longer the trauma, and the less protection, the more pervasive the damage. The field trials confirmed that trauma has its most profound impact during the first decade of life, and that its effects become less pervasive in more mature indi-

TABLE 9.2. Disorders of Extreme Stress Not Otherwise Specified (DESNOS): Proposed Criteria

A. Alterations in regulating affective arousal
   (1) chronic affect dysregulation
   (2) difficulty modulating anger
   (3) self-destructive and suicidal behavior
   (4) difficulty modulating sexual involvement
   (5) impulsive and risk-taking behaviors

B. Alterations in attention and consciousness
   (1) amnesia
   (2) dissociation

C. Somatization

D. Chronic characterological changes
   (1) alterations in self-perception: chronic guilt and shame; feelings of self-blame, of ineffectiveness, and of being permanently damaged
   (2) alterations in perception of perpetrator: adopting distorted beliefs and idealizing the perpetrator
   (3) alterations in relations with others:
      (a) an inability to trust or maintain relationships with others
      (b) a tendency to be revictimized
      (c) a tendency to victimize others

E. Alterations in systems of meaning
   (1) despair and hopelessness
   (2) loss of previously sustaining beliefs

viduals: Overwhelming experiences clearly had a different impact on people at different stages of development. Early and prolonged interpersonal trauma resulted, not in nonspecific character changes, but in the psychological problems captured in the DESNOS syndrome. DESNOS was eventually incorporated in the DSM-IV under the "Associated Features and Disorders" section (APA, 1994, p. 488). The ICD-10 created a separate category to accommodate enduring personality changes after catastrophic experience (F62.0) which includes (1) permanent hostility and distrust, (2) social withdrawal, (3) feelings of emptiness and hopelessness, (4) increased dependency and problems with modulation of aggression, (5) hypervigilance and irritability, and (6) feelings of alienation (World Health Organization, 1992, pp. 136–138).

TREATMENT IMPLICATIONS

If one understands the role of trauma in the psychopathology of DESNOS patients, much of their symptomatology can be explained as manifestations of adaptations to traumatic experiences appropriate to the developmental level at which the trauma occurred. Young children, like BPD patients, engage in preoperational thinking. The characteristic BPD defense of "splitting" can be understood as the persistence of preoperational thinking, in which the same objects cannot have different qualities at the same time. Thus, under stress, these patients fall back to the stage of cognitive development in which children are as yet incapable of ambivalence (van der Kolk, Hostetler, Herron, & Fisler, 1994). The histories of real trauma in the lives of these patients could help clinicians understand that their disturbed interpersonal relationships are based on a repetition of earlier actual experiences: lack of affect modulation, decreased capacity for true (guilty as opposed to rageful) depression, poor superego integration, lack of anxiety tolerance, poor impulse control, and poorly developed sublimatory channels.

If it is true that traumatized people tend to become fixated at the emotional and cognitive level at which they were traumatized—as was observed by Janet, Kardiner, and many subsequent students of trauma—they will tend to use the same means to deal with contemporary stresses that they used at the stage of development at which the trauma first occurred. This understanding should help in effective treatment of people with histories of severe and complex trauma. Since safe attachments appear to be the primary way in which children learn to regulate internal state changes (Putnam, 1988), the negotiation of interpersonal safety needs to be the first focus of treatment. Mental health professionals working with chronically traumatized patients become all too familiar with the patients' compulsion to repeat the trauma in the therapeutic relationship, and with their skill in enlisting therapists' help in recreating the context in which their trauma happened, whether it be their families of origin or some other traumatic situation. So the therapists often become rescuers, victims, or victimizers.

These are the patients who are force-fed, thrown into seclusion, medicated against their will, and/or transferred without warning, and who generally become the focus of therapists' rage and frustrations. These seem to be the patients who show up in emergency rooms, are maltreated, and return shortly afterwards, seemingly oblivious to the lessons from the previous encounter. It is the task of mental health professionals to understand what trauma is being reenacted and to take steps not to participate in these dramas. With their histories of interpersonal violations, these patients need to be approached with the greatest care, lest the abusive relationships be recreated (by the patients or their therapists). Since many of these patients have not learned to negotiate with people who are in a position to hurt them, they tend not to give clear signals when the reality of the therapeutic relationship itself becomes a violation. These are the patients who are most at risk of being abused by their therapists and by the medical profession in general (Gutheil, 1989; Herman, 1992a).

Therapists treating patients who exhibit affect dysregulation, who repetitively attempt suicide or engage in chronic self-destructive behavior, and who repeatedly seek medical help for problems for which no organic basis can be found need to be prepared to deal with issues of trauma, neglect, and abandonment, both in the past and as reexperienced in current relationships. With these patients, therapists must anticipate that painful emotions related to interpersonal safety, anger, and emotional needs may give rise to dissociative episodes, which may in turn be accompanied by increased self-destructive behavior. The work of therapy must clarify how current stresses are experienced as the return of past traumas, and how small disruptions in present relationships are seen as repetitions of prior abandonments. As features of this treatment, it is essential that the therapists provide validation, support, and avoidance of participation in a reenactment of the traumas (van der Kolk, 1989; Perry et al., 1990).

Fear needs to be tamed in order for people to be able to think and be conscious of their needs. A person's bodily response of fear can be mitigated by safety of attachments, by security of meaning schemes, and by a body whose reactions to environmental stress can be predicted and controlled. One of the mysteries of the mind is that as long as trauma is experienced in the form of speechless terror, the body continues to react to conditioned stimuli as a return of the trauma, without the capacity to define alternative courses of action. However, when the triggers are identified and the individual gains the capacity to attach words to somatic experiences, these experiences appear to lose some of their terror (Harber & Pennebaker, 1992). Thus, the task of therapy is both to create the capacity to be mindful of current experience, and to create symbolic representations of past traumatic experiences, with the goals of taming the associated terror and of desomatizing the memories.

REFERENCES

Abueg, F. R., & Fairbank, J. A. (1992). Behavioral treatment of posttraumatic stress disorder and co-occurring substance abuse. In P. A. Saigh (Ed.), *Posttraumatic stress disorder: A behavioral approach to assessment and treatment* (pp. 111–146). Boston: Allyn & Bacon.

Ainsworth, M. D. S. (1967). *Infancy in Uganda: Infant care and the growth of attachment.* Baltimore: Johns Hopkins University Press.

American Psychiatric Association (APA). (1980). *Diagnostic and statistical manual of mental disorders* (3rd ed.). Washington, DC: Author.

American Psychiatric Association (APA). (1994). *Diagnostic and statistical manual of mental disorders* (4th ed.). Washington, DC: Author.

Andreasen, N. J. C., Norris, A. S., & Hartford, C. E. (1971). Incidence of long term psychiatric complications in severely burnt adults. *Annals of Surgery, 174,* 785–793.

Archibald, H., & Tuddenham, R. (1956). Persistant stress reaction after combat. *Archives of General Psychiatry, 12,* 475–481.

Bernstein, E. M., & Putnam, F. W. (1986). Development, reliability, and validity of a dissociation scale. *Journal of Nervous and Mental Disease, 174,* 727–735.

Bowlby, J. (1984).Violence in the family as a disorder of the attachment and caregiving systems. *American Journal of Psychoanalysis, 44,* 9–27.

Briere, J. (1988). Long-term clinical correlates of childhood sexual victimization. *Annals of the New York Academy of Sciences, 528,* 327–334.

Briere, J., & Runtz, M. (1988). Symptomatology associated with childhood sexual victimization in a nonlineal adult sample. *Child Abuse and Neglect, 12,* 51–59.

Briquet, P. (1859). *Traité clinique et thérapeutique de l'hystérie.* Paris: Ballière.

Browne, A., & Finkelhor, D. (1986). Impact of child sexual abuse: A review of the research. *Psychological Bulletin, 99,* 66–77.

Burgess, A. W., Hartman, C. R., McClausland, M. P., & Powers, P. (1984). Response patterns in children and adolescents expoited through sex rings and pornography. *American Journal of Psychiatry, 141,* 656–662.

Burgess, A. W., Hartman, C. R., & McCormick, A. (1987). Abused to abuser: Antecedents of socially devient behavior. *American Journal of Psychiatry, 144,* 1431–1436.

Cicchetti, D., & Beeghly, M. (1987). Symbolic development in maltreatment of youngsters: An organizational psychopathology perspective. *Journal of Consulting and Clinical Psychology, 60,* 174–184.

Cicchetti, D., & White, J. (1990). Emotion and developmental psychopathology. In N. Stein, B., Leventhal, & T. Trebasso (Eds.), *Psychological and biological approaches to emotion* (pp. 359–382). Hillsdale, NJ: Erlbaum.

Cole, P., & Putnam, F. W. (1992). Effect of incest on self and social functioning: A developmental psychopathology perspective. *Journal of Consulting and Clinical Psychology, 60,* 174–184.

Coons, P. M., Bowman, E. S., & Milstein, V. (1988). Multiple personality disorder: A clinical investigation of 50 cases. *Journal of Nervous and Mental Disease, 176,* 519–527.

Crittenden, P. M. (1994). Peering into the black box: An exploratory treatise on the development of the self in children. In D. Cicchetti & S. L. Troth (Eds.), *Disorders and dysfunctions of the self: Rochester Symposium on developemental psychotherapy* (Vol. 5, pp. 79–148). Rochester, NY: University of Rochester Press.

Demitrack, M. A., Putnam, F. W., Brewerton, T. D., Brandt, H. A., & Gold, P. W. (1990). Relation of clinical variables to dissociative phenomena in eating disorders. *American Journal of Psychiatry, 147,* 1184–1188.

Dutton, D., & Painter, S. L. (1981). Traumatic bonding: The development of emotional attachments in battered women and other relationships of intermittent abuse. *Victimology, 6,* 139–168.

Favazza, A. R. (1987). *Bodies under siege.* Baltimore: Johns Hopkins University Press.

Favazza, A. R. (1989). Why patients mutilate themselves. *Hospital and Community Psychiatry, 40,* 137–145.

Ferenczi, S. (1955). The confusion of tongues between the adult and the child: The language of tenderness and the language of passion. In *Final contributions to the problems and methods of psychoanalysis.* New York: Basic Books. (Original work presented 1932)

Field, T. M. (1985). Attachment as psychobiological attunement: Being on the same wavelength. In M. Reite & T. M. Fields (Eds.), *The psychobiology of attachment and separation.* Orlando, FL: Academic Press.

Field, T. M., & Reite, M. (1984). Children's responses to separation from mother during the birth of another child. *Child Development, 55,* 530–541.

Finkelhor, D., & Browne, A. (1984). The traumatic impact of child sexual abuse: A conceptualization. *American Journal of Orthopsychiatry*, 55, 530–541.

Fish-Murray, C. C., Koby, E. V., & van der Kolk, B. A. (1987). Evolving ideas: The effect of abuse on children's thought. In B. A. van der Kolk (Ed.), *Psychological trauma* (pp. 89–110). Washington, DC: American Psychiatric Press.

Folsom, V. L., Krahn, D. D., Canum, K. K., Gold, L., & Silk, K. R. (1989). *Sex abuse: Role in eating disorder.* Paper presented at the 142nd Annual Meeting of the American Psychiatric Association, Washington, DC.

Frieze, I. (1983). Investigating the causes and consequences of marital rape. *Journal of Women in Culture and Society*, 8, 532–553.

Freud, S. (1955). Beyond the pleasure principle. In J. Strachey (Ed. and Trans.), *The standard edition of the complete psychological works of Sigmund Freud* (Vol. 18, pp. 3–64). London: Hogarth Press. (Original work published 1920)

Freud, S. (1962). The aetiology of hysteria. In J. Strachey (Ed. and Trans.), *The standard edition of the complete psychological works of Sigmund Freud* (Vol. 3, pp. 189–221). London: Hogarth Press. (Original work published 1896)

Freud, S. (1964). Moses and monotheism. In J. Strachey (Ed. and Trans.), *The standard edition of the complete psychological works of Sigmund Freud* (Vol. 23, pp. 3–137). London: Hogarth Press. (Original work published 1939)

Gardner, D. L., & Cowdry, R. W. (1985). Suicidal and parasuicidal behavior in borderline personality disorder. *Psychiatric Clinics of North America*, 8, 389–403.

Gelinas, D. J. (1983). The persistent negative effects of incest. *Psychiatry*, 46, 312–332.

Goodwin, J., Cheeves, K., & Connel, V. (1990). Borderline and other severe symptoms in adult survivors of incestuous abuse. *Psychiatric Annals*, 20, 22–32.

Graff, H., & Mallin, R. (1967). The syndrome of wrist cutter. *American Journal of Psychiatry*, 124, 36–42.

Green, A. H. (1978). Self-destructive behavior in battered children. *American Journal of Psychiatry*, 141, 520–525.

Green, A. H. (1983). Dimension of psychological trauma in abused children. *American Journal of Psychiatry*, 22, 231–237.

Gross, R. J., Doerr, H., Caldirola, D., Guzinski, G. M., & Ripley, H. S. (1980). Borderline syndrome and incest in chronic pelvic pain patients. *International Journal of Psychiatric Medicine*, 10, 79–89.

Groth, A. N. (1979). Sexual trauma in the life histories of sex offenders. *Victimology*, 4, 6–10.

Grunebaum, H. U., & Klerman, G. L. (1967). Wrist slashing. *American Journal of Psychiatry*, 124, 527–534.

Gutheil, T. G. (1989). Borderline personality disorder, boundary violations and patient–therapist sex: Medico-legal pitfalls. *American Journal of Psychiatry*, 146, 597–602.

Hall, R. C. W., Tice, L., Beresford, T. P., Wooley, B., & Hall, A. K. (1989). Sexual abuse in patients with anorexia and bulimia. *Psychosomatics*, 30, 73–79.

Harber, K. D., & Pennebaker, J. W. (1992). Overcoming traumatic memories. In S. A. Christianson (Ed.), *The handbook of emotion and memory: Research and theory* (pp. 359–386). Hillsdale, NJ: Erlbaum.

Herman, J. L. (1992a). *Trauma and recovery.* New York: Basic Books.

Herman, J. L. (1992b). Complex PTSD: A syndrome in survivors of prolonged and repeated trauma. *Journal of Traumatic Stress, 5,* 377–391.

Herman, J. L., Perry, J. C., & van der Kolk, B. A. (1989). Childhood trauma in borderline personality disorder. *American Journal of Psychiatry, 146,* 490–495.

Herman, J. L., & van der Kolk, B. A. (1987). Traumatic origins of borderline personality disorder. In B. A. van der Kolk (Ed.), *Psychological trauma.* Washington, DC: American Psychiatric Press.

Hernandez, J. T., & DiClemente, R. J. (1992). Emotional and behavioral correlates of sexual abuse among adolescents: Is there a difference according to gender? *Journal of Adolescent Health, 13,* 658–662.

Herzog, D. B., Staley, J. E., Carmody, S., Robbins, W. M., & van der Kolk, B. A. (1993). Childhood sexual abuse in anorexia nervosa and bulimia nervosa: A pilot study. *Journal of the American Academy of Child and Adolescent Psychiatry, 32,* 962–966.

Hilberman, E. (1980). Overview: The wife-beater's wife reconsidered. *American Journal of Psychiatry, 137,* 974–975.

Irwin, H. J. (1994). Proneness to dissociation and traumatic childhood events. *Journal of Nervous and Mental Disease, 182,* 456–460.

Janet, P. (1889). *L'automatisme psychologique.* Paris: Alcan.

Janoff-Bulman, R. (1992). *Shattered assumptions: Towards a new psychology of trauma.* New York: Free Press.

Jellinek, J. M., & Williams, T. (1987). Post-traumatic stress disorder and substance abuse: Treatment problems, strategies, and recommendations. In T. Williams (Ed.), *Post-traumatic stress disorder: A handbook for clinicians* (pp. 103–117). Cincinnati, OH: Disabled American Veterans.

Kardiner, A. (1941). *The traumatic neuroses of war.* New York: Hoeber.

Keane, T. M., Gerardi, R. J., Lyons, J. A., & Wolfe, J. (1988). The interrelationship of substance abuse and posttraumatic stress disorder: Epidemiological and clinical considerations. In M. Galanter (Ed.), *Recent developments in alcoholism* (Vol. 6, pp. 27–48). New York: Plenum Press.

Keane, T. M., & Kaloupek, D. G. (1982). Imaginal flooding in the treatment of posttraumatic stress disorder. *Journal of Consulting and Clinical Psychology, 50,* 138–140.

Keane, T. M., & Wolfe, J. (1990). Comorbidity in post-traumatic stress disorder: An analysis of community and clinical studies. *Journal of Applied Social Psychology, 20,* 1776–1788.

Kempe, R.S., & Kempe, C.H. (1978). *Child abuse.* Cambridge, MA: Harvard University Press.

Kernberg, O. (1975). *Borderline conditions and pathological narcissism.* New York: Jason Aronson.

Khantzian, E. J. (1985). The self-medication hypothesis of addictive disorders: Focus on heroin and cocaine dependence. *American Journal of Psychiatry, 142,* 1259–1264.

Kluft, R. P. (Ed.). (1990). *Incest-related syndromes of adult psychopathology.* Washington, DC: American Psychiatric Press.

Kluft, R. P. (1991). Multiple personality disorder. In A. Tasman & A. Goldfinger (Eds.), *American Psychiatric Press review of psychiatry* (Vol. 10, pp. 161–188). Washington, DC: American Psychiatric Press.

Kraemer, G. W. (1985). Effects of differences in early social experiences on primate neurobiological–behavioral development. In M. Reite & T. M. Fields (Eds.), *The psychobiology of attachment and separation* (pp. 135–161). Orlando, FL: Academic Press.

Kroll, J., Habenicht, M., & McKenzie, R. (1989). Depression and posttraumatic stress disorder among Southeast Asian refugees. *American Journal of Psychiatry, 146,* 1592–1597.

Krystal, H. (Ed.). (1968). *Massive psychic trauma.* New York: International Universities Press.

Krystal, H. (1978). Trauma and affects. *Psychoanalytic Study of the Child, 33,* 81–116.

Kulka, R. A., Schlenger, W. E., Fairbank, J. A., Hough, R. L., Jordan, B. K., & Marmar, C. R. (1990). *Trauma and the Vietnam War generation: Report of findings from the National Vietnam Veterans' Readjustment Study.* New York: Brunner/Mazel.

Lacey, J. H. (1990). Incest, incestuous fantasy, and indecency: A clinical catchment-area study of normal-weight bulimic women. *British Journal of Psychiatry, 157,* 399–403.

Lacey, J. H., & Evans, C. D. H. (1986). The impulsivist: A multi-impulsive personality disorder. *British Journal of Addiction, 81,* 641–649.

Leibenluft, E., Gardner, D. L., & Cowdry, R. W. (1987). The inner experience of the borderline self-mutilator. *Journal of Personality Disorders, 1,* 317–324.

Lewis, D. O., Lovely, R., Yeager, C., & Della Femina, D. (1989). Toward a theory of the genesis of violence: A follow up study of delinquents. *Journal of the American Academy of Child and Adolescent Psychiatry, 28,* 431–436.

Lewis, D. O., Pincus, J. H., Bard, B., Richardson, E., Prichep, L. S., Feldman, M., & Yeager, C. (1988). Neuropsychiatric, psychoedeucational, and family characteristics of 14 juveniles condemned to death in the US. *American Journal of Psychiatry, 145,* 584–589.

Linehan, M. M. (1993). *Cognitive-behavioral treatment of borderline personality disorder.* New York: Guilford Press.

Lisak, D. (1993). Men as victims: Challenging cultural myths. *Journal of Traumatic Stress, 6,* 577–580.

Litz, B. T., & Keane, T. M. (1989). Information processing in anxiety disorders: Application to the understanding of post-traumatic stress disorder. *Clinical Psychology Review, 9,* 243–257.

Loewenstein, R. J. (1990). Somatoform disorders in victims of incest and child abuse. In R. P. Kluft (Ed.), *Incest-related syndromes of adult psychopathology* (pp. 75–112). Washington, DC: American Psychiatric Press.

Lyons-Ruth, K. (1991). Rapprochment or approchement: Mahler's theory reconsidered from the vantage point of recent research in early attachment relationships. *Psychoanalytic Psychology, 8,* 1–23.

Mai, F. M., & Mersky, H. (1980). Briquet's treatise on hysteria: A synopsis and commentary. *Archives of General Psychiatry, 37,* 1401–1405.

Marmar, C. R., Weiss, D. S., Schlenger, W. E., Fairbank, J. A., Jordan, K., Kulka, R. A., & Hough, R. L. (1994). Peritraumatic dissociation and posttraumatic stress in male Vietnam theater veterans. *American Journal of Psychiatry, 151,* 902–907.

McFarlane, A. C. (1988). Recent life events and psychiatric disorder in children: The interaction with preceding extreme adversity. *Journal of Clinical Psychiatry, 29*(5), 677–690.

McFarlane, A. C., Atchinson, M., Rafalowicz, E., & Papay, P. (1994). Physical symptoms in posttraumatic stress disorder. *Journal of Psychosomatic Research, 38,* 715–726.

McFarlane, A. C., Weber, D. L., & Clark, C. R. (1993). Abnormal stimulus processing in PTSD. *Biological Psychiatry, 34,* 311–320.

Mezey, G., & King, M. (1989). The effects of sexual assault on men: A survey of 22 victims. *Psychological Medicine, 19,* 205–209.

Mezey, G. C., & Taylor, P. J. (1988). Psychological reactions of women who have been raped. *British Journal of Psychiatry, 152,* 330–339.

Nadelson, C. C., Notman, M. T., Zackson, H., & Gornick, J. (1982). A follow-up study of rape victims. *American Journal of Psychiatry, 139,* 1266–1270.

Noyes, R., & Kletti, R. (1977). Depersonalization in response to life threatening danger. *Comprehensive Psychiatry, 18,* 375–384.

Oates, R. K. (1984). Personality development after physical abuse. *Archives of General Psychiatry, 59,* 147–150.

Ogata, S. N., Silk, K. R., Goodrick, S., Lohr, N., Westen, D., & Hill, E. (1989). Childhood and sexual abuse in adult patients with borderline personality disorder. *American Journal of Psychiatry, 147*(8), 1008–1013.

Palmer, R. L., Oppenheimer, R., Dignon, A., Chaloner, D. A., & Howells, K. (1990). Childhood sexual experiences with adults reported by women with eating disorders: An extended series. *British Journal of Psychiatry, 156,* 699–703.

Paris, J., & Zweig-Frank, H. (1992). A critical review of the role of childhood sexual abuse in the etiology of borderline personality disorder. *Canadian Journal of Psychiatry, 37,* 125–128.

Pattison, E. M., & Kahan, J. (1983). The deliberate self-harm syndrome. *American Journal of Psychiatry, 140,* 867–872.

Pearlman, K. W., & Saakvitne, L. A. (1995). *Trauma and the therapist.* New York: Norton.

Pelcovitz, D., van der Kolk, B. A., Roth, S., Mandel, F., Kaplan, S., & Resick, P. (in press). Development and validation of the Structured Interview for Disorders of Extreme Stress. *Journal of Traumatic Stress.*

Perry, J. C., Herman, J. L., van der Kolk, B. A., & Hoke, L. A. (1990). Psychotherapy and psychological trauma in borderline personality disorder. *Psychiatric Annals, 20,* 33–43.

Piaget, J. (1962). *Play, dreams, and imitation in childhood.* New York: Norton.

Pitman, R. K. (1995, September). *Psychophysiological responses in PTSD populations.* Paper presented at the 2nd International Congress on New Directions in the Affective Disorders, Jerusalem.

Pitman, R. K., Orr, S., & Shalev, A. (1993). Once bitten, twice shy: Beyond the conditioning model of PTSD. *Biological Psychiatry, 33,* 145–146.

Pope, H. G., Jr., & Hudson, J. I. (1983). Is childhood sexual abuse a risk factor for bulimia nervosa? *American Journal of Psychiatry, 150*(2), 357–358.

Pribor, E. F., Yutzy, S. H., Dean, T., & Wetzel, R. D. (1993). Briquet's syndrome, dissociation, and abuse. *American Journal of Psychiatry, 150,* 1507–1511.

Putnam, F. W. (1988). The switch process in multiple personality disorder. *Dissociation, 1,* 24–32.

Putnam, F. W. (1989). *Diagnosis and treatment of multiple personality disorder.* New York: Guilford Press.

Putnam, F. W. (1995, June). *Developmental pathways of sexually abused girls.* Paper presented at the Harvard Trauma Conference, Boston, MA.

Putnam, F. W., Guroff, J. J., Silberman, E. K., et al. (1986). The clinical phenomenology of multiple personality disorder: Review of 100 recent cases. *Journal of Clinical Psychiatry, 47,* 285–293.

Putnam, F. W., Loewenstein, R. J., Silberman, E. K., & Post, R. M. (1984). Multiple personality disorder in a hospital setting. *Journal of Clinical Psychiatry, 45,* 172–175.

Pynoos, R. S., Frederick, C. J., Nader, K., Arroyo, W., Steinberg, A., Nunez, F., & Fairbanks, L. (1987). Life threat and posttraumatic stress in school age children. *Archives of General Psychiatry, 44,* 1057–1063.

Pynoos, R. S., & Nader, K. (1988). Children's memory and proximity to violence. *Journal of the American Academy of Child and Adolescent Psychiatry, 28,* 236–244.

Rauch, S. L., van der Kolk, B. A., Fisler, R. E., Alpert, N. M., Orr, S. P., Savage, C. R., Fischman, A. J., Jenike, M. A., & Pitman, R. K. (in press). A symptom provocation study of posttraumatic stress disorder using positron emission tomography and script-driven imagery. *Archives of General Psychiatry.*

Reite, M., Seiler, C., & Short, R. (1978). Loss of your mother is more than loss of a mother. *American Journal of Psychiatry, 135,* 370–371.

Ross, C. A. (1995, May). *Dissociative disorders: Scientific state of the art.* Paper presented at the meeting of the International Society for the Study of Dissociation, Amsterdam.

Ross, C. A., Heber, S., Norton, G. R., & Andreason, G. (1989). Somatic symptoms in multiple personality disorder. *Psychosomatics, 30,* 154–160.

Ross, C. A., Miller, S. D., Reagor, P., Bjornson, L., Fraser, G. A., & Anderson, G. (1990). Multicenter structured interview data on 102 cases of multiple personality disorder from four centers. *American Journal of Psychiatry, 147*(5), 596–601.

Roy, A. (Ed). (1985). Self-destructive behavior [Special issue]. *Psychiatric Clinics of North America, 8*(2).

Russell, D. (1986). *The secret trauma.* New York: Basic Books.

Rutter, M., & Hersov, L. (1985). *Child and adolescent psychiatry: Modern approaches* (2nd ed.). Oxford: Blackwell Scientific.

Sanders, B., & Giolas, M. H. (1991). Dissociation and childhood trauma in psychologically disturbed adolescents. *American Journal of Psychiatry, 148,* 50–54.

Saxe, G. N., Chinman, G., Berkowitz, R., Hall, K., Lieberg, G., Schwartz, J., & van der Kolk, B. A. (1994). Somatization in patients with dissociative disorders. *American Journal of Psychiatry, 151,* 1329–1335.

Saxe, G., van der Kolk, B. A., Hall, K., Schwartz, J., Chinman, G., Hall, M. D., Lieberg, G., & Berkowitz, R. (1993). Dissociative disorders in psychiatric inpatients. *American Journal of Psychiaty, 150*(7), 1037–1042.

Shalev, A. Y., & Rogel-Fuchs, N. Y. (1993). Psychophysiology of PTSD: From sulfur fumes to behavioral genetics. *Journal of Nervous and Mental Disease, 55*(5), 413–423.

Simpson, C.A., & Porter, G.L. (1981). Self-mutilation in children and adolescents. *Bulletin of the Menninger Clinic, 45,* 428–438.

212 ADAPTATIONS TO TRAUMA

Spiegel, D. (1988a). Dissociating damage. *American Journal of Clinical Hypnosis, 29,* 123–131.

Spiegel, D. (1988b). Dissociation and hypnosis in posttraumatic stress disorder. *Journal of Traumatic Stress, 1,* 17–33.

Stern, D. (1983). *The role and the nature of empathy in the mother–infant interaction.* Paper presented at the Second World Congress on Infant Psychiatry, Cannes, France.

Stone, M. H. (1987). A psychodynamic approach: Some thoughts on the dynamics and therapy of self-mutilating borderline patients. *Journal of Personality Disorders, 1,* 347–349.

Sullivan, H. S. (1940). *Conceptions of modern psychiatry.* New York: Norton.

Terr, L. C. (1983). Chowchilla revisited: The effects of psychic trauma four years after a school-bus kidnapping. *American Journal of Psychiatry, 140,* 1543–1550.

Terr, L. C. (1988). What happens to early memories of trauma? *Journal of the American Academy of Child and Adolescent Psychiatry, 1,* 96–104.

Tichener, J. L. (1986). Post-traumatic decline: A consequence of unresolved destructive drives. In C. Figley (Ed.), *Trauma and its wake* (Vol. 2, pp. 5–19). New York: Brunner/Mazel.

van der Hart, O., Steele, K., Boon, S., & Brown, P. (1993). The treatment of traumatic memories: Synthesis, realization, and integration. *Dissociation, 6,* 162–180.

van der Hart, O., van der Kolk, B. A., & Boon, D. (1996). In D. Bremner & C. Marmar (Eds.), *Trauma, memory, and dissociation.* Washington, DC: American Psychiatric Press.

van der Kolk, B. A. (1987). *Psychological trauma.* Washington, DC: American Psychiatric Press.

van der Kolk, B. A. (1988). The trauma spectrum: The interaction of biological and social events in the genesis of the trauma response. *Journal of Traumatic Stress, 1,* 273–290.

van der Kolk, B. A. (1989). The compulsion to repeat the trauma. *Psychiatric Clinics of North America, 12,* 389–411.

van der Kolk, B. A., & Ducey, C. (1989). The psychological processing of traumatic experience: Rorschach patterns in PTSD. *Journal of Traumatic Stress, 2*(3), 259–274.

van der Kolk, B. A., & Fisler, R. (1994). Childhood abuse and neglect and loss of self-regulation. *Bulletin of the Menninger Clinic, 58,* 145–168.

van der Kolk, B. A., Hostetler, A., Herron, N., & Fisler, R. (1994). Trauma and the development of borderline personality disorder. *Psychiatric Clinics of North America, 17*(4), 715–730.

van der Kolk, B. A., Pelcovitz, D., Roth, S., Mandel, F. S., McFarlane, A., & Herman, J. L. (in press). Dissociation, affect dysregulation and somatization. *American Journal of Psychiatry.*

van der Kolk, B. A., Perry, C., & Herman, J. L. (1991). Childhood origins of self-destructive behavior. *American Journal of Psychiatry, 148,* 1665–1671.

van der Kolk, B. A., Roth, S., Pelcovitz, D., & Mandel, F. (1993). *Complex PTSD: Results of the PTSD field trials for DSM-IV.* Washington, DC: American Psychiatric Association.

van der Kolk, B. A., & van der Hart, O. (1989). Pierre Janet and the breakdown of adaptation in psychological trauma. *American Journal of Psychiatry, 146,* 1530–1540.

Walker, E. A., Katon, W. J., Neraas, K., Jemelka, R. P., & Massoth, D. (1992). Dissociation in women with chronic pelvic pain. *American Journal of Psychiatry, 149,* 534–537.

Walker, L. (1979). *The battered women.* New York: Harper & Row.

Werner, E. E. (1989). High-risk children in young adulthood:A longitudinal study from birth to 32 years. *American Journal of Psychiatry, 59,* 72–81.

Widom, C. S. (1987). The cycle of violence. *Science, 244,* 160–165.

World Health Organization. (1992). *ICD-10: International statistics classification of diseases and related health problems* (10th revision). Geneva: Author.

Zanarini, M. C., Gunderson, J. G., Marino, M. F., Schwartz, E. O., & Frankenburg, F. R. (1989). Childhood experience of borderline patients. *Comprehensive Psychiatry, 30,* 18–25.

CHAPTER 10

The Body Keeps the Score

Approaches to the Psychobiology of Posttraumatic Stress Disorder

BESSEL A. VAN DER KOLK

GENERAL BACKGROUND: THE INTERRELATED SYSTEMS OF THE BRAIN

Paul MacLean (1985) defined the brain as a detecting, amplifying, and analyzing device for maintaning an individual in his or her internal and external environment. Different systems in the brain are involved in different functions, ranging all the way from the visceral regulation of blood glucose levels, oxygen intake, and temperature balance to the categorization of incoming information necessary for making complex, long-term decisions affecting both the individual and various social systems. In the course of evolution, the human brain has developed three interdependent subanalyzers, each with different anatomical and neurochemical substrates: (1) the brainstem and hypothalamus, which are primarily associated with the regulation of internal homeostasis; (2) the limbic system, which is charged with maintaining the balance between the internal world and external reality; and (3) the neocortex, which is responsible for analyzing and interacting with the external world.

Parts of this chapter are adapted from van der Kolk (1994). Copyright 1994 by Mosby–Year Book, Inc. Adapted by permission.

It is generally thought that the circuitry of the brainstem and hypothalamus is most innate and stable; that the limbic system contains both innate circuitry and circuitry modifiable by experience; and that the structure of the neocortex is most affected by environmental input (DeMasio, 1995). If this is true, trauma would be expected to have its most profound effects on neocortical functions, and to have the least influence on basic regulatory functions. However, the current state of knowledge about how trauma affects biological systems cannot yet support such a hierarchy. Trauma seems to affect people on multiple levels of biological functioning.

Together, the brainstem/hypothalamus, the limbic system, and the neocortex control a host of regulatory functions:

1. They control internal vegatative functions, the rhythms of life—rest/sleeping and activity; feeding; reproductive cycles; and the most elemental forms of care of offspring.

2. They monitor relations with the outside world and assess what is new, dangerous, or gratifying. To accomplish this assessment, the brain needs to take in and categorize new information, and to integrate it with previously stored knowledge. In this process, it needs to attend to relevant information and ignore irrelevant data. After the meaning of an incoming signal has been categorized, the brain needs to "formulate" (usually unconsciously) an appropriate plan of action, weighing short-term and long-term consequences. This assessment in turn needs to be followed by an appropriate response, and then by a letting go after the challenge has passed.

3. In addition to this, the organism needs to be able to engage in routine tasks without being distracted by irrelevant stimuli, and to be able to explore new options without getting disorganized. This involves the complex capacity to distinguish relevant from irrelevant stimuli, and to select only relevant stimuli in attaining one's goals. In order to be able to do all this, the organism needs to be able to learn from experience.

4. It has been proposed that much of the human brain's evolution over the past few million years has resulted in the development of the capacity to form highly complex collaborative social relationships that allow for social systems with highly specialized but interdependent divisions of labor, based on the ability to adhere to complex social rules (Donald, 1991).

These complicated functions of the mind/brain are accomplished by multiple layers of interconnected clusters of neurons with specialized functions. The modern tendency to attempt to reduce disruptions of these various functions to abnormalities of one particular neurotransmitter system, or to dysfunction in one particular anatomical location, reflects an overly simplistic understanding of the reality of human psychopathology. However, it is likely that I will commit some of these same sins of oversimplification in this chapter as well.

Brain, body, and mind are inextricably linked, and it is only for heuristic reasons that we can still speak of them as if they constitute separate entities. Alterations in any one of these three will intimately affect the other two. For example, emotions and perceptions are both psychological functions and part and parcel of the neural machinery for biological regulation. Their core consists of homeostatic controls—drives and instincts. Mental processes are products of the brain and body, which continuously interact with each other through nerve impulses and through chemicals carried by the bloodstream: neurohormones and other neuromodulators.

The organism receives information from the environment via its sensory input. After analyzing this input, it responds with movement either of the whole body or of parts of the body, such as limbs or vocal cords. A large number of complex brain structures mediate between sensory input and motor output: the sensory association cortices, the brainstem, the thalamus, the basal ganglia, the limbic system, the cerebellum, and the neocortex. Together, these constitute a great collection of systems for processing information, utilizing both innate and acquired knowledge about the body, the brain itself, and the environment.

The innate neural patterns that are necessary for the maintanance of the internal homeostasis, and that thus are fundamental for survival, are carried by cicuits of the brainstem and hypothalamus. The maintenance of these elemental functions, such as regulating temperature, fighting alien microorganisms, and maintaining blood sugar levels, is mediated by the interactions between these structures and the endocrine glands (the pituitary, thyroid, and adrenal glands), as well as via their action on the immune system. The hypothalamus and interrelated stuctures are regulated not only by neural and chemical signals from other brain regions, but also by chemical signals arising in various bodily systems.

The biological regulation mediated by the hypothalamus and brainstem is complemented by the regulation of the limbic system. For example, activity of the pituitary gland, which controls the production of hormones in the thyroid and adrenal glands, is partially controlled by input from the limbic system and even the neocortex. The limbic system, according to MacLean (1985), has three principal functions. The first two are oral and genital functions, necessary for self-preservation and procreation; and the third principal function involves parental care, audiovocal behavior, and play. The neocortex is primarily oriented toward the external world, and is involved in problem solving, learning, and complex stimulus discriminations. In addition, it plays a critical role by mediating the transcription of subjective states into communicable language to self and others. A well-functioning neocortex is necessary for reasoning strategies to attain personal goals, for weighing a range of options for action, for predicting the outcome of one's actions, and for deciding which sensory stimuli are relevant and which are not. In these discriminatory functions, it is assisted by a well-functioning septo-hippocampal system. Obviously, people with posttraumatic stress disorder (PTSD) have a great deal of trouble carrying out a host of these functions.

THE PSYCHOBIOLOGICAL SYMPTOMATOLOGY OF PTSD

Abram Kardiner (1941), who first systematically defined posttraumatic stress for U.S. audiences, noted that sufferers from "traumatic neuroses" become enduringly vigilant for and hyperreactive to environmental threat. He emphasized that "the nucleus of the neurosis is a physioneurosis. . . . The traumatic syndrome is ever present and unchanged." Kardiner noted that physiological hyperarousal occurs not only in response to auditory stimuli, but to temperature, pain, and sudden tactile stimuli as well: "These patients cannot stand being slapped on the back abruptly; they cannot tolerate a misstep or a stumble. From a physiologic point of view there exists a lowering of the threshold of stimulation; and from a psychological point of view a state of readiness for fright reactions" (p. 95). The problem of explosive aggressive reactions recurs throughout Kardiner's work. He stressed that his patients' aggressive outbursts were foreign to their premorbid personalities and impossible to control: "The aggressiveness of the traumatic neurotic is not deliberate or premeditated. His aggression is always impulsive; nor is it capable of being long sustained. Entirely episodic, it often alternates with moods of extreme tenderness" (p. 97).

In *Men under Stress*, Grinker and Spiegel (1945) catalogued the physical symptoms of soldiers in acute posttraumatic states: flexor changes in posture, hyperkinesis, "violently propulsive gait," tremor at rest, mask-like faces, cogwheel rigidity, gastric distress, urinary incontinence, mutism, and a violent startle reflex. They noted the similarity between many of these symptoms and those of diseases of the extrapyramidal motor system. Today we can understand them as the result of stimulation of biological systems, particularly of ascending amine projections. Contemporary research on the biology of PTSD, generally uninformed by this earlier research, confirms that there are persistent and profound alterations in stress hormone secretion in people with PTSD. These findings have profound implications for understanding the nature of the disorder and for designing appropriate treatment.

Physiological Arousal

Starting with Kardiner (1941), and closely followed by Lindemann (1944), a vast literature on combat trauma, crimes, rape, kidnapping, natural disasters, accidents, and imprisonment has demonstrated that the trauma response is complex: Hypermnesia, hyperreactivity to stimuli, and traumatic reexperiencing coexist with psychic numbing, avoidance, amnesia, and anhedonia (American Psychiatric Association [APA], 1987, 1994; Horowitz, 1978). Over time, we have come to understand that PTSD is only one manifestation of psychological distress to trauma (see Chapters 4, 8, and 9, this volume), and that the development of a chronic trauma-based disorder is qualitatively different from a simple exaggeration of the normal stress response. In affected individuals, a cascade of biobehavioral changes occurs that results in the eventual development of what we call PTSD. It also is clear that we are not dealing with simple conditioning: Many people who do not suffer from PTSD, but who have been exposed to an extreme stressor, will again become distressed when they are once again confronted with the tragedy. Pitman, Orr, and Shalev (1993) pointed out that the critical issue in PTSD is that the stimuli that cause people to overreact may not be conditioned *enough*; a variety of triggers not directly related to the traumatic experience may come to precipitate extreme reactions.

Almost all persons who have been exposed to extreme stress develop intrusive symptoms, but only some of them also develop avoidance and hyperarousal. It is thought that the persistence of intrusive and repetitious thoughts, by means of the process of kindling, sets up a chronically disordered pattern of arousal. A patient is victimized by having memories of the event, not by the event itself (McFarlane, 1988). In recent years, dissociation at the moment of the trauma has been shown to be an important concomitant for the development of full-blown PTSD. Although the precise relationships among dissociation, numbing, and hyperarousal remain unclear, several studies have indicated a progression from extreme arousal to dissociation (see Chapter 13, this volume).

As I have noted in Chapter 9, traumatized people seem to try to compensate for their chronic hyperarousal by "shutting down"—on a behavioral level, by avoiding stimuli that remind them of the trauma, and on a psychobiological level, by emotional numbing to both trauma-related and everyday experience (Litz & Keane, 1989). Over time, people with chronic PTSD come to suffer from numbed responsiveness to the environment, punctuated by intermittent hyperarousal in response to emotionally arousing stimuli. Thus, they come to suffer both from generalized hyperarousal and from physiological emergency reactions to specific reminders (APA, 1987, 1994).

Loss of Emotions as Signals

Chronic physiological arousal, and the resulting failure to regulate autonomic reactions to internal or external stimuli, affect people's capacity to utilize emotions as signals. The psychological function of emotions is to alert people to pay attention to what is happening, so that they can take adaptive action

(Krystal, 1978). Ordinarily, people stop having an emotional response when they have realigned their expectations of what is supposed to happen with what is actually happening—either by taking action that adjusts the given situation to their expectations, or by changing their expectations to fit better with what is actually going on (Horowitz, 1986). Krystal (1978) first noted that the emotions of people with PTSD do not seem to serve their usual alerting function—namely, as warning signals to take adaptive action. In PTSD, emotional arousal and goal-directed action are often disconnected from each other. As a result, people who suffer from PTSD no longer use arousal as a cue to pay attention to incoming information. Instead, they tend to go immediately from stimulus to response without first being able to figure out the meaning of what is going on; they respond with fight-or-flight reactions. This causes them to freeze, or, alternatively, to overreact and intimidate others in response to minor provocations (van der Kolk & Ducey, 1989).

After having been chronically aroused, without being able to do much to change this level of arousal, persons with PTSD may (correctly) experience just having feelings as being dangerous. Because of their difficulties using emotions to help them think through situations and come up with adaptive solutions, emotions merely become reminders of their inability to affect the outcome of their life. In PTSD, extreme feelings of anger and helplessness can be understood as the reliving of memories of the trauma; like other memories of the trauma, they become reminders that are to be avoided.

In the remainder of this chapter, I discuss specific psychobiological abnormalities in PTSD. These are summarized in Table 10.1.

PSYCHOPHYSIOLOGICAL EFFECTS OF TRAUMA

Abnormal psychophysiological reactions in PTSD occur on two very different levels: (1) in response to specific reminders of the trauma, and (2) in response to intense but neutral stimuli (e.g., loud noises), signifying a loss of stimulus discrimination.

Conditioned Responses to Specific Stimuli

The present paradigm implies that people with PTSD suffer from heightened physiological arousal in response to sounds, images, and thoughts related to specific traumatic incidents. A large number of studies have confirmed that people with PTSD, but not eposed controls without PTSD, respond to such reminders with significant increases in heart rate, skin conductance, and blood pressure (Dobbs & Wilson, 1960; Malloy, Fairbank, & Keane, 1983; Kolb &

TABLE 10.1. Psychobiological Abnormalities in PTSD

I. Psychophysiological effects
  A. Extreme autonomic responses to stimuli reminiscent of the trauma
  B. Hyperarousal to intense but neutral stimuli (loss of stimulus discrimination)
    1. Nonhabituation of the acoustic startle response
    2. Response below threshold to sound intensities
    3. Reduced electrical pattern in cortical event-related potentials

II. Neurohormonal effects
  A. Norepinephrine (NE), other catecholamines
    1. Elevated urinary catecholamines
    2. Increased plasma NE metabolite response to yohimbine
    3. Down-regulation of adrenergic receptors
  B. Glucocorticoids
    1. Decreased resting glucocorticoid levels
    2. Decreased glucocorticoid response to stress
    3. Down-regulation of glucocorticoid receptors
    4. Hyperresponsivenes to low-dose dexamethasone
  C. Serotonin
    1. Decreased serotonin activity in traumatized animals
    2. Best pharmacological responses to serotonin uptake inhibitors
  D. Endogenous opioids
    1. Increased opioid response to stimuli reminiscent of trauma
    2. Conditionability of stress-induced analgesia
  E. Various hormones: Memory effects
    1. NE, vasopressin: Consolidation of traumatic memories
    2. Oxytocin, endogenous opioids: Amnesias

III. Neuroanatomical effects
  A. Decreased hippocampal volume
  B. Activation of amygdala and connected structures during flashbacks
  C. Activation of sensory areas during flashbacks
  D. Decreased activation of Broca's area during flashbacks
  E. Marked right-hemispheric lateralization

IV. Immunological effects
  A. Increased CD45 RO/RA ratio (see Conclusions and Future Directions, p. 571)

Multipassi, 1982; Blanchard, Kolb, & Gerardi, 1986; Pitman, Orr, Forgue, de Jong, & Claiborn, 1987). The highly elevated autonomic responses to reminders of traumatic experiences that happened years (and sometimes decades) ago indicate the intensity and timelessness with which these memories continue to affect current experience (Pitman et al., 1993).

Recent research has shown that medications that stimulate autonomic nervous system (ANS) arousal may precipitate visual images and affect states associated with prior traumatic experiences in people with PTSD, but not in controls. In patients with PTSD, the injection of such drugs as lactate (Rainey et al., 1987) and yohimbine (Southwick et al., 1993) tends to precipitate panic attacks, flashbacks (exact reliving experiences) of earlier trauma, or both. In our own laboratory, approximately 20% of PTSD subjects responded with a flashback of a traumatic experience when they were presented with acoustic startle stimuli (van der Kolk, 1994).

The strength of these autonomic responses is generally understood in the light of Peter Lang's work (Lang, 1979; see Chapter 13), which has shown that emotionally laden mental images are accompanied by increased ANS activity. Lang proposed that emotional memories are stored as "associative networks" consisting of sensory elements of the experience; these are reactivated when a person is confronted with situations that stimulate a sufficient number of the elements making up these networks. Currently, a decrease in physiological arousal in response to trauma-related images has become widely accepted as one standard of positive treatment outcome (Keane & Kaloupek, 1982). Shalev, Orr, Peri, Schreiber, and Pitman (1992) have shown that desensitization to particular trauma-related mental images does not necessarily generalize to recollections of other traumatic events as well.

Hyperarousal to Intense but Neutral Stimuli (Loss of Stimulus Discrimination)

Kolb (1987) was the first to propose that excessive stimulation of the central nervous system (CNS) at the time of the trauma may result in permanent neuronal changes that have a negative effect on learning, habituation, and stimulus discrimination. These neuronal changes do not depend on actual exposure to reminders of the trauma for expression. The abnormal startle response characteristic of PTSD (APA, 1994) is one example of this phenomenon. Despite the fact that an abnormal acoustic startle response (ASR) has been seen as a cardinal feature of the trauma response for over half a century, systematic explorations of the ASR in PTSD have just begun. The ASR consists of a characteristic sequence of muscular and autonomic responses elicited by sudden and intense stimuli (Shalev & Rogel-Fuchs, 1993; Davis, 1984).

Several studies have demonstrated abnormalities in habituation to the ASR in PTSD (Shalev et al., 1992; Ornitz & Pynoos, 1989; Butler et al., 1990; Ross, Ball, & Cohen, 1989). Shalev et al. (1992) found that both CNS- and ANS-mediated elements of the ASR failed to habituate in 93% of the PTSD group, compared with 22% of the control subjects. Interestingly, people who previously met criteria for PTSD, but no longer do so, continue to show failure of habituation of the ASR (Fisler & van der Kolk, 1995; Pitman & Orr, 1995). This raises the question of whether abnormal ASR habituation is a marker of, or a vulnerability factor for, developing PTSD.

The failure of the ASR to habituate suggests that traumatized people have difficulty in evaluating sensory stimuli and mobilizing appropriate levels of physiological arousal (Shalev & Rogel-Fuchs, 1993). Thus, the fact that people with PTSD cannot properly integrate memories of the trauma, and instead get mired in a continual reliving of the past, is mirrored physiologically in the misinterpretation of innocuous stimuli (such as the ASR) as potential threats. Another example of this phenomenon is recorded in traumatized people's cortical event-related potentials (ERPs) in response to noises.

Paige, Reid, Allen, and Newton (1990) demonstrated significant differences between PTSD patients and controls in the pattern of ERPs in response to a stimulus pulse of white noise. The PTSD patients were more sensitive to sounds; they responded to sound intensities that were at or below threshold for most normal subjects. Moreover, the cortical ERPs elicited by auditory stimuli in PTSD patients showed a reduced rather than the expected augmented electrical pattern. Paige et al. interpreted these findings to mean that PTSD patients are "reducers" in whom inhibitory feedback loops are activated to dampen a tonic state of hyperarousal. Using ERPs, McFarlane, Weber, and Clark (1993) found that people with PTSD (1) were unable to differentiate relevant from irrelevant stimuli; (2) attended less to affectively neutral but existentially relevant events; and (3) as a consequence of this relative lack of responsiveness, needed to apply more effort than nontraumatized people to respond to current experience (as reflected in delayed reaction times). These studies suggest that people with PTSD have difficulty neutralizing stimuli in their environment in order to attend to relevant tasks. To compensate, they tend to shut down. However, the price for shutting down is decreased involvement in ordinary, everyday life.

NEUROHORMONAL EFFECTS OF TRAUMA

Background: Neurohormones and Their Roles in the Stress Response

PTSD develops following exposure to events that are intensely distressing. Intense stress is accompanied by the release of endogenous, stress-responsive neurohormones, such as the catecholamines (e.g., epinephrine and norepinephrine [NE]), serotonin, hormones of the hypothalamic–pituitary–adrenal (HPA) axis (e.g., cortisol and other glucocorticoids, vasopressin, oxytocin), and endogenous opioids. These stress hormones help the organism mobilize the energy required to deal with the stress, in ways ranging from increased glucose release to enhanced immune function. In a well-functioning organism, stress produces rapid and pronounced hormonal responses. However, chronic and persistent stress inhibits the effectiveness of the stress response and induces desensitization (Axelrod & Reisine, 1984).

Much still remains to be learned about the specific roles of the different neurohormones in the stress response. NE is secreted by the locus coeruleus and distributed through much of the CNS, particularly the neocortex and the limbic system, where it plays a role in memory consolidation and where it helps initiate fight-or-flight behaviors. Adrenocorticotropic hormone (ACTH) is released from the anterior pituitary and activates a cascade of reactions, eventuating in release of glucocorticoids from the adrenals. The precise interrelation between HPA axis hormones and the catecholamines in the stress response is not entirely clear, but it is known that stressors that activate NE neurons also increase concentrations of corticotropin-releasing factor (CRF) in the locus coeruleus (Dunn & Berridge, 1987), while intracerebral ventricular infusion of CRF increases NE in the forebrain (Valentino & Foote, 1988). There is evidence that corticosteroids normalize catecholamine-induced arousal in limbic midbrain structures in response to stress (Bohus & DeWied, 1978), thereby modulating the secetion of other stress hormones.

At least two hormonal systems in particular have been implicated in the modulation of the stress response: the glucocorticoid system and serotonin.

Glucocorticoids

Glucocorticoids and catecholamines modulate each other's effects. In acute stress, cortisol helps regulate stress hormone release via a negative feedback loop to the hippocampus, hypothalamus, and pituitary (Munck et al., 1984). Yehuda, Southwick, Mason, and Giller (1990) have proposed that cortisol's function is to shut off all the other biological reactions that have been initiated by the stress response, and hence that it is basically an "antistress" hormone. Thus, these authors propose that simultaneous activation of catecholamines and glucocorticoids stimulates active coping behaviors, whereas increased arousal in the presence of low glucocorticoid levels provokes undifferentiated fight-or-flight reactions.

Chronic exposure to stress affects both acute and chronic adaptation: It permanently alters how an organism deals with its environment on a day-to-day basis, and it interferes with how it copes with subsequent acute stress (Yehuda et al., 1993). Whereas acute stress activates the HPA axis and increases glucocorticoid levels, organisms adapt to chronic stress by activating a negative feedback loop that results in (1) decreased resting glucocorticoid levels in chronically stressed organisms (Meany, Aitken, Viau, Sharma, & Sarieau, 1989), (2) decreased glucocorticoid secretion in response to subsequent stress (Yehuda, Giller, Southwick, Lowy, & Mason, 1991; Yehuda et al., 1995), and (3) increased concentration of glucocorticoid receptors in the hippocampus (Sapolsky, Krey, & McEwen, 1984). Yehuda et al. (1995) have suggested that increased concentration of glucocorticoid receptors could facilitate a stronger glucocorticoid negative feedback, resulting in a more sensitive HPA axis and a faster recovery from acute stress.

Serotonin

Serotonin systems also appear to modulate NE responsiveness and arousal (Depue & Spoont, 1986; Gerson & Baldessarini, 1980). Low serotonin in animals is related to an inability to modulate arousal, as exemplified by an exaggerated startle response (Gerson & Baldessarini, 1980; Depue & Spoont, 1986), and increased arousal in response to novel stimuli, handling, or pain (Depue & Spoont, 1986). Depue and Spoont (1986) characterize the phenomena produced in animals by serotonin depletion as hyperirritability, hyperexcitability, and hypersensitivity— an "exaggerated emotional arousal and/or aggressive display (though not necessarily attack) to relatively mild stimuli" (p. 55). These behaviors bear a striking resemblance to those observed in people with PTSD. Decreased serotonin function has also been correlated with hostility, impulsivity, and self-directed aggression in patients with depression and with borderline personality disorder (Asberg, Traskman, & Thoren, 1976; Brown, Goodwin, Ballenger, Goyer, & Major, 1979; Coccaro, Siever, Klar, & Maurer, 1989); the latter diagnostic group has frequent histories of severe childhood trauma (Herman, Perry, & van der Kolk, 1989).

The degree to which neurotransmitter levels are affected by social factors is illustrated by studies of nonhuman primates showing that serotonin levels are highly correlated with position in the social hierarchy, and that enviromental changes can profoundly affect both social hierarchies and the serotonin levels of the animals within those hierarchies (Raleigh, McGuire, & Brammer, 1984).

Serotonin mediates a behavioral inhibition system in the brain that helps suppress behaviors motivated by emergencies or by previous reward (Depue & Spoont, 1986; Gray, 1987; Soubrie, 1986). Furthermore, serotonin reuptake inhibitors have been found to be the most effective pharmacological treatment both of obsessive thinking in people with obsessive–compulsive disorder (Jenike et al., 1990), and of involuntary preoccupation with traumatic memories in people with PTSD (van der Kolk et al., 1994; van der Kolk & Saporta, 1991). It is likely that serotonin plays a role in the capacity to monitor the environment flexibly and to respond with behaviors that are situation-appropriate, instead of reacting to internal stimuli that are irrelevant to current demands. Stress-induced serotonin dysfunction may lead to impaired functioning of the behavioral inhibition system; this may be related to various behavioral problems seen in PTSD, including impulsivity, aggressive outbursts, compulsive reenactment of trauma-related behavior patterns, and a seeming inability to learn from past mistakes.

Specific Neuroendocrine Abnormalities in PTSD

Since there is an extensive literature on the effects of inescapable stress on the biological stress response of other species, such as monkeys and rats, much of the biological research on people with PTSD has focused on testing the applicability of the animal research findings (van der Kolk, Greenberg, Boyd, & Krystal, 1985; Krystal et al., 1989; Foa, Zinbarg, & Rothbaum, 1992). People with PTSD, like chronically and inescapably shocked animals, seem to suffer from a persistent activation of the biological stress response upon exposure to stimuli reminiscent of the trauma. The most thoroughly studied systems are catecholamines, glucocorticoids, serotonin, and endogenous opioids.

Catecholamines

Neuroendocrine studies of Vietnam veterans with PTSD have found good evidence for chronically increased sympathetic nervous system activity in PTSD. One study (Kosten, Mason, Giller, Ostroff, & Harkness, 1987) found elevated 24-hour excretions of urinary NE and epinephrine in PTSD combat veterans, compared with patients with other psychiatric diagnoses. Although Pitman and Orr (1990a) did not replicate these findings in 20 veterans and 15 combat controls, the mean urinary NE excretion values in their combat controls (58.0 (μg/day) were substantially higher than those previously reported in normal populations. The expected compensatory down-regulation of adrenergic receptors in response to increased levels of NE was confirmed by a study that found decreased platelet alpha$_2$-adrenergic receptors in combat veterans with PTSD, compared with normal controls (Perry, Giller & Southwick, 1987). Another study also found an abnormally low alpha$_2$-adrenergic receptor-mediated adenylate cyclase signal transduction (Lerer, Bleich, & Kotler, 1987). Southwick et al. (1993) used yohimbine injections (0.4 mg/kg), which activate noradrenergic neurons by blocking the alpha$_2$-adrenergic autoreceptor, to study noradrenergic neuronal dysregulation in Vietnam veterans with PTSD. Yohimbine precipitated panic attacks in 70% of subjects and flashbacks in 40%. Subjects responded with larger increases in a plasma NE metabolite than controls showed. Yohimbine precipitated significant increases in all PTSD symptoms. (For a more extensive discussion of catecholamines in PTSD, see Murburg, 1993.)

Corticosteroids

Two studies have shown that veterans with PTSD have low urinary cortisol excretion, even when they have comorbid major depressive disorder (Yehuda et al., 1990). One study failed to replicate this finding (Pitman & Orr, 1990b). In a series of studies, Yehuda et al. (1990, 1991) found increased numbers of lymphocyte glucocorticoid receptors in Vietnam veterans with PTSD. Interestingly, the number of glucocorticoid receptors was proportional to the severity of PTSD symptoms. Heidi Resnick and her colleagues (Resnick, Yehuda, Pitman, & Foy, 1995) studied the acute cortisol response to trauma from blood samples from 20 recent rape victims. Three months later, a prior trauma history was taken, and the subjects were evaluated for the presence of PTSD. Victims with a prior history of sexual abuse were significantly more likely to have developed PTSD 3 months after the rape than rape victims who did not develop PTSD. Cortisol levels shortly after the rape were correlated with histories of prior assaults: The mean initial cortisol level of individuals with a prior assault history was 15 μg/dl, compared to 30 μg/dl in individuals without such a history. These findings can be interpreted to mean that prior exposure to traumatic events results either in a blunted cortisol response to subsequent trauma, or in a quicker return of cortisol to baseline following stress. The fact that Yehuda et al. (1995) also found subjects with PTSD to be hyperresponsive to low doses of dexamethasone argues for an enhanced sensitivity of HPA axis feedback in traumatized patients.

Serotonin

Although the role of serotonin in PTSD has received less systematic attention than that of the glucocorticoids, the potential importance of serotonin in PTSD is illustrated by the facts that inescapably shocked animals are found to have decreased CNS serotonin levels (Valzelli, 1982), and that serotonin reuptake blockers are singularly effective pharmacological agents in the treatment of PTSD. Decreased serotonin in humans has repeatedly been correlated with impulsivity and aggression (Brown et al., 1979; Mann, 1987; Coccaro et al., 1989). The literature tends to assume readily that these relationships are based on genetic traits. However, studies of impulsive, aggressive, and suicidal patients seem to find at least as robust an association between those behaviors and histories of childhood trauma (e.g., Green, 1978; van der Kolk, Perry, & Herman, 1991; Lewis, 1992). It is likely that both temperament and experience affect relative CNS serotonin levels (van der Kolk, 1987).

In order to test serotonergic contributions to trauma-related symptomatology, Southwick et al. (1990) administered 1 mg/kg of metacholorophenylpiperazine (m-CPP), a serotonin agonist, to 26 Vietnam veterans with PTSD. Thirty-one percent of the subjects experienced a panic attack, and 27% had a flashback. These figures are comparable to the effects of the injection of yohimbine, which acts solely on the noradrenergic system. There was almost no overlap between the subjects who had these reactions to m-CPP and those who reacted to yohimbine. This suggests that multiple neurotransmitters are involved in these complex PTSD symptoms.

Endogenous Opioids

Stress-induced analgesia (SIA) has been described in experimental animals following a variety of inescapable stressors, such as electric shock, fighting, starvation, and a cold-water swim (Akil, Watson, & Young, 1983). In severely stressed animals, opiate withdrawal symptoms can be produced either by termination of the stressful stimulus or by naloxone injections. Stimulated by the findings that fear activates the secretion of endogenous opioid peptides, and that SIA can become conditioned to subsequent stressors and to previously neutral events associated with the noxious stimulus, we tested the hypothesis that in people with PTSD, reexposure to a stimulus resembling the original trauma will cause an endogenous opioid response that can be indirectly measured as naloxone-reversible analgesia (van der Kolk, Greenberg, Orr, & Pitman, 1989; Pitman, van der Kolk, Orr, & Greenberg, 1990). We found that two decades after the original trauma, people with PTSD developed opioid-mediated anal-gesia in response to a stimulus resembling the traumatic stressor, which we correlated with a secretion of endogenous opioids equivalent to 8 mg of mor-phine. Self-reports of emotional responses suggested that endogenous opioids were responsible for a relative blunting of the emotional response to the trau-matic stimulus.

Endogenous Opioids, Dissociation, and Stress-Induced Analgesia. When young animals are isolated, and older ones attacked, they respond initially with aggression (hyperarousal–fight–protest); if that does not produce the required results, they respond with withdrawal (numbing–flight–despair). Fear-induced attack or protest patterns in the young serve to attract protection, and in mature animals to prevent or counteract the predator's activity. When an animal is attacked, pain inhibition can be useful in helping the animal to defend itself, because attending to pain would get in the way of effective self-defense. In addition, grooming or licking wounds might attract opponents and stimu-late further attack (Siegfried, Frischknecht, & Nunez de Souza, 1990). Thus defending oneself against outside aggressors and tending to one's wounds can-not be accomplished at the same time. Nature provides protection against pain by means of SIA. During World War II, Beecher (1946), after observing that 75% of severely wounded soldiers on the Italian front did not request morphine, speculated that "strong emotions can block pain." Today, we can reasonably attribute this phenomenon to the release of endogenous opioids (van der Kolk et al., 1989; Pitman et al.,1990).

Endogenous opioids, which inhibit pain and reduce panic, are secreted after prolonged exposure to severe stress. Siegfried et al. (1990) have observed that memory is impaired in animals when they can no longer actively influence the outcome of a threatening situation. They showed that both the freezing response and panic interfere with effective memory processing; correspond-ingly, excessive endogenous opioids and NE both interfere with the storage of experience in explicit memory. Freezing/numbing responses may serve the function of allowing organisms not to "consciously experience" or not to remember situations of overwhelming stress (which would also keep them from learning from experience). The dissociative reactions in people in response to trauma may be analogous to this complex of behaviors that occurs in ani-mals after prolonged exposure to severe uncontrollable stress.

DEVELOPMENTAL LEVEL AFFECTS THE PSYCHOBIOLOGICAL EFFECTS OF TRAUMA

Although most studies on PTSD have been done on adults (particularly on war veterans), in recent years a small prospective literature has been emerging that documents the differential effects of trauma at various age levels. Anxiety disorders, chronic hyperarousal, and behavioral disturbances have been regularly described in traumatized children (e.g., Bowlby, 1969; Cicchetti, 1985; Terr, 1991). In addition to the reactions to discrete, one-time traumatic incidents documented in these studies, intrafamilial abuse is increasingly recognized to produce complex posttraumatic syndromes (Cole & Putnam, 1992), which involve chronic affect dysregulation, destructive behavior against self and others, learning disabilities, dissociative problems, somatization, and distortions in concepts about self and others (van der Kolk, 1988; Herman, 1992). The field trials for DSM-IV showed that this conglomeration of symptoms tended to occur together and that the severity of this syndrome was proportional to the age of onset of the trauma and its duration (van der Kolk et al., 1993; see Chapter 9, this volume).

Although current research on traumatized children is outside the scope of this chapter, it is important to recognize that various neurobiological abnormalities are beginning to be identified in this population. Frank Putnam's group's prospective but still largely unpublished studies (personal communications, 1991–1995) are showing major neuroendocrine disturbances in sexually abused girls compared with normals, particularly in corticosteroid and thyroid functions (DeBellis, Burke, Trickett, & Putnam, in press). Research on the psychobiology of childhood trauma can be profitably informed by the vast literature on the psychobiological effects of trauma and deprivation in non-human primates (Reite & Fields, 1985).

The ability of trauma to disrupt the functional integration of widespread cortical and subcortical regions is suggested by the findings of an electro-encephalographic (EEG) study of sexually abused children (Teicher, Glod, Survey, & Swett, in press). In these children, there was a loss of the normal synchronization between the electrical activity of the different cortical areas. This indicates a loss of function associated with the integration of distributed cortical activity. There is some evidence to suggest that the dominant hemisphere is more sensitive to cortico-cortical uncoupling: Thatcher, Walker, and Giudice (1987) and Teicher et al. (in press) found that the EEG disruption was particularly prominent in the left hemisphere. This finding mirrors the clinical observation that abused children have significant problems in the dominant- hemishere function of language development (see Chapter 9, this volume). The problems that abused children have as adults recalling historical information are probably also clinical correlates of this problem (see Chapter 12, this volume).

Trauma, Neurohormones, and Memory Consolidation

When people are under severe stress, they secrete endogenous stress hormones that affect how their memories are laid down. On the basis of animal models, it has been widely assumed that massive secretion of neurohormones at the time of the trauma plays a role in the long-term potentiation (and thus the overconsolidation) of traumatic memories. Long-term potentiation helps the organism evaluate the importance of subsequent sensory input according to the relative strength of associated memory traces. This phenomenon appears to be largely mediated by NE input to the amygdala (LeDoux, 1990; Ademac, 1978). In traumatized organisms, the capacity to access relevant memories appears to have gone awry; they tend to access memory traces of the trauma at the expense of other memories, and to "remember" the trauma whenever aroused. Although NE seems to be the principal hormone involved in producing long-term potentiation, other neurohormones secreted under particular stressful circumstances, such as endorphins and oxytocin, actually inhibit memory consolidation (Zager & Black, 1985; Pitman, Orr, & Lasko, 1993). Excessive NE or vasopressin release at the time of the trauma could well play a role in memories' being excessively consolidated, whereas other neurohormones, such as endogenous opioids or oxytocin, are likely to play a role in creating the amnesias that are often seen in PTSD (APA, 1987, 1994). It is of interest that childbirth, which can be extraordinarily stressful, only rarely results in posttraumatic problems (Moleman, van der Hart, & van der Kolk, 1992). Oxytocin may play a protective role that prevents the overconsolidation of memories surrounding childbirth.

Physiological arousal in general can trigger trauma-related memories; conversely, trauma-related memories precipitate generalized physiological arousal. It is likely that the frequent reliving of a traumatic event in flashbacks or nightmares causes a re-release of stress hormones, which further kindle the strength of the memory trace (van der Kolk et al., 1985). Such a positive feedback loop could cause subclinical PTSD to escalate into clinical PTSD (Pitman et al., 1993), in which the memories appear so strong and powerful that Pitman and Orr (1990a) have called them "the black hole" in the mental life of the PTSD patient. They attract all associations to themselves, and sap current life of its significance.

TRAUMA AND THE CENTRAL NERVOUS SYSTEM

Background: Structures and Functions of the Limbic System

The limbic system is thought to be the part of the CNS that maintains and guides the emotions and behavior necessary for self-preservation and survival of the species (MacLean, 1985). During both waking and sleeping states, signals from the sensory organs continuously travel to the thalamus; from there, they are distributed to the cortex (where they affect thinking), to the basal ganglia (where they affect movement), and to the limbic system (where they affect memories and emotions) (Papez, 1937). Most processing of sensory input occurs outside of conscious awareness, and only novel, significant, or threatening information is selectively passed on to the neocortex for further attention.

People with PTSD tend to overinterpret sensory input as a recurrence of past trauma. Both the previously discussed ERP studies, and recent studies that have shown limbic system abnormalities in brain imaging studies of patients with PTSD (e.g., Saxe, Vasile, Hill, Bloomingdale, & van der Kolk, 1992; Bremner et al., 1995), may begin to shed light on these attentional problems in people with PTSD. Two particular areas of the limbic system have been implicated in the processing of emotionally charged memories: the amygdala and the hippocampus (see Table 10.2). Before I discuss their possible involvement in the pathophysiology of PTSD, a brief review of their functions may be useful.

The Amygdala

Of all areas in the CNS, the amygdala is most clearly implicated in the evaluation of the emotional meaning of incoming stimuli (LeDoux, 1986). Several investigators have proposed that the amygdala assigns free-floating feelings of significance to sensory input, which the neocortex then further elaborates and imbues with personal meaning (MacLean, 1985; LeDoux, 1986; Ademac, 1991; O'Keefe & Bouma, 1969). Moreover, the amygdala is thought to integrate internal representations of the external world in the form of memory images with emotional experiences associated with those memories (Calvin, 1990). After assigning meaning to sensory information, the amygdala guides emotional behavior by projections to the hypothalamus, hippocampus, and basal forebrain (LeDoux, 1986; Ademac, 1991; Squire & Zola-Morgan, 1991; Pitman, 1989).

TABLE 10.2. Functions of Limbic Structures and Effects of Lesions

Hippocampus	Amygdala
Functions of limbic structures	
Categories of experience	Conditioning of fear responses
Creation of a spatial map	Attachment of affect to neutral stimuli
Storage of simple memory	Establishment of associations between
Creation of summary sketch/index	sensory modalities
Effects of lesions	
Declarative memory lost	Loss of fear responses
Skill-based memory spared	Meaningful social interaction lost
Immediate memory spared	Declarative memory intact

The Hippocampus

The hippocampal system, which is anatomically adjacent to the amygdala, is thought to record in memory the spatial and temporal dimensions of experience. It plays an important role in the categorization and storage of incoming stimuli in memory. The hippocampus is especially vital to short-term memory—the holding in mind of a piece of information for a few moments, after which it either comes to reside in more permanent memory or is immediately forgotten. Proper functioning of the hippocampus is necessary for explicit or declarative memory (Squire & Zola-Morgan, 1991). Being able to learn from experience depends, at least in part, on smoothly functioning short-term memory processes.

The hippocampus is involved in the evaluation of how incoming stimuli are spatially and temporally related with one another and with previously stored information. It also determines whether the new stimuli involve reward, punishment, novelty, or nonreward (Ademac, 1991; Gray, 1987). Decreased hippocampal functioning causes behavioral disinhibition and hyperresponsiveness to environmental stimuli (Altman, Brunner, & Bayer, 1973; O'Keefe & Nadel, 1978). The neurotransmitter serotonin plays a crucial role in the capacity of the septo-hippocampal system to activate inhibitory pathways that prevent the initiation of emergency responses until it is clear that they will be of use (Gray, 1987).

In animals, stress-induced corticosterone (Pfaff, Silva, & Weiss, 1971) decreases hippocampal activity. High levels of circulating glucocorticoids have a significant negative effect on memory, which is thought to be a function of the fact that sustained activation of the glucocorticoid system under conditions of prolonged stress eventually leads to cell death in the hippocampus (Sapolsky, Hideo, Rebert, & Finch, 1990, McEwen, Gould, & Sakai, 1992). This phenomenon has been well demonstrated in patients with Cushing's disease, a hormonal condition in which tumors in the adrenal or pituitary glands, or corticosteroid drugs used for a prolonged time, cause the adrenal glands to secrete high levels of ACTH and of cortisol (Bremner et al., 1995). These patients suffer from serious short-term memory problems. Magnetic resonance imaging studies of patients with Cushing's disease have shown atrophy and shrinkage of the hippocampus; cortisol levels are proportional to the level of shrinkage (Starkman, Gebarski, Berent, & Schteingart, 1992).

"Emotional Memory May Be Forever"

In animals, high-level stimulation of the amygdala interferes with hippocampal functioning (Ademac, 1991). This implies that intense emotions may inhibit the proper evaluation and categorization of experience. In mature animals, one-time intense stimulation of the amygdala will produce lasting changes in neuronal excitability and enduring behavioral changes in the direction of either fight or flight (LeDoux, Romanski, & Xagoraris, 1991). In kindling experiments with animals, Ademac, Stark-Ademac, and Livingston (1980) showed that following an increase in the amplitude of amygdala and hippocampal seizure activity, permanent changes in limbic physiology caused lasting changes in defensiveness and in predatory aggression. Preexisting "personality" played a significant role in the behavioral effects of amygdala stimulation in cats: Animals that were temperamentally insensitive to threat and prone to attack became more aggressive, whereas in highly defensive animals different pathways were activated, increasing behavioral inhibition (Ademac et al., 1980).

In a series of experiments, LeDoux and colleagues utilized repeated electrical stimulation of the amygdala to produce conditioned fear responses. They found that cortical lesions prevented the extinction of these responses. This led the authors to conclude that, once formed, the subcortical traces of the conditioned fear response are indelible, and that "emotional memory may be forever" (LeDoux et al., 1991, p. 24). This conclusion is in line with Lawrence Kolb's (1987) speculation that patients with PTSD suffer from impaired cortical control over subcortical areas responsible for learning, habituation, and stimulus discrimination. Decreased inhibitory control may occur under a variety of circumstances: under the influence of drugs and alcohol, during sleep (as in nightmares), with aging, and after exposure to strong reminders of the traumatic past. It is conceivable that traumatic sensations may then be revived, not in the distorted fashion of ordinary recall, but as affect states, somatic sensations, or visual images (nightmares or flashbacks) that are timeless and unmodified by further experience (see Chapter 12, this volume). The concept of indelible subcortical emotional responses, held in check to varying degrees by cortical and septo-hippocampal activity, has led to the speculation that delayed-onset PTSD may be the expression of subcortically mediated emotional responses that escape cortical (and possibly hippocampal) inhibitory control (van der Kolk & van der Hart, 1991; Pitman et al., 1993; Charney, Deutch, Krystal, Southwick, & Davis, 1993; Shalev et al., 1992).

Specific Limbic System Abnormalities in PTSD

The Hippocampus

A recent series of studies indicates that people with PTSD have decreased hippocampal volume. Bremner et al. (1995) found that Vietnam combat veterans with PTSD had an 8% reduction in the volume of their right hippocampus, compared with vets who suffered no such symptoms. Stein et al. (1994) found a 7% reduction in hippocampus volume in women with PTSD who had suffered repeated childhood sexual abuse, whereas Gurvitz, Shenton, and Pitman (1995) found that Vietnam veterans with the most intense combat exposure and with the most severe PTSD had an average shrinkage of 26% in the left hippocampus and 22% in the right hippocampus, compared with vets who saw combat but had no symptoms.

Shrinkage in the hippocampus suggests a loss of cell mass. Whether the loss results from the atrophy of dendrites or from actual cell death is not yet known. On a test of verbal memory, Bremner et al.'s veterans performed 40% worse than did people of comparable age and education. Exposure to trauma is not the only explanation for these findings; it is conceivable that people with a smaller hippocampus are most vulnerable to developing PTSD. However, a more likely explanation is that the shrinkage in the hippocampus is due to the effects of heightened levels of cortisol, which is known to be toxic to the hippocampus.

The Amygdala

We recently collaborated in a positron emission tomography study of patients with PTSD, in which they were exposed to vivid, detailed narratives of their own traumatic experiences (Rauch et al., in press). We collected narratives from these subjects with PTSD, and then read these accounts back to them; when this precipitated marked autonomic responses and triggered flashbacks, a scan was made. For comparison, the subjects also wrote and were exposed to narratives that invoked a neutral scene. During exposure to the scripts of their traumatic experiences, these subjects demonstrated heightened activity only in the right hemisphere—in the paralimbic belt, parts of the the limbic system connected with the amygdala. Most active were the amygdala itself, the insular cortex, the posterior orbito-frontal cortex, the anterior cingulate cortex, and the anterior temporal cortex. Activation of these structures was accompanied by heightened activity in the right visual cortex, reflecting the visual reexperiencing of their traumas that these patients reported. Perhaps most significantly, Broca's area "turned off." We believe that this reflects the tendency in PTSD to experience emotions as physical states rather than as verbally encoded experiences. Our findings suggest that PTSD patients' difficulties with putting feelings into words are mirrored in actual changes in brain activity.

Lateralization

A striking finding in our study (Rauch et al., in press) was the marked lateralization of activity in the right hemisphere, which is thought to be involved in evaluating the emotional significance of incoming information and in regulating autonomic and hormonal responses to these incoming stimuli. In contrast, Broca's area—the part of the left hemisphere that is responsible for translating personal experiences into communicable language—showed a significant decrease in oxygen utilization during exposure to traumatic reminders. This probably means that during activation of a traumatic memory, the brain is "having" its experience: The person may feel, see, or hear the sensory elements of the traumatic experience. He or she may also be physiologically prevented from translating this experience into communicable language. When PTSD victims are having their traumatic recall, they may suffer from speechless terror in which they may be literally "out of touch with their feelings."

Our findings lend support to LeDoux's (1992) hypothesis that emotional memories can be established without any conscious evaluation of incoming information by the neocortex, and that a high degree of activation of the amygdala and related structures can facilitate the generation of emotional responses and sensory impressions based on fragments of information, rather than full-blown perceptions of objects and events. On the basis of his animal work, LeDoux has proposed that intense stimulation of the amygdala may uncouple emotional responses to particular stimuli from the subjective perceptions, and that intense affective stimulation may thus inhibit proper evaluation and categorization of experience.

Our data revealed marked assymetry in lateralization in the direction of the right hemisphere while the traumatic memories were activated. It is now generally understood that whereas the left hemisphere is specialized for cognitive analysis and language production, the right hemisphere plays a central role in the perception and expression of emotion, particularly of negative emotion (e.g., Silberman & Weingartner, 1986; Tomarken, Davidson, Wheeler, & Ross, 1992). The right hemisphere is thought to be able to maintain a social–emotional system that can independently recall and act on certain memories and perceptions without active participation of the left hemisphere (Joseph, 1988). Our data provide a possible neurobiological underpinning of our (van der Kolk & Ducey, 1989) comments on the psychological processing in men with PTSD: "These patients are unable to integrate the immediate affective experience with the cognitive structuring of experience. Lack of integration resulted in extreme reactivity to the environment without intervening reflection" (p. 272). It remains to be seen whether gaining a greater capacity to attach semantic representations to traumatic reliving experiences will decrease activation of the amygdala and sensory association areas during exposures to reminders of the trauma.

REFERENCES

Ademac, R. E. (1978). Normal and abnormal limbic system mechanisms of emotive biasing. In K. E. Livingston & O. Hornykiewicz (Eds.), *Limbic mechanisms*. New York: Plenum Press.

Ademac, R. E. (1991). Partial kindling of the ventral hippocampus: Identification of changes in limbic physiology which accompany changes in feline aggression and defense. *Physiology and Behavior, 49,* 443–454.

Ademac, R. E., Stark-Ademac, & C., Livingston, K. E. (1980). The development of predatory aggression and defense in the domestic cat. *Neurological Biology, 30,* 389–447.

Akil, H., Watson, S. J., & Young, E. (1983). Endogenous opioids: Biology and function. *Annual Review of Neuroscience, 7,* 223–255.

Altman, J., Brunner, R. L., & Bayer, S. A. (1973). The hippocampus and behavioral maturation. *Behavioral Biology, 8,* 557–596.

American Psychiatric Association (APA). (1987). *Diagnostic and statistical manual of mental disorders* (3rd ed., rev.). Washington, DC: Author.

American Psychiatric Association (APA). (1994). *Diagnostic and statistical manual of mental disorders* (4th ed.). Washington, DC: Author.

Asberg, M., Traskman, L., & Thoren, R. (1976). 5-HIAA in the cerebrospinal fluid: A biochemical suicide predictor. *Archives of General Psychiatry, 33,* 93–97.

Axelrod, J., & Reisine, T. D. (1984). Stress hormones, their interaction and regulation. *Science, 224,* 452–459.

Beecher, H. K. (1946). Pain in men wounded in battle. *Annals of Surgery, 123,* 96–105.

Blanchard, E. B., Kolb, L. C., & Gerardi, R. J. (1986). Cardiac response to relevant stimuli as an adjunctive tool for diagnosing post traumatic stress disorder in Vietnam veterans. *Behavior Therapy, 17,* 592–606.

Bohus, B., & DeWied, D. (1978). Pituitary–adrenal system hormones and adaptive behavior. In I. Chester-Jones & I. W. Henderson (Eds.), *General, comparative, and clinical endocrinology of the adrenal cortex* (Vol. 3). New York: Academic Press.

Bowlby, J. (1969). *Attachment and loss* (Vol. 1). New York: Basic Books.

Bremner, J. D., Randall, P., Scott, T. M., Bronen, R. A., Seibyl, J. P., Southwick, S. M., Delaney, R. C., McCarthy, G., Charney, D. S., & Innis, R. B. (1995). MRI-based measures of hippocampal volume in patients with PTSD. *American Journal of Psychiatry, 152,* 973–981.

Brown, G. L., Goodwin, F. K., Ballenger, J. C., Goyer, P. F., & Major, L. F. (1979). Aggression in humans correlates with cerebrospinal fluid metabolites. *Psychiatry Research, 1,* 131–139.

Butler, R. W., Braff, D. L., Jenkins, M. A., Sprock, J., Geyer, M. A., & Rausch, J. L. (1990). Physiological evidence of exaggerated startle response in a subgroup of Vietnam veterans with combat-related PTSD. *American Journal of Psychiatry, 147*(10), 1308–1312.

Calvin, W. H. (1990). *The cerebral symphony.* New York: Bantam Books.

Charney, D. S., Deutch, A. Y., Krystal, J. H., Southwick, S. M., & Davis, M. (1993). Psychobiologic mechanisms of post-traumatic stress disorder. *Archives of General Psychiatry, 50,* 294–305.

Cicchetti, D. (1985). The emergence of developmental psychopathology. *Child Development, 55,* 1–7.

Coccaro, E. F., Siever, L. J., Klar, H. M., & Maurer, G. (1989). Serotonergic studies in patients with affective and personality disorders. *Archives of General Psychiatry, 46,* 587–598.

Cole, P. M., & Putnam, F. W. (1992). Effect of incest on self and social functioning: A developmental psychopathology perspective. *Journal of Consulting and Clinical Psychology, 60,* 174–184.

Davis, M. (1984). The mammalian startle response. In R. C. Eaton (Ed.), *Neural mechanisms of startle behavior.* New York: Plenum Press.

DeBellis, M., Burke, L., Trickett, P., & Putnam, F. (in press). Antinuclear antibodies and thyroid function in sexually abused girls. *Journal of Traumatic Stress.*

DeMasio, A. (1995). *Descartes' error.* New York: Grosset/Putnam.

Depue, R. A., & Spoont, M. R. (1986). Conceptualizing a serotonin trait: A behavioral dimension of constraint. *Annals of the New York Academy of Sciences, 487,* 47–62.

Dobbs, D., & Wilson, W. P. (1960). Observations on the persistence of traumatic war neurosis. *Journal of Nervous and Mental Disease, 21,* 40–46.

Donald, M. (1991). *Origins of the modern mind.* Cambridge, MA: Harvard University Press.

Dunn, A. J., & Berridge, C. W. (1987). Corticotropin-releasing factor administration elicits stresslike activation of cerebral catecholamine systems. *Pharmacology, Biochemistry and Behavior, 27,* 685–691.

Fisler, R., & van der Kolk, B. A. (1995). [Unpublished raw data.]

Foa, E., Zinbarg, R., & Rothbaum, B. O. (1992). Uncontrollability and unpredictability in post-traumatic stress disorder: An animal model. *Psychological Bulletin, 112*(2), 218–238.

Gerson, S. C., & Baldessarini, R. J. (1980). Motor effects of serotonin in the central nervous system. *Life Sciences, 27,* 1435–1451.

Gray, J. F. (1987). *The neuropsychology of anxiety: An enquiry into the functions of the septo-hippocampal system.* New York: Oxford University Press.

Green, A. H. (1978). Self-destructive behavior in battered children. *American Journal of Psychiatry, 135,* 579–582.

Grinker, R. R., & Spiegel, J. J. (1945). *Men under stress.* Philidelphia: Blakiston.

Gurvitz, T. V., Shenton, M. E., & Pitman, R. K. (1995). *Reduced hippocampal volume on magnetic resonance imaging in chronic post-traumatic stress disorder.* Paper presented at the annual meeting of the International Society for Traumatic Stress Studies, Miami.

Herman, J. L. (1992). Complex PTSD: A syndrome in survivors of prolonged and repeated trauma. *Journal of Traumatic Stress, 5,* 377–391.

Herman, J. L., Perry, J. C., & van der Kolk, B. A. (1989). Childhood trauma in borderline personality disorder. *American Journal of Psychiatry, 146,* 490–495.

Horowitz, M. J. (1978). *Stress response syndromes* (2nd ed.). New York: Jason Aronson.

Horowitz, M. J. (1986). Stress-response syndromes: A review of posttraumatic and adjustment disorders. *Hospital and Community Psychiatry, 37*(3), 241–249.

Jenike, M. A., Baer, L., Summergrad, P., Minichiello, W. E., Holland, A., & Seymour, K. (1990). Sertraline in obsessive–compulsive disorder: A double blind study. *American Journal of Psychiatry, 147,* 923–928.

Joseph, R. (1988). Dual mental functioning in a split-brain patient. *Journal of Clinical Psychology, 44*(5), 770–779.

Kardiner, A. (1941). *The traumatic neuroses of war.* New York: Hoeber.

Keane, T. M., & Kaloupek. D. G. (1982). Imaginal flooding in the treatment of posttraumatic stress disorder. *Journal of Consulting and Clinical Psychology, 50,* 138–140.

Kolb, L. C. (1987). Neurophysiological hypothesis explaining posttraumatic stress disorder. *American Journal of Psychiatry, 144,* 989–995.

Kolb, L. C., & Multipassi, L. R. (1982). The conditioned emotional response: A subclass of chronic and delayed post traumatic stress disorder. *Psychiatric Annals, 12,* 979–987.

Kosten, T. R., Mason, J. W., Giller, E. L., Ostroff, R. B., & Harkness, L. (1987). Sustained urinary norepinephrine and epinephrine elevation in PTSD. *Psychoneuroendocrinology, 12,* 13–20.

Krystal, H. (1978). Trauma and affects. *Psychoanalytic Study of the Child, 33,* 81–116.

Krystal, J. H., Kosten, T. R., Southwick, S., Mason, J. W., Perry, B. D., & Giller, E. L. (1989). Neurobiological aspects of PTSD: Review of clinical and preclinical studies. *Behavior Therapy, 20,* 177–198.

Lang, P. J. (1979). A bio-informational theory of emotional imagery. *Psychophysiology, 16,* 495–512.

LeDoux, J. E. (1986). Sensory systems and emotion: A model of affective processing. *Integrative Psychiatry, 4,* 237–243.

LeDoux, J. E. (1990). Information flow from sensation to emotion: Plasticity of the neutral computation of stimulus value. In M. Gabriel & J. Moore (Eds.), *Learning computational neuroscience: Foundations of adaptive networks.* Cambridge, MA: MIT Press.

LeDoux, J. E. (1992). Emotion as memory: Anatomical systems underlying indelible neural traces. In S.-A. Christianson (Ed.), *Handbook of emotion and memory.* Hillsdale, NJ: Erlbaum.

LeDoux, J. E., Romanski, L., & Xagoraris, A. (1991). Indelibility of subcortical emotional memories. *Journal of Cognitive Neuroscience, 1,* 238–243.

Lerer, B., Bleich, A., & Kotler, M. (1987). Post traumatic stress disorder in Israeli combat veterans: Effect of phenelzine treatment. *Archives of General Psychiatry, 44,* 976–981.

Lewis, D. O. (1992). From abuse to violence: Psychophysiological consequences of maltreatment. *Journal of the American Academy of Child and Adolescent Psychiatry, 31,* 383–391.

Lindemann, E. (1944). Symptomatology and management of acute grief. *American Journal of Psychiatry, 101,* 141–148.

Litz, B. T., & Keane, T. M. (1989). Information processing in anxiety disorders: Application to the understanding of post-traumatic stress disorder. *Clinical Psychology Review, 9,* 243–257.

MacLean, P. D. (1985). Brain evolution relating to family, play, and the separation call. *Archives of General Psychiatry, 42,* 405–417.

Malloy, P. F., Fairbank, J. A., & Keane, T. M. (1983). Validation of a multimethod assessment of post traumatic stress disorders in Vietnam veterans. *Journal of Consulting and Clinical Psychology, 51,* 4–21.

Mann, J. D. (1987). Psychobiologic predictors of suicide. *Journal of Clinical Psychiatry, 48,* 39–43.

McEwen, B. S., Gould, E. A., & Sakai, R. R. (1992). The vulnerability of the hippocampus to protective and destructive effects of glucocorticoids in relation to stress. *British Journal of Psychiatry, 160,* 18–24.

McFarlane, A. C. (1988). The longitudinal course of posttraumatic morbidity: The range of outcomes and their predictors. *Journal of Nervous and Mental Disease, 176,* 30–39.

McFarlane, A. C., Weber, D. L., & Clark, C. R. (1993). Abnormal stimulus processing in PTSD. *Biological Psychiatry, 34,* 311–320.

Meaney, M. J., Aitken, D. H., Viau, V., Sharma, S., & Sarieau, A. (1989). Neonatal handling alters adrenocortical negative feedback sensitivity and hippocampal Type II glucocorticoid binding in the rat. *Neuroendocrinology, 50,* 597–604.

Moleman, N., van der Hart, O., & van der Kolk, B.A. (1992). The partus stress reaction: A neglected etiological factor in post-partum psychiatric disorders. *Journal of Nervous and Mental Disease, 180,* 271–272.

Murburg, M. (Ed.). (1993). *Catecholamine function in posttraumatic stress disorder.* Washington, DC: American Psychiatric Press.

O'Keefe, J., & Bouma, H. (1969). Complex sensory properties of certain amygdala units in the freely moving cat. *Experimental Neurology, 23,* 384–398.

O'Keefe, J., & Nadel, L. (1978). *The hippocampus as a cognitive map.* Oxford: Clarendon Press.

Ornitz, E. M., & Pynoos, R. S. (1989). Startle modulation in children with post traumatic stress disorder. *American Journal of Psychiatry, 146,* 866–870.

Paige, S., Reid, G., Allen, M., & Newton, J. (1990). Psychophysiological correlates of PTSD. *Biological Psychiatry, 58,* 329–335.

Papez, J. W. (1937). A proposed mechanism of emotion. *Archives of General Psychiatry, 38,* 725–743.

Perry, B. D., Giller, E. L., & Southwick, S. M. (1987). Altered plasma alpha-2 adrenergic receptor affinity states in PTSD. *American Journal of Psychiatry, 144,* 1511–1512.

Pfaff, D. W., Silva, M. T., & Weiss, J. M. (1971). Telemetered recording of hormone effects on hippocampal neurons. *Science, 172,* 394–395.

Pitman, R. K. (1989). Post traumatic stress disorder, hormones and memory. *Biological Psychiatry, 26,* 221–223.

Pitman, R. K., & Orr, S. P. (1990a). The black hole of trauma. *Biological Psychiatry, 26,* 221–223.

Pitman, R. K., & Orr, S. P. (1990b). Twenty-four hour urinary cortisol and catecholamine excretion in combat-related post-traumatic stress disorder. *Biological Psychiatry, 27,* 245–247.

Pitman, R. K., & Orr, S. P. (1995). [Unpublished raw data.]

Pitman, R. K., Orr, S. P., Forgue, D. F., de Jong, J., & Claiborn, J. M. (1987). Psychophysiologic assessment of posttraumatic stress disorder imagery in Vietnam combat veterans. *Archives of General Psychiatry, 44,* 970– 975.

Pitman, R., Orr, S. P., & Lasko, N. B. (1993). Effects of intranasal vasopressin and oxytocin on physiologic responding during personal combat imagery in Vietnam veterans with posttraumatic stress disorder. *Psychiatry Research, 48,* 107–117.

Pitman, R. K., Orr, S. P., & Shalev, A. (1993). Once bitten, twice shy: Beyond the conditioning model of PTSD. *Biological Psychiatry, 33,* 145–146.

Pitman, R. K., van der Kolk, B. A., Orr, S. P., & Greenberg, M. S. (1990). Naloxone reversible stress induced analgesia in post traumatic stress disorder. *Archives of General Psychiatry, 47,* 541–547.

Rainey, J. M., Aleem, A., Ortiz, A., Yaragani, V., Pohl, R., & Berchow, R. (1987). Laboratory procedure for the inducement of flashbacks. *American Journal of Psychiatry, 144,* 1317–1319.

Raleigh, M. J., McGuire, M. T., & Brammer, G. L. (1984). Social and environmental influences on blood serotonin concentrations in monkeys. *Archives of General Psychiatry, 41,* 505–510.

Rauch, S. L., van der Kolk, B. A., Fisler, R. E., Alpert, N. M., Orr, S. P., Savage, C. R., Fischman, A. J., Jenike, M. A., & Pitman, R. K. (in press). A symptom provocation study of posttraumatic stress disorder using positron emission tomography and script-driven imagery. *Archives of General Psychiatry.*

Reite, M., & Fields, T. M. (Eds.). (1985). *The psychobiology of attachment and separation.* Orlando, FL: Academic Press.

Resnick, H., Yehuda, R., Pitman, R. K., & Foy, D. W. (1995). Effect of previous trauma on acute plasma cortisol level following rape. *American Journal of Psychiatry, 152,* 1675–1677.

Ross, R. J., Ball, W. A., & Cohen, M. E. (1989). Habituation of the startle response in post traumatic stress disorder. *Journal of Neuropsychiatry, 1,* 305–307.

Sapolsky, R. M., Hideo, E., Rebert, C. S., & Finch, C. E. (1990). Hippocampal damage associated with prolonged glucocorticoid exposure in primates. *Journal of Neuroscience, 10,* 2897–2902.

Sapolsky, R. M., Krey, L., & McEwen, B. S. (1984). Stress down-regulates corticosterone receptors in a site specific manner in the brain. *Endocrinology, 114,* 287–292.

Saxe, G. N., Vasile, R. G., Hill, T. C., Bloomingdale, K., & van der Kolk, B. A. (1992). SPECT imaging and multiple personality disorder. *Journal of Nervous and Mental Disease, 180,* 662–663.

Shalev, A. Y., Orr, S. P., Peri, T., Schreiber, S., & Pitman, R. K. (1992). Physiologic responses to loud tones in Israeli patients with post-traumatic stress disorder. *Archives of General Psychiatry, 49,* 870–875.

Shalev, A. Y., & Rogel-Fuchs, Y. (1993). Psychophysiology of PTSD: From sulfur fumes to behavioral genetics [Review]. *Journal of Nervous and Mental Disease, 55*(5), 413–423.

Siegfried, B., Frischknecht, H. R., & Nunez de Souza, R. (1990). An ethological model for the study of activation and interaction of pain, memory, and defensive systems in the attacked mouse: Role of endogenous opioids. *Neuroscience and Biobehavioral Reviews, 14,* 481–490.

Silberman, E. K., & Weingartner, H. (1986). Hemispheric lateralization of functions related to emotion. *Brain and Cognition, 5,* 322–353.

Soubrie, P. (1986). Reconciling the role of central serotonin neurons in human and animal behavior. *Behavioral and Brain Sciences, 9,* 319–364.

Southwick, S. M., Morgan, C. A., Bremner, J. D., Nagy, L., Krystal, J. H., & Charney, D. S. (1990, December). *Yohimbine and M-CPP effects in PTSD patients.* Poster presented at the Annual Meeting of the American College of Neuropharmacology, Puerto Rico.

Southwick, S. M., Krystal, J. H., Morgan, A., Johnson, D., Nagy, L., Nicolaou, A., Henninger, G. R., & Charney, D. S. (1993). Abnormal noradrenergic function in post traumatic stress disorder. *Archives of General Psychiatry, 50,* 266–274.

Squire, L. R., & Zola-Morgan, S. (1991). The medical temporal lobe memory system. *Science, 253,* 2380–2386.

Starkman, M. N., Gebarksi, S. S., Berent, S., & Schteingart, D. E. (1992). Hippocampal formation volume, memory of dysfunction, and cortisol levels in patients with Cushing's syndrome. *Biological Psychiatry, 32,* 756–765.

Stein, M. B., Hannah, C., Koverola, C., Yehuda, R., Torchia, M., & McClarty, B. (1994, December 15). *Neuroanatomical and neuroendocrine correlates in adulthood of severe sexual abuse in childhood.* Paper presented at the 33rd annual meeting of the American College of Neuropsychopharmacology, San Juan, PR.

Teicher, M. H., Glod, C. A., Survey, J., & Swett, C. (in press). Early childhood abuse and limbic system satings in adult psychiatric outpatients. *Journal of Neuropsychiatry and Clinical Neuroscience.*

Terr, L. C. (1991). Childhood traumas: An outline and overview. *American Journal of Psychiatry, 148,*10–20.

Thatcher, R. W., Walker, R. A., & Giudice, S. (1987). Human cerebral hemisphere development at different rates and ages. *Science, 236,* 1110–1113.

Tomarken, A. J., Davidson, R. J., Wheeler, R. E., & Ross, R. C. (1992). Individual differences in anterior brain asymmetry and fundamental dimensions of emotion. *Journal of Personality and Social Psychology, 64,* 676–687.

Valentino, R. J., & Foote, S. L. (1988). Corticotropin releasing hormone increases tonic, but not sensory-evoked activity of noradrenergic locus coeruleus in unanesthetized rats. *Journal of Neuroscience, 8,* 1016–1025.

Valzelli, L. (1982). Serotonergic inhibitory control of experimental aggression. *Psychopharmacological Research Communications, 12,* 1–13.

van der Kolk, B. A. (1987). *Psychological trauma.* Washington, DC: American Psychiatric Press.

van der Kolk, B.A. (1988). The trauma spectrum: The interaction of biological and social events in the genesis of the trauma response. *Journal of Traumatic Stress, 1,* 273–290.

van der Kolk, B. A. (1994). The body keeps the score: Memory and the evolving psychobiology of PTSD. *Harvard Review of Psychiatry, 1,* 253–265.

van der Kolk, B. A., Dreyfuss, D., Michaels, M., Shera, D., Berkowitz, B., Fisler, R., & Saxe, G. (1994). Flouxetine in posttraumatic stress disorder. *Journal of Clinical Psychiatry, 55*(12), 517–522.

van der Kolk, B. A., & Ducey, C. P. (1989). The psychological processing of traumatic experience: Rorschach patterns in PTSD. *Journal of Traumatic Stress, 2,* 259–274.

van der Kolk, B. A. Greenberg, M. S., Boyd, H., & Krystal, J. H. (1985). Inescapable shock, neurotransmitters and addiction to trauma: Towards a psychobiology of post traumatic stress. *Biological Psychiatry, 20,* 314–325.

van der Kolk, B. A., Greenberg, M. S., Orr, S. P., & Pitman, R. K. (1989). Endogenous opioids and stress induced analgesia in post traumatic stress disorder. *Psychopharmacology Bulletin, 25,* 108–112.

van der Kolk, B. A., Perry, J. C., & Herman, J. L. (1991). Childhood origins of self-destructive behavior. *American Journal of Psychiatry, 148,* 1665–1671.

van der Kolk, B. A., Roth, S., & Pelcovitz, D. (1993). *Field trials for DSM-IV, post traumatic stress disorder: II. Disorders of extreme stress.* Washington, DC: American Psychiatric Association.

van der Kolk, B. A., & Saporta, J. (1991). The biological response to psychic trauma: Mechanisms and treatment of intrusion and numbing. *Anxiety Research, 4,* 199–212.

van der Kolk, B. A., & van der Hart, O. (1991). The intrusive past: The flexibility of memory and the engraving of trauma. *American Imago, 48,* 425–454.

Yehuda, R., Giller, E. L., Southwick, S. M., Lowy, M. T., & Mason, J. W. (1991). Hypothalamic–pituitary–adrenal dysfunction in posttraumatic stress disorder. *Biological Psychiatry, 30,* 1031–1048.

Yehuda, R., Kahana, B., Binder-Byrnes, K., Southwick, S., & Mason, J., & Giller, E. L. (1995). Low urinary cortisol excretion in Holocaust survivors with post traumatic stress disorder. *American Journal of Psychiatry, 152,* 982–986.

Yehuda, R., Southwick, S. M., Krystal, J. H., Bremner, D., Charney, D. S., & Mason, J. W. (1993). Enhanced suppression of cortisol following dexamethasone administration in post traumatic stress disorder. *American Journal of Psychiatry, 150,* 83–86.

Yehuda, R., Southwick, S. M., Mason, J. W., & Giller, E. L. (1990). Interactions of the hypothalamic–pituitary–adrenal axis and the catecholaminergic system of the stress disorder. In E. L. Giller (Ed.), *Biological assessment and treatment of PTSD.* Washington, DC: American Psychiatric Press.

Zager, E. L., & Black, P. M. (1985). Neuropeptides in human memory and learning processes. *Neurosurgery, 17,* 355–369.

Assessment of Posttraumatic Stress Disorder in Clinical and Research Settings

ELANA NEWMAN
DANNY G. KALOUPEK
TERENCE M. KEANE

Since posttraumatic stress disorder (PTSD) became an official part of the diagnostic nomenclature in 1980, the development of reliable and valid instruments to measure the effects of trauma exposure has been the goal of an extensive set of investigations. In general, these efforts have been quite successful and have provided a firm quantitative foundation for the diagnosis, assessment, and broad spectrum evaluation of PTSD. The aim of this chapter is to describe the available structured and semistructured interviews, self-report measures, and other means of assessing PTSD in adults, and to detail the strengths and weaknesses of particular assessment methods. A related aim is to enumerate the assessment goals and explain the rationale and implementation of the multimethod assessment strategy for PTSD. We begin this undertaking with a brief overview of considerations that influence the context and methods for diagnostic assessment of potentially traumatized individuals.

ASSESSMENT TARGETS, GOALS, AND COMPLICATIONS

The level of required detail and confidence in the diagnoses will vary by assessment purpose. For example, in clinical settings PTSD assessment may be useful in devising a comprehensive treatment plan for an individual, or it may serve as a screen for early intervention or further PTSD evaluation. As we describe in more detail below, we advocate the most comprehensive multimodal assessment strategy possible for a given context. Ideally, this will include a semistructured clinical interview assessing lifetime exposure to potentially traumatic events, PTSD, and other disorders, as well as self-report measures, psychophysiological assessment, and collateral assessment. However, since this level of detail is not always necessary, this chapter describes the challenges and principles involved in selecting suitable PTSD assessment techniques for a given purpose.

For the purposes of this chapter, we focus on the assessment of PTSD according to the symptom and duration criteria defined by the revised third edition or, when possible, the fourth edition of the *Diagnostic and Statistical Manual of Mental Disorders* (DSM III-R or DSM-IV; American Psychiatric Association [APA], 1987, 1994). Given these criteria, one of the basic tasks in assessing PTSD is firmly establishing the presence of specific symptoms of the disorder. To state this another way, a clinician cannot simply infer PTSD on the basis of exposure to a high-magnitude stressor. Of the many individuals exposed to such stressors during their lives, only a minority ultimately develop PTSD (e.g., Breslau, Davis, Andreski, & Peterson, 1991). Several studies have found that exposure to a potentially traumatic event is a risk factor for the development of numerous mental health problems, among which PTSD is just one possibility (e.g., Burnam et al., 1988; Keane & Wolfe, 1990; Shore, Tatum, & Vollmer, 1986). It is evident that exposure to highly stressful events does not imply that an individual will necessarily develop the debilitating symptoms of PTSD. Consequently, it is incumbent upon the clinician to examine exposed individuals for all symptom criteria, including intrusions, numbing, avoidance, and hyperarousal, within the specified time frame (APA, 1980, 1987, 1994).

Survey data indicate that after an individual experiences one high-magnitude stressor, there is an increased probability that he or she will be exposed to two or more such stressors over the lifespan (e.g., Breslau et al., 1991; Kilpatrick, Saunders, Veronen, Best, & Von, 1987). Accordingly, it seems wise to routinely explore the possibility that several significant stressors have been experienced by any adult who presents for a clinical assessment related to trauma. This perspective is further justified by evidence that exposure to one traumatic event increases both the risk of exposure to future potentially traumatic events and the probability of developing PTSD in reaction to these events (e.g., Helzer, Robins, & McEvoy, 1987; Kulka et al., 1990).

Background knowledge about the physical, social, and political circumstances in which potentially traumatic events occur can provide critical contextual information for evaluating psychological reactions such as reexperiencing symptoms. Clearly, such symptoms as avoidance or hypervigilance are manifested differently for particular types of potentially traumatic events; the clinician must therefore consider the nature of the event and its interaction with gender, race, class, and culture. In addition, the nature of the relationship between symptom and stressor may be obvious, or it may be complex and difficult to discern. For example, nightmares may obviously recapitulate the potentially traumatic events, or a complex relationship may be found, such as that which occurs when people who have been exposed to potentially traumatic events place themselves in risky situations in efforts to promote mastery. Clinical strategies that can help identify these complex relationships include careful questioning about symptom content, initial symptom onset, and external cues associated with the symptoms, as well as a careful examination of the individual's demographic characteristics.

The temporal stability (or instability) of posttraumatic symptoms can also be a valuable target of assessment. Different sets of symptoms may appear in different phases of the disorder, at various times across the lifespan, or in response to other developmental markers or stressors (Keane, 1989). Clinically, we have noted that anniversaries of traumatic events, life transitions, and family holidays appear to influence symptom presentation. Similarly, emerging research data provide support regarding the fluctuating longitudinal course of PTSD. For example, 50 Australian bush firefighters were assessed at 4, 8, 11, 29, and 42 months after a traumatic event. The firefighters demonstrated variations in intrusion, avoidance, and hyperarousal symptoms; however, the overall pattern suggested that intrusion symptoms may be frequent at onset, but decrease in later phases of the disorder (McFarlane, 1988).

In addition to a careful evaluation of PTSD symptoms, a necessary goal of assessment is to evaluate the presence of other psychological disorders. Levels of comorbidity in PTSD populations are quite high in both community and clinical populations (e.g., Boudewyns, Albrecht, Talbert, & Hyer, 1991; Davidson & Fairbank, 1993; Davidson, Hughes, & Blazer, 1991; Keane & Wolfe, 1990; Jordan et al., 1991), with substance abuse, affective disorders, and other anxiety disorders as the most common comorbid diagnoses across all PTSD populations (Davidson & Fairbank, 1993). Similarly, high rates of concurrent personality disorders are noted among individuals with PTSD (e.g., Faustman & White, 1989; Southwick, Yehuda, & Giller, 1993). The use of a diagnostic interview assessing all Axis I and Axis II disorders is effective for detecting such comorbid disorders. In addition, general psychometric assessments of psychopathology, health, distress, and social and functional impairment can provide important data on comorbid symptom severity. Measures such as the Symptom Checklist 90—Revised (SCL-90-R; Derogatis, 1977), the General Health Questionnaire (Goldberg, 1972), the Social Adjustment Scale—Revised (Weissman & Bothwell, 1976), and the Global Assessment of Functioning Scale (APA, 1994) may provide information on functional impairment and symptom severity.

A careful lifetime history of the individual's adjustment before and after traumatic events can provide evidence about the potential interactions between PTSD and other comorbid disorders. For example, a substance-abuse disorder in a traumatized individual may reflect an effort to self-medicate against intrusive thoughts and feelings, numbness, and psychological distress. Comorbid disorders may also reflect preexisting vulnerability. Two studies have demonstrated that those with preexisting disorder are at greater risk of developing PTSD after exposure to a stressor (Breslau et al., 1991; Resnick, Kilpatrick, Best, & Kramer, 1992).

MULTIMETHOD ASSESSMENT

A comprehensive assessment strategy aims to gather data about the person's life context, symptoms, beliefs, strengths, weaknesses, and coping repertoire. The challenge in the clinical assessment of PTSD is to combine appropriate measures so as to distinguish individuals who, once exposed to potentially traumatic events, have gone on to develop the disorder from those who have not. In many settings there is the additional consideration of wanting the most comprehensive and diagnostically accurate assessment involving the fewest number of measures, so that efficiency is maximized.

Multiple measures are recommended in assessing PTSD, for several reasons. First, no existing single measure can function as a definitive indicator of PTSD (Keane, Wolfe, & Taylor, 1987; Malloy, Fairbank, & Keane, 1983; Kulka et al., 1988). Among the reasons for this lack of an absolute criterion is the fact that a respondent may have difficulty with a particular test format, may experience fatigue or attentional difficulties at one testing occasion, or may demonstrate response bias on a particular test. The impact of extraneous factors such as these is diminished when a range of assessment approaches is used. Second, various assessment formats have different relative strengths. For example, interviewers can increase comprehension by rephrasing questions to insure that a respondent understands them. On the other hand, the interviewer format may decrease the accuracy of response, by virtue of the reluctance some people may feel about revealing certain experiences to another person directly. Self-report instruments, by contrast, can yield information that is less influenced by a respondent's direct interpersonal communications with the evaluator, although flexibility to aid comprehension or gather qualitative information is lost. Observational and physiological data can provide information that is less subject to respondent biases, but measurement is often more complex and costly. Thus, multimodal assessment offers the potential ability to overcome the psychometric limitations of any one type of instrument (cf. Keane et al., 1987).

For a fuller understanding of the psychometric advantages of multimethod assessment, definitions of terms relating to diagnostic performance may be useful. "Diagnostic utility" is the general extent to which a particular test index can accurately predict that a person belongs or does not belong in a specified category. Diagnostic utility is measured in terms of sensitivity, specificity, and efficiency. "Sensitivity" is the probability that those with the diagnosis will be correctly identified by the test score (i.e., will score above the cutoff score of a particular test); "specificity" is the probability that those without the diagnosis will be correctly identified (i.e., will score below the cutoff score). "Efficiency" is the overall probability that true cases and noncases will be categorized appropriately. Sensitivity, specificity, and efficiency are quantified as percentages (0–100%), or alternatively as decimal fractions ranging from 0 to 1.

The diagnostic utility of different PTSD measures appears to vary across populations. For example, studies (e.g., Green, 1991; Kulka et al., 1991) indicate that a PTSD structured interview may demonstrate good psychometric performance for clinical populations, but may not always do so for community populations (and vice versa). This variation occurs at least in part because the base rates for disorders in a population can affect how accurately PTSD is detected (e.g., Green, 1991; Kulka et al., 1991). In addition, PTSD measures that have been developed and applied only within specific trauma populations (e.g., the PTSD Symptom Scale Interview [PSS-I] and PTSD Symptom Scale Self-Report [PSS-S] with sexual assault victims; Foa, Riggs, Dancu, & Rothbaum, 1993) may not perform equally well across all trauma groups because of specific item phrasing, population-specific scoring criteria, and variations from the base rates for the disorder relative to the populations upon which the instruments were validated.

Batteries of tests can be combined to maximize the predictive power of the entire assessment by incorporating measures with varying levels of specificity and sensitivity. It is advantageous to combine measures that can collectively offer high sensitivity and high specificity. For example, tests with especially high specificity may be valuable, independent of sensitivity, in order to efficiently screen out those who do not have PTSD. Likewise, tests which demonstrate excellent sensitivity can cast a broad net for possible cases, and additional assessment methods can then be applied to enhance specificity and overall efficiency.

Discrepancies often emerge among indicators when multiple measures are used to assess PTSD. Apparent contradictions may result from measurement discrepancies (e.g., differing time frames for two instruments) or from the varying presentations of the disorder over time. Alternatively, some measures may focus on one dimension of the disorder, while others focus on different dimensions. Clinical judgment assists in reconciling the discordance among measures insofar as clinical interpretation is concerned. For example, when a self-report measure is not indicative of PTSD and an interview is, pertinent evidence can be sought to reconcile these differences. Possibilities include examining the onset of functional impairment, psychophysiological evidence of hyperarousal, and any evidence of a minimizing or overreporting response style on validity indicators such as those contained in the Minnesota Multiphasic Personality Inventory—2 (MMPI-2).

In research, analysis of discrepancies in terms of modality, overall response bias, influence of other disorders, and areas of functional impairment can be pursued, and statistical algorithms can be developed to reconcile differences across measures. The National Vietnam Veterans Readjustment Study (NVVRS) offers a systematic and logical approach for using data to mimic the process of clinical decision making when multiple sources of information are being used (Kulka et al., 1990; Schlenger et al., 1992). In this investigation, a statistical algorithm was developed and applied to reconcile those cases where disagreements among PTSD indicators occurred. Resolution of caseness was thus possible for virtually all subjects in this large-scale epidemiological study.

Since our approach to assessment of PTSD advocates the use of multiple measures drawn from different categories of available instruments, the following review details several approaches for assessing PTSD, including structured and semistructured diagnostic interviews, self-report checklists, empirically derived psychometric measures, psychophysiological assessment, and collateral measures. Although the majority of the measures are published and have been standardized on trauma-exposed populations, several unpublished and/or unvalidated measures are included in this chapter because of their special features. As each assessment instrument is described below, information is provided on (1) the psychometric characteristics of the measure, (2) the samples with which the instrument has been used, (3) the approximate administration time, and (4) relative strengths and limitations. Evidence is generally not available to support direct comparisons among measures; instead, each is evaluated on the basis of content, structure, and clinical and diagnostic utility. All the data reported are based on DSM-III-R criteria for PTSD (APA, 1987), or, when indicated, on DSM-III criteria (APA, 1980).

STRUCTURED AND SEMISTRUCTURED DIAGNOSTIC INTERVIEWS

A comprehensive structured or semistructured interview instrument is recommended to insure that all PTSD symptomatology is reviewed in detail (e.g., Green, 1990; Resnick, Kilpatrick, & Lipovsky, 1991; Weiss, 1993; Wolfe & Keane, 1993). The semistructured format has the particular advantage of providing organization and consistency, while allowing interviewees to discuss their experiences using their own words and metaphors. Clinical skill is required on the part of the interviewer with respect to interpreting, clarifying, guiding, pacing, reflecting, and listening to responses during the interview. Finally, attention to behavioral indices of PTSD, such as avoidance, hypervigilance, emotional detachment, and startle response to noises, can assist clinical decision making.

Table 11.1 lists the salient features of those structured or semistructured interviews and self-report measures available for assessing PTSD. The table summarizes the following: (1) the edition of the DSM to which the measure is referenced; (2) the types of information the measure assesses; (3) whether administration of the instrument requires advanced training; and (4) the populations with which the measure has been used. Modality and approximate time of administration, and psychometric findings, are also noted. Measures of sensitivity, specificity, interrater reliability, test–retest reliability, and internal consistency are included when these are available from the published literature.

Structured Clinical Interview for DSM-III-R

The PTSD module of the Structured Clinical Interview for DSM-III-R (SCID; Spitzer, Williams, Gibbon, & First, 1990) is the most widely used semistructured interview in PTSD studies across a range of trauma populations. It has demonstrated excellent reliability across clinicians and is highly correlated with other psychometric measures of PTSD, such as the Keane PTSD scale of the MMPI-2 (PK) and the Mississippi Scale for Combat-Related PTSD (e.g., Kulka et al., 1990). Diagnostically, it also has good sensitivity and excellent specificity (Kulka et al., 1990). The advantages of the SCID PTSD module include its widespread application, its use across diverse clinical populations, and its psychometric properties. One of the disadvantages of the SCID is that it only rates the presence, absence, and subthreshold presence of PTSD symptoms and the overall PTSD diagnosis (yes–no). Thus, if the aim is to monitor the change of PTSD symptom severity over time, the SCID does not offer sufficient resolution to identify small changes. In addition, the SCID measures lifetime PTSD based on the respondent's memory of his or her "worst ever" experience with each symptom, regardless of when it occurred. This may result in an inaccurately high estimate of lifetime PTSD, because all symptoms experienced by the individual may not have occurred concurrently.

Diagnostic Interview Schedule

The Diagnostic Interview Schedule (DIS; Robins, Helzer, Croughan, & Ratliff, 1981a), which has been primarily used in community studies, is a semistructured interview that a trained technician can administer. Despite the popularity of the PTSD section of the DIS in studies of disaster, there is surprisingly little evidence substantiating its diagnostic performance. In a review of PTSD assessment instruments, Watson (1990) described two studies on veterans indicating that the DIS correlated well with previously established psychometric measures of PTSD in clinical settings. However, data from the NVVRS indicated that the DIS may be less accurate in identifying PTSD in community samples, where the disorder is less prevalent; despite an excellent specificity, the DIS had poor sensitivity, identifying only one of five PTSD cases diagnosed by expert clinicians using other PTSD measures (Kulka et al., 1991). Although one study did show adequate 3-week test–retest reliability (Breslau & Davis, 1987), questions about the diagnostic sensitivity of the DIS (e.g., Keane & Penk, 1989; Kulka et al., 1990) suggest a need for additional psychometric evaluation in field studies. The major advantage of the DIS is the fact that it has been used in most community-based studies; this facilitates comparisons across findings and over time. In addition, the use of a lay interviewer makes it less costly to obtain diagnostic information. The major disadvantages of the DIS are its questionable sensitivity and its use of dichotomous (yes–no) ratings, which limit its ability to detect ranges of symptoms and changes over time. Furthermore, the DIS requires the interviewee to associate each PTSD symptom directly with a specific traumatic event. This requirement may inadvertently reduce endorsement of PTSD symptoms, because some traumatized individuals are unable to attribute symptomatology to specific life experiences (e.g., childhood sexual abuse).

Structured Interview for PTSD

The Structured Interview for PTSD (SI-PTSD; Davidson, Smith, & Kudler, 1989), designed as an alternative to the SCID and DIS, uses ratings that are directly tied to the severity and frequency of particular behaviors for each symptom (e.g., nightmares are rated by frequency and disruption caused, including anchors such as ability to share a bed with a partner). Another unique aspect of the SI-PTSD is that it rates "constricted affect" on the basis of observation rather than through questioning of the respondent. The authors report that when the SI-PTSD was compared with the SCID module for PTSD, it had excellent diagnostic sensitivity and good specificity. The SI-PTSD has fair test–retest reliability over a 2-week interval, excellent internal consistency, and good interrater reliability. Thus far, the SI-PTSD has been validated only with veterans, although further validity data are currently being collected in a study that includes both civilian and combat veteran populations and utilizes DSM-III-R criteria (R. D. Smith, personal communication, October 21, 1993). The advantages of the SI-PTSD include applicability as both a dichotomous and a continuous measure, use of clear criteria to rate symptom severity, and good psychometric properties. One of the disadvantages of the SI-PTSD is that, like the SCID, it uses the problematic "worst ever" convention to assess lifetime PTSD.

PTSD Interview

The PTSD Interview (Watson, Juba, Manifold, Kucula, & Anderson, 1991) is a brief interview that asks subjects to rate their own symptom severity on a 7-point Likert scale. This instrument had excellent test–retest reliability at a 1-week interval, excellent internal reliability, and good interrater agreement in a clini-

TABLE 11.1. Assessments Resulting in Formal PTSD Diagnosis

Test	Diagnostic version	Modality	Associated features	Frequency and intensity	Approximate administration time in minutes	Requires advanced clinical training	Continuous or dichotomous measures	Community or clinical
SCID	DSM-III DSM-III-R DSM-IV	Interview	No	No	25	Yes	Dichotomous	Community Clinical
DIS	DSM-III-R DSM-IV	Interview	No	No	15	No	Dichotomous	Community Clinical
SI-PTSD	DSM-III	Interview	No	No	20	Yes	Both	Clinical
PTSD-I	DSM-III-R	Interview	No	No	10	No	Both	Clinical
ADIS ADIS-R	DSM-III-R	Interview	Yes	No	20	No	Dichotomous	Community
SCAN	ICD-10	Interview	No	No	5	Yes	Dichotomous	Clinical
CAPS	DSM-III-R	Interview	Yes	Yes	60	Yes	Both	Clinical
PSS-I	DSM-III-R	Interview	No	No	10	No	Both	Both
PCL	DSM-III-R	Self-report	No	No	10	No	Both	Both
PSS-S	DSM-III-R	Self-report	No	No	10	No	Both	Both
MPSS-R	DSM-III-R	Self-report	No	Yes	10	No	Both	Both
PENN	DSM-III-R	Self-report	No	No	10	No	Both	Clinical
DUTCH	DSM-III-R	Self-Report	No	No	10	No	Both	Community

Note.—, not reported; n/a, not applicable; Com., community sample; Clin., clinical sample; SCID, Structured Clinical Interview for DSM-III-R; DIS, Diagnostic Interview Schedule; SI-PTSD, Structured Interview for PTSD; PTSD-I, PTSD Interview; ADIS, Anxiety Disorders Interview Schedule; ADIS-R, Anxiety Disorders Interview Schedule—Revised; SCAN, Schedules for Clinical Assessment in Neuropsychiatry; CAPS, Clinician-Administered PTSD Scale; PSS-I, PTSD Symptom Scale Interview; PCL, PTSD Checklist; PSS-S, PTSD Symptom Scale Self-Report; MPSS-R, Modified PTSD Symptom Scale; PENN, Penn Inventory for Posttraumatic Stress; Dutch, Dutch PTSD Scale.
[a]6 of the 81 veterans were staff members.

cal sample of 61 Vietnam veterans. When the DIS was used as the criterion, the PTSD Interview had excellent sensitivity and specificity. The advantages of the PTSD Interview are its brevity, ability to be used by a lay interviewer, its psychometric performance, and the use of a continuous rating for PTSD. The primary disadvantages result from its questionnaire-like format and reliance on the interviewee's responses, which may be biased because of inaccurate self-appraisal or other shortcomings of self-report methods.

Trauma type	Gender(s) used in psychometric studies	Sensitivity	Specificity	Efficiency	Interrater reliability (kappa)	Evidence of test–retest reliability	Internal consistency (alpha)
Combat Crime Disaster Overall	Both	0.81	0.98	—			
Accident Combat Overall	Both	Com. = .22 Clin. = .81–.89 .23–.89	Com. = .98 Clin. = .92–.94 .92–.98	0.64			
Combat	Men	0.96	0.8	—			
Vietnam veterans[a]	Men	0.89 0.92	0.94 0.91	—			
Veterans	Men Both	1	0.94	—			
—	—	—	—	—			
Combat	Men	0.84	0.95	0.89			
Sexual assault	Women	0.88	0.96	—			
Combat	Men	0.82	0.83	—			
Sexual assault	Women	0.62	1	—			
Mixed	Both	Com. = .63 Clin. = .70	Com. = .92 Clin. = .92	—	n/a	—	.96, .97
Accidents Combat Psychiatric patients	Men	.90–.97	.61–1	0.94	n/a	—	
Dutch resistance fighters	Both	0.84	0.79	0.82	n/a	0.91	0.88

Anxiety Disorders Interview Schedule–Revised

The Anxiety Disorders Interview Schedule—Revised (ADIS-R; DiNardo & Barlow, 1988) is a structured diagnostic interview that focuses on the anxiety and mood disorders, although it also contains abbreviated sections that assess other disorders. When two independent interviewers assessed combat veterans over a maximum 10-day interval, initial interrater reliability of the ADIS PTSD module was good (Blanchard, Gerardi, Kolb, & Barlow, 1986). However, in a community sample examined over an interval of 0–44 days, the module was less stable (DiNardo, Moras, Barlow, Rapee, & Brown, 1993). Importantly, the findings in the second study were based on so few cases of PTSD ($n = 11$) that the results need to be interpreted cautiously; it is unclear whether the poor reliability reflects the small sample size, changes from the original ADIS, or the diagnostic performance of the ADIS-R in a community or field sample. An advantage of the ADIS-R may be the inclusion of questions about panic symptoms—a consideration that may be most useful when the relationship between panic disorder and PTSD needs to be explored. Disadvantages of the ADIS-R include provisional psychometric data, a lack of explicit behavioral anchors for coding the presence or absence of PTSD symptoms, and a lack of specific prompts for the interviewer. Other disadvantages are a lack of continuous measurement of PTSD or PTSD symptoms and inadequate explorations of the lifetime presence of PTSD.

Composite International Diagnostic Interview

The Division of Mental Health of the World Health Organization constructed the Composite International Diagnostic Interview (CIDI) for paraprofessionals to use with community samples (Robins, Helzer, Croughan, Williams, & Spitzer, 1981b; Robins et al., 1988). Although the CIDI is based on the *International Classification of Diseases*, 10th revision (ICD-10) criteria for psychiatric disorders, it can reportedly be scored according to DSM-III-R criteria. The CIDI has undergone field trial testing, but no data are currently published on its reliability and validity when used to assess PTSD.

Schedules for Clinical Assessment in Neuropsychiatry

The Division of Mental Health of the World Health Organization constructed a second international interview, the Schedules for Clinical Assessment in Neuropsychiatry (SCAN; Wing et al., 1990; Sartorius et al., 1993), for mental health professionals to use with clinical populations. The SCAN is also based on the ICD-10 criteria for psychiatric disorders but can be scored according to DSM-III-R criteria. The SCAN segment on PTSD is optional, but administration takes only 5 minutes because it assesses only 7 of the 17 PTSD symptoms recognized by DSM. The SCAN module phrases questions about current symptoms in terms of the last 6 months—an approach that diverges from the DSM-III-R time frame of 1 month. In the SCAN field trials, the PTSD interrater agreement was adequate either when one clinician observed another or when a patient was interviewed and presented to other assessors in a case conference. However, so few patients received a primary diagnosis of PTSD (Sartorius et al., 1993) that further evaluation of the SCAN's sensitivity is warranted. An advantage of the SCAN is its potential to provide some useful information about PTSD across cultures, traumas, and languages for those who use the ICD system of diagnosis. However, the SCAN has several disadvantages. First, because the PTSD module is optional, PTSD diagnoses may be missed because of mere oversight. In addition, when the PTSD module is used alone, several DSM-III-R

PTSD symptoms are not assessed. Moreover, because the time span for current symptoms is designated as the last 6 months, the SCAN may overdiagnose current cases, given that a patient with "current" PTSD can have been symptom-free for the past 5 months or more. Other disadvantages include the lack of standardized content, detailed probes, and standard behavioral anchors for the interviewer to determine the presence and absence of symptoms. A final disadvantage is the limited psychometric information on the PTSD module.

Clinician-Administered PTSD Scale

The Clinician-Administered PTSD Scale (CAPS; Blake et al., 1990, 1995; Weathers, 1993; Weathers et al., 1996a) was designed to address the limitations of other structured PTSD interviews. It has specific criteria for both intensity and frequency of symptoms; thus, an individual who has occasional intense symptoms can meet diagnostic criteria, as well as a person who has more frequent but less intense symptoms. In addition, the CAPS items address both the 17 primary PTSD symptoms and 13 associated features. Each item has clear behavioral anchors for ratings of both symptom intensity and frequency, and the time frame of 1 month for current symptoms is consistent with DSM-III-R and DSM-IV criteria. It also uses a "worst ever" 1-month time period—a feature that eliminates the potential for inflated lifetime rates. In addition, the CAPS information can generate both continuous and dichotomous indices of PTSD. Studies to date indicate that the CAPS has excellent test–retest reliability and good interrater reliability when two independent clinicians assessed the same combat veteran 2 or 3 days apart. In addition, the measure has good convergent validity with standard measures of PTSD, such as the Mississippi Scale for Combat-Related PTSD ($r = .91$), PK PTSD subscale of the MMPI-2 ($r = .77$), and the SCID ($r = .89$) When used as a continuous measure with a cutoff score of 65 for diagnosis of combat veterans, the CAPS had good sensitivity, excellent specificity, and good overall efficiency. Its strong psychometric properties, its use of a "worst ever" 1-month time period for establishing lifetime PTSD rates, its inclusion of intensity and frequency ratings, and its clear behavioral anchors for diagnosing PTSD symptoms make the CAPS an excellent choice for use in research and clinical settings. Its major drawbacks are the length of time required for administration and the lack of validation with nonveterans.

PTSD Symptom Scale Interview

The PSS-I (Foa et al., 1993) is a 17-item semistructured interview that can be used by lay interviewers to assess the severity of PTSD symptoms over the prior 2 weeks. Administering this measure to 118 women, including both those who were and were not survivors of sexual assault, the authors reported excellent interrater reliability, good internal consistency, good sensitivity, and excellent specificity. Its test–retest reliability over 1 month was also good. The advantages of the PSS-I include its brevity, promising psychometric qualities, and ability to be scored as a continuous measure. The disadvantages of the PSS-I include its lack of explicit behavioral anchors for ratings and the unavailability of a lifetime diagnosis. Moreover, it has only been validated with female sexual and criminal assault survivors, and its 2-week time frame differs from that employed in the DSM-III-R and DSM-IV.

SELF-REPORT PTSD CHECKLISTS

Several self-report PTSD checklists have been developed as a time- and cost-efficient means for collecting PTSD information. These checklists can be important tools in the multimethod assessment process because they provide relatively inexpensive information about how respondents view their symptoms, in a context that is not influenced by direct interaction with an interviewer. Unfortunately, none of the measures described below includes validity indices that measure cooperativeness, defensiveness, symptom exaggeration, symptom underestimation, confusion, or random responding to questions. The following brief descriptions and Table 11.1 provide an overview of these measures.

PTSD Checklist

The PTSD Checklist (Weathers, Litz, Herman, Huska, & Keane, 1993) is a 17-item checklist that provides a continuous measure of PTSD. It has good sensitivity and specificity relative to a cutoff score of 50 with this veteran population. In addition, it has shown positive correlation with other standard measures of PTSD (Mississippi Scale, $r = .93$; PK PTSD scale of the MMPI-2, $r = .77$; Impact of Event Scale [IES], $r = .90$). The advantages of the PTSD Checklist include its brevity and demonstrated psychometric properties. Its main disadvantage is that it has only been validated with male combat veterans.

PTSD Symptom Scale Self-Report

The PSS-S (Foa et al., 1993) is a 17-item self-report measure that consists of the same items as the PSS-I (described earlier). The PSS-S was validated relative to the SCID PTSD diagnosis on 118 women, 46 of whom were sexually assaulted. The strengths of the PSS-S include its brevity, its high degree of specificity, and its continuous format. Its disadvantages include the lack of validity data with other trauma-exposed samples and its somewhat limited ability to identify those with PTSD; moreover, its truncated time frame does not converge with the time frame used in DSM. This feature may be an advantage for looking at change over time, but it is a disadvantage for establishing DSM diagnoses.

Modified PTSD Symptom Scale Self-Report

The Modified PTSD Symptom Scale Self-Report (MPSS-S; Falsetti, Resnick, Resick, & Kilpatrick, 1993) is a modification of the PSS-S that includes both frequency and intensity ratings over a 2-week time period. In the clinical sample of people exposed to various types of trauma, the MPSS-S had fair sensitivity and specificity when a summed frequency and intensity cutoff score of 71 was used (S. A. Falsetti, personal communication, November 24, 1993). Although it is unclear whether the addition of the severity and intensity ratings has improved the instrument's diagnostic accuracy relative to that of the PSS-S, it may improve the quality of data collection and the ability of the measure to detect change over time. The use of a 2-week time frame has the same disadvantage of departing from the DSM criteria.

Penn Inventory for Posttraumatic Stress

The Penn Inventory (Hammerberg, 1992) is a 26-item questionnaire that has shown somewhat lower specificity than the Mississippi Scale, but similar sensitivity and overall efficiency, when a cutoff score of 35 has been used. The advantages of the Penn Inventory are questions that apply to all trauma types and validation with several male populations (accident survivors, combat veterans, and veteran psychiatric patients). To date, it has not been validated with women.

Dutch PTSD Scale

The Dutch PTSD Scale (Hovens et al., 1993) consists of 28 items designed for use with Dutch World War II resistance fighters. Although the instrument's intial psychometric performance is promising, thus far it has only been used with elderly war veteran populations. It is also of limited applicability because questions are phrased with reference to wartime experiences.

EMPIRICALLY DERIVED PSYCHOMETRIC MEASURES OF PTSD

This section reviews measures that have been rationally developed rather than formally based on the diagnostic criteria for PTSD. Each measure has been empirically tested for its ability to differentiate between those individuals who do and do not qualify for a clinical PTSD diagnosis. Table 11.2 summarizes important features, such as approximate administration time; type of rating

TABLE 11.2. Empirically Derived Psychometric Measures of PTSD

Test	Approximate administration time in minutes	Separate measure of or part of another instrument	Continuous or dichotomous measure	Clinical or community	Trauma types	Gender(s) used in psychometric studies	Sensitivity	Specificity	Efficiency	Evidence of test-retest reliability	Internal consistency (alpha)
Mississippi	15	Separate	Both	Both	Combat Civilian	Both	.77–.93	.83–.89	0.9	0.97	0.94
MMPI-PK	20	Both	Both	Both	Combat Airline crash Car accident Crime	Both	0.57–0.90	0.55–0.95	.87	.86–.94 .86–.89	.95–.96 .85–.87
MMPI-PS	90	Part of MMPI	Both	Both	Combat	Both	0.82	0.88	—	.88–.92.	89–.91
CR-PTSD	25	Part of SCL-90-R	Both	Com.	Crime	Women	0.75	0.9	0.89	—	—
Green PTSD	25	Part of SCL-90-R	Both	Com.	Accident	Both	0.78	0.82	—	—	—
WZ-PTSD	25	Part of SCL-90-R	Both	Both	Combat	Men	0.87–90	0.65–0.72	0.81–0.82	—	0.97
IES	10	Separate	Both				0.91	0.61		Intr. = .89 Avod. = .79	Intr. = .78 Avod.= .82
TSI	30	Separate	Continuous	Clinical	Interpersonal and non-interpersonal PTEs	Both	—	—	—	—	0.87 .74–.90

Note. —, not reported; Mississippi, Mississippi Scale for Combat-Related PTSD; MMPI-PK, Keane PTSD Scale; MMPI-PS, Schlenger and Kulka PTSD Scale; CR-PTSD, Crime-Related PTSD Scale; Green PTSD, Green's Disaster PTSD Scale; WZ-PTSD, War Zone-Related PTSD Scale; IES, Impact of Event Scale; TSI, Trauma Symptom Inventory; PTE, potentially traumatizing event; Com., community sample; Intr., intrusions; Avod., avoidance.

(dichotomous vs. continuous); sample with which the measure was validated; and indices of sensitivity, specificity, test–retest reliability, and internal consistency. In addition, the table lists whether the measure is embedded in another instrument or is administered independently.

Mississippi Scale for Combat-Related PTSD

The Mississippi Scale (Keane, Caddell, & Taylor, 1988) consists of 35 items and is one of the most widely used PTSD measures (e.g., Kulka, et al., 1990; McFall, Smith, MacKay, & Tarver, 1990). Combined with the SCID, this measure functioned as a primary PTSD indicator in the NVVRS, and it performed as the best self-report measure of the disorder (e.g., Kulka et al., 1990, 1991). Several versions of the Mississippi Scale have been developed to make it applicable to other populations. For the NVVRS, versions were created for civilians and female veterans. Two abbreviated versions of the scale also show promising correlations (.95 and .90 respectively) with the original scale (Fontana & Rosenheck, 1994; Wolfe, Keane, Kaloupek, Mora, & Wine, 1993b). Overall, the Mississippi Scale seems to function as a very good indicator of PTSD, although not every symptom of the disorder is directly assessed.

Keane PTSD Scale of the MMPI/MMPI-2

The PK scale of the MMPI (Keane, Malloy, & Fairbank, 1984) contains 49 MMPI items that differentiated PTSD and non-PTSD veteran patients. Although the sensitivity and specificity of PK has varied from study to study, it appears to have moderate or better psychometric quality in most studies (e.g., Graham, 1993; Keane et al., 1984; Koretzsky & Peck, 1990; Kulka et al., 1991; McFall et al., 1989; Watson, 1990). It is important to keep in mind that optimal cutoff scores ranging from 8.5 to 30 have been identified across a variety of populations, studies, and assessment circumstances (e.g., Graham, 1993; Koretzsky & Peck, 1990; McCaffrey, Hickling, & Marazzo, 1989; Orr et al., 1990; Query, Megran, & McDonald, 1986; Sloan, 1988; Sutker, Bugg, & Allain, 1991a; Watson, Kucula, & Manifold, 1986). Accordingly, Lyons and Keane (1992) emphasize the importance of selecting local norms for PK and discuss the methodology involved in selecting appropriate cutoff scores for each trauma population. For the MMPI-2, the Keane PTSD scale was revised solely by deleting the three item repetitions. This 46-item measure remains psychometrically sound, and its performance appears to be comparable to that of the original scale (Litz et al., 1991; Graham, 1993). Importantly, the PK scale seems to work as well when it is applied as a separate measure as it does when it is imbedded in the MMPI-2 (Herman, Weathers, Litz, & Keane, 1995). Overall, the PK scale appears to be a good psychometric scale that can be especially useful for archival analysis of trauma-related symptoms in data sets that were not originally designed to examine PTSD. Although it may provide a reasonable screening index for the disorder when it is used alone, use of other convergent PTSD measures is advisable when PTSD status is sought.

Schlenger and Kulka PTSD Scale of the MMPI-2

Schlenger and Kulka (1989) also developed a PTSD scale of the MMPI-2, the MMPI-PS, for use in the NVVRS to differentiate among Vietnam veterans who had PTSD, other psychiatric disorders, and no psychiatric disorders. The PS consists of 75 items, 45 of which overlap with the PK scale (Graham, 1993; Schlenger & Kulka, 1989). There are no known advantages of the PS over the PK. Further research on the psychometric characteristics of this new scale is needed to determine its unique merits.

SCL-90-R Scales

Several authors have derived PTSD scales from the items that make up the SCL-90-R (Derogatis, 1977). These efforts are valuable because such scales can be incorporated into many research and clinical protocols that already contain the SCL-90-R, without the addition of dedicated PTSD measures. In addition, because the SCL-90-R has been widely used for a number of years in clinical and research settings, PTSD scales for this instrument should permit archival analysis of data sets that were not originally designed to examine PTSD.

Saunders, Arata, and Kilpatrick (1990) have developed a 28-item Crime-Related PTSD scale, and Green (1991) and her colleagues have developed a 12-item SCL-90-R PTSD subscale for disaster survivors. Green (1991) has added an important caveat with respect to the SCL-90-R scales that she and Saunders have developed: She notes that there is no evidence that either scale has greater predictive validity than the Global Severity Index of the SCL-90-R. The ability to outperform nonspecific distress ratings is a criterion that probably should be applied to all psychometric measures of PTSD, not just those derived from the SCL-90-R.

A 25-item War-Zone-Related PTSD scale was developed by Weathers et al. (1996b). Interestingly, only 11 of the 25 items overlap with the 28 items of the Crime-Related PTSD scale. Twice it has been demonstrated that this measure can clearly outperform the Global Severity Index. The War-Zone-Related PTSD scale appears to be a solid PTSD measure that may be useful in many settings, although its applicability to non-war-related stress has yet to be examined.

Impact of Event Scale

The IES (Horowitz, Wilner, & Alvarez, 1979; Zilberg, Weiss, & Horowitz, 1982) has 15 items and is one of the most widely used PTSD-related scales, having been applied across several different trauma samples (e.g., Horowitz et al., 1979; Kulka et al., 1990; Schwarzwald, Solomon, Weisenberg, & Mikulincer, 1987; Zilberg et al., 1982). The IES assesses the extent of avoidance/numbing and intrusive symptoms, rather than the full range of PTSD symptoms. Green (1991) has noted that two different scoring systems have been used in published studies on the IES; thus, caution is necessary when one is comparing results across studies. This simple measure is easy to administer and widely used across sites and samples, but is limited by its exclusive emphasis on the intrusive and avoidant facets of PTSD.

Trauma Symptom Inventory

The Trauma Symptom Inventory (TSI; Briere, Elliott, Harris, & Cotman, 1995) is a new 100-item scale designed to assess the frequency of several posttrauma symptoms occurring over a 6-month period. The TSI has 10 clinical scales that assess the domains of anxiety/arousal, anger/irritability, depression, defensive avoidance, dissociation, dysfunctional sexual behavior, intrusive experiences, impaired self-reference, sexual concerns, and tension-reducing external behaviors. In addition, two validity scales are proposed to assess response style, although the clinical and psychometric utility of these scales is still under investigation. The specificity and sensitivity of the TSI have yet to be established. Important features of the TSI include its validity scales and its focus on several aspects of posttrauma functioning not captured in other scales.

PSYCHOMETRIC MEASUREMENT OF EXPOSURE TO POTENTIALLY TRAUMATIC EVENTS

Considerable debate has surrounded the question of how to identify events as sufficient in nature and scope to satisfy Criterion A for the disorder. Stressors have been categorized by event types, by survivors' subjective appraisal of the experience, and by salient aspects of exposure (e.g., extent of physical injury and ability to escape) that have been hypothesized as causal for PTSD (Sutker, Uddo-Crane, & Allain, 1991b). The DSM-IV has included some of these dimensions in the new Criterion A definition, which specifies that a traumatic event must involve actual or threatened injury to oneself or others, and must engender concomitant feelings of fear, helplessness, or horror.

Comprehensive assessment methods that can accommodate exposure to multiple stressors, intensity of exposure, and unique qualitative features of particular stressors have evolved as conceptualizations of potentially traumatic events have advanced. Early measures focused on detailed evaluation of particular subtypes of potentially traumatic events and salient aspects of such experiences (e.g., sexual abuse—Herman & van der Kolk, 1990; Russell, 1986; Wyatt, 1985; combat—Figley & Stretch, 1986; Foy, Sipprelle, Rueger, & Carroll, 1984; Keane et al., 1989a; Gallops, Laufer, & Yager, 1981; Watson, Juba, & Anderson 1989; Watson, Kucula, Manifold, Vassar, & Juba, 1988; Wilson & Kraus, 1985). Although these delimited efforts have been successful, a means for assessing the full range of potential Criterion A events has remained elusive for several reasons. Respondents with PTSD often have difficulty recalling aspects of traumatic events (Green, 1993) because of such factors as amnesia (e.g., Briere & Conte, 1993), avoidance of trauma-related material (e.g., Mollica & Caspi-Yavin, 1991), and dissociation (e.g., Kirby, Chu, & Dill, 1993). Alternatively, survivors of trauma may not disclose traumatic events for fear of disbelief and blame by others, shame, or stigma (Kilpatrick, 1983). The measurement of traumatic stressors has also been influenced by societal stereotypes, in that researchers have defined certain potentially traumatic events quite narrowly because of cultural misconceptions and avoidance of the reality of violence in our society (e.g., Resnick et al., 1991). Sexual abuse of men is an example of a topic researchers and clinicians have failed to address adequately until recent years (e.g., Briere, Evans, Runtz, & Wall, 1988; Lisak, 1993; Watkins & Bentovim, 1992). A similar claim can be made with respect to violence based upon race, ethnicity, religion, and sexual orientation (Berrill & Herek, 1990; Berrill, 1990).

There are no published instruments that assess a range of trauma exposure types and that have also been subjected to psychometric validation. With the exception of the Potential Stressful Events Interview (PSEI; Falsetti, Resnick, Kilpatrick, & Freedy, 1994; Kilpatrick, Resnick, & Freedy, 1991) and the Evaluation of Lifetime Stressors (ELS; Krinsley et al., 1994), none of the published assessment tools corresponds to the new transactional model of the DSM-IV, which incorporates the objective *and* subjective elements of an experience. The following brief review identifies several of the most popular current measures of trauma exposure, and Table 11.3 provides a summary of their psychometric properties, administration time, and populations with which the measures have been used. When available, evidence for test–retest reliability is also reported. These latter findings must be evaluated cautiously, as clinical experience suggests that initial trauma interviews can facilitate future reporting of exposure to other potentially traumatic events; therefore, formal test–retest reliability may not always be an adequate or meaningful reflection of a measure's performance.

Combat Exposure Scale

The Combat Exposure Scale (Keane et al., 1989a) has seven items and was developed for use in psychiatric settings to assess exposure to potentially traumatic combat events, especially those related to service in Vietnam. The scale has demonstrated good internal consistency and excellent test–retest reliabil-

TABLE 11.3. Psychometric Measurement of Trauma Exposure

Test	Modality	Trauma type assessed	Approximate administration time in minutes	Gender(s) used in psychometric validation	Evidence of test–reliability	Internal consistency (kappa)	DSM-IV criteria
CES	Self-report	Combat	5	Men	0.97	0.85	No
WWTSS	Self-report	Military	10	Women	0.91	0.89	No
HTQ	Interview	Torture	40	Both	0.23 (personal injury)[a] 0.9 (murder of family)	—	Yes
TSS	Interview	Multiple	10	—	—	—	—
PSEI	Interview	Multiple	25–90	Both	—	—	Yes
ETI	Interview	Childhood	60	—	—	—	No
ELS	Self-report Interview	Multiple	45–90	Both	—	—	Yes

Note. —, not reported; CES, Combat Exposure Scale; WWTSS, Women's War-Time Stressor Scale; PSEI, Potential Stressful Events Interview; HTQ, Harvard Trauma Questionnaire; ETI, Early Trauma Interview; ELS, Evaluation of Lifetime Stressors; TSS, Traumatic Stress Schedule. [a]Test–retest reliability for one week varied based on traumatic event; overall the authors report that higher consistency was found for personal trauma (e.g., torture) rather than for general events (e.g., lack of water).

ity at a 1-week interval. Its primary limitation is its narrow content of war-zone-related stress experiences.

Women's War-Time Stressor Scale

Wolfe, Furey, and Sandecki (1989) created a 27-item scale to assess psychosocial stressors that may be unique for women veterans. Preliminary analysis of this scale yielded excellent internal consistency, test–retest reliability within 12–18 months, and good concordance with measures of PTSD (Wolfe, Brown, Furey, & Levin, 1993a). Its primary limitations as a trauma exposure instrument are its exclusive focus on military events and its questionable applicability to men.

Harvard Trauma Questionnaire

The Harvard Trauma Questionnaire (Mollica, Wyshak, & Lavelle, 1987; Mollica & Caspi-Yavin, 1991) is a guided interview that begins by assessing 17 trauma experiences specific to Indochinese refugees. The second interview section includes an open-ended question about the refugees' perceived worst experiences, so that salient aspects of the stressor can be delineated. The third section elicits 30 symptoms related to torture and trauma, 16 of which overlap with the DSM-III-R criteria. One strength of the measure is that it is available in English and three Indochinese languages. Perhaps more important is that it represents an effort to assess trauma exposure and symptoms cross-culturally—a task few investigators have undertaken to date.

Traumatic Stress Schedule

The Traumatic Stress Schedule (Norris, 1990) is a short screening device with nine general questions to be administered by a lay interviewer. These questions inquire about robbery, physical assault, rape, serious motor vehicle accident, additional bereavement, injury or property loss, evacuation, and other stressful or life change within any time frame the interviewer specifies. Each respondent's endorsement of an event is assessed by 12 further questions pertaining to scope, threat to life and physical integrity, blame, intrusions, nightmares, and avoidance symptoms. The measure functions as a screening device that may be useful in epidemiological studies. Its flexibility may make it useful for many purposes, but it may also result in a lack of standardization, preventing comparisons across studies that use it. No psychometric data are available.

Potential Stressful Events Interview

The PSEI (Falsetti et al., 1994; Kilpatrick et al., 1991) is a structured interview that addresses exposure to sexual and physical assaults, combat, disaster, witnessing serious injury or death, traumatic grief due to homicide of a close friend or family member, and robbery, as well as financial and interpersonal stress and family illness. The interview is based on the experience of Kilpatrick and his colleagues in developing interviews such as the Incident Report Interview for community and clinical epidemiological studies (e.g., Kilpatrick et al., 1989). Used as part of the DSM-IV field trials (Kilpatrick et al., in press), the PSEI has demonstrated many strengths, including well-defined behavioral anchors for identifying events, the use of explicit terminology, measurement of appraisal variables, and concordance with DSM-IV definitions of stressors. The explicit terminology can also be a potential disadvantage, in that technical phrasing may impede reporting among some interviewees. To date, no psychometric data have been published on the reliability and validity of the PSEI.

New Developments

Other instruments to detect trauma histories are under development. The Early Trauma Interview (ETI; Kriegler et al., 1992) is an interview designed to focus on exposure to natural disasters and sexual, emotional, and physical abuse during the respondent's childhood. Each question asks about perpetrator, victim's age, and frequency of the experience across three developmental periods. The respondent's appraisal of the impact of each type of potentially traumatic event is assessed for both the time of occurrence and at the time of assessment. Psychometric evaluation of the ETI is currently underway.

Expanding on work with the ETI, Krinsley et al. (1994) have developed the ELS, a clinically sensitive, two-stage approach to assessing lifespan trauma. A screening questionnaire and a follow-up interview assess exposure to the full range of potentially traumatic events, including emotional, physical, and sexual abuse. Although the psychometric properties of the ELS instruments are also currently under investigation, they have some noteworthy features aimed at overcoming obstacles to valid retrospective assessment. Among these features are empirical indicators of family environments associated with childhood trauma (e.g., discord; childhood friends not invited into the home), response options that allow for uncertainty in initial endorsements, a combination of formats so that information disclosure is maximized, and an emphasis on clinical sensitivity regarding the progression and phrasing of questions.

NEW FRONTIERS

Psychophysiological Assessment

The most frequently applied methods for assessment of psychopathology are clinical interviews, psychometric tests, and physiological or biological measures. Typical psychophysiological and biological tests offer a unique perspective because of their non-self-report nature, which helps to minimize the impact of response sets or bias. Psychophysiological measures typically include heart rate, blood pressure, muscle tension, skin conductance level and response, and peripheral temperature. As applied to PTSD, psychophysiological assessment has assumed the form of challenge tests (e.g., Blanchard, Kolb, Pallmeyer, & Gerardi, 1982; McNally et al., 1987; Malloy et al., 1983; Pallmeyer, Blanchard, & Kolb, 1985; Pitman, Orr, Forgue, de Jong, & Claiborn, 1987; Shalev, Orr, & Pitman, 1992). Most studies conducted in the context of PTSD have presented either standardized or idiographic (personalized) cues of potentially traumatic experiences while measuring responses across one or more channels. For example, evaluation of a vehicular accident survivor might involve the recording of physiological reactivity for such measures as blood pressure and heart rate, as the subject views a depiction of such an accident.

Individuals who have developed PTSD often manifest elevations across multiple measurement channels when they are exposed to cues of the traumatic experience. Psychophysiological assessments permit at least three types of data to be gathered simultaneously: physiological activity measures, subjective ratings, and observations of the individual's behavior. Both subjective and physiological measures have been found to distinguished PTSD veterans' reactions to trauma-related cues (e.g., combat photos, taped scripts of their traumatic experiences) from their reactions to neutral cues, and from the reactions of other groups of trauma-exposed subjects without PTSD (e.g., Blanchard et al., 1986; Malloy et al., 1983; Pitman et al., 1987). Research on the psychophysiological assessment of PTSD has also expanded recently to include a broader range of traumatized subjects (e.g., Shalev, Orr, & Pitman, 1993), and this is an area of increasing theoretical and empirical interest (see Resnick et al., 1991). Findings indicate that although physiological reactivity has good specificity, estimates of sensitivity are somewhat more variable (Gerardi, Keane, & Penk, 1989). Studies are underway to determine the extent to which this assessment approach is useful in discriminating PTSD from non-PTSD cases in various trauma-exposed populations (e.g., Keane, Kolb, & Thomas, 1989b).

Collateral Assessment

Collateral assessment of PTSD can also provide important information about the disorder, especially about its impact on functioning. Individuals with PTSD may have difficulty reporting on their condition because of denial, amnesia, avoidance, minimization, and/or cognitive impairment. Therefore, collateral reports from spouses, partners, family members, or friends can provide valuable information to clinicians and researchers. Prior records, such as medical, school, legal, and military documents, may also serve to corroborate and amplify patients' reports of PTSD symptoms and prior functioning. Furthermore, discrepancies between reports can help an evaluator understand the impact a traumatized person is having on others and ways in which the individual interprets personal symptoms and experiences. Finally, collateral reports can provide supplementary data that may not be observable under other assessment conditions.

Few psychometrically sound instruments have been developed for collateral assessment of PTSD. The most noteworthy effort thus far appears to be the Spouse/Partner (S/P) Mississippi Scale, which was developed for the NVVRS to ascertain partners' observations and perceptions of the veterans; it is based on the content of the original Mississippi Scale (Keane et al., 1988). The instrument has a "don't know" category to prevent artificially low scores when a partner is not aware of certain information. In preliminary research on 222 partners of veterans, the 35-item S/P Mississippi Scale demonstrated excellent reliability (Cronbach's alpha = .93), adequate sensitivity (.68), and good specificity (.86) when compared to a PTSD SCID diagnosis (Caddell, Fairbank, Schlenger, Jordan, & Weiss, 1991). Another preliminary study (Niles, Herman, Segura-Schultz, Joaquim, & Litz, 1993) explored the overall concordance of symptom reports between 54 spouses and veterans. A moderate correlation ($r = .54$) was found between total scores for veterans and spouses, and item-level analyses revealed that the more observable symptoms of PTSD (e.g., reexperiencing, avoidance, and hyperarousal) were jointly reported by the veterans and spouses, whereas the more subjective symptoms (e.g., emotional numbing, guilt) were less reliably identified by spouses (Niles et al., 1993).

THE ASSESSMENT PROCESS

As in any clinical endeavor, establishing safety is an integral part of the assessment process. First, the individual must be in a physically safe environment, so that any additional stress of the assessment will not put the individual in danger. For example, the assessment of a currently abused, incarcerated, or homeless person may be contraindicated in those instances when the person's physical and psychological safety is dependent on PTSD symptoms of avoidance and hypervigilance for survival in his or her particular environment (e.g., Herman, 1992). Second, safety is a central concern within the assessment, because a thorough assessment of PTSD requires that an individual identify and describe traumatic memories, feelings, and symptoms, which are often accompanied by strong emotional reactions. Psychological safety, which includes trust in the clinician and the associated ability to communicate extreme feelings and reactions, can mitigate any potential that an assessment will increase self-destructive behavior (e.g., substance abuse, suicidal behavior, or other self-injury). The interviewer's sensitivity in the form and pacing of the process can foster this safe atmosphere.

Similarly, it is important for the individual being assessed to understand the goal of assessment, whether it is to be comprehensive or brief. When the diagnostic contract is being set up, it is often helpful to discuss the roles and responsibilities of both the evaluator and the person being assessed, so that issues such as cancellations, attendance, and the like can be easily negotiated. Limits of confidentiality for all assessments, but especially for forensic evaluations, need to be clearly understood and documented.

Establishing a clinical rapport for PTSD assessment is essential and at times quite challenging. Exposure to potentially traumatic events can evoke a range of emotions that impede the assessment process. These emotions include mistrust, hypervigilance about being controlled, shame, anger, and an avoidant response style that can affect the assessment process and the validity of the data obtained. Although empirical data on these factors are sparse, clinical experience suggests that the interviewer's flexibility, respect for the respondent, and careful monitoring of the process can markedly reduce these difficulties. Clinical strategies that may facilitate the assessment process include using "normalizing" responses, as well as giving the participant choices and opportunities to feel in control of the process. Normalizing responses include all explicit and implicit communications indicating that others have experienced similar reactions. This can be communicated by anticipating or predicting reactions, reflecting, and/or phrasing open-ended questions in terms of experience with others who have been exposed to potentially traumatic experiences. Similarly, pacing can be achieved by offering individuals choices about scheduling, answering questions, and anticipating potential distress. For example, we have found it helpful to predict or discuss potential distress or reactions that the respondent may experience after the session, and, if appropriate, to discuss ways of managing those reactions as a means of preparing the individual to manage any potential difficulties.

SUMMARY AND FUTURE DIRECTIONS

Several techniques for assessing PTSD have been reviewed, including self-report questionnaires, structured and semistructured interviews, empirically derived psychometric measures, psychophysiological approaches, and collateral evaluations. Within each domain, the strengths and weaknesses of particular assessment instruments have been outlined. The ideal battery for clinical assessment purposes should include a variety of measures drawn from the different approaches, so as to maximize case identification and functional understanding of connections among events, behaviors, and symptoms. When time and resources permit and detailed information is needed, we advocate the use of a clinical semistructured interview for PTSD and comorbid disorders; a psycho-physiological assessment; and supplementary rating scales and collateral information from family members or others. In most cases, consideration of purpose, target population, and available resources can be used to guide selection of instruments for a test battery. For example, when studying the impact of psychotherapy, clinicians and researchers may be more interested in selecting validated measures whose time frames coincide with treatment intervals rather than traditional DSM time frames. In epidemiological research, time constraints and the use of lay interviewers may weigh heavily as considerations regarding instrument selection. In all cases, it is clear that the goals of PTSD assessment are best achieved through the use of multiple reliable and valid instruments to assess PTSD and concomitant disorders.

Although the field of instrumentation for assessment of PTSD has become increasingly sophisticated and complex, continued advancements are necessary to facilitate growth in our clinical understanding of trauma. Foremost among our needs are assessment techniques that are validated across trauma types so that cross-trauma comparisons can be made. In an effort to facilitate consistency across studies of disasters, a panel of experts (Baum et al., 1993) has recommended that researchers apply the following measures for studies of community disasters: the SCL-90-R (Derogatis, 1977), the MMPI-2 (Butcher, Dahlstrom, Graham, & Kaemmer, 1989), the Beck Depression Inventory (Beck, Ward, Mendelson, Mock, & Erbaugh, 1961), the Center for Epidemiologic Studies Depression Scale (Radloff, 1977), the State–Trait Anxiety Inventory (Spielberger, Gorsuch, & Lushene, 1970), the Zung Depression Scale (Zung, 1965), and the Family Environment Scale (Moos & Moos, 1986). Similar efforts across laboratories and clinics, as well as across all trauma types, await empirical efforts to develop accurate assessment tools whose results are comparable across settings and situations.

Given the rapid advancement of PTSD assessment over the last few years, it is likely that assessment procedures will continue to advance systematically. This chapter has provided a review of the currently available instrumentation, and also proposes a technical framework for both the researcher and practitioner to evaluate and design more complete measures to be used in PTSD assessments.

REFERENCES

American Psychiatric Association (APA). (1980). *Diagnostic and statistical manual of mental disorders* (3rd ed.). Washington, DC: Author.

American Psychiatric Association (APA). (1987). *Diagnostic and statistical manual of mental disorders* (3rd ed., rev.). Washington, DC: Author

American Psychiatric Association (APA). (1994). *Diagnostic and statistical manual of mental disorders* (4th ed.). Washington, DC: Author.

Baum, A., Solomon, S. D., Ursano, R. J., Bickman, L., Blanchard, E., Green, B. L., Keane, T. M., Laufer, R., Norris, F., Reid, J., Smith, E. M., & Steinglass, P. (1993). Emergency/disaster studies: Practical, conceptual and methodological issues. In J. P. Wilson & B. Raphael (Eds.), *International handbook of traumatic stress syndromes* (pp. 125–133). New York: Plenum Press.

Beck, A. T., Ward, C. H., Mendelson, M., Mock, J., & Erbaugh, J. (1961). An inventory for measuring depression. *Archives of General Psychiatry, 4,* 53–63.

Berrill, K. T. (1990). Anti-gay violence and victimization in the United States. *Journal of Interpersonal Violence, 5,* 274–294.

Berrill, K. T., & Herek, G. M. (1990). Primary and secondary victimization in anti-gay hate crimes. *Journal of Interpersonal Violence, 5,* 401–413.

Blake, D. D., Weathers, F. W., Nagy, L. N., Kaloupek, D. G., Gusman, F., Charney, D. S., & Keane, T. M. (1995). The development of a clinician-administered PTSD scale. *Journal of Traumatic Stress, 8,* 75–90.

Blake, D. D., Weathers, F. W., Nagy, L. N., Kaloupek, D. G., Klauminser, G., Charney, D. S., & Keane, T. M. (1990). A clinician rating scale for assessing current and lifetime PTSD: The CAPS-1. *The Behavior Therapist, 18,* 187–188.

Blanchard, E. B., Gerardi, R. J., Kolb, L. C., & Barlow, D. H. (1986). The utility of the Anxiety Disorders Interview Schedule in the diagnosis of post-traumatic stress disorder (PTSD) in Vietnam veterans. *Behaviour Research and Therapy, 24,* 577–580.

Blanchard, E. B., Kolb, L. C., Pallmeyer, T. P., & Gerardi, R. (1982). A psychophysiological study of post traumatic stress disorder in Vietnam veterans. *Psychiatric Quarterly, 54,* 220–229.

Boudewyns, P. A., Albrecht, J. W., Talbert, F. S., & Hyer, L. A. (1991). Comorbidity and treatment outcome of inpatients with chronic combat-related PTSD. *Hospital and Community Psychiatry, 42,* 847–849.

Breslau, N., & Davis, G. C. (1987). Posttraumatic stress disorder: The etiologic specificity of wartime stressors. *American Journal of Psychiatry, 144,* 578–583.

Breslau, N., Davis, G. C., Andreski, P., & Peterson, E. (1991). Traumatic events and posttraumatic stress disorder in an urban population of young adults. *Archives of General Psychiatry, 48,* 216–222.

Briere, J. (1995). *Professional manual for the Trauma Symptom Inventory.* Odessa, FL: Psychological Assessment Resources.

Briere, J., & Conte, J. (1993). Self-reported amnesia for abuse in adults molested as children. *Journal of Traumatic Stress, 6,* 21–31.

Briere, J., Elliott, D. M., Harris, K., & Cotman, A. (1995). The Trauma Symptom Inventory: Reliability and validity in a clinical sample. *Journal of Interpersonal Violence, 10,* 387–401.

Briere, J., Evans, D., Runz, M., & Wall, T. (1988). Symptomatology in men who were molested as children: A comparison study. *American Journal of Orthopsychiatry, 58,* 467–461.

Burnam, M. A., Stein, J. A., Golding, J. M., Siegel, J., Sorenson, S. B., Forsythe, A. B., & Telles, C. A. (1988). Sexual assault and mental disorders in community population. *Journal of Consulting and Clinical Psychology, 56,* 843–851.

Butcher, J. N., Dahlstrom, W. G., Graham, J. R., & Kaemmer, B. (1989). *Manual for the restandardization of the Minnesota Multiphasic Personality Inventory: MMPI-2, and interpretative and administrative guide.* Minneapolis: University of Minnesota Press.

Caddell, J. M., Fairbank, J. A., Schlenger, W. E., Jordan, B. K., & Weiss, D. S. (1991, August). *Psychometric properties of Spouse's Mississippi Scale for Combat-Related PTSD.* Paper presented at the annual convention of the American Psychological Association, San Francisco.

Davidson, J. R. T., & Fairbank, J. A. (1993). The epidemiology of posttraumatic stress disorder. In J. R. T. Davidson & E. B. Foa (Eds.), *Posttraumatic stress disorder: DSM-IV and beyond* (pp. 147–169). Washington, DC: American Psychiatric Press.

Davidson, J. R. T., Hughes, D., & Blazer, D. (1991). Posttraumatic stress disorder in the community: An epidemiological study. *Psychological Medicine, 21,* 1–9.

Davidson, J. R. T., Smith, R. D., & Kudler, H. S. (1989). Validity and reliability of the DSM III criteria for posttraumatic stress disorder: Experience with a structured interview. *Journal of Nervous and Mental Disease, 177,* 336–341.

Derogatis, L. R. (1977). *The SCL-90 manual: Vol. 1. Scoring, administration and procedures for the SCL-90.* Baltimore: Johns Hopkins University School of Medicine, Clinical Psychometrics Unit.

DiNardo, P. A., & Barlow, D. H. (1988). *Anxiety Disorders Interview Scale—Revised.* Albany, NY: Center for Phobia and Anxiety Disorders.

DiNardo, P. A., Moras, K., Barlow, D. H., Rapee, R. M., & Brown, T. A. (1993). Reliability of DSM-III-R anxiety disorder categories: Using the Anxiety Disorders Interview Schedule—Revised (ADIS-R). *Archives of General Psychiatry, 50,* 251–256.

Falsetti, S. A., Resnick, H. S., Kilpatrick, D. G., & Freedy, J. R. (1994). A review of the Potential Stressful Events Interview: A comprehensive assessment instrument of high and low magnitude stressors. *The Behavior Therapist, 17,* 66–67.

Falsetti, S. A., Resnick, H. S., Resick, P. A., & Kilpatrick, D. G. (1993). The Modified PTSD Symptom Scale: A brief self-report measure of posttraumatic stress disorder. *The Behavior Therapist, 16,* 161–162.

Faustman, W. O., & White, P. A. (1989). Diagnostic and psychopharmacological treatment characteristics of 536 inpatients with posttraumatic stress disorder. *Journal of Nervous and Mental Disease, 177,* 154–159.

Figley, C. R., & Stretch, R. H. (1980). Vietnam Veterans Questionnaire Combat Exposure Scale. In *Vietnam Veterans Questionnaire: Instrument development* (Final Report). West Lafayette, IN: Purdue University.

Foa, E. B., Riggs, D. S., Dancu, C. V., & Rothbaum, B. O. (1993). Reliability and validity of a brief instrument for assessing post-traumatic stress disorder. *Journal of Traumatic Stress. 6, 459–474.*

Fontana, A., & Rosenheck, R. (1994). A short form of the Mississippi Scale for Measuring Change in Combat Related PTSD. *Journal of Traumatic Stress, 7,* 407–414.

Foy, D., Sipprelle, R. C., Rueger, D. B., & Carroll, E. (1984). Etiology of posttraumatic stress disorder in Vietnam veterans: Analysis of premilitary, military and combat exposure influences. *Journal of Consulting and Clinical Psychology, 52,* 79–87.

Gallops, M., Laufer, R. S., & Yager, T. (1981). Revised Combat Scale. In R. S. Laufer & T. Yager (Eds.), *Legacies of Vietnam: Comparative adjustments of veterans and their peers* (Vol. 3, p. 125). Washington, DC: U.S. Government Printing Office.

Gerardi, R., Keane, T. M., & Penk, W. (1989). Utility: Sensitivity and specificity in developing diagnostic tests of combat-related post-traumatic stress disorder. *Journal of Clinical Psychology, 45,* 691–703.

Goldberg, D. P. (1972). *The detection of psychiatric illness by questionnaire.* London: Oxford University Press.

Graham, J. R. (1993). *MMPI-2: Assessing personality and psychopathology.* New York: Oxford University Press.

Green, B. L. (1990). Defining trauma: Terminology and generic stressor dimensions. *Journal of Applied Social Psychology, 20,* 1632–1642.

Green, B. L. (1991). Evaluating the effects of disasters. *Psychological Assessment: A Journal of Consulting and Clinical Psychology, 3,* 538–546.

Green, B. L. (1993). Identifying survivors at risk: Trauma and stressors across events. In J. P. Wilson & B. Raphael (Eds.), *International handbook of traumatic stress syndromes.* New York: Plenum Press.

Hammerberg, M. (1992). Penn Inventory for Posttraumatic Stress Disorders: Psychometric properties. *Psychological Assessment: A Journal of Consulting and Clinical Psychology, 4,* 67–76.

Helzer, J. E., Robins, L. N., & McEvoy, L. (1987). Post-traumatic stress disorder in the general population: Findings of the Epidemiologic Catchment Area survey. *New England Journal of Medicine, 317,* 1630–1634.

Herman, D. S., Weathers, F. W., Litz, B. T., & Keane, T. M. (1995). *The PK scale of the MMPI-2: Reliability and validity of the embedded and stand-alone versions.* Manuscript submitted for publication.

Herman, J. L. (1992). *Trauma and recovery.* New York: Basic Books.

Herman, J. L., & van der Kolk, B. A. (1990). *Traumatic Antecedents Questionnaire.* Unpublished manuscript.

Horowitz, M. J., Wilner, N. R., & Alvarez, W. (1979). Impact of Event Scale: A measure of subjective distress. *Psychosomatic Medicine, 41,* 208–218.

Hovens, J. E., Falger, P. R. J., Op den Velde, W., Mweijer, P., de Grown, J. H. M., & van Duijn, H. (1993). A self-rating scale for the assessment of posttraumatic stress disorder in Dutch resistance veterans of World War II. *Journal of Clinical Psychology, 49,* 196–203.

Jordan, B. K., Schlenger, W. E., Fairbank, J. A., Marmar, C., Weiss, D., Hough, R. L., & Kulka, R. (1991). Lifetime and current prevalence of specific psychiatric disorders among Vietnam veterans. *Archives of General Psychiatry, 48,* 207–215.

Keane, T. M. (1989). Post-traumatic stress disorders: Current status and future directions. *Behavior Therapy, 20,* 149–153.

Keane, T. M., Caddell, J. M., & Taylor, K. L. (1988). Mississippi Scale for Combat-Related Posttraumatic Stress Disorder: Three studies in reliability and validity. *Journal of Consulting and Clinical Psychology, 56,* 85–90.

Keane, T. M., Fairbank, J. A., Caddell, J. M., Zimering, R. T., Taylor, K. L., & Mora, C. A. (1989a). Clinical evaluation of a measure to assess combat exposure. *Psychological Assessment: A Journal of Consulting and Clinical Psychology, 1,* 53–55.

Keane, T. M., Kolb, L. C., & Thomas, R. T. (1989b). [A psychophysiological study of chronic post-traumatic stress disorder]. Unpublished raw data, VA Cooperative Study Programs.

Keane, T. M., Malloy, P. F., & Fairbank, J. A. (1984). Empirical development of an MMPI subscale for the assessment of combat-related posttraumatic stress disorder. *Journal of Consulting and Clinical Psychology, 52,* 888–891.

Keane, T. M., & Penk, W. (1988). The prevalence of post-traumatic stress disorder [Letter to the editor]. *New England Journal of Medicine, 318,* 1690–1691.

Keane, T. M., & Wolfe, J. (1990). Comorbidity in post-traumatic stress disorder: An analysis of community and clinical studies. *Journal of Applied Social Psychology, 20,* 1776–1788.

Keane, T. M., Wolfe, J., & Taylor, K. L. (1987). Post-traumatic stress disorder: Evidence for diagnostic validity and methods of psychological assessment. *Journal of Clinical Psychology, 43,* 32–43.

Kilpatrick, D. G. (1983). Rape victims: Detection, assessment, and treatment. *The Clinical Psychologist, 36,* 92–95.

Kilpatrick, D. G., Resnick, H. S., & Freedy, J. R. V. (1991). *Potential Stressful Events Inventory.* Charleston: Crime Victims Treatment and Research Center, Medical University of South Carolina.

Kilpatrick, D. G., Resnick, H. S., Freedy, J. R. V., Pelcovitz, D., Resick, P., Roth, S., & van der Kolk, B. (in press). The posttraumatic stress disorder field trial: Emphasis on Criterion A and overall PTSD diagnosis. In *DSM-IV sourcebook.* Washington, DC: American Psychiatric Press.

Kilpatrick, D. G., Saunders, B. E., Amick-McMullan, A., Best, C. L., Veronen, L. J., & Resnick, H. S. (1989). Victim and crime factors associated with the development of crime-related post-traumatic stress disorder. *Behavior Therapy, 20,* 199–214.

Kilpatrick, D. G., Saunders, B. E., Veronen, L. J., Best, C. L., & Von, J. M. (1987). Criminal victimization: Lifetime prevalence, reporting to police, and psychological impact. *Crime and Delinquency, 33,* 479–489.

Kirby, J. S., Chu, J. A., & Dill, D. D. (1993). Correlates of dissociative symptomatology in patients with physical and sexual abuse histories. *Comprehensive Psychiatry, 34,* 258–263.

Koretzky, M. B., & Peck, A. H. (1990). Validation and cross-validation of the PTSD subscale of the MMPI with civilian trauma victims. *Journal of Clinical Psychology, 46,* 296–300.

Kriegler, J., Blake, D., Schnurr, P., Bremner, D., Zaidi, L. Y., & Krinsley, K. (1992). *Early Trauma Interview.* Unpublished manuscript.

Krinsley, K., Weathers, F., Vielhauer, M., Newman, E., Walker, E., & Young, L. (1994). *Evaluation of Lifetime Stressors Questionnaire and Interview.* Unpublished manuscript. (Available from K. Krinsley, National Center for Posttraumatic Stress Disorder, Boston Department of Veterans Affairs Medical Center [116-B], 150 South Huntington Ave., Boston, MA 02130)

Kulka, R. A., Schlenger, W. E., Fairbank, J. A., Hough, R. L., Jordan, B. K., Marmar, C. R., & Weiss, D. S. (1988). *National Vietnam Veterans Readjustment Study (NVVRS): Description, current status, and initial PTSD prevalence estimates.* Research Triangle Park, NC: Research Triangle Institute.

Kulka, R. A., Schlenger, W. E., Fairbank, J. A., Jordan, B. K., Hough, R. L., Marmar, C. R., & Weiss, D. S. (1990). *Trauma and the Vietnam War generation: Report of findings from the National Vietnam Veterans Readjustment Study.* New York: Brunner/Mazel.

Kulka, R. A., Schlenger, W. E., Fairbank, J. A., Jordan, B. K., Hough, R. L., Marmar, C. R., & Weiss, D. S. (1991). Assessment of posttraumatic stress disorder in the community: Prospects and pitfalls from recent studies of Vietnam veterans. *Psychological Assessment: A Journal of Consulting and Clinical Psychology, 3*, 547–560.

Lisak, D. (1993). Men as victims: Challenging cultural myths. *Journal of Traumatic Stress, 6*, 577–580.

Litz, B. T., Penk, W., Walsh, S., Hyer, L., Blake, D. D., Marx, B., Keane, T. M., & Bitman, D. (1991). Similarities and differences between Minnesota Multiphasic Personality Inventory (MMPI) and MMPI-2 applications to the assessment of post-traumatic stress disorder. *Journal of Personality Assessment, 57*, 238–254.

Lyons, J. A., & Keane, T. M. (1992). Keane PTSD scale: MMPI and MMPI-2 update. *Journal of Traumatic Stress, 5*, 111–117.

Malloy, P. F., Fairbank, J. A., & Keane, T. M. (1983). Validation of a multimethod assessment of posttraumatic stress disorders in Vietnam veterans. *Journal of Consulting and Clinical Psychology, 83*, 488–494.

McCaffrey, R. J., Hickling, E. J., & Marazzo, M. J. (1989). Civilian-related posttraumatic stress disorder: Assessment-related issues. *Journal of Clinical Psychology, 45*, 76–79.

McFall, M. E., Smith, D. E., MacKay, P. W., & Tarver, D. J. (1990). Reliability and validity of Mississippi Scale for Combat-Related Posttraumatic Stress Disorder. *Psychological Assessment: A Journal of Consulting and Clinical Psychology, 2*, 114–121.

McFarlane, A. C. (1988). The longitudinal course of post-traumatic morbidity. *Journal of Nervous and Mental Disease, 176*, 30–39.

McNally, R. J., Luedke, D. L., Besyner, J. K., Peterson, R. A., Bohm, K., & Lips, O. J. (1987). Sensitivity to stress-relevant stimuli in post-traumatic stress disorder. *Journal of Anxiety Disorders, 1*, 105–116.

Mollica, R. F., & Caspi-Yavin, Y. (1991). Measuring torture and torture-related symptoms. *Psychological Assessment: A Journal of Consulting and Clinical Psychology, 3*, 581–587.

Mollica, R. F., Wyshak, G., & Lavelle, J. (1987). The psychosocial impact of war trauma and torture on Southeast Asian refugees. *American Journal of Psychiatry, 144*, 1567–1572.

Moos, R. H., & Moos, B. S. (1986). *Family Environment Scale manual* (2nd ed.). Palo Alto, CA: Consulting Psychologists Press.

Niles, B., Herman, D. S., Segura-Schultz, S., Joaquim, S. G., & Litz, B. (1993, October). *The Spouse/Partner Mississippi Scale: How does it compare?* Paper presented at the Ninth Annual Meeting of the International Society for Traumatic Stress Studies, San Antonio, TX.

Norris, F. H. (1990). Screening for traumatic stress: a scale for use in the general population. *Journal of Applied Social Psychology, 20*, 1704–1718.

Orr, S., Clairborn, J. M., Altman, B., Forgue, D. F., de Jong, J. B., Pitman, R. K., & Herz, L. R. (1990). Psychometric profile of PTSD, anxious and healthy Vietnam veterans: Correlations with psychophysiological responses. *Journal of Consulting and Clinical Psychology, 58*, 329–335.

Pallmeyer, T. P., Blanchard, E. B., & Kolb, L. C. (1985). The psychophysiology of combat-induced post-traumatic stress disorders in Vietnam veterans. *Behaviour Research and Therapy, 24*, 645–652.

Pitman, R. K., Orr, S. P., Forgue, D. F., de Jong, J. B., & Claiborn, J. M. (1987). Psychophysiologic assessment of posttraumatic stress disorder imagery in Vietnam combat veterans. *Archives of General Psychiatry, 44*, 970–975.

Query, W. T., Megran, J., & McDonald, G. (1986). Applying posttraumatic stress disorder MMPI subscale to World War II POW veterans. *Journal of Clinical Psychology, 42,* 315–317.

Radloff, L. S. (1977). The CES-D scale: A self-report depression scale for research in the general population. *Applied Psychological Measurement, 1,* 385–401.

Resnick, H. S., Kilpatrick, D. G., Best, C. L., & Kramer, T. L. (1992). Vulnerability–stress factors in development of posttraumatic stress disorder. *Journal of Nervous and Mental Disease, 180,* 424–430.

Resnick, H. S., Kilpatrick, D. G., & Lipovsky, J. A. (1991). Assessment of rape-related posttraumatic stress disorder: Stressor and symptom dimensions. *Psychological Assessment: A Journal of Consulting and Clinical Psychology, 3,* 561–572.

Robins, L. N., Helzer, J. E., Croughan, J. L., & Ratliff, K. S. (1981a). National Institute of Mental Health Diagnostic Interview Schedule: Its history, characteristics, and validity. *Archives of General Psychiatry, 38,* 381–389.

Robins, L. N., Helzer, J. E., Croughan, J. L., Williams, J. B. W., & Spitzer, R. L. (1981b). *NIMH Diagnostic Interview Schedule, Version III* (DHHS Publication No. ADM-T-42-3). Washington, DC: U.S. Government Printing Office.

Robins, L. N., Wing, J., Wittchen, H. U., Helzer, J. E., Babor, F., Burke, J., Farmern, A., Jablenski, A., Pickens, R., Reiger, M. A., Sartorius, N., & Towle, L. H. (1988). The Composite International Diagnostic Interview. *Archives of General Psychiatry, 45,* 1069–1071.

Russell, D. E. H. (1986). *The secret trauma: Incest in the lives of girls and women.* New York: Basic Books.

Sartorius, N., Kaelber, C. T., Cooper, J. E., Roper, M. T., Rae, D. S., Gulbinat, W., Ustun, T. B., & Regierm, D. A. (1993). Progress toward achieving a common language in psychiatry. *Archives of General Psychiatry, 50,* 115–124,

Saunders, B. E., Arata, C. M., & Kilpatrick, D. G. (1990). Development of a crime-related post-traumatic stress disorder scale for women within the Symptom Checklist-90—Revised. *Journal of Traumatic Stress, 3,* 439–448.

Schlenger, W. E., & Kulka, R. A. (1989). *PTSD scale development for the MMPI-2.* Research Triangle Park, NC: Research Triangle Institute.

Schlenger, W. E., Kulka, R. A., Fairbank, J. A., Hough, R. L., Jordan, B. K., Marmar, C. R., & Weiss, D. S. (1992). The prevalence of post-traumatic stress disorder in the Vietnam generation: A multimodal, multisource assessment of psychiatric disorder. *Journal of Traumatic Stress, 5,* 333–363.

Schwarzwald, J., Solomon, Z., Weisenberg, M., & Mikulincer, M. (1987). Validation of the Impact of Event Scale for psychological sequelae of combat. *Journal of Consulting and Clinical Psychology, 55,* 251–256.

Shalev, A. Y., Orr, S. P., & Pitman, R. K. (1992). Psychophysiologic responses during script-driven imagery as an outcome measure in posttraumatic stress disorder. *Journal of Clinical Psychiatry, 532,* 324–326.

Shalev, A. Y., Orr, S. P., & Pitman, R. K. (1993). Psychophysiologic assessment of traumatic imagery in Israeli, civilian patients with posttraumatic stress disorder. *American Journal of Psychiatry, 150,* 620–624.

Shore, J. H., Tatum, E. L., & Vollmer, W. M. (1986). Psychiatric reactions to disaster: The Mount St. Helens experience. *American Journal of Psychiatry, 143,* 590–595.

Sloan, P. (1988). Post-traumatic stress in survivors of an airplane crash-landing: A clinical and exploratory research intervention. *Journal of Traumatic Stress, 1,* 211–229.

Southwick, S. M., Yehuda, R., & Giller, E. L. (1993). Personality disorders in treatment-seeking combat veterans with post-traumatic stress disorder. *American Journal of Psychiatry, 150,* 1020–1023.

Spielberger, C. D., Gorsuch, R. L., & Lushene, R E. (1970). *Manual for the State–Trait Anxiety Inventory (self-evaluating questionnaire).* Palo Alto, CA: Consulting Psychologists Press.

Spitzer, R. L., Williams, J. B., Gibbon, M., & First, M. B. (1990). *Structured Clinical Interview for DSM-III-R—Patient edition (SCID-P).* New York: Biometrics Research Department, New York State Psychiatric Institute.

Sutker, P. B., Bugg, F., & Allain, A. N. (1991a). Psychometric prediction of PTSD among POW survivors. *Psychological Assessment: A Journal of Consulting and Clinical Psychology, 3,* 105–110.

Sutker, P. B., Uddo-Crane, M., & Allain, A. N. (1991b). Clinical and research assessment of posttraumatic stress disorder: A conceptual overview. *Psychological Assessment: A Journal of Consulting and Clinical Psychology, 3,* 520–530.

Watkins, B., & Bentovim, A. (1992). The sexual abuse of male children and adolescents: A review of current research. *Journal of Child Psychology and Psychiatry, 33,* 197–248.

Watson, C. G. (1990). Psychometric posttraumatic stress disorder techniques: A review. *Psychological Assessment: A Journal of Consulting and Clinical Psychology, 2,* 460–469.

Watson, C. G., Juba, M. P., & Anderson, P. E. D. (1989). Validities of five combat scales. *Psychological Assessment: A Journal of Consulting and Clinical Psychology, 1,* 98–102.

Watson, C. G., Juba, M. P., Manifold, V., Kucula, T., & Anderson, P. E. D. (1991). The PTSD Interview: Rationale descriptions, reliability, and concurrent validity of a DSM-III based technique. *Journal of Clinical Psychology, 47,* 179–188.

Watson, C. C., Kucula, T., & Manifold, V. (1986). A cross-validation of the Keane and Penk MMPI scales as measures of post-traumatic stress disorder. *Journal of Clinical Psychology, 42,* 727–732.

Watson, C. C., Kucula, T., Manifold, V., Vassar, P., & Juba, M. (1988). Differences between post-traumatic stress disorder patients with delayed and undelayed onsets. *Journal of Nervous and Mental Disease, 176,* 568–572.

Weathers, F. M. (1993). *Empirically derived scoring rules for the Clinician Administered PTSD Scale.* Unpublished manuscript.

Weathers, F. W., Blake, D. D., Krinsley, K. E., Haddad, W. H., Huska, J. A., & Keane, T. M. (1996a). *The reliability and validity of the Clinician-Administered PTSD Scale.* Manuscript submitted for publication.

Weathers, F. W., Litz, B. T., Herman, D. S., Huska, J. A., & Keane, T. M. (1993, October). *The PTSD Checklist: Reliability, validity and diagnostic utility.* Paper presented at the annual meeting of the International Society for Traumatic Stress Studies, San Antonio, TX.

Weathers, F. W., Litz, B. T., Keane, T. M., Herman, D. S., Steinberg, H. R., Huska, J. A., & Kraemer, H. C. (1996b). The utility of the SCL-90-R for the diagnosis of war-zone-related post-traumatic stress disorder. *Journal of Traumatic Stress, 9,* 111–128.

Weiss, D. S. (1993). Structured clinical interview techniques. In J. W. Wilson & B. Raphael (Eds.), *International handbook of traumatic stress syndromes* (pp. 179–188). Plenum Press: New York.

Weissman, M. M., & Bothwell, S. (1976). Assessment of social adjustment by patient self-report. *Archives of General Psychiatry, 33,* 1111–1114.

Wilson, J., & Kraus, G. E. (1985). Predicting post-traumatic stress disorders among Vietnam veterans. In W. E. Kelly (Ed.), *Posttraumatic stress disorder and the war veteran patient* (pp. 102–147). New York: Brunner/Mazel.

Wing, J. K., Babor, T., Crugha, T., Burke, J., Cooper, J. E., Giel, R., Jablenski, A., Regier, D., & Sartorius, N. (1990). SCAN: Schedules for Clinical Assessment in Neuropsychiatry. *Archives of General Psychiatry, 47,* 589–593.

Wolfe, J., Brown, P. J., Furey, J., & Levin, K. B. (1993a). Development of a war-time stressor scale for women. *Psychological Assessment, 5,* 330–335.

Wolfe, J., Furey, J., & Sandecki, R. (1989). Women's Military Exposure Scale (Available from J. Wolfe, National Center for Posttraumatic Stress Disorder, Boston Department of Veterans Affairs Medical Center [116B], 150 South Huntington Ave., Boston MA 02130)

Wolfe, J., & Keane, T. M. (1993). New perspectives in the assessment and diagnosis of combat-related post-traumatic stress disorder. In J. Wilson & B. Raphael (Eds), *International handbook of traumatic stress syndromes.* New York: Plenum Press.

Wolfe, J., Keane, T. M., Kaloupek, D. G., Mora, C. A., & Wine, P. (1993b). Patterns of positive readjustment in Vietnam combat veterans. *Journal of Traumatic Stress, 6,* 179–193.

Wyatt, G. E. (1985).The sexual abuse of Afro-American and white American women in childhood. *Child Abuse and Neglect, 9,* 231–240.

Zilberg, N. J., Weiss, D. S., & Horowitz, M. J. (1982). Impact of Event Scale: A cross validation study and some empirical evidence supporting a conceptual model of stress response syndromes. *Journal of Consulting and Clinical Psychology, 50,* 407–414.

Zung, W. (1965). A self-rating depression scale. *Archives of General Psychiatry, 12,* 63–70.

PART IV

MEMORY: MECHANISMS AND PROCESSES

CHAPTER 12

Trauma and Memory

BESSEL A. VAN DER KOLK

Traumatic memory plays an important role in certain neuroses and psychoses. While some doctors never trouble their heads about traumatic memories, and are not even aware of the fact that they exist, and while others fancy them everywhere, there is room for people to take a middle course, and to detect the existence of traumatic memories in specific cases.
—JANET (1919/1925, Vol. 1, p. 670)

The nature and reliability of traumatic memories have been controversial issues in psychiatry for over a century. Traumatic memories are difficult to study, since the profoundly upsetting emotional experiences that give rise to posttraumatic stress disorder (PTSD) cannot be approximated in a laboratory setting; even viewing a movie depicting actual executions fails to precipitate posttraumatic symptoms in normal college students (R. K. Pitman, personal communication, 1994). If "trauma" is defined as an inescapably stressful event that overwhelms people's existing coping mechanisms, it is questionable whether findings of memory distortions in normal subjects exposed to videotaped stresses in the laboratory can serve as meaningful guides to understanding traumatic memories. Clearly, there is little similarity between witnessing a simulated car accident on a television screen, and being the responsible driver in a car crash in which one's own children are killed. Whereas response to stress involves homeostatic mechanisms that lead to self-conservation and resource reallocation (e.g., Selye, 1956), PTSD involves a unique combination of hyperarousal, learned conditioning, and shattered meaning propositions. Shalev (Chapter 4, this volume) has proposed that this complexity is best understood as the co-occurrence of

Parts of this chapter are adapted from van der Kolk and Fisler (1995). Copyright 1995 by Plenum Publishing Corp. Adapted by permission.

several interlocking pathogenic processes, including (1) an alteration of neu-robiological processes affecting stimulus discrimination (expressed as increased arousal and decreased attention), (2) the acquisition of conditioned fear responses to trauma-related stimuli, and (3) altered cognitive schemata and social apprehension.

Without the option of simulating trauma in the laboratory, there are only limited options for the exploration of traumatic memories: (1) collecting retrospective reports from traumatized individuals, (2) making post hoc observations, or (3) provoking traumatic memories and flashbacks in a laboratory setting. Surprisingly, since the early part of this century, very few published systematic studies have used patients' own reports to explore the nature of traumatic memories. Provocation studies of traumatic memories have been done in psychophysiology laboratories (e.g., Pitman, Orr, Forgue, de Jong, & Claiborn, 1987; Rauch et al., in press), and in tests where patients with PTSD are given drugs altering the neurotransmitter functions that seem to promote access to trauma-related memories (Rainey et al., 1987; Southwick et al., 1993).

In this chapter, I first review the studies that have collected data on people's memories of highly stressful and of traumatic experiences, and examine the differences between these two types of memories. I next review the evidence implicating dissociation as the central pathogenic mechanism that gives rise to PTSD, and that causes traumatic memories to be retrieved (at least initially) in the form of mental imprints of sensory and affective elements of the traumatic experience. I then present the research findings concerning the alterations in brain structure and function in PTSD that seem to play a role in these abnormal memory processes. I conclude the chapter with further discussion about the nature of traumatic memories, as contrasted with memories of ordinary events.

MEMORIES OF STRESSFUL EVENTS VERSUS TRAUMATIC EXPERIENCES

Background: The Complexity of Memory Systems

Contemporary memory research has demonstrated the existence of a great complexity of memory systems within each individual. Most of these memory functions take place outside of conscious awareness, and each seems to operate with a relative degree of independence from the others. The two main memory systems can be summarized very briefly as follows:

1. "Declarative" (also known as "explicit") memory refers to conscious awareness of facts or events that have happened to the individual (Squire & Zola-Morgan, 1991). This form of memory functioning is seriously affected by lesions of the frontal lobe and of the hippocampus, which have also been implicated in the neurobiology of PTSD (van der Kolk, 1994).

2. "Nondeclarative," "implicit," or "procedural" memory refers to memories of skills and habits, emotional responses, reflexive actions, and classically conditioned responses. Each of these implicit memory subsystems is associated with particular areas in the central nervous system (CNS) (Squire, 1994). Schacter (1987) has referred to scientific descriptions of traumatic memories (e.g., the descriptions by Pierre Janet) as examples of implicit memory.

The Stability and Accuracy
of Memories of Stressful Events

At least since 1889, when Pierre Janet first wrote about the relationship between trauma and memory, it has been widely accepted that what is now called declarative or explicit memory is an active and constructive process. What a person remembers depends on existing mental schemata; once an event or a particular bit of information is integrated into existing mental schemes, it will no longer be available as a separate, immutable entity, but will be distorted both by associated experiences and by the person's emotional state at the time of recall (Janet, 1889; van der Kolk & van der Hart, 1991). As Schachtel (1947) defined it: "Memory as a function of the living personality can be understood as a capacity for the organization and reconstruction of past experiences and impressions in the service of present needs, fears, and interests" (p. 3). However, accuracy of memory is affected by the the emotional valence of an experience. Studies of people's subjective reports of personally highly significant events generally find that their memories are unusually accurate, and that they tend to remain stable over time (Bohannon, 1990; Christianson, 1992; Pillemer, 1984; Yuille & Cutshall, 1986). It appears that evolution favors the consolidation of personally relevant information. For example, Yuille and Cutshall (1989) interviewed 13 out of 22 witnesses to a murder 4–5 months after the event. All witnesses had provided information to the police within 2 days after the murder. These witnesses were found to have very accurate recall, with little apparent decline over time. The authors concluded that emotional memories of such shocking events are "detailed, accurate and persistent" (p. 181). They suggested that witnessing real "traumas" leads to "quantitatively different memories than innocuous laboratory events" (p. 181).

Researchers have also studied the accuracy of memories for culturally significant events, such as the murder of President Kennedy and the explosion of the space shuttle *Challenger*. Brown and Kulik (1977) first called memories for such events "flashbulb memories." Although people report that these experiences are etched accurately in their minds, research has shown that even those memories are subject to some distortion and disintegration over time. For example, Neisser and Harsch (1992) found that people changed their recollections of the *Challenger* disaster considerably after a number of years. However, these investigators did not measure the personal significance that their subjects attached to this event. Clinical observations of people who suffer from PTSD suggest that there are significant differences between flashbulb memories and the posttraumatic perceptions characteristic of PTSD. As of early 1995, I could find no published accounts in the scientific literature of intrusive traumatic recollections of traumatic events in patients suffering from PTSD that had become distorted over time, either in an experimental or in a clinical setting.

The Apparent Uniqueness of Traumatic Memories

The *Diagnostic and Statistical Manual of Mental Disorders* (DSM) definition of PTSD recognizes that trauma can lead to extremes of retention and forgetting: Terrifying experiences may be remembered with extreme vividness, or may totally resist integration. In many instances, traumatized individuals report a combination of both. Whereas people seem to assimilate familiar and expectable experiences easily, and whereas memories of ordinary events disintegrate in clarity over time, some aspects of traumatic events appear to become fixed in the mind, unaltered by the passage of time or by the intervention of subsequent experience. For example, in our own research on posttraumatic nightmares, subjects claimed that they saw the same traumatic scenes over and over again without modification over a 15-year period (van der Kolk, Blitz, Burr, & Hartmann, 1984). For the past century, many students of trauma have noted that the imprints of traumatic experiences seem to be qualitatively different from memories of ordinary events. Starting with Janet, accounts of the memories of traumatized patients consistently mention that emotional and perceptual elements tend to be more prominent than declarative components (e.g., Grinker & Spiegel, 1945; Kardiner, 1941; Terr, 1993). These recurrent observations of the apparent immutability of traumatic memories have given rise to the notion that traumatic memories may be encoded differently from memories for ordinary events—perhaps because of alterations in the focusing of attention, or perhaps because extreme emotional arousal interferes with hippocampal memory functions (Christianson, 1992; Heuer & Rausberg, 1992; Janet, 1889; LeDoux, 1992; McGaugh, 1992; Nilsson & Archer, 1992; Pitman, Orr, & Shalev, 1993; van der Kolk, 1994).

AMNESIAS AND THE RETURN OF DISSOCIATED MEMORIES

Global Memory Impairment

Although amnesias following adult trauma have been well documented, the mechanisms for such memory impairment remain insufficiently understood. This issue becomes even more complicated when it concerns childhood trauma, since children have fewer mental capacities for constructing a coherent narrative out of traumatic events. More research is needed to explore the consistent clinical observation that adults who were chronically traumatized as children suffer from generalized impairment of memories for both cultural and autobiographical events. It is likely that their autobiographical memory gaps and their continued reliance on dissociation make it very hard for these patients to reconstruct a precise account of both their past and their current reality. The combination of lack of autobiographical memory, continued dissociation, and meaning schemes that include victimization, helplessness, and betrayal is likely to make these individuals vulnerable to suggestion and to the construction of explanations for their trauma-related affects that may bear little relationship to the actual realities of their lives.

Research on Traumatic Amnesias and Delayed Memory Retrieval

Whereas vivid intrusions of traumatic images and sensations are the most dramatic expressions of PTSD, the loss of recollections for traumatic experiences is also well documented. The complexity of memory loss for trauma, and the psychological elaboration of the experience itself, are illustrated by a very early case in the psychiatric literature. Charcot (1887) described the case of Lelog, who was in a traffic accident with a horse-drawn wagon, after which his legs were paralyzed. Although Lelog fell to the ground and was unconscious, there were no neurological signs indicating a somatic cause of the paralysis. Instead, it was discovered that as he fell and just before he lost consciousness, he saw the wheels of the cart approaching him, and strongly believed that he would be run over. This fantasy was dissociated and gave rise to his paralysis (quoted in van der Hart, Steele, Boon, & Brown, 1993). Janet (1893) described another case of a woman who reenacted her traumatic experience without having any conscious recollection of what had happened to her (van der Kolk & van der Hart, 1991). Early in my own work with traumatized patients, we described the case of a woman who had lost all memory of having been involved in the Cocoanut Grove nightclub fire in Boston, but who kept reenacting her experience on its anniversary (van der Kolk & Kadish, 1987). I also described the case of a Vietnam veteran who set up the police to recreate a shootout with him on the anniversary of his buddy's death, for which he had no conscious recollection (van der Kolk, 1989).

For over 100 years, there have been numerous descriptions of traumatized patients who suffer from amnesias for traumatic experiences. In the detailed case reports, the role of dissociation in those amnesias is usually easy to detect. For example, in his book *The Traumatic Neuroses of War* (1941), Kardiner described a patient who had a complete amnesia for all the events preceding an accident. The story was reconstructed by the patient from fragments related to him. During the month of unconsciousness he was said to have set fire to the hospital several times. Since then, the patient had been subject to lapses of unconsciousness lasting for twelve hours to eleven days. He was later told that he was taken to a hospital and that he was fully awake during these lapses, was active, smoked, read, and talked but was not his conscious self. He was also told that he did not appear to be in his "right mind." These major lapses of unconsciousness occurred at intervals for five years. Since that time he had only minor ones. They usually began with a feeling of paralysis in one extremity, either an arm or a leg. Sometimes it was only an attack of vertigo. (p. 63)

Kardiner noted that fragments of his patients' dissociated memories often returned in dissociative fugue states. For example, when triggered by a sensory stimulus, patients would become agitated and assaultive, using language that would have been appropriate to being caught up in the midlle of a military assault. Many patients, while riding the subway in New York City, had flashbacks to being back in the trenches (especially upon entering a tunnel). In other cases, people had panic attacks in response to stimuli reminiscent of the trauma, while failing to make a conscious connection between how they felt, and the prior traumatic experience.

Today it is generally accepted that the memory system is made up of networks of related information, and that activation of one aspect of such a network facilitates the retrieval of associated memories (Collins & Loftus, 1975; Leichtman, Ceci, & Ornstein, 1992). Emotions and sensations seem to be the critical cues for the retrieval of information along these associative pathways. This means that the emotions attached to any particular experience play a major role in determining what cognitive schemes will be activated. In this regard, it is relevant that many people with histories of trauma, such as rape, spouse battering, and child abuse, seem to function quite well, as long as feelings related to traumatic memories are not stirred up. However, after exposure to specific emotnal or sensory triggers, they may feel or act as if they were being traumatized all over again. These triggers are not necessarily intrinsically frightening; any affect or sensation related to a particular traumatic experience may serve as a cue for the retrieval of associated sensations, including fear, longing, intimacy, and sexual arousal.

Amnesias for traumatic experiences, with delayed recall for all or parts of the trauma, have been noted after natural disasters and accidents (Janet, 1889; Madakasira & O'Brian, 1987; van der Kolk & Kadish, 1987; Wilkinson, 1983); war-related traumas (Archibald & Tuddenham, 1965; Grinker & Spiegel, 1945; Hendin, Haas, & Singer, 1984; Kardiner, 1941; Kubie, 1943; Myers, 1915; Sargant & Slater, 1941; Sonnenberg, Blank, & Talbott, 1985; Southard, 1919; Thom & Fenton, 1920); kidnapping, torture, and concentration camp experiences (Goldfeld, Mollica, Pesavento, & Faraone, 1988; Kinzie, 1993; Niederland, 1968); physical and sexual abuse (Briere & Conte, 1993; Burkett & Bruno, 1993; Janet, 1893; Loftus, Polensky, & Fullilove, 1994; Williams, 1994); and committing murder (Schacter, 1986). A recent general population study by Diana Elliott and John Briere (1995) showed that total amnesia for traumatic events occurred in a certain proportion of victims after every conceivable traumatic experience (except for witnessing the death of one's child), and that in addition, a substantially higher proportion of victims had significant amnesia for particular details of these traumatic experiences. For reasons that are not at all clear, childhood sexual abuse seems to result in the highest degree of total amnesia prior to memory retrieval, with figures ranging from 19% (Loftus et al., 1994) to 38% (Williams, 1994). Amnesias for emotional and cognitive material seem to be age- and dose-related: The younger a person was at the time of the trauma, and the more prolonged the trauma was, the greater the likelihood of significant amnesia (Briere & Conte, 1993; Herman & Shatzow, 1987; van der Kolk et al., 1996).

Trauma and Dissociation

Christianson (1984) noted that when people feel threatened, they experience a significant narrowing of consciousness, and remain focused on only the central perceptual details. As people are being traumatized, this narrowing of consciousness sometimes seems to evolve into a complete amnesia for the experience. More than 85 years ago, Janet (1909) claimed: "Forgetting the event which precipitated the emotion . . . has frequently been found to accompany intense emotional experiences in the form of continuous and retrograde amnesia. . . . [This is] an exaggerated form of a general disturbance of memory which is characteristic of all emotions" (p. 1607). He also noted that when people become too upset, memories cannot be transformed into a neutral narrative; a person is "unable to make the recital which we call narrative memory, and yet he remains confronted by [the] difficult situation" (Janet, 1919/1925, Vol. 1, p. 660). This results in "a phobia of memory" (Vol. 1, p. 661), which prevents the integration of traumatic events and splits off the traumatic memories from ordinary consciousness. Janet claimed that the memory traces of the trauma linger as what he called "unconscious fixed ideas," which cannot be "liquidated" as long as they have not been translated into a personal narrative. When this occurs, they instead continue to intrude as terrifying perceptions, obsessional preoccupations, and somatic reexperiences such as anxiety reactions (see van der Kolk & van der Hart, 1991).

Similar observations have been made by other clinicians treating traumatized individuals. For example, Grinker and Spiegel (1945) noted that some combat soldiers develop excessive responses under stress and that these are responsible for the transformation of stress into a permanent disorder. "Fear and anger in small doses are stimulating and alert the ego, increasing efficacy. But, when stimulated by repeated psychological trauma, the intensity of the emotion heightens until a point is reached at which the ego loses its effectiveness and may become altogether crippled" (p. 82). Grinker and Spiegel described these soldiers as suffering from severe anxiety states, accompanied by confusion, mutism, and stupor. In civilian trauma victims, Horowitz (1986) described an "acute catastrophic stress reaction" characterized by panic, cognitive disorganization, disorientation, and dissociation. Recent research (Holen, 1993; Marmar et al., 1994; Spiegel, 1991) has shown that having dissociative experiences at the moment of the trauma is the most important long-term predictor for the ultimate development of PTSD. Carlson and Rosser-Hogan (1991) found a strong relationship among severity of the trauma, dissociative symptoms, and PTSD in Cambodian refugees. Bremner et al. (1992) found that Vietnam veterans with PTSD reported having experienced higher levels of dissociative symptoms during combat than men who did not develop PTSD. Koopman, Classen, and Spiegel (1994) found that dissociative symptoms early in the course of a natural disaster predicted PTSD symptoms 7 months later. A prospective study of 51 injured trauma survivors in Israel (Shalev, Orr, & Pitman, 1993) found that peritraumatic dissociation explained 29.4% of the variance in PTSD symptoms at a 6-month follow-up, over and above the effects of gender, education, age, and event severity, as well as of the intrusion, avoidance anxiety, and depression that followed the event. Peritraumatic dissociation was also the strongest predictor of PTSD status 6 months after the event. (For a fuller discussion of the importance of dissociation in PTSD, see Chapter 13, this volume.)

Althouh dissociation may be adaptive under extreme conditions, the lack of integration of traumatic memories is thought to be the pathogenic agent leading to the development of complex biobehavioral changes, of which PTSD is the clinical manifestation. This observation was first made by Janet, and has been confirmed by a subsequent century of clinical and research data. Janet proposed that intense arousal ("vehement emotion") seems to interfere with proper information processing and the storage of information in narrative (explicit) memory. He and subsequent students of this issue noted that during conditions of high arousal, "explicit memory" may fail. The traumatized individual is left in a state of "speechless terror" in which words fail to describe what has happened. However, although the individual may be unable to produce a coherent narrative of the incident, there may be no interference with implicit memory; the person may "know" the emotional valence of a stimulus and be aware of associated perceptions, without being able to articulate the reasons for feeling or behaving in a particular way. Janet proposed that traumatic memories are split off (dissociated) from consciousness, and instead are stored as sensory perceptions, obsessional ruminations, or behavioral reenactments (Nemiah, 1995; van der Kolk & van der Hart, 1989, 1991). Janet's student Piaget (1962) described how an active failure of semantic memory leads to the organization of memory on somatosensory or iconic levels. He pointed out: "It is precisely because there is no immediate accommodation that there is complete dissociation of the inner activity from the external world. As the external world is solely represented by images, it is assimilated without resistance (i.e., unattached to other memories) to the unconscious ego."

These and subsequent observations of other traumatized populations suggest that what may most complicate the capacity to communicate about traumatic experiences is that memories of trauma may have no verbal (explicit) component whatsoever. Instead, the memories may have been organized on an implicit or perceptual level, without any accompanying narrative about what happened. Recent symptom provocation neuroimaging studies of people with PTSD support this clinical observation: During the provocation of traumatic memories, there is a decrease in activation of Broca's area—the part of the brain most centrally involved in the transformation of subjective experience into speech (Rauch et al., in press). Simultaneously, the areas in the right hemisphere that are thought to process intense emotions and visual images show significantly increased activation. (See Chapter 10, this volume, for further discussion.)

The Perceptual Organization of Traumatic Experience

Numerous commentators on trauma—for example, Janet (1889; see also van der Kolk & van der Hart, 1991), Kardiner (1941), and Terr (1993)—keep noting that trauma is organized in memory on a perceptual level. Having listened to the narratives of traumatic experiences from hundreds of traumatized children and adults over many years, my colleagues and I keep hearing both adults and children describe how traumatic experiences are initially organized on a nonverbal level. Clinical experience and our reading of a century of observations by clinicians dealing with a variety of traumatized populations have led us to postulate that memories of the trauma tend, at least initially, to be experienced as fragments of the sensory components of the event: as visual images; olfactory, auditory, or kinesthetic sensations; or intense waves of feelings that patients usually claim to be representations of elements of the original traumatic event. What is intriguing is that patients consistently claim that their perceptions are exact representations of sensations at the time of the trauma. For example, when Southwick et al. (1993) injected yohimbine into Vietnam veterans with PTSD, half of their subjects reported trauma-related perceptions that they reported to be "just like it was" (i.e., in Vietnam).

In a recent study, we (van der Kolk & Fisler, 1995) designed and tested an instrument, the Traumatic Memory Inventory (TMI), that provides a structured way of recording whether and how memories of traumatic experiences are retrieved differently from memories of personally significant but nontraumatic events. In order to examine the retrieval of traumatic memories in a systematic way, the TMI specifically inquires about sensory, affective, and narrative ways of remembering; about triggers for unbidden recollections of traumatic memories; and about ways of mastering. Questions on the TMI cover the following:

1. Nature of the trauma(s).
2. Duration.
3. Whether the subject has always been aware that the trauma happened, and if not, when and where the subject became conscious of the trauma.
4. Circumstances under which the subject first experienced intrusive memories, and circumstances under which they occur presently.
5. Sensory modalities in which memories were/are experienced: (a) as a story, (b) as an image ("What did you see?"), (c) in sounds ("What did you hear?"), (d) as a smell ("What did you smell?"), (e) as feelings in the body ("What did you feel? Where?"), (f) as emotions ("What did you feel? What was it like?"). These data are gathered for the subject's recollection of the trauma (a) initially, (b) while the subject was most bothered by the sensory experiences, and (c) currently.
6. Nature of flashbacks.
7. Nature of nightmares.
8. Precipitants of flashbacks and nightmares.
9. Ways of mastering intrusive recollections (e.g., by eating, working, taking drugs or alcohol, cleaning, etc.).
10. Confirmation: records (court or hospital), direct witness, relative who went through same trauma, other.

We then asked each subject the same questions about a personally highly significant experience (e.g., a wedding or the birth of a child), and collected the same information. Subjects considered most questions related to the non-traumatic memories nonsensical. None had olfactory, visual, auditory, or kinesthetic reliving experiences related to these events, and they denied having vivid dreams or flashbacks about them. The subjects also claimed not to have had periods in their lives when they had amnesias for any of these events; nor did any of them report having photographic recollections of any of them. Environmental triggers did not suddenly bring back vivid and detailed memories of ordinary experiences, and none of the subjects felt a need to make special efforts to suppress memories of them.

When asked about their traumatic memories, all of our subjects reported that they initially had no narrative memories for the events; they could not tell a story about what had happened, regardless of whether they always knew that the trauma had happened, or whether they retrieved memories of the trauma at a later date. All these subjects, regardless of the age at which the trauma occurred, claimed that they initially "remembered" the trauma in the form of somatosensory flashback experiences. These flashbacks occurred in a variety of sensory modalities (visual, olfactory, affective, auditory, and kinesthetic), but initially the different modalities did not occur together. As the trauma came into consciousness with greater intensity, more sensory modalities were activated, and the subjects' capacity to tell themselves and others what actually had happened emerged over time.

This study suggests that there is a dramatic difference between the ways people experience traumatic memories and the ways they experience other significant personal events. It supports the idea that the very nature of a traumatic memory is to be dissociated, and to be stored initially as sensory fragments that have no linguistic components. All of the subjects in this study claimed that they only came to develop a narrative of their trauma over time. Indeed, five of the subjects who claimed to have been abused as children were, even as adults, unable to tell a complete story of what had happened to them. They merely had fragmentary memories to support other people's accounts and their own intuitive feelings that they had been abused.

Thus, the subjects' traumatic experiences were not initially organized in a narrative form, and they seemed to serve no communicative function. It appears that as people become aware of more and more elements of the traumatic experience, they construct a narrative that "explains" what happened to them. This process of weaving a narrative out of disparate sensory elements of an experience is probably not all that dissimilar from how people automatically construct a narrative under ordinary conditions. However, when people have day-to-day, nontraumatic experiences, the sensory elements of the experience are not registered separately in consciousness, but are automatically integrated into a personal narrative.

This study supports Piaget's (1962) notion that when memories cannot be integrated on a semantic/linguistic level, they tend to be organized on more primitive levels of information processing (i.e., as visual images or somatic sensations). Even after considerable periods of time, and even after acquiring a personal narrative for the traumatic experience, most of our subjects reported that these experiences continued to come back as sensory perceptions and as affective states. The persistence of intrusive sensations related to the trauma, even after the construction of a narrative, contradicts the notion that learning to put the traumatic experience into words will reliably help abolish the occurrence of flashbacks—a notion that seems to be a central assumption in a variety of treatment modalities.

Prospective Studies of Traumatized Children

Three studies to date have prospectively followed how children with confirmed trauma histories process their memories over time. In a series of cases involving physical and sexual abuse in three day care centers, Ann Burgess and her colleagues (Burgess, Hartman, & Baker, 1995) followed up 34 children several years after their initial disclosure. All children were below age 2½ at time of disclosure. The material gathered at the time of disclosure included the reports of investigating therapists and parent reports of behavioral changes in their children. At the time of first interview all children presented with symptoms of abuse. Many suffered from such physical problems as herpes, vaginal bleeding, and bruises. Many children demonstrated what had happened to them with their sexualized behavior. All children suffered from mood swings, temper tantrums and difficulty in peer relationships. Follow-up interviews were conducted 5 years later and involved interviews with both parents and children. Parents filled out symptom checklists on themselves and their children; the children were interviewed, observed, and did a Trauma Drawing Series.

The investigators identified four basic levels of memory processing in these children: somatic, behavioral, visual, and verbal. At the time of disclosure all children manifested somatic memories which were defined as evidence of physiological arousal or of physical symptoms closely associated with known elements of the trauma. The physical expressions related to the trauma had decreased between the first and second interviews; at follow-up the somatic memory traces consisted of persistent complaints of anal pain in some children who had had foreign objects inserted in their rectums. Some children would clench their legs and defecate and urinate on the floor. Parents reported that their children had fought off rectal temperature taking. Several children had developed bowel problems; other children who were known to have been forced to engage in fellatio had developed eating problems. None of the children made a connection between their physical complaints and their earlier abuse.

At time of disclosure 75% of the children displayed evidence of behavioral memories; at follow-up 63% had behavioral memories. "Behavioral" memories were defined as spontaneous expressions of trauma-related behaviors in everyday activities, such as sexually provocative play (e.g., "hump the doll"), or sexually inappropriate behavior with peers. At time of disclosure 59% of the children were able to give a verbal account of what had happened to them, with varying degrees of detail. Five children had fragmented verbal memory traces; the rest of the children were unable to verbalize what had happened. Sixty percent of the children drew full, fragmented, or delayed representations of their abuse.

In a comparable group of 20 children (Terr, 1988) who had been traumatized before age 3, Terr found that 15 out of 20 children showed some form of verbal recall; half told a story that closely corresponded with the results of the formal investigation. In their play, 18 of the 20 children displayed fears that were related to their trauma: 16 children in posttraumatic play consisting of compulsive re-enactment of their traumas, 9 children displayed personality changes related to frequent re-enactments or to long-standing grief or rage, and 9 children had trauma-specific fears.

Similar cases have been described by Ted Gaensbauer and his colleagues (Gaensbauer, Chatoor, & Drell, 1995), and others (e.g., James, 1989). These studies suggest that many children, like traumatized adults, are unable to integrate sensations and perceptions related to the trauma into explicit memories.

Instead, the trauma is often reproduced in actions, without conscious awareness that what is played out is an actual reproduction of the past.

PSYCHOBIOLOGICAL ISSUES PERTAINING TO TRAUMATIC MEMORIES

The Role of Neurohormones in Memory Consolidation after Trauma

As I have discussed in Chapter 10 of this volume, when people are under stress, they secrete endogenous stress hormones that affect the strength of memory consolidation. It has been widely assumed from animal models that massive secretion of neurohormones at the time of the trauma plays a role in the ways traumatic experiences are laid down (consolidated) in long-term memory. The critical issue here is the long-term potentiation of memory traces (van der Kolk & van der Hart, 1991; Pitman et al., 1993). Mammals have memory storage mechanisms that modulate how strongly a memory is laid down according to the strength of the accompanying hormonal stimulation (McGaugh, 1989; McGaugh, Weinberger, Lynch, & Granger, 1985). This capacity helps organisms evaluate the importance of sensory input in proportion to how strongly the associated memory traces are laid down: Emotionally significant material, laid down in states of high arousal, is accessed more easily in subsequent states of high arousal. In traumatized organisms, the capacity to access relevant memories appears to have gone awry: They access trauma-related memory traces too readily, and hence they tend to "remember" the trauma too easily—namely when it is irrelevant to current experience (Pitman & Orr, 1990).

In Chapter 10, I have described how the norepinephrine (NE) input to the amygdala determines how strongly a memory trace is laid down (Ademac, 1978; LeDoux, 1990). The role of NE in memory consolidation has been shown to have an inverted-U-shaped function (McGaugh, 1989; McGaugh et al., 1985): Both very low and very high levels of CNS NE activity interfere with memory storage. Generalized physiological arousal can set off trauma-related memories, and trauma-related memories, in turn, can trigger physiological arousal. It is likely that the frequent reliving of a traumatic event in flashbacks or nightmares cause a re-release of stress hormones, and that this further strengthens the memory trace (van der Kolk, Greenberg, Boyd, & Krystal, 1985).

The State-Dependent Nature of Traumatic Memory Recall

Research has shown that under ordinary conditions, people with PTSD often have a fairly good psychosocial adjustment. However, they do not respond to stress the way other people do; under pressure they may feel or act as if they were being traumatized all over again. Thus, high states of arousal seem to selectively promote retrieval of traumatic memories, sensory information, or behaviors associated with prior traumatic experiences (American Psychiatric Association, 1987, 1994). Traumatized animals have also been shown to revert to irrelevant emergency behaviors in response to minor stresses. Rhesus monkeys with histories of severe early maternal deprivation, but not normally raised monkeys, become markedly withdrawn or aggressive in response to emotional or physical stimuli (such as exposure to loud noises or the administration of amphetamines) (Kraemer, 1985). Mitchell, Osbourne, and O'Boyle (1985) found that the response of mice to novel situations depended on whether or not they had been previously exposed to high stress. In states of low arousal, animals tend to be curious and to seek novelty; under ordinary conditions, they will choose the most pleasant of two alternatives. However, during states of high arousal, they avoid novelty and revert to what is familiar, regardless of the outcome. Mitchell and his colleagues found that mice that had been locked in a box in which they were exposed to electric shocks, and then released, returned to those boxes when they were subsequently stressed. The authors concluded that this return to familiar patterns of behavior was nonassociative (i.e., uncoupled from the usual reward systems).

In people, analogous phenomena have been documented. Memories (somatic or symbolic) related to the trauma are elicited by heightened arousal (Solomon, Garb, Bleich, & Grupper, 1987). Information acquired in an aroused or otherwise altered state of mind is retrieved more readily when people are brought back to that particular state of mind (Phillips & LePiane, 1980; Rawlins, 1980). State-dependent memory retrieval may also be involved in dissociative phenomena in which traumatized persons may be wholly or partially amnesic for memories or behaviors enacted while in altered states of mind (van der Kolk & van der Hart, 1989, 1991; Putnam, 1989).

Contemporary biological researchers have shown that medications stimulating autonomic arousal may precipitate visual images and emotional states associated with earlier traumatic experiences in people with PTSD, but not in controls. In subjects with PTSD, the injection of lactate (Rainey et al., 1987) or yohimbine (Southwick et al., 1993) has been found to trigger panic attacks, flashbacks of earlier trauma, or both. I believe that these are examples of state-dependent memory retrieval. In our own laboratory, approximately 20% of PTSD subjects responded with a flashback when they were presented with acoustic startle stimuli; heightened arousal led to the retrieval of sensory elements of the trauma that were ordinarily inaccessible (van der Kolk, 1994).

Functional and Neuronatomical Correlates of PTSD: Their Possible Relationship to Traumatic Memory Processes

I have also noted in Chapter 10 that recent brain imaging studies of patients with PTSD have shown sigificant limbic system involvement. These studies may begin to provide an understanding of the problems with both memory storage and retrieval problems in these patients. Two sets of significant findings have now been demonstrated in the laboratory: (1) decreased hippocampal volume in people with PTSD; and (2) excessive activation of the amygdala and related structures, abnormal lateralization, and decreased Broca's area activity when patients are induced to reexperience their traumas.

1. Three different studies in three different laboratories have shown that people with PTSD have decreased hippocampal volumes, compared with matched controls (Bremner et al., 1995; Stein et al., 1994; Gurvitz, Shenton, & Pitman, 1995). See Chapter 10 for details.

2. We recently conducted positron emission tomography studies of patients with PTSD, in which they were exposed to vivid, detailed narratives they had written about their own traumatic experiences (Rauch et al., in press; again, see Chapter 10 for details). To summarize the findings briefly, during exposure to the traumatic scripts, these subjects demonstrated heightened activity only in the right hemisphere, in the areas that are most involved in emotional arousal—the parts of the limbic system most intimately associated with the amygdala. Because these structures are central sites for the experience of anxiety, they have been called the "worry circuit." Activation of these structures was accompanied by heightened activity in the right visual cortex, reflecting the flashbacks reported by these patients. Perhaps most significantly, Broca's area—the part of the left hemisphere responsible for translating personal experiences into communicable language—"turned off." We believe this to reflect the speechless terror experienced by these patients, and their tendency to experience emotions as physical states rather than as verbally encoded experiences. These findings indicate that PTSD patients' difficulties putting feelings into words are reflected in actual changes in brain activity.

A Neuroanatomical Model for the Failure to Integrate Traumatic Memories

How can we interpret the significance of these findings for understanding the nature of PTSD? Figure 12.1 provides a schematic presentation of the interrelationships among various brain structures involved in the interpretation, storage, and retrieval of information, and provides a scheme of what may occur in people who suffer from PTSD. Sensory information enters the CNS via the sensory organs (e.g., eyes, nose, skin, ears); this information is passed on to the thalamus, where some of it is integrated. The thalamus, in turn, passes this raw sensory information on for further evaluation both to the amygdala and to the prefrontal cortex. The amygdala interprets the emotional valence of the incoming information; it attaches emotional significance to what is coming in (see Chapter 10). The information evaluated by the amygdala is passed on to areas in the brainstem that control the behavioral, autonomic, and neurohormonal response systems. By way of these connections, the amygdala transforms

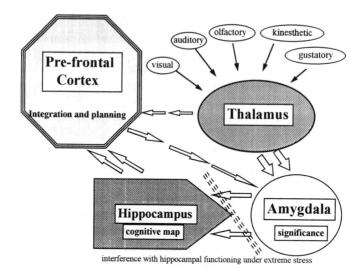

Figure 12.1. Schematic representation of the hypothesized effects of emotional arousal on declarative memory. The thalamus, amygdala, hippocampus, and prefrontal cortex are all involved in the stepwise integration and interpretation of incoming sensory information. This integration can be disrupted by high levels of arousal: Moderate to high activation of the amygdala enhances the long-term potentiation of declarative memory mediated by the hippocampus, while extreme arousal disrupts hippocampal functioning, leaving the memories to be stored as affective states or in sensorimotor modalities, as somatic sensations and visual images. These amygdala-mediated emotional memories are thought to be relatively indelible, but their expression can be modified by feedback from the prefrontal cortex.

sensory stimuli into emotional and hormonal signals, thereby initiating and controlling emotional responses (LeDoux, 1992).

LeDoux proposes that since input from the thalamus arrives at the amygdala before information from the neocortex, this earlier-arriving sensory input from the thalamus "prepares" the amygdala to process the later-arriving information from the cortex. Thus, the emotional evaluation of sensory input precedes conscious emotional experience: People may become autonomically and hormonally activated before they are able to make a conscious appraisal of what they are reacting to. Thus, a high degree of activation of the amygdala and related structures can generate emotional responses and sensory impressions that are based on fragments of information, rather than on full-blown perceptions of objects and events. LeDoux (1992) points out that emotion itself can be a memory, and he advocates that emotion be treated as a memory process rather than as a process that simply influences memory.

Once the amygdala has assigned emotional significance to sensory input, it passes this evaluation on to other brain structures, including the hippocampus, whose task it is to begin organizing this information and integrating it with previously existing information about similar sensory input (see Chapter 10). The strength of the hippocampal activation is affected by the intensity of input from the amygdala: The more significance assigned by the amygdala, the more closely the input will be atended to, and the more strongly the memory will be retained. However, this interaction has an inverted-U-shaped function: In animals, high levels of stimulation of the amygdala interfere with hippocampal functioning (Ademac, 1991; Squire & Zola-Morgan, 1991). This means that very high levels of emotional arousal may prevent the proper evaluation and categorization of experience by interfering with hippocampal function. One can hypothesize that when this occurs, sensory inprints of experience are stored in memory; however, because the hippocampus is prevented from fulfilling its integrative function, these various inprints are not organized into a unified whole. The experience is laid down, and later retrieved, as isolated images, bodily sensations, smells, and sounds that feel alien and separate from other life experiences. Because the hippocampus has not played its usual role in helping to localize the incoming information in time and space, these fragments continue to lead an isolated existence. Traumatic memories are timeless and ego-alien.

Effects of High Levels of Amygdala Activation and Decreased Hippocampal Volume

Two groups of investigators have shown that one-time intense stimulation of the amygdala will produce lasting changes in neuronal excitability and enduring behavioral changes in the direction of either fight or flight (LeDoux, Romanski, & Xagoraris, 1991; Ademac, Stark-Ademac, & Livingston, 1980). In kindling experiments with animals, Ademac et al. (1980) have shown that permanent changes in limbic physiology can cause lasting changes in defensiveness and in predatory aggression. An animal's preexisting "personality" determines in large part the effects of high levels of amygdala stimulation: Fearless animals become still more aggressive, while shy and withdrawn animals become even more so. Thus, in animals, previous personality characteristics can be exaggerated by trauma; it is likely that this is true for people as well.

The twice-replicated finding that people with chronic PTSD have decreased hippocampal volume may explain some of the behavioral abnormalities seen in people with chronic PTSD. In animals, decreased hippocampal functioning causes behavioral disinhibition; it is likely that this sets the stage for the animal to interpret incoming stimuli in the direction of emergency (fight-or-flight) responses. If the same is true for people, this may explain why patients with PTSD have difficulties with "taking in" and processing arousing information, as well as with learning from such experiences. Their altered biology may cause them to react to newly arousing stimuli as a threat, and to react with aggression or withdrawal, depending on their premorbid personalities. Their decreased functioning in Broca's area during this time may make it dificult for them to "understand" what is going on; they experience intense emotions without being able to name their feelings. Their bodies are aroused, and fragments of memories may be activated, but they are unable to form a clear mental construct of what they are experiencing. Needing to reestablish their internal homeostasis, they use their muscles. Discharge via the smooth muscles leads to psychosomatic reactions, whereas discharge through the striated muscles leads to action. Both of these solutions are likely to have adverse consequences, and neither gives a person much chance to learn from experience.

CONCLUSIONS

When people receive sensory input, they generally automatically synthesize this incoming information into their large store of preexisting information. If an event is personally significant, they will generally transcribe these sensations into a narrative, without conscious awareness of the processes by which they translate sensory impressions into a personal story. Our research shows that in contrast with the way people seem to process ordinary information, traumatic experiences are initially imprinted as sensations or feeling states, and are not collated and transcribed into personal narratives. Our interviews with trauma-tized people, as well as our brain imaging studies of them, seem to confirm that traumatic memories come back as emotional and sensory states with little verbal representation. This failure to process information on a symbolic level, which is essential for proper categorization and integration with other experi-ence, is at the very core of the pathology of PTSD.

We (van der Kolk & van der Hart, 1991) have writen earlier about Janet's clear distinctions between traumatic and ordinary memory. According to Janet, traumatic memory consists of images, sensations, affective states, and behav-iors that are invariable and do not change over time. He suggested that these memories are highly state-dependent and cannot be evoked at will. They also are not condensed in order to fit social expectations. In contrast, narrative (explicit) memory is semantic and symbolic; it is social and adapted to the needs of both the narrator and the listener; and it can be expanded or contracted, according to social demands.

The irony is that although the sensory perceptions reported in PTSD may well reflect the actual imprints of sensations that were recorded at the time of the trauma, all narratives that weave sensory imprints into socially communi-cable stories are subject to condensation, embellishment, and contamination. Although trauma may leave an indelible imprint, once people start talking about these sensations and try to make meaning of of them, they are transcribed into ordinary memories—and, like all ordinary memories, they are then prone to distortion. People seem to be unable to accept experiences that have no meaning; they will try to make sense of what they are feeling. Once people become conscious of intrusive elements of the trauma, they are likely to try to fill in the blanks and complete the picture.

Like all stories that people construct, our autobiographies contain elements of truth, of things that we wish had happened, but did not, and elements that are meant to please the audience. The stories that people tell about their traumas are as vulnerable to distortion as people's stories about anything else. However, the question of whether the brain is able to "take pictures," and whether some smells, images, sounds, or physical sensations may be etched onto the mind and remain unaltered by subsequent experience and by the passage of time, still remains to be answered.

REFERENCES

Ademac, R. E. (1978). Normal and abnormal limbic system mechanisms of emotive biasing. In K. E. Livingston & O. Hornykiewicz (Eds.), *Limbic mechanisms.* New York: Plenum Press.

Ademac, R. E. (1991). Partial kindling of the ventral hippocampus: Identification of changes in limbic physiology which accompany changes in feline aggression and defense. *Physiology and Behavior, 49,* 443–454.

Ademac, R. E., Stark-Ademac, C., & Livingston, K. E. (1980). The development of predatory aggression and defense in the domestic cat. *Neurological Biology, 30,* 389–447.

American Psychiatric Association. (1987). *Diagnostic and statistical manual of mental disorders* (3rd ed., rev.). Washington, DC: Author.

American Psychiatric Association. (1994). *Diagnostic and statistical manual of mental disorders* (4th ed.). Washington, DC: Author.

Archibald, H. C., & Tuddenham, R. D. (1965). Persistent stress reaction after combat. *Archives of General Psychiatry, 12,* 475–481.

Bohannon, J. N. (1990, February). *Arousal and memory: Quantity and consistency over the years.* Paper presented at the Conference on Affect and Flashbulb Memories, Emory University, Atlanta, GA.

Bremner, J. D., Randall, P., Scott, T. M., Bronen, R. A., Seibyl, J. P., Southwick, S. M., Delaney, R. C., McCarthy, G., Charney, D. S., & Innis, R. B. (1995). MRI-based measures of hippocampal volume in patients with PTSD. *American Journal of Psychiatry, 152,* 973–981.

Bremner, J. D., Southwick, S. M., Brett, E., Fontana, A., Rosenheck, R., & Charney, D. S. (1992). Dissociation and posttraumatic stress disorder in Vietnam combat veterans. *American Journal of Psychiatry, 149,* 328–332.

Briere, J., & Conte, J. (1993). Self-reported amnesia for abuse in adults molested as children. *Journal of Traumatic Stress, 6*(1), 21–31.

Brown, R., & Kulik, J. (1977). Flashbulb memories. *Cognition, 5,* 73–99.

Burgess, A. W., Hartmann, C. R., & Baker, T. (1995). Memory representations of childhood sexual abuse. *Journal of Psychosocial Nursing, 33*(9), 9–16.

Burkett, E., & Bruno, F. (1993). *A gospel of shame.* New York: Viking.

Carlson, E. B., & Rosser-Hogan, R. (1991). Trauma experiences, posttraumatic stress, dissociation, and depression in Cambodian refugees. *American Journal of Psychiatry, 148,* 1548–1551.

Charcot, J. M. (1887). *Leçons sur les maladies du système nerveux faites à la Salpêtrière [Lessons on the illnesses of the nervous system held at the Salpêtrière]* (Vol. 3). Paris: Progrès Médical en A. Delahaye & E. Lecrosnie.

Christianson, S.-A. (1984). The relationship between induced emotional arousal and amnesia. *Scandinavian Journal of Psychology, 25,* 147–160.

Christianson, S.-A. (1992). Emotional stress and eyewitness memory: A critical review. *Psychological Bulletin, 112,* 284–309.

Collins, A. M., & Loftus, E. F. (1975). A spreading activation theory of semantic processing. *Psychological Bulletin, 82,* 407–428.

Demitrack, M. A., Putnam, F. W., Brewerton, T. D., Brandt, H. A., & Gold, P. W. (1990). Relation of clinical variables to dissociative phenomena in eating disorders. *American Journal of Psychiatry, 147,* 1184–1188

Elliott, D. M., & Briere, J. (1995, November). *Epidemiology of memory and trauma.* Paper presented at the annual meeting of the International Society on Traumatic Stress Studies, Chicago.

Goldfeld, A. E., Mollica, R. F., Pesavento, B. H., & Faraone, S. V. (1988). The physical and psychological sequelae of torture: Symptomatology and diagnosis. *Journal of the American Medical Association, 259,* 2725–2729.

Grinker, R. R., & Spiegel, J. P. (1945). *Men under stress.* Philadelphia: Blakiston.

Gurvitz, T. V., Shenton, M. E., & Pitman, R. K. (1995). *Reduced hippocampal volume on magnetic resonance imaging in chronic posttraumatic stress disorder.* Paper presented at the annual meeting of the International Society on Traumatic Stress Studies, Miami.

Hendin, H., Haas, A. P., & Singer, P. (1984). The reliving experience in Vietnam veterans with posttraumatic stress disorder. *Comprehensive Psychiatry, 25,* 165–173.

Herman, J. L., & Shatzow, E. (1987). Recovery and verification of memories of childhood sexual trauma. *Psychoanalytic Psychology, 4,* 1–14.

Heuer, F., & Rausberg, D. (1992). Emotion, arousal, and memory for detail. In S.-A. Christianson (Ed.), *The handbook of emotion and memory* (pp.151–206). Hillsdale, NJ: Erlbaum.

Holen, A. (1993). The North Sea oil rig disaster. In J. P. Wilson & B. Raphael (Eds.), *International handbook of traumatic stress syndromes.* New York: Plenum Press.

Janet, P. (1889). *L'automatisme psychologique.* Paris: Alcan.

Janet, P. (1893). L'amnésie continué. *Revue Générale des Sciences, 4,* 167–179.

Janet, P. (1909). *Les névroses.* Paris: Flammarion.

Janet, P. (1925). *Psychological healing* (Vols. 1–2). New York: Macmillan. (Original work published 1919)

Kardiner, A. (1941). *The traumatic neuroses of war.* New York: Hoeber.

Kinzie, J. D. (1993). Posttraumatic effects and their treatment among Southeast Asian refugees. In J. P. Wilson & B. Raphael (Eds.), *International handbook of traumatic stress syndromes* (pp. 311–319). New York: Plenum Press.

Koopman, C., Classen, C., & Spiegel, D. (1994). Predictors of posttraumatic stress symptoms among survivors of the Oakland/Berkeley, California firestorm. *American Journal of Psychiatry, 151,* 888–894.

Kraemer, G. W. (1985). Effects of differences in early social experiences on primate neurobiological–behavioral development. In M. Reite & T. M. Fields (Eds.), *The psychology of attachment and separation* (pp. 135–161). Orlando, FL: Academic Press.

Kubie, L. S. (1943). Manual of emergency treatment for acute war neuroses. *War Medicine, 4,* 582–599.

LeDoux, J. E. (1990). Information flow from sensation to emotion: Plasticity of the neutral computation of stimulus value. In M. Gabriel & J. Moore (Eds.), *Learning computational neuroscience: Foundations of adaptive networks* (pp. 3–51). Cambridge, MA: MIT press.

LeDoux, J. E. (1992). Emotion as memory: Anatomical systems underlying indelible neural traces. In S.-A. Christianson (Ed.), *Handbook of emotion and memory* (pp. 269–288). Hillsdale, NJ: Erlbaum.

LeDoux, J. E., Romanski, L., & Xagoraris, A. (1991). Indelibility of subcortical emotional memories. *Journal of Cognitive Neuroscience, 1,* 238–243.

Leichtman, M. D., Ceci, S., & Ornstein, P. A. (1992). The influence of affect on memory: Mechanism and development. In S.-A. Christianson (Ed.), *Handbook of emotion and memory* (pp. 181–199). Hillsdale, NJ: Erlbaum.

Loftus, E. F., Polensky, S., & Fullilove, M. T. (1994). Memories of childhood sexual abuse: Remembering and repressing. *Psychology of Women Quarterly, 18,* 67–84.

Madakasira, S., & O'Brian, K. (1987). Acute posttraumatic stress disorder in victims of a natural disaster. *Journal of Nervous and Mental Disease, 175,* 286–290.

Marmar, C. R., Weiss, D. S., Schlenger, W. E., Fairbank, J. A., Jordan, K., Kulka, R. A., & Hough, R. L. (1994). Peritraumatic dissociation and post-traumatic stress in male Vietnam theater veterans. *American Journal of Psychiatry, 151,* 902–907.

McGaugh, J. L. (1989). Involvement of hormonal and neuromodulatory systems in the regulation of memory storage. *Annual Review of Neuroscience, 2,* 255–287.

McGaugh, J. L. (1992). Affect, neuromodulatory systems, and memory storage. In S. A. Christianson (Ed.), *Handbook of emotion and memory* (pp. 245–268). Hillsdale, NJ: Erlbaum.

McGaugh, J. L., Weinberger, N. M., Lynch, G., & Granger, R. H. (1985). Neural mechanisms of learning and memory: Cells, systems and computations. *Naval Research Reviews, 37,* 15–29.

Mitchell, D., Osbourne, E. W., & O'Boyle, M. W. (1985). Habituation under stress: Shocked mice show non-associative learning in a T-maze. *Behavioral and Neural Biology, 43,* 212–217.

Myers, C. S. (1915, January). A contribution to the study of shell-shock. *Lancet,* 316–320.

Neisser, U., & Harsch, N. (1992). Phantom flashbulbs: False recollections of hearing the news about *Challenger.* In E. Winograd & U. Niesser (Eds.), *Affect and accuracy in recall* (pp. 9–31). New York: Cambridge University Press.

Nemiah, J. (1995). Early concepts of trauma, dissociation, and the unconscious: Their history and current implications. In J. D. Bremner & C. R. Marmar (Eds.), *Trauma, memory, and dissociation.* Washington, DC: American Psychiatric Press.

Niederland, W. G. (1968). Clinical observations on the "survivor syndrome." *International Journal of Psycho-Analysis, 49,* 313–315.

Nilsson, L. G., & Archer, T. (1992). Biological aspects of memory and emotion: Affect and cognition. In S.-A. Christianson (Ed.), *Handbook of emotion and memory* (pp. 289–306). Hillsdale, NJ: Erlbaum.

Phillips, A. G., & LePiane, F. G. (1980). Disruption of conditioned taste aversion in the rat by stimulation of amygdala: A conditioned effect, not amnesia. *Journal of Comparative and Physiological Psychology, 94,* 664–674.

Piaget, J. (1962). *Play, dreams, and imitation in childhood.* New York: Norton.

Pillemer, D. B. (1984). Flashbulb memories of the assassination attempt on President Reagan. *Cognition, 16,* 63–80.

Pitman, R. K., & Orr, S. (1990). The black hole of trauma. *Biological Psychiatry, 26,* 221–223.

Pitman, R. K., Orr, S. P., Forgue, D. F., de Jong, J., & Clairborn, J. M. (1987). Psychophysiologic assessment of posttraumatic stress disorder imagery in Vietnam combat veterans. *Archives of General Psychiatry, 17,* 970–975.

Pitman, R. K., Orr, S., & Shalev, A. (1993). Once bitten, twice shy: Beyond the conditioning model of PTSD. *Biological Psychiatry, 33,* 145–146.

Putnam, F. W. (1989). *Diagnosis and treatment of multiple personality disorder.* New York: Guilford Press.

Rainey, J. M., Aleem, A., Ortiz, A., Yaragani, V., Pohl, R., & Berchow, R. (1987). Laboratory procedure for the inducement of flashbacks. *American Journal of Psychiatry, 144,* 1317–1319.

Rauch, S., van der Kolk, B. A., Fisler, R., Alpert, N. M., Orr, S. P., Savage, C. R., Fischman, A. J., Jenike, M. A., & Pitman, R. K. (in press). A symptom provocation study of posttraumatic stress disorder using positron emission tomography and script-driven imagery. *Archives of General Psychiatry.*

Rawlins, J. N. P. (1980). Associative and non-associative mechanisms in the development of tolerance for stress: The problem of state dependent learning. In S. Levine & H. Ursin (Eds.), *Coping and health.* New York: Plenum Press.

Sargant, W., & Slater, E. (1941). Amnesic syndromes in war. *Proceedings of the Royal Society of Medicine, 34,* 757–764.

Schachtel, E. G. (1947). On memory and childhood amnesia. *Psychiatry, 10,* 1–26.

Schacter, D. L. (1986). Amnesia and crime: How much do we really know? *American Psychologist, 41*(3), 286–295.

Schacter, D. L. (1987). Implicit memory: History and current status. *Journal of Experimental Psychology: Learning, Memory, and Cognition, 13,* 510–518.

Selye, H. (1956). *The stress of life.* New York: McGraw-Hill.

Shalev, A. Y., Orr, S. P., & Pitman, R. K. (1993). Psychophysiologic assessment of traumatic imagery in Israeli civilian patients with posttraumatic stress disorder. *American Journal of Psychiatry, 150,* 620–624.

Solomon, A., Garb, R., Bleich, A., & Grupper, D. (1987). Reactivation of combat-related post-traumatic stress disorder. *American Journal of Psychiatry, 144,* 51–55.

Sonnenberg, S. M., Blank, A. S., & Talbott, J. A. (1985). *The trauma of war: Stress and recovery in Vietnam veterans.* Washington, DC: American Psychiatric Press.

Southard, E. E. (1919). *Shell-shock and other neuropsychiatric problems.* Boston: W. W. Leonard.

Southwick, S. M., Krystal, J. H., Morgan, A., Johnson, D., Nagy, L., Nicolaou, A., Henninger, G. R., & Charney, D. S. (1993). Abnormal noradrenergic function in posttraumatic stress disorder. *Archives of General Psychiatry, 50,* 266–274.

Spiegel, D. (1991). Dissociation and trauma. In A. Tasman & S. M. Goldfinger (Eds.), *American Psychiatric Press annual review of psychiatry* (Vol. 10). Washington, DC: American Psychiatric Press.

Squire, L. R. (1994). Declarative and nondeclarative memory; Multiple brain systems supporting learning and memory. In D. L. Schacter & E. Tulving (Eds.), *Memory systems.* Cambridge, MA: MIT Press.

Squire, L. R., & Zola-Morgan, S. (1991). The medial temporal lobe memory system. *Science, 153,* 2380–2386.

Stein, M. B., Hannah, C., Koverola, C., Yehuda, R., Torchia, M., & McClarty, B. (1994, December 15). *Neuroanatomical and neuroendocrine correlates in adulthood of severe sexual abuse in childhood.* Paper presented at the 33rd Annual Meeting of the American College of Neuropsychopharmacology, San Juan, PR.

Terr, L. C. (1988). What happens to early memories of trauma? *Journal of the American Academy of Child and Adolescent Psychiatry, 1,* 96–104.

Terr, L. (1993). *Unchained memories.* New York: Basic Books.

Thom, D. A., & Fenton, N. (1920). Amnesias in war cases. *American Journal of Insanity, 76,* 437–448.

van der Hart, O., Steele, K., Boon, S., & Brown, P. (1993). The treatment of traumatic memories: Synthesis, realization, and integration. *Dissociation, 6,* 162–180.

van der Kolk, B. A. (1989). The compulsion to repeat trauma: Revictimization, attachment and masochism. *Psychiatric Clinics of North America, 12,* 389–411.

van der Kolk, B. A. (1994). The body keeps the score: Memory and the evolving psychobiology of posttraumatic stress. *Harvard Review of Psychiatry, 1*(5), 253–265.

van der Kolk, B. A., Blitz, R., Burr, W. A., & Hartmann, E. (1984). Nightmares and trauma: Lifelong and traumatic nightmares in Veterans. *American Journal of Psychiatry, 141,* 187–190.

van der Kolk, B. A., & Fisler, R. (1995). Dissociation and the fragmentary nature of traumatic memories: Review and experimental confirmation. *Journal of Traumatic Stress, 8*(4), 505–525.

van der Kolk, B. A., Greenberg, M. S., Boyd, H., & Krystal, J. H. (1985). Inescapable shock, neurotransmitters and addiction to trauma: Towards a psychobiology of post traumatic stress. *Biological Psychiatry, 20,* 314–325.

van der Kolk, B .A., & Kadish, W. (1987). Amnesia, dissociation, and the return of the repressed. In B. A. van der Kolk, *Psychological trauma.* Washington, DC: American Psychiatric Press.

van der Kolk, B. A., Pelcovitz, D., Ross, S., Mandel, F., McFarlane, A. C., & Herman, J. L. (in press). Dissociation, affect dysregulation, and somatization: The complexity of adaptation to trauma. *American Journal of Psychiatry.*

van der Kolk, B. A., & van der Hart, O. (1989). Pierre Janet and the breakdown of adaptation in psychological trauma. *American Journal of Psychiatry, 146,* 1530–1540.

van der Kolk, B. A., & van der Hart, O. (1991). The intrusive past: The flexibility of memory and the engraving of trauma. *American Imago, 48*(4), 425–454.

Wilkinson, C. B. (1983). Aftermath of a disaster: The collapse of the Hyatt Regency Hotel skywalks. *American Journal of Psychiatry, 140,* 1134–1139.

Williams, L. (1994). Adult memories of childhood abuse. *Journal of Consulting and Clinical Psychology, 62*(6), 1167–1176.

Yuille, J. C., & Cutshall, J. L. (1986). A case study of eyewitness memory of a crime. Journal of *Applied Psychology, 71,* 318–323.

Yuille, J. C., & Cutshall, J. L. (1989). Analysis of the statements of victims, witnesses and suspects. In J. C. Yuille (Ed.), *Credibility assessment.* Dordrecht: The Netherlands: Kluwer.

CHAPTER 13

Dissociation and Information Processing in Posttraumatic Stress Disorder

BESSEL VAN DER KOLK
ONNO VAN DER HART
CHARLES R. MARMAR

When all sides are assailed by prospects of disaster the soul of man never confronts the totality of its wretchedness. The bitter drug is divided into separate draughts for him; today he takes on part of his woe; tomorrow he takes more; and so on; till the last drop is drunk.

—HERMAN MELVILLE, *PIERRE*

THE COGNITIVE ORGANIZATION OF TRAUMATIC EXPERIENCE

What causes people to become overwhelmed and to convert a stressful experience into a personal trauma? As long as people are able to imagine some way of staving off the inevitable, or as long as they feel taken care of by someone stronger than themselves, psychological and biological systems seem to be protected against becoming overwhelmed. Much of human activity seems to involve the development of notions of how the world functions and the creation of more or less predictable stable social environments for protection. Developmentally, these processes start with children's reliance on external caregivers who supply basic security. As children grow, they gradually develop

303

more autonomy by expanding their knowledge about the way things work and by developing skills that help them cope with external threats. Over time, predictability and controllability also involves making commitments to people, institutions, and value systems that provide a sense of meaning, belonging, and protection against threat (Erikson, 1963).

Feelings of security and predictability depend on a person's being able to rely on a balance of internal and external resources. When the person does not have enough resources to deal with outside threat, and external agents fail to come to the rescue, the inability to take appropriate action to eliminate the threat may well set up an acute stress reaction (see Chapter 5, this volume). In the early chapters of this book, we have examined the many variables that contribute to people's becoming overwhelmed and developing lasting alterations in their psychological and biological makeup. In this chapter, we look at the mental processes involved in these alterations.

Human beings are meaning-making creatures. As they develop, they organize their world according to a personal theory of reality, some of which may be conscious, but much of which is an unconscious integration of accumulated experience (Janet, 1889; Freud, 1920/1955; Horowitz, 1986; Harber & Pennebaker, 1992). Thus, cognitive schemata allow people to make sense out of emotionally arousing experiences, and serve as buffers against their becoming overwhelmed (Epstein, 1991; Janoff-Bulman, 1992). These internal schemata also function as filters that select the relevant perceptual input for further encoding and categorization, and thus constitute the pathways along which people analyze ongoing experiences (van der Kolk & Ducey, 1989; see Chapter 12, this volume).What constitutes a trauma is highly personal and depends on preexisting mental schemata. For example, an emergency medical technician is much less likely to react to witnessing an injured person with panic than someone who is unprepared.

Coping can be roughly divided into two general categories: (1) problem-focused coping (channeling resources to solve the stress-creating problem), and (2) emotion-focused coping (easing the tension aroused by the threat through intrapsychic activity, such as denying or changing one's attitude toward the threatening circumstances) (Lazarus, 1966; Solomon, Mikulincer, & Avitzur, 1988). Of these two coping styles, problem-focused coping would, on the surface, appear to be superior. And, indeed, it is associated with lower rates of posttraumatic stress disorder (PTSD) in combat soldiers (see Chapter 5). However, different styles of coping can be useful under different conditions. Although being assertive often helps people escape from danger, it may be dangerous when a person is being tortured, when a child is being physically or sexually abused, or when an individual is a witness to violence. There are situations in which people simply are unable to affect the outcome of events: In the context of child abuse, rape, or political torture, active resistance is likely to provoke retaliation from the perpetrator. In such cases, "passive" coping is not maladaptive; sometimes "spacing out" and disengaging can help people survive.

INFORMATION PROCESSING IN PTSD

Three critical problems affect information processing in people who suffer from PTSD. First, they overinterpret current stimuli as reminders of the trauma; minor stimuli come to have the power to activate intrusive recollections of the trauma (see Chapter 1, this volume). Second, they suffer from generalized hyperarousal and difficulty in distinguishing between what is relevant and what is not (see Chapters 4 and 10, this volume). Third, after dissociating at the moment of the trauma, many traumatized individuals continue to use dissociation as a way of dealing both with trauma-related intrusions and with other ongoing stressful life experiences.

Hyperarousal and Problems with Stimulus Discrimination

Earlier in this century, Abram Kardiner (1941) first pointed out that people with PTSD develop serious distortions in the ways they process information because they narrow their attentional focus onto sources of potential threat. They remain on guard for the return of the trauma, and thus stay in a physiological state of chronic overarousal. This hyperarousal creates a vicious cycle: State-dependent memory retrieval causes increased access to traumatic memories and involuntary intrusions of the trauma, which lead in turn to even more arousal. In an apparent effort to avoid feelings that could trigger memories of the trauma, many patients start organizing their lives around avoiding emotional engagement. Such attempts at control can take many different forms: Some people may simply avoid people or situations that serve as triggers, while others ingest drugs or alcohol to numb awareness of distressing emotional states. Many learn to use dissociation to banish unpleasant experiences from conscious awareness. However, in the long run, all these attempts to ward off memories of the trauma interfere with these people's capacity to live their lives.

Adults and children with PTSD not only have difficulty mastering distressing emotions; they also have trouble attending to neutral or pleasurable stimuli. Several studies that have measured the physiological arousal of PTSD patients have shown that they are more sensitive to sounds than normal subjects (see Chapter 10). McFarlane, Weber, and Clark (1993), using event-related potentials, found that people with PTSD had trouble differentiating relevant from irrelevant stimuli. They attended less to emotionally neutral but existentially relevant events, and they needed to apply more effort than nontraumatized people to respond to ordinary experience. This problem with focusing on what really matters amplifies the central role of the trauma in these patients' lives. Their inattention prevents them from getting pleasure out of what is happening in the here and now, and interferes with building up specific skills and feelings of mastery. Their difficulties in "knowing" what they feel, and in imagining a range of options without getting intensely emotionally aroused, also get in the way of their being able to integrate and resolve the trauma itself. Although they tend to be overwhelmed by diffuse emotions, they are often quite unaware of what precisely these intense feelings are all about. Because of this inability to identify what they are feeling, it is difficult for them to do anything about it (Krystal, 1978; van der Kolk & Ducey, 1989).

This difficulty in managing emotions interferes with the capacity to work through ordinary problems and conflicts as well. Because people with PTSD either shun emotional entanglements or fail to modulate the extent of their involvement, they often fail to build up a store of restitutive, gratifying experiences. Hence, they are deprived of precisely those psychological rewards that allow most people to cope with the injuries of everyday life. This keeps them preoccupied with the trauma at the expense of getting satisfaction out of daily life, which could help them overcome the central role of the trauma in their lives.

Dissociation

Dissociation is a way of organizing information. In recent years, psychiatry has rediscovered that dissociative processes play a critical role in the development of trauma-related psychological problems (e.g., Briere & Conte, 1993; Spiegel & Cardeña, 1991; Marmar et al., 1994b; Shalev, Peri, Caneti, & Schreiber, 1996). Dissociation occurs both at the time of the traumatic event (Bremner et al., 1992; Marmar et al., 1994b; Noyes & Kletti, 1977), and posttraumatically, as a long-term consequence of traumatic exposure (Bremner, Steinberg, Southwick, Johnson, & Charney, 1993; Cardeña & Spiegel, 1993; Chu & Dill, 1990; Saxe et al., 1993).

"Dissociation" refers to a compartmentalization of experience: Elements of a trauma are not integrated into a unitary whole or an integrated sense of self. The British psychiatrist Charles Samuel Myers, who coined the term "shell-shock" during World War I, proposed that the essence of traumatization is that individuals are unable to integrate it into their normal personality states. Instead, these traumatic memories are characteristically stored separately from other memories, in discrete personality states: ". . . the normal has been replaced by what we may call the 'emotional personality.' Gradually or suddenly an 'apparently normal' personality returns—normal save for the lack of all memory of events directly connected with the shock [i.e., trauma], normal save for the manifestation of other ('somatic') hysteric disorders indicative of mental dissociation" (1940, p. 67). Kardiner also noted the central role of dissociation in his traumatized war veterans: During dissociative fugue states, "[a] subject acts as if the original traumatic situation were still in existence and engages in protective devices which failed on the original occasion" (1941, p. 82). Triggered by a sensory stimulus, a patient might lash out, employing language suggestive of his trying to defend himself during a military assault. While riding the subway in New York and entering tunnels, many of Kardiner's patients had flashbacks to being back in the trenches.

The word "dissociation" is currently utilized to refer to three distinct but related mental phenomena (van der Hart, van der Kolk, & Boon, 1996).

Primary Dissociation

Many children and adults, when confronted with overwhelming threat, are unable to integrate the totality of what is happening into consciousness. Sensory and emotional elements of the event may not be integrated onto personal memory and identity, and remain isolated from ordinary consciousness; the experience is split into its isolated somatosensory elements, without integration into a personal narrative (van der Kolk & Fisler, 1995). This fragmentation is accompanied by ego states that are distinct from the normal state of consciousness. This condition, "primary dissociation," is characteristic of PTSD, in which the most dramatic symptoms are expressions of dissociated traumatic memories—intensely upsetting intrusive recollections, nightmares, and flashbacks.

Secondary Dissociation

Once an individual is in a traumatic (dissociated) state of mind, further disintegration of elements of the personal experience can occur. A "dissociation between observing ego and experiencing ego" (Fromm, 1965) has often been described in traumatized individuals, such as incest survivors, traffic accident victims, and combat soldiers (Gelinas, 1983; Noyes, Hoenck, & Kupperman, 1977). They report mentally leaving their bodies at the moment of the trauma and observing what happens from a distance. These distancing maneuvers of "secondary dissociation" allow individuals to observe their traumatic experience as spectators, and to limit their pain or distress; they are protected from awareness of the full impact of the event. Whereas primary dissociation limits people's cognitions regarding the reality of their traumatic experience, and enables them to go on temporarily as if nothing happened (e.g., Christianson & Nilsson, 1984, 1989; Spiegel, Hunt, & Dondershine, 1988), secondary dissociation puts people out of touch with the feelings and emotions related to the trauma; it anesthetizes them. In recent publications, secondary dissociation has been labeled "peritraumatic dissociation" (Marmar et al., 1994b).

Tertiary Dissociation

When people develop distinct ego states that contain the traumatic experience, consisting of complex identities with distinct cognitive, affective, and behavioral patterns, we call this "tertiary dissociation." Some ego states may contain the pain, fear, or anger related to particular traumatic experiences, while other ego states that remain unaware of the trauma and its concomitant affects, and continue to perform the routine functions of daily life. Examples are the multiple dissociated identity (alter) fragments in dissociative identity disorder (DID), some of which experience different aspects of one or more traumatic incidents, while others stay unaware of these unbearable experiences. To the extent that their dissociative amnesia allows them to, these patients typically report chronic and intense sexual, physical, and psychological abuse that started at a very early age (Putnam, Guroff, Silberman, Barban, & Post, 1986; Loewenstein & Putnam, 1990; Boon & Draijer, 1993).

THE HISTORY OF DISSOCIATION IN PSYCHIATRY

Because the early investigators of dissociative processes produced such careful documentation in their case histories, and because their understanding of dissociative phenomena and their treatment approaches remain as lucid and relevant today as they were a century ago, we dwell at some length on the historical aspects of the relationships between trauma and dissociation. The concept of dissociation was first discussed in a systematic fashion in the 1880s, in the work of Frederic Myers in England, and that of Jean-Martin Charcot, Gilles de la Tourette, and Pierre Janet in France. Myers was probably the first to demonstrate the degree of dissociation of memories, faculties, and sensibilities in patients with multiple personalities. Charcot noted that "by reason of the easy dissociation of mental unity, certain centers of the psychic organ may be put into play without the other regions of the psychic organ being made aware of it and called upon to take part in the process" (quoted in van der Hart, 1993). Gilles de la Tourette used the concept of dissociation to describe the abolition of certain physical sensations in hysterical patients (see van der Hart, 1993). Finally, Janet became the first systematic investigator of the relationship between dissociation and psychological trauma during his work at the psychiatric hospital in Le Havre and subsequently at the Salpêtrière in Paris (Janet, 1889; van der Kolk & van der Hart, 1989, 1991).

Janet believed dissociation to be the critical factor that determines the eventual adaptation to a traumatic experience. Trying to account for what causes people to dissociate, Janet wrote: "I was led to recognize in many subjects the role of one or several events in their past life. These events, which were accompanied by a vehement emotion and a destruction of the psychological system, had left traces. The remembrance of these events absorbed a great deal of energy and played a part in the persistent weakening" (1932, p. 128). According to Janet, the intensity of a "vehement emotion" depends both on the emotional state of the victim at the time of the event and on the cognitive appraisal of the situation.

Thus, the intensity of the emotional reaction—determined by the meaning attributed to the event, rather than by the event itself—eventually accounts for the resulting psychopathology: "The individual, when overcome by vehement emotions, is not himself. Forgetting the event which precipitated the emotion has frequently been found to accompany intense emotional experiences in the form of continuous and retrograde amnesia" (Janet, 1909b, p. 1607). In such cases, the person is "unable to make the recital which we call narrative memory, and yet he remains confronted by [the] difficult situation" (Janet, 1919/1925, Vol. 1, p. 660). The resulting "phobia of memory" (Janet, 1919/1925, Vol. 1, p. 661) prevents the integration ("synthesis") of traumatic events and splits off the traumatic memories from ordinary consciousness (Janet, 1898, p. 145). As long as these split-off memory traces have not been translated into a personal narrative, they will continue to intrude as terrifying perceptions, obsessional preoccupations, and somatic reexperiences (see van der Kolk & van der Hart, 1991).

Janet noted that somatosensory elements of the trauma may come back into consciousness when a person is confronted with reminders of the trauma. Thus, the trauma may be reexperienced as physical sensations (such as panic attacks), visual images (such as flashbacks and nightmares), obsessive ruminations, or behavioral reenactments (Janet, 1904). For example, Janet (1889) described the case of a young woman whose blindness in the left eye could be traced back to her having been forced to sleep in the same bed with a child who had impetigo on the left side of her face. Although the dominant personality had not experienced the event, a split-off part of consciousness encoded it outside of usual awareness. Janet also described how, even though dissociation fulfills no further useful function and lacks continued adaptive value, it often remains a way of coping with subsequent stress. This further cements the power of subconscious traumatic memories over current behavior. He described how people who continue to dissociate in the face of stress become emotionally constricted and cannot experience a full range of affects within what we would call today the same ego state (Janet, 1909a). The most extreme example of this is what is now called DID, in which fixed ideas develop into entirely separate identities (Janet, 1909b; van der Kolk & van der Hart, 1991).

William James (1894), reviewing Janet's work in the *Psychological Review*, added that two Viennese physicians, Josef Breuer and Sigmund Freud, were in the process of confirming many of Janet's findings. When Freud visited Charcot, he adopted many of the ideas then current at the Salpêtrière (e.g., Breuer & Freud, 1893–1895/1955; see also MacMillan, 1990, and Chapter 3, this volume). Although Breuer originally emphasized verbal over emotional expression of feelings, Breuer and Freud found that during Breuer's hypnotic explorations of the celebrated patient Anna O.'s multiple hysterical symptoms, a vivid reliving of traumatic events combined with the associated affects led to the resolution of her symptoms. Breuer's technique emphasized bringing the pathogenic traumatic memories into conscious awareness, verbalizing the distressing emotions related to those events, and discharging the emotions in a process that Breuer and Freud termed "catharsis" (abreaction).

We (van der Kolk & van der Hart, 1991) and Nemiah (1996) have pointed out some fundamental theoretical differences between Janet's approach and Freud's. From a psychoanalytic point of view, traumatic memories are actively extruded from consciousness by ego mechanisms of defense that protect the individual from painful memories. From Janet's point of view, individuals who dissociate do so not because of active repression, but rather because their mental capacities are weakened by "vehement emotions," which impair their ability to integrate mental contents. The traumatized individual is incapable of integrating the memories of the trauma into personal consciousness. Janet (1904, 1919/1925) called this a "phobia" for traumatic memories. This formulation stands in marked contrast to the psychoanalytic notion of active extrusion through repression. Like most contemporary specialists in the treatment of dissociative disorders, Janet believed that abreaction in itself is not curative. Because of the very nature of dissociative psychopathology, many such patients regularly enter states in which they partially or completely reexperience the trauma, without any resolution whatsoever. Controlling dissociation and integrating the traumatic experience must be the goal.

Following these initial contributions, interest in the relationship of trauma and dissociation waned. The Boston psychiatrist Morton Prince (1911), who specializd in the treatment of dissociative disorders, bemoaned the fact that with the advent of psychoanalysis the study of dissociation was inundated, like clams in the New England tides. Psychiatry as a profession followed Freud in his reformulation of the nature of symptom formation and psychological conflicts in hysteria. Although he initially conceived of hysterics as "suffering from reminiscences," Freud's further clinical inquiries led him to the conclusion that alleged memories of early traumatic events were in fact recovered memories not of actual trauma, but of eroticized fantasies occurring in the course of childhood sexual development.

During both World Wars, psychiatry was again powerfully confronted with the issue of dissociation. During World War I and its aftermath, British psychiatrists treating war casualties had an ongoing discussion about the repressed or dissociated nature of traumatic memories, and hence about the relative therapeutic value of abreaction versus the integration of the dissociated memories into personal awareness (van der Hart & Brown, 1992). Jung (1921–1922) participated in this discussion by claiming that the discharge of excess emotion in therapy did not work. He also recognized that abreaction is not only useless, but often actually harmful. Jung concurred with McDougall (1926) and Myers (1940) that the critical issue in posttraumatic stress is psychological dissociation. He claimed that a traumatic memory creates a dissociation of the psyche: "It is removed from the control of the will and therefore possesses the quality of psychical autonomy" (p. 15). "Support and understanding of the therapist increases the patient's level of awareness and consciously enables him once again to bring the autonomous dissociated traumatic memory under volitional control."

As we have already noted (see Chapter 3, this volume), after World War II the hard-earned knowledge about these processes disappeared, until clinicians rediscovered the relationship between trauma and the dissociative disorders in the mid-1980s (e.g., Spiegel, 1984; Putnam, 1985).

CONTEMPORARY VIEWS ON TRAUMA AND DISSOCIATIVE PROCESSES

In the *Diagnostic and Statistical Manual of Mental Disorders,* fourth edition (DSM-IV; American Psychiatric Association, 1994), the new diagnosis of acute stress disorder (ASD) focuses on dissociation in the immediate aftermath of trauma. Either while experiencing or after experiencing the traumatic event, the individual has at least three of the following dissociative symptoms: (1) a feeling of detachment, numbing, or lack of emotional responsiveness; (2) decreased awareness of surroundings; (3) derealization; (4) depersonalization; and (5) inability to remember a significant aspect of the trauma. Thus, dissociation of a traumatic experience happens while the trauma is still going on. There is little evidence for an active process of pushing away the overwhelming experience; the uncoupling seems to have other mechanisms.

Both ASD and PTSD seem to originate in the individual's capacity to access dissociative states (Spiegel & Cardeña, 1991). People who have earlier learned to use this mode of coping with threat seem to be particularly vulnerable to using it again during acute stress. This prevents them from being fully aware of what is happening to them, and thus from "owning" the experience; dissociating the experience means that they cannot learn from it. Failure to integrate the trauma in the acute stage makes people vulnerable to the later development of PTSD (see Chapter 5, this volume).

In the long run, people may adapt to the combination of dissociation and other ways of coping with the trauma by developing a wide spectrum of mental disorders. Depending on the developmental level at which the trauma occurs, the trauma's severity and chronicity, and on the individual's temperament and posttrauma environment, a traumatized individual may develop any of a variety of Axis I and II disorders (see Chapters 7 and 9, this volume). In some individuals, the dissociated fragments of a traumatic experience may be buried without markedly interfering with their overall functioning, whereas others organize the totality of their personality around dealing with the aftermath of the trauma. This may be particularly the case in patients with borderline personality disorder (BPD; Herman, Perry, & van der Kolk, 1989). Although high levels of dissociation have been noted in patients with somatization disorder, BPD, and PTSD (van der Kolk et al., in press), the DSM-III created a separate category for dissociative disorders to capture the phenomena associated with people's switching into alternate states of consciousness (which are characterized by "a disruption in the usually integrated functions of consciousness, memory, identity, or perception of the environment"; American Psychiatric Association, 1994, p. 477). The DSM thereby created a category for describing a way of processing information, without capturing the various personality organizations that are part and parcel of the adaptation to trauma (van der Kolk et al., in press; see Chapter 9, this volume).

CLINICAL AND RESEARCH ISSUES

Primary Dissociation: The Fragmented Nature of Traumatic Memories

As we have seen, trauma is often first organized in memory on a perceptual level (see Chapter 12, this volume). "Memories" of the trauma are initially experienced as fragments of the sensory components of the event—as visual images; olfactory, auditory, or kinesthetic sensations; or intense waves of feelings that patients usually claim to be representations of elements of the original traumatic event. The Traumatic Memory Inventory (TMI) is one way of measuring this fragmented (dissociated) nature of traumatic memories (van der Kolk & Fisler, 1995). The TMI is a 60-item structured interview that provides a systematic assessment of the circumstances and means of retrieval of a traumatic memory, compared with retrieval of a memory of a personally highly emotionally significant but nontraumatic event. In one study (van der Kolk & Fisler, 1995), all subjects, regardless of the age at which the trauma occurred and whether they had periods of amnesia or not, reported that the trauma initially came into consciousness in the form of somatosensory flashback experiences. These flashbacks occurred in a variety of modalities. Initially, these sensory modalities did not occur together; however, as the trauma came into consciousness with greater intensity, more sensory modalities were activated.

Over time, this increasing spectrum of sensory modalities was accompanied by the gradual emergence of a personal narrative.

Thus, the imprints of traumatic experiences are initially dissociated, and retrieved as sensory fragments that have little or no linguistic component. As traumatized people become aware of more and more elements of their experience, they construct a narrative that "explains" what happened to them, utilizing the memory fragments that are available to them. This process of weaving a narrative out of disparate sensory elements of an experience is probably not all that dissimilar from how people automatically construct a narrative under ordinary conditions, or from the process that occurs in effective therapy of PTSD (see Chapter 22). In contrast, day-to-day, nontraumatic experiences are not registered in consciousness as separate sensory elements of the experience, but are automatically integrated into a coherent personal narrative.

Secondary Dissociation (Peritraumatic Dissociation)

As noted earlier, survivors of childhood abuse, victims of traffic accidents, and traumatized combat soldiers frequently suffer from secondary dissociation—a "dissociation between observing ego and experiencing ego" (Fromm, 1965). Trauma victims often report alterations in the experience of time, place, and person, which conferred a sense of unreality on the event as it was occurring. Dissociation during trauma may take the form of altered time sense; time may be experienced as either slowed down or accelerated. Many victims experience depersonalization, out-of-body experiences, bewilderment, confusion, disorientation, altered pain perception, altered body image, tunnel vision, and immediate dissociative experiences. Marmar and his colleagues have called these acute dissociative responses to trauma "peritraumatic dissociation" (Marmar et al., 1994b; Marmar, Weiss, & Metzler, in press-a; Weiss, Marmar, Metzler, & Ronfeldt, 1995).

Although clinical reports of peritraumatic dissociation date back nearly a century, it has not been systematically investigated until fairly recently. Noyes and Kletti (1977) surveyed 101 survivors of automobile accidents and physical assault: 72% reported experiencing feelings of unreality and altered passage of time during the event, 57% automatic movement, 52% sense of detachment, 56% depersonalization, 34% detachment from the body, and 30% derealization. Hillman (1981) reported on the experiences of 14 correctional officers held hostage during a violent prison riot, who described employing time distortion and psychogenic anesthesia to protect themselves against overwhelming pain. Wilkinson (1983) investigated the psychological responses of survivors of the Hyatt Regency Hotel skywalk collapse, in which 114 people died and 200 were injured. Survivors commonly reported depersonalization and derealization experiences at the time of the collapse. Siegel (1984) studied 31 kidnapping victims and terrorist hostages, and reported that during the hostage experience 25.8% experienced alterations in body imagery and sensations, depersonalization, and disorientation, and 12.9% had out-of-body experiences.

In recent years, studies of a variety of traumatized populations have shown that dissociation during the trauma is a significant predictor of the subsequent development of PTSD. Holen (1993) found this in survivors of a North Sea oil rig disaster; Cardeña and Spiegel (1993) in 100 graduate students following the 1989 Loma Prieta, California, earthquake; and Koopman, Classen, and Spiegel (1994) in survivors of the Oakland/Berkeley, California, fires. In clinical populations, Carlson and Rosser-Hogan (1991) found a strong relationship among severity of the trauma, dissociative symptoms, and PTSD in Cambodian refugees. Bremner et al. (1992) found that Vietnam veterans with PTSD reported having experienced higher levels of dissociative symptoms during combat than men who did not develop PTSD. A prospective study of 51 injured trauma survivors in Israel (Shalev et al., 1996) found that peritraumatic dissociation explained 29.4% of the variance in PTSD symptoms at 6-month follow-up, over and above the effects of demographic variables, event severity, and other types of symptoms during the week following the event. Peritraumatic dissociation was also the strongest predictor of PTSD status at follow-up.

These research findings were at first surprising, given the predominant clinical belief that dissociative responses to trauma at the time of occurrence of life-threatening or otherwise terrifying events conferred a sense of distance and safety on the victims. For example, adult survivors of childhood incest often report that during the experience of sexual abuse they left their bodies and viewed the assault from above, with a feeling of detachment and compassion for the helpless little children who were being sexually assaulted. Although the use of out-of-body and other peritraumatic dissociative responses at the time of trauma may defend against even more catastrophic states of helplessness and terror, dissociation at the time of trauma is one of the most important risk factors for the subsequent development of chronic PTSD.

The Peritraumatic Dissociative Experiences Questionnaire

On the basis of these early research observations on peritraumatic dissociation as a risk factor for chronic PTSD, Marmar and his colleagues embarked on a series of studies to develop a reliable and valid measure of peritraumatic dissociation. This measure, the Peritraumatic Dissociative Experiences Questionnaire (PDEQ), consists of nine items addressing dissociative experiences at the time of the traumatic event: moments of losing track or blanking out; finding the self acting on "automatic pilot"; sense of time changing during the event; the event's seeming unreal, as in a dream or play; feeling as if floating above the scene; feeling disconnected from the body or experiencing body distortion; confusing what was happening to the self and others; not being aware of things happening during the event that normally would have been noticed; and not feeling pain associated with physical injury.

Using the PDEQ, Marmar et al. (1994b) investigated the relationship of peritraumatic dissociation to posttraumatic stress in 251 male Vietnam theater veterans. The total score on the PDEQ was strongly associated with level of posttraumatic stress symptoms, level of stress exposure, and general dissociative tendencies. This study showed that the greater the dissociation during traumatic stress exposure, the greater the likelihood of meeting criteria for current PTSD. These findings were replicated in 367 emergency services personnel exposed to traumatic critical incidents, including police, firefighters, emergency medical technicians/paramedics, and California Department of Transportation workers (Weiss et al., 1995; Marmar, Weiss, Metzler, Ronfeldt, & Foreman, 1996). These 367 included 154 workers who helped to deal with the 1989 Interstate 880/Nimitz Freeway collapse during the Loma Prieta earthquake. Various predictors of current symptomatic distress were measured, including level of critical incident exposure, social support, psychological traits, locus of control, general dissociative tendencies, and peritraumatic dissociation. After both exposure and adjustment were controlled for, symptomatic distress could be predicted by social support, experience on the job, locus of control, general dissociative tendencies, and dissociative experiences at the time of the critical incident. The two dissociative variables, total score on the Dissociative Experiences Scale (DES; Bernstein & Putnam, 1986) and total score on the PDEQ, strongly predicted level of symptoms.

These results were further replicated in studies of 60 adult men and women who lived close to the epicenter of the 1994 Los Angeles area Northridge earthquake (Marmar, Weiss, Metzler, & Ronfeldt, 1994a) and in female Vietnam theater veterans (Tichenor, Marmar, Weiss, Metzler, & Ronfeldt, 1994). The findings have been even further strengthened by two independent studies. Bremner et al. (1992) reported a strong relationship of peritraumatic dissociation with posttraumatic stress response in a sample of Vietnam veterans. In the first prospective study with the PDEQ (Shalev et al., 1996), ratings at 1 week predicted stress symptomatology at 5 months. Although retrospective ratings of peritraumatic dissociation months, years, or decades after the occurrence of traumatic events are subject to possible bias (i.e., greater current distress may result in greater recollection of dissociation at the time of the trauma's occurrence), the prospective findings of Shalev et al.'s study support the use of retrospective ratings of peritraumatic dissociation.

Mechanisms for Peritraumatic Dissociation

The findings that relate peritraumatic dissociation to subsequent PTSD raise important questions concerning the mechanisms that underlie peritraumatic dissociation. As we have seen, clinical observations concerning the psychological factors underlying trauma-related dissociation date back to the early contributions of Charcot (1887), Janet (1889), and Breuer and Freud (1893–1895/1955). Contemporary psychological studies of peritraumatic dissociation have focused on individual differences in the threshold for dissociation. We have noted earlier that adult victims who dissociate during a traumatic event may be more likely to have experienced childhood or adolescent traumatic events, which have lowered their threshold for dissociation. The neurobiology and neuropharmacology of anxiety may be able to offer important clues concerning the underlying mechanisms for peritraumatic dissociation (see Chapter 10, this volume). The study of Southwick et al. (1993) with yohimbine challenges suggests that in individuals with PTSD, flashbacks occur in response to high states of arousal. Patients with panic disorder frequently report dissociative reactions at the height of their anxiety attacks (Krystal, Woods, Hill, & Charney, 1991). Moleman, van der Hart, and van der Kolk (1992) reported a progression from panic to dissociated states in women with complicated childbirths who later developed PTSD. These studies suggest that the relationship between peritraumatic dissociation and PTSD may be mediated by high levels of anxiety during the trauma. Contemporary research may yet prove Janet right in his claim that "vehement emotions" form the basis of dissociative phenomena.

Marmar, Weiss, Metzler, and Delucchi (in press-b) found the following factors to be associated with greater levels of peritraumatic dissociation: younger age, higher levels of exposure, greater subjective perceived threat, poorer general psychological adjustment, poorer identity formation, lower levels of ambition and prudence as defined by the Hogan Personality Inventory, greater external locus of control, and greater use of escape/avoidance and emotion-focused coping. Taken together, these findings suggest that people with less work experience, more vulnerable personality structures, greater reliance on the external world for a sense of security, and greater use of maladaptive coping strategies are more vulnerable to peritraumatic dissociation (see Chapters 5 and 19, this volume).

Tertiary Dissociation: The Development of Dissociative Disorders

It has been repeatedly observed that once people have learned to dissociate in response to trauma, they tend to continue to do so in the face of subsequent stress. Continued dissociation may not only interfere with the conscious processing of current information; it also prevents the exploration of alternative ways of coping, and thus interferes with general adaptation. Even if tuning out potentially frightening stimuli helps to keep a person from feeling overwhelmed, in the long run trauma victims are in danger of having difficulties with active problem-solving strategies; that is, they may consolidate a helpless and passive social stance (Wolfe, Keane, & Kaloupek, 1993). The utilization of dissociative responses on a day-to-day basis is best measured by the DES (Bernstein & Putnam, 1986), and the encapsulation of traumatic experiences in separate states of consciousness is best measured by the Dissociative Disorders Interview Scale (DDIS; Ross et al., 1992), or the Structured Clinical Interview for DSM-III-R Dissociative Disorders (SCID-D; Steinberg, Rounsaville, & Cicchetti, 1990).

Dissociation and the Sense of Self

Many clinicians who treat traumatized individuals with PTSD have noted that in response to certain apparently neutral stimuli, some traumatized individuals behave as though they were being traumatized all over again, and experience a state of mind that seems to have been present at the time of the trauma, even if they do not explicitly recall the traumatic event when they behave that way (e.g., Kardiner, 1941; Spiegel, 1993). Traumatized individuals can contain their dissociated memories in an ego state of which they ordinarily are not aware; McDougall (1926) proposed that traumatic memories are always "part of some personality" (p. 543). Earlier in this chapter, we have noted Myers's (1940), observation that following a traumatic event, an "apparently normal" personality alternates with an "emotional" personality that seems to act as the container of traumatic experiences and reactions. In recent years, research such as that by Nissen, Ross, Willingham, MacKenzie, and Schacter (1988) has shown that even in patients who suffer from full-blown DID, the dissociations between implicit and explicit memory stores of normal and dissociative states, and among the stores of different dissociative states, are not absolute; some degree of co-consciousness among different ego states is common.

Dissociation allows people to maintain their existing schemata, while separate states of mind process the traumatic event. As a result, traumatic memory structures may contain trauma-related cognitions and self-schemata that differ from one another and from the habitual state, since they rely on divergent life experiences. That is, cognitive schemata—which involve schemata of the self—vary with the state a person is in. The dissociative patient in his or her normal state may insist, "I was not abused," whereas the dissociated cognitive system contains beliefs such as "I am weak, helpless, and unworthy" or "I am strong and aggressive." Accordingly, actual cognition will depend on the state that is reactivated.

If the trauma can be contained in a separate ego state, a part of a person's personality can continue to develop with relatively little interference from the traumatic memory. If the aspect of the personality that contains the traumatic memory remains fixated at the level of mental development at which the trauma occurred, this would imply that trauma has different long-term consequences at different stages of development. For example, people who were traumatized when they were 3 years old may continue to process intense emotional states with the developmental capacities of young children, whereas people traumatized at a later age will utilize different mechanisms to cope with further stressful experiences (van der Kolk, Hostetler, Herron, & Fisler, 1994).

As we have seen in Chapter 9, trauma, if it first befalls someone who already is an adult, tends to produce PTSD as currently defined. However, trauma at earlier ages tends to give rise to much more complex symptomatology, which can at least in part be understood as the result of a developmental fixation at earlier stages of psychological maturation.

Dissociative Psychopathology and Other Psychiatric Disorders

The phenomenology of DID patients illustrates that in the context of being traumatized, fragmentation may occur on many different levels. Not only can the memory of the trauma itself be fragmented; the ego identity that is engaged in the act of remembering can be split into multiple dissociated fragments as well. Some of these will carry the awareness for different aspects of one or more traumatic incidents, while others will stay unaware of these unbearable experiences. Studies have consistently found a highly significant relationship between childhood trauma and the development of DID (formerly known as multiple personality disorder). Coons and Milstein (1986) reported that 85% of a series of 20 patients with multiple personality disorder had documented histories of childhood abuse, while Frischholz (1985) and Putnam et al. (1986) reported rates of severe childhood abuse in more than 90% of their subjects. Usually, the severity of the childhood trauma in these chronically dissociated patients was truly extraordinary: severe and prolonged physical and/or sexual abuse, life threats, and a total lack of a subjective sense of safety secondary to abuse by the primary caretaker.

However, DID is not the only psychiatric condition in which high levels of dissociation are found in conjunction with prior histories of trauma. High levels of both trauma and dissociation have been found in BPD (e.g., Herman et al., 1989; Ogata et al., 1990), somatization disorder (Saxe et al., 1994), major depression, and PTSD (Bremner et al., 1992, 1993; Spiegel et al., 1988), as well as in patients with dissociative disorders themselves (Bernstein & Putnam, 1986; Boon & Draijer, 1993; Saxe et al., 1993). Prospectively, dissociation is a predictor both of self-mutilation and of suicide attempts (van der Kolk, Perry, & Herman, 1991).

The studies by Chu and Dill (1990) and Saxe et al. (1993) (see Chapter 9) have shown that dissociative disorders are quite common in psychiatric inpatients in the United States. The prevalence estimates of dissociative disorders in general and DID in particular derived from Saxe et al.'s study were 15% and 4%, respectively. However, clinicians are rarely trained to diagnose these patients properly: A chart review in the Saxe et al. (1993) study revealed that dissociative experiences such as amnesia, depersonalization, autonomous behavior, and numbing were recognized in only approximately 17% of the patients who suffered from them. The diagnosis of both PTSD and a dissociative disorder was made in only 8% of the patients who met diagnostic criteria for those conditions. Although very high proportions of patients reported sexual and physical abuse upon specific questioning (100% reported sexual abuse and 86% reported physical abuse, respectively), these experiences were only recorded in the patients' medical records some of the time (58% and 25%, respectively).

PRINCIPLES OF TREATMENT

The treatment of both acute and chronic trauma has three principal components: helping patients to (1) control and master physiological and biological stress reactions; (2) process and come to terms with the horrifying, overwhelming experience; and (3) reestablish secure social connections and personal as well as interpersonal efficacy. As long as traumatized people dissociate, and are plagued by involuntary intrusions of fragments of the trauma, the emphasis in treatment needs to be on self-regulation and on rebuilding. Early exploration and abreaction of traumatic experiences, without first establishing a sense of stability, are likely to lead to very negative therapeutic outcomes. This means that initial therapy needs to focus on security and predictability, and on encouraging active engagement in adaptive action.

Only a limited number of people with acute stress reactions go on to develop PTSD. The people who are able to overcome their initial reactions are most likely those who are able to restabilize their physiology, and who are able to take action that affects the outcome of the traumatic event. Outcome studies of acute interventions increasingly question the utility of emotional "working through" in the initial phases of treatment (see Chapters 18 and 20, this volume). Given the paucity of controlled studies, we are left with the clinical impression that the initial response to trauma should consist of reconnecting with ordinarily supportive networks, and of engaging in activities that reestablish a sense of mastery.

To date, no controlled clinical trials have been reported for psychosocial or pharmacological interventions specifically targeting trauma-related dissociation. Contemporary writers essentially follow the same stages that were outlined in Janet's (1919/1925) psychotherapeutic approach to patients with dissociative disorders (see Braun, 1986; Brown & Fromm, 1986; Kluft, 1987; Herman, 1992; van der Hart, Brown, & van der Kolk, 1989; van der Hart et al., 1996):

1. Stabilization, symptom-oriented treatment, and preparation for approaching traumatic memories.
2. Identification, exploration, and modification of traumatic memories.
3. Relapse prevention, relief of residual symptomatology, personality reintegration, and rehabilitation.

Each of these stages (the first two of which are briefly discussed below) requires different therapeutic techniques. In uncomplicated cases, traumatic memories and the psychological charge associated with them can be "near the surface" and are often accessible to nonhypnotic interventions. Simply discussing these patients' experiences in a safe setting, and encouraging them to share personal reminders of the trauma (e.g., pictures or a diary) with the therapist, can lead to resolution. Patients with chronic dissociative problems require more complex approaches, the details of which are beyond the scope of this chapter. These approaches involve a stepwise process of reexperiencing and verbalizing traumatic memories, starting with the least threatening ones and working toward assimilation of the most traumatic ones (Putnam, 1989; Kluft, 1991; van der Hart et al., 1996). In the treatment of these patients, particular attention needs to be paid to trauma-related concepts of the self (or fragments of self) as they are activated in the transference. This is critical for helping a patient process perceived threats in the relationship with the therapist without resorting to dissociation (e.g., Horowitz, 1986; Marmar, 1991, Pearlman & Saakvitne, 1995).

Stabilization

A sense of physical security depends on the knowledge that the trauma will not return. This means that active steps need to be taken to insure that traumatized patients are both physically and emotionally in a safe environment. In this context, the prime goal of treatment is to facilitate the patients' gaining control over the transitions in their dissociative mental states; this will permit a retreat from terror and a gradual integration. Since dissociative responses occur in reaction to intense emotional reminders, initial treatment needs to focus on defining problems and setting goals. Since dissociative states often involve autohypnosis, patients need to be helped to "ground" themselves. This includes assistance in identifying their sensations ("What do you see, hear, smell, and feel in your body?"), attending to objects in the present, and labeling emotions. Many traumatized individuals can use physical touch to help ground them; this may involve increasing awareness of bodily sensations, but also the use of prearranged touch between a helper and a patient (i.e., touching a hand or shoulder). In patients with histories of sexual abuse and other violations of personal boundaries, the meaning of touching needs to be clearly spelled out, understood, and agreed to before it is introduced in the treatment. Interventions that involve touching need to be properly timed, after a secure relationship in which a patient can confidently register reactions has been established.

Since dissociation involves the loss of a continuous sense of time, schedules, regular appointments, and routines are essential. Because fatigue and stress probably exacerbate dissociative episodes, establishing regular sleep–wake cycles, acitivity–rest schedules, and mealtimes is important. These patients often anxiously try to avoid feelings through impulsive action, which only aggravates the sense of ongoing threat and instability. Treatment needs to focus on helping patients think through the consequences of their actions. Many of these patients develop unstable social lives, which often become the source of unpleasant surprises. Hence, the social support structure needs to be analyzed, and the patients must be helped to find consistent and reliable people and organizations on whom they can rely when they feel "spaced out" and out of control. Whatever aspect of stabilization is being focused upon, the emphasis always needs to be on the patients' gaining a sense of control and mastery.

Although hypnosis is not a useful tool to uncover the "truth" in forensic settings, it can be of enormous benefit in the treatment of dissociative patients. van der Hart and Spiegel (1993) advocate the use of hypnosis as (1) a way of creating a safe mental state in which patients can learn to gain control over the unbidden intrusion of traumatic memories, and (2) an approach to the treatment of trauma-induced dissociative states presenting as hysterical psychosis. Exercise can also be immensely helpful in enhancing people's sense of control over their bodily sensations. Identifying triggers of dissociative episodes is a critical element of treatment.

Dealing with Traumatic Memories

The essence of the treatment of traumatic memories can be described as follows: (1) overcoming the phobia of the dissociated sense of self associated with the trauma, as well as the fear and shame associated with thinking about the trauma; (2) overcoming the phobia of the dissociated traumatic memories, which must be uncovered and transformed from intrusive reexperiencing of trauma-related feelings and sensations to a trauma-related narrative within a personal stream of consciousness; and (3) overcoming the phobia of life itself, which includes the fear of being revictimized, and the feeling that the victim will be unable to take charge of his or her own destiny (van der Hart, Steele, Boon, & Brown, 1993; van der Hart et al., 1996; see Chapter 18, this volume, for a more detailed discussion). A traumatic memory cannot be adequately processed if its affective and sensory–motor elements remain isolated from the rest of the memory (van der Hart & Op den Velde, 1991). For adequate processing to occur, all dissociated aspects must be integrated. One of the reasons why reliving a trauma in nightmares and flashbacks is not an effective means of memory processing is that some fragments of the event remain dissociated from other elements of what has to become an integrated, semantically represented, autobiographical memory.

Much remains to be learned before a definitive canon of treatment of dissociative disorders can be articulated. The systematic exploration and validation of existing treatment methods for both acutely and chronically traumatized patients need to be informed by an improved understanding of the psychological and neurobiological factors underlying dissociation. In this regard, we hope that contemporary advances in the understanding of the core mechanisms and processes involved in adaptation to trauma, as we have attempted to describe in this book, will open up better ways of treating patients who respond to exposure to a trauma by dissociating.

REFERENCES

American Psychiatric Association. (1994). *Diagnostic and statistical manual of mental disorders* (4th ed.). Washington, DC: Author.

Bernstein, E. M., & Putnam, F. W. (1986). Development, reliability, and validity of a dissociation scale. *Journal of Nervous and Mental Disease, 174,* 727–735.

Boon, S., & Draijer, N. (1993). Multiple personality disorder in the Netherlands: A clinical investigation of 71 patients. *American Journal of Psychiatry, 150,* 489–494.

Braun, B. G. (1986). Issues in the psychotherapy of multiple personality disorder. In B. G. Braun (Ed.), *Treatment of multiple personality disorder* (pp. 3–28). Washington, DC: American Psychiatric Press.

Bremner, J. D., Southwick, S., Brett, E., Fontana, A., Rosenheck, R., & Charney, D. S. (1992). Dissociation and posttraumatic stress disorder in Vietnam combat veterans. *American Journal of Psychiatry, 149,* 328–332.

Bremner, J. D., Steinberg, M., Southwick, S. M., Johnson, D. R., & Charney, D. S. (1993). Use of the Structured Clinical Interview for DSM-IV Dissociative Disorders for systematic assessment of dissociative symptoms in posttraumatic stress disorder. *American Journal of Psychiatry, 150*(7), 1011–1014.

Breuer, J., & Freud, S. (1955). Studies on hysteria. In J. Strachey (Ed. and Trans.), *The standard edition of the complete psychological works of Sigmund Freud* (Vol. 2, pp. 1–305). London: Hogarth Press. (Original work published 1893–1895)

Briere, J., & Conte, J. (1993). Self-reported amnesia for abuse in adults molested as children. *Journal of Traumatic Stress, 6,* 21–32.

Brown, D. P., & Fromm, E. (1986). *Hypnotherapy and hypnoanalysis.* Hillsdale, NJ: Erlbaum.

Cardeña, E., & Spiegel, D. (1993). Dissociative reactions to the Bay Area earthquake. *American Journal of Psychiatry, 150,* 474–478.

Carlson, E. B., & Rosser-Hogan, R. (1991). Trauma experiences, posttraumatic stress, dissociation, and depression in Cambodian refugees. *American Journal of Psychiatry, 148,* 1548–1551.

Charcot, J. M. (1887). *Leçons sur les maladies du système nerveux faites à la Salpêtrière* [*Lessons on the illnesses of the nervous system held at the Salpêtrière*] (Vol. 3). Paris: Progrès Médical en A. Delahaye & E. Lecrosnie.

Christianson, S.-A., & Nilsson, L.-G. (1984). Functional amnesia as induced by a psychological trauma. *Memory and Cognition, 12,* 142–155.

Christianson, S.-A., & Nilsson, L.-G. (1989). Hysterical amnesia: A case of aversively motivated isolation of memory. In T. Archer & L.-G. Nilsson (Eds.), *Aversion, avoidance and anxiety* (pp. 289–310). Hillsdale, NJ: Erlbaum.

Chu, J. A., & Dill, D. L. (1990). Dissociative symptoms in relation to childhood physical and sexual abuse. *American Journal of Psychiatry, 147,* 887– 892.

Coons, P. M., & Milstein, V. (1986). Psychosexual disturbances in multiple personality. *Journal of Clinical Psychiatry, 47,* 106–110.

Epstein, S. (1991). The self-concept, the traumatic neurosis, and the structure of personality. In D. Ozer, J. M. Healy, Jr., & A. J. Stewart (Eds.), *Perspectives in personality* (Vol. 3, Part A, pp. 63–98). London: Jessica Kingsley.

Erikson, E. H. (1963). *Childhood and society* (2nd ed.). New York: Norton.

Freud, S. (1955). Beyond the pleasure principle. In J. Strachey (Ed. and Trans.), *The standard edition of the complete psychological works of Sigmund Freud* (Vol. 18, pp. 3–64). London: Hogarth Press. (Original work published 1920)

Frischholz, E. J. (1985). The relationship among dissociation, hypnosis, and child abuse in the development of multiple personality disorder. In R. P. Kluft (Ed.), *Childhood antecedents of multiple personality* (pp. 99–126). Washington, DC: American Psychiatric Press.

Fromm, E. (1965). Hypnoanalysis: Theory and two case excerpts. *Psychotherapy: Theory, Research, and Practice, 2,* 127–133.

Gelinas, D. (1983). The persisting negative effects of incest. *Psychiatry, 46,* 312–332.

Harber, K. D., & Pennebaker, J. W. (1992). Overcoming traumatic memories. In S.-A. Christianson (Ed.), *The handbook of emotion and memory: Research and theory* (pp. 359–386). Hillsdale, NJ: Erlbaum.

Herman, J. L. (1992). *Trauma and recovery.* New York: Basic Books.

Herman, J. L., Perry, J. C., & van der Kolk, B. A. (1989). Childhood trauma in borderline personality disorder. *American Journal of Psychiatry, 146,* 490–495.

Hillman, R. G. (1981). The psychopathology of being held hostage. *American Journal of Psychiatry, 138,* 1193–1197.

Holen, A. (1993). The North Sea oil rig disaster. In J. P. Wilson & B. Raphael (Eds.), *International handbook of traumatic stress syndromes* (pp. 471–479). New York: Plenum Press.

Horowitz, M. J. (1986). *Stress response syndromes* (2nd. ed.). New York: Jason Aronson.

James, W. (1894). Book review of Janet's *Etat mentale des hystériques* and of J. Breuer & S. Freud's *Über den Psychischen Mechanismus Hysterischer Phänomene. Psychological Review, 1,* 195–199.

Janet, P. (1889). *L'automatisme psychologique.* Paris: Alcan.

Janet, P. (1898). *Névroses et idées fixes* (Vol. 1). Paris: Alcan.

Janet, P. (1904). L'amnésie et la dissociation des souvenirs par l'émotion [Amnesia and the dissociation of memories by emotions]. *Journal de Psychologie, 1*, 417–453.

Janet, P. (1909a). *Les névroses.* Paris: Flammarion.

Janet, P. (1909b). Problèmes psychologiques de l'emotion. *Revue Neurologique, 17*, 1551–1687.

Janet, P. (1925). *Psychological healing* (2 vols.). New York: Macmillan. (Original work published 1919)

Janet, P. (1932). *La force et la faiblesse psychologiques.* Paris: Maloine.

Janoff-Bulman, R. (1992). *Shattered assumptions: Towards a new psychology of trauma.* New York: Free Press.

Jung, C. G. (1921–1922). The question of the therapeutic value of abreaction. *British Journal of Medical Psychology, 2*, 13–22.

Kardiner, A. (1941). *The traumatic neuroses of war.* New York: Hoeber.

Kluft, R. P. (1987). An update on multiple personality disorder. *Hospital and Community Psychiatry, 38*(4), 363–373.

Kluft, R. P. (1991). Multiple personality disorder. In A. Tasman & A. Goldfinger (Eds.), *American Psychiatric Press review of psychiatry* (Vol. 10, pp. 161–188). Washington, DC: American Psychiatric Press.

Koopman, C., Classen, C., & Spiegel, D. (1994). Predictors of posttraumatic stress symptoms among survivors of the Oakland/Berkeley, California, firestorm. *American Journal of Psychiatry, 151*, 888–894.

Krystal, H. (1978). Trauma and affects. *Psychoanalytic Study of the Child, 33*, 81–116.

Krystal, J. H., Woods, S., Hill, C., & Charney, D. S. (1991). Characteristics of panic attack subtypes: Assessment of spontaneous panic, situational panic, sleep panic, and limited symptom attacks. *Comprehensive Psychiatry, 32*, 474–480.

Lazarus, R. S. (1966). *Psychological stress and the coping process.* New York: McGraw-Hill.

Loewenstein, R. J., & Putnam, F. W. (1990). The clinical phenomenology of males with multiple personality disorder. *Dissociation, 3*, 135–143.

MacMillan, M. (1990). Freud and Janet on organic and hysterical paralyses: A mystery solved? *International Review of Psychoanalysis, 17*, 189–203.

Marmar, C. R. (1991). Brief dynamic psychotherapy of post-traumatic stress disorder. *Psychiatric Annals, 21*, 405–414.

Marmar, C. R., Weiss, D. S., & Metzler, T. J. (in press-a). The Peritraumatic Dissociative Experiences Questionnaire. In J. P. Wilson & T. M. Keane (Eds.), *Assessing psychological trauma and PTSD: A practitioner's handbook.* New York: Guilford Press.

Marmar, C. R., Weiss, D. S., Metzler, T. J., & Delucchi, K. (in press-b). Characteristics of emergency services personnel related to peritraumatic dissociation during critical incident exposure. *American Journal of Psychiatry.*

Marmar, C. R., Weiss, D. S., Metzler, T. J., & Ronfeldt, H. M. (1994a). Predicting symptomatic distress in emergency services personnel. *Journal of Consulting and Clinical Psychology.*

Marmar, C. R., Weiss, D. S., Metzler, T. J., Ronfeldt, H. M., & Foreman, C. (1996). Stress response of emergency services personnel to the Loma Prieta earthquake Interstate 880 freeway collapse and control traumatic incidents. *Journal of Traumatic Stress, 9*, 63.

Marmar, C. R., Weiss, D. S., Schlenger, W. E., Fairbank, J. A., Jordan, K., Kulka, R. A., & Hough, R. L. (1994b). Peritraumatic dissociation and posttraumatic stress in male Vietnam theater veterans. *American Journal of Psychiatry, 151,* 902–907.

McDougall, W. (1926). *An outline of abnormal psychology.* London: Methuen.

McFarlane, A. C., Weber, D. L., & Clark, C. R. (1993). Abnormal stimulus processing in PTSD. *Biological Psychiatry, 34,* 311–320.

Melville, H. (1984). *Selections.* New York: Viking Press.

Moleman, N., van der Hart, O., & van der Kolk, B. A. (1992). The partus stress reaction: A neglected etiological factor in post-partum psychiatric disorders. *Journal of Nervous and Mental Disease, 180,* 271–272.

Myers, C. S. (1940). *Shell shock in France 1914–18.* Cambridge, England: Cambridge Unversity Press.

Nemiah, J. C. (1996). Early concepts of trauma, dissociation, and the unconscious: Their history and current implications. In J. D. Bremner & C. R. Marmar (Eds.), *Trauma, memory, and dissociation.* Washington, DC: American Psychiatric Press.

Nissen, M. J., Ross, J. L., Willingham, D. B., MacKenzie, T. B., & Schacter, D. L. (1988). Memory and awareness in a patient with multiple personality disorder. *Brain and Cognition, 8,* 117–134.

Noyes, R., Hoenck, P. R., & Kupperman, B. A. (1977). Depersonalization in accident victims and psychiatric patients. *Journal of Nervous and Mental Disease, 164,* 401–407.

Noyes, R., & Kletti, R. (1977). Depersonalization in response to life-threatening danger. *Comprehensive Psychiatry, 18,* 375–384.

Ogata, S. N., Silk, K. R., Goodrich, S., Lohr, N. E., Westen, D., & Hill, E. M. (1990). Childhood sexual and physical abuse in adult patients with borderline personality disorder. *American Journal of Psychiatry, 147,* 1008–1013.

Pearlman, K. W., & Saakvitne, L. A. (1995). *Trauma and the therapist.* New York: Norton.

Prince, M. (1911). *The dissociation of personality.* New York: Longmans, Green.

Putnam, F. W. (1985). Dissociation as a response to extreme trauma. In R. P. Kluft (Ed.), *Childhood antecedents of multiple personality* (pp. 65–97). Washington, DC: American Psychiatric Press.

Putnam, F. W. (1989). *Diagnosis and treatment of multiple personality disorder.* New York: Guilford Press.

Putnam, F. W., Guroff, J. J., Silberman, E. K., Barban, L., & Post, R. M. (1986). The clinical phenomenology of multiple personality disorder. *Journal of Clinical Psychiatry, 47,* 285–293.

Ross, C. A., Anderson, G., Fraser, G. A., Reagor, P., Bjornson, L., & Miller, S. D. (1992). Differentiating multiple personality disorder and dissociative disorder not otherwise specified. *Dissociation, 5,* 87–91.

Saxe, G. N., Chinman, G., Berkowitz, R., Hall, K., Lieberg, G., Schwartz, J., & van der Kolk, B. A. (1994). Somatization in patients with dissociative disorders. *American Journal of Psychiatry, 151,* 1329–1335.

Saxe, G. N., van der Kolk, B. A., Berkowitz, R., Chinman, G., Hall, K., Lieberg, G., & Schwartz, J. (1993). Dissociative disorders in psychiatric inpatients. *American Journal of Psychiatry, 150,* 1037–1042.

Shalev, A. P., Peri, T., Caneti, L., & Schreiber, S. (1996). Predictors of PTSD in injured trauma survivors: A prospective study. *American Journal of Psychiatry, 153,* 219–225.

Siegel, R. K. (1984). Hostage hallucinations. *Journal of Nervous and Mental Disease, 172,* 264–272.

Solomon, Z., Mikulincer, M., & Avitzur, E. (1988). Coping, locus of control, social support, and combat-related posttraumatic stress disorder: A prospective study. *Journal of Personality and Social Psychology, 55,* 279–285.

Southwick, S. M., Krystal, J. H., Morgan, C. A., Johnson, D., Nagy, L. M., Niculaou, A., Heninger, G. R., & Charney, D. S. (1993). Abnormal noradrenergic function in posttraumatic stress disorder. *Archives of General Psychiatry, 50,* 266–274.

Spiegel, D. (1984). Multiple personality disorder as a post-traumatic stress disorder. *Psychiatric Clinics of North America, 7,* 101–110.

Spiegel, D. (1993). Dissociation and trauma. In M. D. Lutherville (Ed.), *Dissociative disorders: A clinical review.* Baltimore: Sidran Press.

Spiegel, D., & Cardeña, E. (1991). Disintegrated experience: The dissociative disorders revisited. *Journal of Abnormal Psychology, 100,* 366–378.

Spiegel, D, Hunt, T., & Dondershine, H. E. (1988). Dissociation and hypnotizability in post traumatic stress disorder. *American Journal of Psychiatry, 145,* 301–305.

Steinberg, M., Rounsaville, B., & Cicchetti, D. V. (1990). The Structured Clinical Interview for DSM-III-R Dissociative Disorders: Preliminary report on a new diagnostic instrument. *American Journal of Psychiatry, 147,* 76–82.

Tichenor, V., Marmar, C. R., Weiss, D. S., Metzler, T. J., & Ronfeldt, H. M. (1994). *The relationship of peritraumatic dissociation and posttraumatic stress: Findings in female Vietnam theatre veterans.* Unpublished manuscript.

van der Hart, O. (1993). *Trauma, memory and dissociation* [In Dutch]. Lisse, The Netherlands: Swets & Zeitlinger.

van der Hart, O., & Brown, P. (1992). Abreaction re-evaluated. *Dissociation, 5*(4), 127–140.

van der Hart, O., Brown, P., & van der Kolk, B. A. (1989). Pierre Janet's treatment of post-traumatic stress. *Journal of Traumatic Stress, 2,* 356–380.

van der Hart, O., & Op den Velde, W. (1991). Traumatische herinneringen [Traumatic memories]. In O. van der Hart (Ed.), *Trauma, dissociatie en hypnose* [Trauma, dissociation, and hypnosis] (pp. 71–90). Lisse, The Netherlands: Swets & Zeitlinger.

van der Hart, O., & Spiegel, D. (1993). Hypnotic assessment and treatment of trauma-induced psychoses: The early psychotherapy of H. Breukink and modern views. *International Journal of Clinical and Experimental Hypnosis, 41,* 191–209.

van der Hart, O., Steele, K., Boon, S., & Brown, P. (1993). The treatment of traumatic memories: Synthesis, realization, and integration. *Dissociation, 6,* 162–180.

van der Hart, O., van der Kolk, B. A., & Boon, S. (1996). The treatment of dissociative disorders. In J. D. Bremner & C. R. Marmar (Eds.), *Trauma, memory and dissociation.* Washington, DC: American Psychiatric Press.

van der Kolk, B.A., & Ducey, C. (1989). The psychological processing of traumatic experience: Rorschach patterns in PTSD. *Journal of Traumatic Stress, 2*(3), 259–274.

van der Kolk, B.A., & Fisler, R. (1995). Dissociation and the fragmentary nature of traumatic memories: Review and experimental confirmation. *Journal of Traumatic Stress, 8,* 505–525.

van der Kolk, B. A., Hostetler, A., Herron, N., & Fisler, R. E. (1994). Trauma and the development of borderline personality disorder. *Psychiatric Clinics of North America, 17*(4), 715–730.

van der Kolk, B. A., Pelcovitz, D., Roth, S., Mandel, F., McFarlane, A. C., & Herman, J. L. (in press). Dissociation, affect dysregulation and somatization: The complexity of adaptation to trauma. *American Journal of Psychiatry.*

van der Kolk, B. A., Perry, C., & Herman, J. L. (1991). Childhood origins of self-destructive behavior. *American Journal of Psychiatry, 148,* 1665–1671.

van der Kolk, B. A., & van der Hart, O. (1989). Pierre Janet and the breakdown of adaptation in psychological trauma. *American Journal of Psychiatry, 146,* 1530–1540.

van der Kolk, B. A., & van der Hart, O. (1991). The intrusive past: The flexibility of memory and the engraving of trauma. *American Imago, 48,* 425–454.

van der Kolk, B. A., van der Hart, O., & Brown, P. (1989). Pierre Janet and psychological trauma: The centenary of the publication of *L'automatisme psychologique. Journal of Traumatic Stress, 2*(4), 365–378.

Weiss, D. W., Marmar, C. R., Metzler, T. J., & Ronfeldt, H. M. (1995). Predicting symptomatic distress in emergency services personnel. *Journal of Consulting and Clinical Psychology, 63,* 361–368.

Wilkinson, C. B. (1983). Aftermath of a disaster: The collapse of the Hyatt Regency Hotel skywalks. *American Journal of Psychiatry, 140,* 1134–1139.

Wolfe, J., Keane, T. M., & Kaloupek, D. G. (1993). Patterns of positive readjustment in Vietnam combat veterans. *Journal of Traumatic Stress, 6,* 179–193.

DEVELOPMENTAL, SOCIAL, AND CULTURAL ISSUES

Traumatic Stress in Childhood and Adolescence

Recent Developments and Current Controversies

ROBERT S. PYNOOS
ALAN M. STEINBERG
ARMEN GOENJIAN

The past two decades have produced increased knowledge about the reactions of children and adolescents exposed to traumatic stress. Research from around the world has encompassed studies of children exposed to intrafamilial, interpersonal, and community violence; political violence; natural and human-made disasters; serious accidents; and life-threatening medical illnesses. This chapter reviews the evolution of this field of research, and highlights important recent developments and selected areas of current interest and controversy.

Over the past decade, there has been increasing awareness of the extent to which children are exposed to and are victims of intrafamilial violence. Recently, the significant risk of exposure of young children to community violence within the United States has also been documented. There is enhanced appreciation of the extent to which children are exposed to terrorism, war, atrocities against civilians, ethnic or religious violence, and political oppression and torture. Whereas the morbidity and mortality rates associated with natural disasters are decreasing in the more industrialized countries, in developing countries death, injury, and destruction are often widespread, with large numbers of affected child survivors (Weisaeth, 1993).

As we have come to appreciate more fully the extent to which children are exposed to traumatic situations, the severity of their subsequent acute distress, and the potential serious long-term psychiatric sequelae, there is an urgent need to embed both research and clinical practice within a sound developmental framework. This framework recognizes the fundamental interrelationship of trauma and development. It applies to the whole spectrum of child and adolescent traumatic stress, including the risk of exposure; the subjective experience of traumatic situations; the nature of, and response to, acute distress; the construction and evolution of traumatic memory and narrative; the neurobiology of traumatic stress; the nature, severity, and course of trauma-related psychopathology; the influence of child intrinsic factors on resistance, resilience, and adjustment; the mediation of traumatic stress through parental function, peer relationships, and school milieu; and strategies of prevention and intervention.

From the earliest account of an adolescent's experience of a catastrophic disaster, the eruption of Mount Vesuvius, in the *Letters* of Pliny the Younger (100–113 A.D./1931); through the autobiographical description of intrafamilial abuse and societal violence provided by Maxim Gorky in *My Childhood* (1913/1965); to the powerful literary rendering of the Holocaust by Elie Wiesel in *Night* (1958/1960) and the trenchant autobiographical account of childhood rape by Maya Angelou in *I Know Why the Caged Bird Sings* (1969), authors have reflected on the formative influences of traumatic experiences in childhood. Indeed, it is a common assumption that personal creativity and character are often born out of early tragedy. We have reached a point in childhood traumatic stress studies at which, by incorporating new knowledge and methodology from the rapidly expanding field of developmental psychology, we can begin to enrich our understanding of the developmental impact of traumatic stress—including its effects on the acquisition of developmental competencies, the achievement of developmental transitions, moral development, and emerging personality.

We would propose that the critical link between traumatic stress and personality is the formation of trauma-related expectations as these are expressed in the thoughts, emotions, behaviors, and biology of the developing child. By their very nature and degree of personal impact, traumatic experiences can skew expectations about the world, the safety and security of interpersonal life, and the child's sense of personal integrity. These expectancies, as Bowlby (1973) noted, contribute to the child's inner plans of the world, shape concepts of self and others, and lead to forecasts about the future that can have a profound influence on current and future behavior. Outcome measures of childhood traumatic stress to date have been narrowly restricted to symptoms of posttraumatic stress disorder (PTSD). More recently, other comorbid psychiatric conditions, including depression and separation anxiety disorder, have been assessed (Goenjian et al., 1995). The concept of traumatic expectations implies that outcome considerations must also include proximal and distal developmental disturbances, changes in life trajectory, risks to later physical health, and vulnerability to future life stresses.

OVERVIEW OF THE FIELD

Progress in childhood traumatic stress studies has accelerated over the past decade. Studies of children and adolescents have benefited from numerous scientific advances in the understanding of traumatic stress in adulthood. At the same time, the enriched knowledge of childhood trauma is contributing to an increased understanding of the interplay of child and adult trauma, including how the reverberations of childhood trauma may compromise adult functioning (particularly recovery after traumatic stress in adulthood).

The field of childhood traumatic stress studies has itself passed through several stages of development. Its infancy was characterized by efforts to develop psychologically and clinically sound approaches to interviewing children exposed to traumatic situations. These early clinical descriptive studies had to overcome the scientific and social reluctance to engage children directly. They assembled the first collective evidence about the heightened level of children's mental activity during and after traumatic exposure, the complexity of their traumatic experiences, and the seriousness of their resultant distress. At the same time, they helped to bring attention to children who witnessed extreme violence, including parental suicide, parental homicide, and rape. Alongside these studies, social questions began to emerge about the reliability of children's eyewitness accounts and suggestibility, which in turn have spurred increased efforts to understand the processes of memory, learning, and the co-construction of traumatic narrative among young children.

In the second stage, researchers began to organize the complex phenomenology of children's distress under the emerging rubric of "PTSD" and to describe more precisely how these symptoms are manifested in children and adolescents. These efforts required the construction of valid and reliable means of assessment. The assessment of specific PTSD-related reactions superseded the previous use of general measures of global anxiety. These interview techniques and structured and self-report instruments then became available for use in more systematic community and population-based studies. These latter studies advanced the scientific methodology in child trauma research, introducing the use of a "dose of exposure" model. This model allowed for more rigorous investigation of factors that predict or mediate the severity and course of posttrauma reactions among children and adolescents.

These studies have documented the following: (1) Children experience the full range of posttraumatic stress symptoms; (2) level of exposure is strongly associated with severity and course of posttraumatic stress reactions; (3) grief, posttraumatic stress, depressive, and separation anxiety reactions are independent of but interrelated with one another; and (4) positive correlations are to be expected between parent and child distress in response to shared traumatic experiences. Important specific findings also began to emerge, including the formation of incident-specific new fears (Dollinger, O'Donnell, & Staley, 1984); the importance of guilt and exaggerated startle reactions as risk factors for increased severity and chronicity of PTSD (Pynoos et al., 1993a); and the isolation of specific symptoms (e.g., persistent sleep disturbance) that are associated with adverse outcomes (e.g., interference with learning) (Pynoos et al., 1987). The use of continuous scales rather than categorical diagnostic classifications for evaluating posttraumatic stress and depressive reactions may provide better information for risk assessment, stratification of interventions, and monitoring course of recovery (Pynoos et al., 1993a).

A third stage of research has emerged, which encompasses three broad areas. The first focuses on more in-depth examination of etiological and mediating factors suggested by findings from the earlier cohort studies. For example, some studies have more clearly delineated specific objective and subjective features of traumatic experiences associated with risk for PTSD and other reactions (Yule, 1993; Freedy, Kilpatrick, & Resnick, 1993; Berkovitz, Wang, Pynoos, James, & Wong, 1994). Others have more closely examined the role of parental symptoms and responsiveness—for example, the relationship of maternal trauma-related avoidance and increased child posttraumatic distress (Bat-Zion & Levy-Shiff, 1993; Stuber, Nader, Yasuda, Pynoos, & Cohen, 1991).

A second area has expanded the scope of research and clinical attention beyond a singular focus on PTSD. These foci include (1) the role of traumatic reminders and secondary adversities; (2) comorbid conditions; (3) specific developmental consequences; (4) the impact on emerging personality and moral development; (5) serial or repeated traumatic experiences; (6) the interplay of traumatic experiences within a background of neglect or abuse and parental psychopathology; (7) the role of child intrinsic factors, such as temperament, intelligence, or prior successful coping; and (8) the link of PTSD and second-ary disorders to specific familial predispositions. A third area encompasses preliminary investigations of biological alterations associated with posttraumatic stress symptoms in children and adolescents. These studies are beginning to examine alterations in peripheral autonomic functioning (Perry, 1994); in the modulation of neurophysiological functioning—for example, the startle reflex (Ornitz & Pynoos, 1989); and in baseline levels and responsiveness of stress hormones (De Bellis et al., 1994; Goenjian et al., in press). Biological studies in children require careful attention to the maturation of biological systems under investigation and to the potential for interference with normal physiological development.

The accumulated knowledge from around the world has paved the way for implementing rigorous public mental health intervention programs for children exposed to violence, disaster, and traumatic bereavement. We have seen initial utilization of these new approaches in the UNICEF Psychosocial

Program (Kuterovac, Dyregrov, & Stuvland, 1994; Stuvland, 1993) instituted throughout the former Yugoslavia even as the war there continues, and in the Armenian Relief Society's Psychiatric Outreach Program after the 1988 earthquake in Armenia (Goenjian, 1993). These newer approaches include systematic school-based screening of children for degree of exposure and presence of posttrauma reactions, in conjunction with provision of acute psychological assistance. The screening information is used to define at-risk populations, to guide case-finding and outreach efforts, to plan the timing of interventions with different at-risk groups, and to select appropriate treatment techniques. Periodic additional screening (which incorporates further assessments of traumatic reminders and secondary stresses faced by children and their families) monitors the course of recovery, permits prompt recognition of exacerbations resulting from unanticipated occurrences or intercurrent traumas or adversities, and permits evaluation of the efficacy of interventions.

These programs include the use of individual, group, family, classroom, and community interventions. They involve the selective and integrated use of the following therapeutic modalities:

1. Psychoeducational approaches
2. Social skills training
3. Psychodynamic therapy
4. Cognitive-behavioral therapy
5. Pharmacological therapies
6. Educational assistance
7. Remedial interventions to address developmental disturbances

At the same time, we are seeing more efforts to design and implement preventive interventions aimed at reducing rates of exposure; risk of acute psychiatric morbidity after exposure; incidence of comorbid conditions; interference with normal developmental progression, academic performance, and family functioning; and the onset of behavioral and conduct disturbances associated independently with additional risks. In the United States, representative programs include the Yale Child Study Center's Program on Child Development and Community Policing (Marans & Cohen, 1993) and the Charles Drew University Center for the Study of Violence and Social Change–UCLA Trauma Psychiatry Program. The former has trained community-based police officers in traumatic stress and child development, in order to increase responsiveness to children exposed to violence, to minimize this exposure, and to facilitate prompt psychological intervention and referral. The latter program is systematically screening at-risk elementary school children, both for behavioral and academic disturbances and for their exposures to intra- and extrafamilial violence, traumatic injury, and loss. This program provides a three-stage school-based intervention, utilizing individual therapy, group therapy, and mentorship components. In Great Britain, a team of clinicians and researchers has implemented a nationwide prevention–intervention program for children exposed to family homicide (Hendriks, Black, & Kaplan, 1993).

These types of programs will usher in a new era of much-needed prevention–intervention outcome research. Findings from this stage of clinical research will have important public health and mental health implications, as this new knowledge is employed to promote more effective public policy and utilization of societal resources. For example, our increasing clinical knowledge about adolescents exposed to violence is stimulating a rethinking of approaches to violence prevention. There is a movement away from a primary reliance on educational approaches to conflict resolution, and toward more therapeutically oriented prevention–intervention strategies that address past and present exposures to violence among adolescents, as well as the developmental impact of these exposures.

A DEVELOPMENTAL APPROACH TO CLINICAL ASSESSMENT AND TREATMENT

We have recently formulated a developmental conceptual model of traumatic stress in childhood, to characterize the complex interactions of child development with traumatic stress and its sequelae (Pynoos, 1993; Pynoos, Steinberg, & Wraith, 1995). Such a model has direct implications for the systematic clinical evaluation and treatment of traumatized children. The evaluation should address the tripartite etiology of distress by rigorously characterizing three interdependent factors: the traumatic experience(s), traumatic reminders, and secondary adversities. Each evaluation should include (1) a clear delineation of the objective features and a thorough description of the child's subjective experience of the traumatic episode(s); (2) a determination of the type and frequency of traumatic reminders (both external and internal cues) and their anticipated future occurrence; and (3) a detailed accounting of current and potential secondary stresses and adversities.

In the past, it has been common for clinicians and researchers alike to use broad categories in classifying a child's traumatic experience. A modern approach includes more precise delineation of the specific objective features of traumatic experiences associated with severer posttraumatic reactions. These include the following:

1. Exposure to direct life threat
2. Injury to self, including extent of physical pain
3. Witnessing of mutilating injury or grotesque death (especially to family members or friends)
4. Perpetrating violent acts against others

5. Hearing unanswered screams for help and cries of distress; smelling noxious odors
6. Being trapped or without assistance
7. Proximity to violent threat
8. Unexpectedness and duration of the experience(s)
9. Extent of violent force and the use of a weapon or injurious object
10. Number and nature of threats during a violent episode
11. Witnessing of atrocities
12. The relationship to the assailant and other victims
13. Use of physical coercion
14. Violation of the physical integrity of the child
15. Degree of brutality and malevolence

All of these factors are strongly associated with the onset and persistence of PTSD in children and adolescents (Gleser, Green, & Winget, 1981; Pynoos et al., 1993a; Yule & Williams, 1990; Pynoos, Sorenson, & Steinberg, 1993b). Exposure to photographs or media presentations of atrocities or the mutilated corpse of a family member or friend constitutes an important secondary source of risk (Nader, Pynoos, Fairbanks, Al-Ajeel, & Asfour, 1993).

Recent studies have begun to examine the contribution of children's subjective perception of threat to severity of posttraumatic distress (Yule, Bolton, & Udwin, 1992; Schwartz & Kowalski, 1991). In our most recent studies (Berkovitz et al., 1994) of children after the 1994 Northridge earthquake in Los Angeles, we found that in addition to objective features such as being trapped or injured, specific subjective experiences during the earthquake—including fear of dying, feeling one's heart beating fast, and feeling very upset about how one acted during the earthquake—were each highly predictive of overall severity of PTSD symptoms at 5 months. Guilt over acts of omission or commission perceived to have endangered others has also been found to predict distress (Pynoos et al., 1987, 1993a; Yule & Williams, 1990). The generation of other negative emotions (e.g., shame and rage) can have a similar impact (Lansky, 1992).

In the following subsections, we discuss the three elements of our model of traumatic stress—the traumatic experience(s), traumatic reminders, and secondary adversities—in greater detail.

A Developmental Analysis of Traumatic Experiences in Childhood

The most recent definitions of a traumatic experience by the American Psychiatric Association (1994) and the World Health Organization (1992) represent improvements over earlier formulations in providing specific subjective and objective criteria. However, the definitions lack reference to developmental considerations. A sophisticated developmental analysis of traumatic experiences is needed for both research and clinical purposes. Although Freud's original formulation of childhood trauma as a breaching of a stimulus barrier is often considered to be representative of his view, he outlined a more intricate developmental definition in "Inhibitions, Symptoms and Anxiety" (1926/1959). There he defined a traumatic situation as one where "external and internal, real and instinctual dangers *converge*" (p. 168; emphasis added). In traumatic situations, the experience of external threat involves an estimation of the extreme magnitude of the threat, the unavailability or ineffectiveness of contemplated or actual protective actions by self or others, and the experience of physical helplessness at irreversible traumatic moments. The experience of internal threat includes a sense of inability to tolerate the affective responses and physiological reactions, as well as a sense of catastrophic personal consequence. The latter includes both dire external and psychodynamic threats.

The experience of external and internal threats is influenced by subjective appraisals and the adequacy of efforts to address the situation and manage the internal responses. These appraisals and efforts at coping vary with the developmental and experiential maturation of the child, especially in regard to the degree of reliance on parents, adult caretakers, siblings, and peers. The internal responses include not only the autonomic or affective reactions, but also the emerging attribution of symbolic meaning and psychosexual interpretation. As Rosenblatt and Thickstun (1977) have noted, the autonomic arousal, which often continues beyond the direct perception of threat, may itself be appraised as a sign of danger; it may thus maintain traumatic expectations, as well as "emergency emotions" (Rado, 1942) and behavior.

Empirical studies of acutely traumatized school-age children and adolescents have increased clinical awareness of the complexity of their traumatic experiences (Pynoos, in press). First, one must understand the context in the child's life that contributes to the acute affective state, cognitive preoccupations, and developmental concerns at the onset of the traumatic stress. Second, a traumatic experience involves intense moment-to-moment perceptual, kinesthetic, and somatic experiences, accompanied by appraisals of external and internal threats. The child is challenged by the intensity and duration of the physiological arousal, affective responses, and psychodynamic threats, while at the same time making continuous efforts to address the situation in behavior, thought, and fantasy, and to manage physiological and emotional reactions.

Third, the vantage point of concern or attention in the child may vary. Children may have their attention drawn away from (or suppress fear for) their own safety when there is imminent danger (or actual injury) to a parent, sibling, or friend, and may experience unalleviated empathic distress (Hoffman, 1979). Alternatively, when there is immediate threat or injury to a child, he or she may experience a moment of unconcern about or even estrangement from other family members who may also be under threat. Adolescents may acutely experience an "existential dilemma" over the conflict of intervening on behalf of others or taking self-protective action. When injury to themselves or other occurs, children may become suddenly preoccupied with concerns about the severity of injury, rescue, and repair. In violent circumstances children may also feel compelled to inhibit wishes to intervene, or to suppress retaliatory impulses, out of fear of provoking counterretaliatory behavior.

Fourth, a more radical change in the child's attention and concerns occurs when his or her physical integrity or autonomy begins to be compromised: The child's attention is then directed more toward fears and fantasies of the nature and extent of psychic and physical harm than toward intervention. The child may try to use self-protective mechanisms to meet the internal threats, including "dissociative responses" that allow the child to feel a physical distancing from what is happening, to feel it is not happening to him or her, to obliterate painful sensations, to control autonomic arousal and anxiety, to protect certain ego functions, and to decrease any sense of active participation (Rose, 1991). During incestuous violation or hostage situations, there may be attempts either to disclaim or to invoke affiliative needs and desires as a means of warding off any sense of active participation or mitigating awareness of the physical menace, psychological abasement, and the accompanying distress (Bernstein, 1990; Strenz, 1982).

Fifth, traumatic stress may include additional traumatic moments that occur after cessation of violence or threat, including staying by an injured or dead family member until help arrives; trying to stop bleeding or giving resuscitation; the arrival and activities of the police or paramedics; and subsequent emergency room care or surgery, and/or waiting for information about the condition of a family member or friend.

Sixth, a traumatic experience is often multilayered. Worry about the safety of a family member or friend, whether in the next room or at a different location, adds an additional source of extreme stress. The danger may also remind a child of a previous situation, renewing prior fears and anxieties that influence the immediate appraisal of threat and exacerbate physiological and psychological responses. Witnessing the death of an attachment figure or peer evokes concurrent acute reactions to the loss, even while the life threat continues.

In addition to underestimating the complexity of children's traumatic experiences, the salient developmental impact is often overlooked in our attention to posttraumatic stress reactions. Commonly, the experience involves a specific failure in evolving developmentally related expectations associated with efforts to appraise and address external dangers. These may include (1) the failure of alarm reactions (Krystal, 1991), social referencing (Emde, 1991), or a protective shield; (2) the inability to resist coercive violation (Murray, 1938); (3) the betrayal of basic affiliative assumptions; (4) the failure of emerging catastrophic emotions to protect against harm (Rangell, 1991); (5) the disruption of a belief in a socially modulated world; and (6) the sense of resignation in having to surrender to an unavoidable moment of danger (Krystal, 1991).

Traumatic Reminders

Traumatic reminders are embedded in the external and internal cues specific to the child's traumatic experience. The frequency of traumatic reminders is dependent both on the nature of the traumatic experience and on the posttrauma environmental circumstances. The role of traumatic reminders is insufficiently appreciated: They contribute to the phasic nature of posttraumatic stress reactions; the appearance of behavioral changes; and, over time, the increased risk of heightened neurophysiological reactivity and slower neurophysiological recovery after arousal. Unanticipated reminders can revoke a sense of unpreparedness that exacerbates fears of recurrence. The treatment of reactivity to traumatic reminders requires identifying the reminders, increasing the child's understanding of the traumatic reference, providing assistance with cognitive discriminations, increasing the child's internal tolerance for expectable reactivity, and utilizing strategies to promote the child's ability to recover after reminders.

The socioenvironmental interventions are threefold. One addresses reducing the impact of traumatic reminders by enhancing a parent's, teacher's, or caretaker's appreciation of the role of traumatic reminders; promoting appropriate communication over the anticipation or occurrence of such reminders; and providing extra assistance to reduce both the intensity and duration of reactivity. The second is to institute appropriate environmental interventions to reduce the frequency of traumatic reminders and to reduce unnecessary reexposures, including graphic depictions. A third is to provide assistance and support to parents, in order to reduce their own reactivity and unnecessary exposures. Parents' reactive behavior to reminders may accentuate children's anxieties and interfere with parenting. In our research after the 1994 Northridge earthquake (Berkovitz et al., 1994), we found that current reactivity to reminders and inability to calm down after reminders were highly predictive of chronic PTSD.

Secondary Adversities

Traumatic situations are frequently associated with both acute and long-term adversities and secondary stresses. These may include medical, surgical, and rehabilitative treatment for acute injuries and subsequent disabilities; relocation, immigration, and resettlement; change in caretaking; change in family finances; alterations in role performance or school performance due to posttraumatic stress reactions; the stress of responding to questions from peers and others; and stigmatization (Pynoos et al., 1993). In both research and clinical settings, there has been inadequate differentiation of the effects of the traumatic experience itself from those related to secondary stresses. Secondary stresses (1) increase the risk of comorbidity; (2) complicate efforts at adjustment; (3) initiate maladaptive coping; and (4) interfere with the availability of social support, family functioning, and reintegration with peers. Secondary adversities for the family are often filtered through compromised parental function to the child.

Therapeutic attention to secondary adversities includes assisting the child in identifying the sources of secondary stresses, addressing the resulting internal emotional conflicts, and enhancing coping skills. Socioenvironmental interventions to minimize adversities and secondary stresses often require a child advocate role.

TRAUMA-RELATED PSYCHOPATHOLOGY

The study of trauma-related psychopathology in children and adolescents is entering a new stage. Efforts continue to refine the measurement of PTSD in children and to develop supplemental observational protocols for use with preschool children and infants. The most recent trend has been to include assessment of symptoms from a wider spectrum of diagnoses and to examine their differential etiologies and interactions. These have included depression, separation anxiety, and complicated grief. Other important areas under investigation include the posttrauma onset of attention-deficit/hyperactivity disorders, phobias, conduct disorders, and substance abuse.

One significant problem in much of the child literature has been a failure to differentiate between posttraumatic stress symptoms and grief reactions, and to consider their interactions. In many of our studies in children and adolescents (Pynoos, 1992; Goenjian et al., 1995), we have found evidence for both complicated grief and bereavement-related depression, as recently described in adults (Prigerson et al., 1995). We have also consistently observed how PTSD complicates the grieving process by repeatedly directing attention to the traumatic circumstances of the death and the surrounding issues (Pynoos, 1992). In doing so, it interferes with efforts to address the loss and to adapt to subsequent life changes.

Our recent findings from an ongoing longitudinal study of children and adolescents in Armenia after the 1988 earthquake (Goenjian et al., 1995) indicate an interactive relationship among PTSD symptoms, depressive symptoms, and separation anxiety disorder. The distress caused by severe and persistent PTSD symptoms exacerbated symptoms of anxious attachment, including increased clinging in an effort to obtain comfort from their caretakers. Fear of recurrence increased children's anxiety about their own and family members' safety, increasing the need for proximity. Conversely, separation anxiety aggravated some PTSD symptoms, particularly arousal symptoms.

Severe and chronic PTSD was found to be a risk factor for the onset of secondary depression. Our findings suggest that this risk arises from two independent sources. As McFarlane (1995) has proposed, the persistence of PTSD symptoms may itself become a primary source of ongoing distress and demoralization for a child and family. The persistence of PTSD symptoms also appears to compromise a child's ability to cope with posttrauma adversities. Independently, the accumulation of secondary adversities places the child at additional risk for depression. In turn, depression can interfere with the resolution of posttraumatic stress symptoms. PTSD, depressive disorder, loss, and secondary adversity constitute a pernicious interactive matrix that strongly influences the adaptation and recovery of children, adolescents, and their families.

PROXIMAL DEVELOPMENTAL DISTURBANCES

Studies of traumatic stress in children have generally been bereft of adequate assessments of resultant developmental disturbances. The assessment should include attention both to the achievement of proximal and distal developmental competencies and to the passage through critical developmental transitions. When equal attention is given to these development risks and to psychopathology, their interactions can be better ascertained, monitored, and addressed. Figure 14.1 outlines key areas of proximal development and stress-related psychopathology.

Advances in child developmental psychology are providing more refined tools to evaluate the impact of traumatic stress on developmental competencies. For example, in recent years, research has elucidated the normal developmental achievement of narrative coherence (i.e., children's ability to organize narrative material into a beginning, middle, and end). Current research among preschool children exposed to both intrafamilial and community violence has indicated interference with this task, resulting in more chaotic narrative construction (Osofsky, 1993). Achievement of this developmental task is essential to subsequent competencies in reading, writing, and communications skills. The use of an incoherent narrative style may interfere with processing subsequent traumatic experiences and may be misconstrued as a dissociative phenomenon.

Developmental studies of the generation of intense negative emotions indicate ways in which childhood traumatic experiences may challenge maturing mechanisms of emotional regulation (Parens, 1991). Fear of affective intensity may interfere with the preschool task of increasing differentiation of

Proximal development

Proximal stress-related psychopathology

Selective attention/cognition/learning
Generation of intense negative emotions
Self-attributions
Autonomous strivings
Perception of self-efficacy
Specific psychodynamic/psychosocial/narcissistic concerns
Impulse control
Moral development
Awareness/sense of historical continuity
Representation of self and others
Biological maturation
Interpersonal and intrafamilial transitions
Ontogenesis of competencies

↔

PTSD
Depression
Phobia
New-onset attention-deficit/hyperactivity disorder
Other anxiety disorders
Sleep disorder
Somatization disorder
Disorders of attachment
Conduct disorder
Dissociative reactions
Eating disturbances
Substance abuse

Figure 14.1. The interaction of proximal stress-related psychopathology with proximal development.

affective states, with school-age children's development of the capacity to elaborate on their affective expression, and with adolescents' efforts to achieve a more sophisticated understanding of the origin and consequences of negative emotions. The achievement of mature emotional regulation rests on the successive acquisition of these skills. Developmentally appropriate emotional regulation is critical to family, peer, and school functioning.

Traumatic experiences can retard or accelerate critical developmental transitions. For example, in child–parent relationships, they can upset the developmental balance between independent and dependent behavior. The mutual sense of a disrupted protective shield may alter a young child's reliance on parental efficacy and assurances of safety or security, and parents' confidence in their own ability to protect their child. A school-age child may increase attachment behaviors because of worries about the safety of family members and self; this can jeopardize the transition to more peer involvement, add frustration to the parent–child relationship, and create embarrassment and shame for the child. Accelerated autonomous strivings may lead to adventuresome pursuits that lie beyond a preadolescent's or early adolescent's developmental capabilities. At the same time, posttraumatic-stress-related estrangement may deter a midadolescent from seeking the counsel of parents at a critical juncture of decision making or risk taking. In late adolescence, there may be either a rapid thrust toward self-sufficiency or, out of concern for other family members' safety and security, postponement of plans to leave home.

Transitions in peer relationships may also be adversely affected. The preschool tasks of cooperation and sharing in relationship to other children may be interfered with by withdrawal, emotional constriction, and disrupted impulse control. Traumatic play may limit the flexibility of play for other developmental purposes, and, for example, disturb preschool coordinated fantasy play (Parker & Gottman, 1989). Posttraumatic symptoms or behavior, or a physical deformity or scar, may acutely disturb a developing close relationship with a best friend, create a sense of isolation from peers, or lead to social ostracism. Reenactment behavior, especially inappropriate sexual or aggressive behavior, may lead to a child's being labeled "deviant" by parents, teachers, and other children. Peer rejection carries important independent risks of secondary developmental consequences and additional psychopathology (Howes, 1987; Rubin, LeMare, & Lollis, 1990). There may be abrupt shifts in an adolescent's interpersonal attachments, including sudden dissolution or heightened attachment, increased identification with a peer group as a protective shield, and involvement in aberrant rather than mainstream relationships (Pynoos & Nader, 1993).

Clinical experience suggests that as children mature, they become increasingly able to envision and appreciate the developmental impact of the traumatic incursions into their lives. Often, during an initial consultation, discussing the developmental impact may be more personally relevant to the adolescent than a review and psychoeducational normalization of symptoms may be. For example, an adolescent soldier from Bosnia, injured and disabled, movingly described to one of us his shattered plans to be the first person from his family to go to college and to pursue his talent in soccer.

Intervention strategies needed to address proximal developmental disturbances differ from those employed in the clinical assessment and treatment of PTSD. For example, we have studied two cases of children who experienced a serious difficulty in learning to read after witnessing a parent's violent death. Therapeutic attention to the trauma-related disturbances in visual information processing needed to be supplemented with remedial educational assistance. Prevention of the secondary repercussion of academic failure, with attendant loss of self-esteem and disturbances in peer relations, reduced the risk of other subsequent developmental disturbances and psychopathology.

After a disaster to which a significant portion of the children within a school have had severe levels of exposure, there may be a measurable decline in academic achievement (Tsui, Dagwell, & Yule, in press). The use of a graduated curriculum to assist the most affected children may be essential during their recovery from posttraumatic and grief reactions. The marginal students may be at greatest academic risk (Yule, 1991), with school failure leading to a significant decrease in self-esteem and increased risk of secondary psychiatric morbidity (Saigh, 1991).

THE REIFICATION OF PTSD AND CHILD DEVELOPMENT

As the reliability and validity of the diagnosis of PTSD in children and adolescents have become better established, the concept of PTSD is becoming reified. The diagnosis is being construed as a type of Platonic form; as a result, the intimate relationship of these symptoms to the particular and complex experience of an individual child is in danger of being lost. For example, we tend to speak of intrusive images as if they are merely reproductions of original photographic negatives of a gruesome scene. In doing so, we risk missing the experiential and clinical significance of these "pictures in the child's mind." Rather, intrusive images constitute memory markers that often capture moments of traumatic helplessness, terror, horror, and utter ineffectiveness— for example, at the occurrence of an irreversible violent injury to a parent. Of special importance is the fact that these memory markers may also indicate "injury" to a developmental expectation (e.g., in young children, of a protective shield) that may have serious developmental consequences.

Traumatic moments, captured in the traumatic imagery, elicit unconscious and conscious fantasies that incorporate wishes for protective intervention. These intervention fantasies are shaped by the child's developmental stage and unique prior experience. Reminders of traumatic moments may selectively reelicit traumatic images, which in turn may be accompanied by renewed traumatic expectations (e.g., of violent escalation or failure of a developmental expectation. These expectations may then have immediate or delayed behavioral expression, influencing both child–parent interactions and peer relationships. Above all, traumatic imagery represents an activity of the child's mind, and incorporates intriguing and subtle modifications over time.

RECENT TRENDS IN CHILDHOOD TRAUMATIC STRESS STUDIES

The most recent trend in childhood traumatic stress studies is to integrate information about various forms of childhood trauma that previously had been pursued in independent lines of inquiry. This trend has been prompted by increased recognition that (1) children exposed to various types of traumatic situations manifest similar PTSD-type reactions; (2) within the same environment, children may be at risk of exposure to a cluster of associated or independent traumas; and (3) over time, children may experience multiple traumatic exposures of different types. The resulting conceptual framework is supplanting earlier ones that typically referred to acute, cumulative strain (Khan, 1963) and to chronic traumatic circumstances, including reference to Type I and Type II traumas (Terr, 1991). As a result of this synthesis of information, methodologies, and intervention techniques, a more complete approach to the assessment and treatment of traumatized children will be available.

Information about acute posttraumatic stress reactions to a single, isolated violent event (e.g., a sniper attack) is being complemented with appreciation of the developmental consequences of living in environments of chronic danger. Discussions of children living in chronic danger must not fail to take into account the immediate and serious nature of a child's posttraumatic stress reactions to an acute violent experience—for example, the responses of a child witness to the murder of an ice cream truck driver, who, in the throes of death, fell upon the child. However, clinicians must also avoid a myopic focus on posttraumatic stress reactions, which would neglect the implications for this child's developing sense of a social contract of her recognizing this unprosecuted killing as part of a pattern of gang-related shootings within her community.

There is also increased awareness of the complicated interactions over time of extrafamilial and intrafamilial trauma (Bell & Jenkins, 1993; Cicchetti & Carlson, 1989; Garbarino, Kostelny, & Dubrow, 1991; Macksoud, Dyregrov, & Raundalen, 1993; Richters & Martinez, 1993). For example, recent disaster studies have documented increases in domestic violence, child abuse, and delinquency during the postdisaster period (Goenjian, 1993). The increased availability of firearms, in part due to concerns over crime, is associated with more gun-related suicides and accidental injuries in the home. Whereas in the past children more often discovered family members after suicide attempts involving drug overdoses, the UCLA Trauma Psychiatry Program is now treating more children who discovered family members after fatal self-inflicted gunshot wounds. In consultations in regions of war, we have also noted cases in which soldiers returning home from war, often traumatized or depressed, have used military weapons to commit suicide, and the aftermath has been witnessed by their children.

Studies of intrafamilial violence are recognizing that there is often a clustering of traumatic exposures. For example, we are beginning to appreciate how in situations of child abuse, additional exposures to spousal abuse and/ or to parental suicidal and homicidal behavior (at different points in the child's life) may influence the form and content of subsequent developmental disturbances. These studies are beginning to elucidate varying ways in which a child's emerging affiliative assumptions are challenged or undermined, along with the developmental consequences.

There should also be an integration of knowledge of childhood traumatic stress with that derived from related fields. Studies of child rearing among parents with identifiable psychopathology (e.g., mood disorders or borderline personality disorder) have often overlooked traumatogenic individual child experiences (e.g., finding an unconscious or injured parent after a suicide attempt) and their psychiatric and developmental sequelae. Conversely, as a child recovers from acute posttraumatic stress reactions after a violent attempted murder–suicide by a manic–depressive father, the child may be challenged by an increased awareness of his or her intersubjective experience of the parent's psychopathology, especially failures to recognize the child's personal boundaries.

A developmental perspective contributes to a more complete characterization of traumatic stress by including consideration of the changing developmental context, even within a particular type of traumatic stress. For example, the nature and circumstances of repeated physical or sexual abuse or witnessing of violence necessarily change over time, as both the child and the circumstances develop. A parent's expressed reason or threat; the child's attribution of meaning; and the content of retaliatory rage, protection, and escape fantasies will vary with developmental maturation (Mones, 1991).

TRAUMATIC MEMORIES AND DEVELOPMENT

There are two trends that are working at opposite poles to restrict the discussion of traumatic memories in childhood. Recent controversies concerning "repressed memories" or "false memory syndromes" in adults, and legal cases involving allegations of widespread sexual exploitation of children at preschools, have resulted in social polarization over the acceptance or dismissal of children's traumatic memories. At the same time, there are efforts to explain traumatic memories in biological terms, such as "malignant memories," "super memories," and "implicit–explicit memories." Both the social polarization and the biological reductionism underrepresent the extraordinary activity of children's minds in the experiencing and remembering of the moment-to-moment aspects of traumatic situations.

The developmental model has important implications for better understanding how children experience, organize, and remember traumatic situations (Pynoos, 1993; Pynoos et al., 1995). The recording, processing, and analyzing of sensory information may vary developmentally according to the specific sensory input, as well as the relative importance of sensory, kinesthetic, and somatic registration. For example, the smell of gunfire during a violent event may be registered with very little processing; this is perhaps related to the underlying neuroanatomy of olfaction (Buck & Axel, 1991). Visual information, however, which utilizes a "visual–spatial pad" (Baddeley, 1984) to represent and manipulate distance and location of a threat, requires more mature ability to discriminate. Because temporal registration in young children appears to require accurate spatial serialization of the event (Baddeley, 1976), they may be especially vulnerable to temporal distortions of the sequence of events during recall.

The emotional content of traumatic memories depends on the maturing capacity for understanding the metacognition of emotions (Saarni & Harris, 1991). The complexity of a traumatic situation may elicit two or more concurrent or successive emotions—for example, fear, sadness, excitement, and anger. The lack of a metacognition of concurrent emotions may interfere with the preschool child's reconstruction of the experience, by requiring either the assignment of concurrent emotions to different portions of the experience or the omission of a competing emotion. Increasing capacity to make affective discriminations, especially among negative emotions (Parens, 1991), permits the more mature child to distinguish among the complex moments.

Developmental maturation also governs a progressive capacity to integrate unimodal sensory information, affective valence, and spatial representation of threat within the interactive neuroprocessing system of the amygdala, hippocampus, and cortical feedbacks. This system tends toward stimulus completion (Rolls, 1989); that is, one sensory, affective, or cognitive reminder tends to elicit the fuller range of associated stimuli, affects, and meanings. As Freud (1900/1953) first proposed, young children are vulnerable to suppression, repression, lack of integration, and fragmentation of frightening memories in an effort to interrupt stimulus completion). In latency, the combined maturation in cortical inhibitory control (Shapiro & Perry, 1976), and capacities for increased contextual discrimination and affective tolerance, reduce the defensive engagement of these protective mechanisms.

The registration and memory of external and internal threats are strongly influenced by developmental and experiential factors. For example, a young child may focus on, and well remember, the facial expression of an approaching assailant (which serves as a measure of the assailant's malevolence) or the cries of distress of a family member. However, when attention shifts to internal threats—for example, once the child is penetrated, injured, or physically coerced—the young child may not have sufficiently mature ego observational capacities to register, locate, and monitor moment-to-moment sensations, feelings, and thoughts.

The nature and content of traumatic memories, including intrusive thoughts, images, traumatic play, and dreams, are in part related to the maturity of both "iconic memory" (integration of isolated pictures into a single percept) and "echoic memory" (the brief sensory story) as components of autobiographical episodic memory (Baddeley, 1984). Typically, the younger the child, the more the recollection is confined to a single image, sound, or smell, usually representing the action most associated by the child with immediate threat or injury.

The organization of memory and strategy of recall differ as children focus on different memory anchor points and their meaning, such as personal life threat, worry about a sibling, or cries of parental distress. Of special importance are significant interactive moments, including not only the moment of harm or protective intervention, but also affective and verbal exchanges. Because of previous life experiences, children may emphasize certain details and attribute special meaning to aspects of the traumatic situation.

Intervention fantasies that occur during the course of a traumatic situation, as well as afterwards, are an integral part of traumatic memory and accompany recall of any particular traumatic moment (Pynoos & Nader, 1993). These include fantasies about (1) altering the precipitating events; (2) interrupting the traumatic action; (3) reversing the lethal or injurious consequences; (4) gaining safe retaliation; and (5) preventing future trauma and loss. They are influenced by maturity, gender, and life experience.

Memory disturbances may reflect specific modifications that occur during remembering (Bjork & Richardson-Klavehn, 1989). Three important mechanisms have been identified. First, as Freud (1900/1953) suggested, highly traumatized children typically "weaken the version" in their reenactment behavior, play, thoughts, and descriptions. Distortions or omissions; reframing of aspects of the experience; misrepresentations of the threat, intentionality, and motivation; and denial of the seriousness of the consequences all reflect efforts to minimize the objective threat and to regulate emotional distress during recall (Pynoos & Nader, 1989). Second, in preschool and school-age children, intervention fantasies may be incorporated into the recounting as if they had occurred. Third, young children have immature strategies of recall (Johnson & Foley, 1984). What appears to be fragmentation or "dissociation" may reflect an inadequate strategy for remembering and integrating the various moments of a traumatic experience.

Children's traumatic narratives typically rely on co-constructions with parents or other adult caretakers. Co-construction can assist a child in clarifying details of the traumatic experience, understanding its context and meaning, and addressing cognitive confusions. Alternatively, adult caretakers may introduce prohibitions and misleading explanations, or may invoke a covert conspiracy of silence (Bowlby, 1979; Cain & Fast, 1972; Kestenberg, 1972). Of special note, co-construction can address "pathogenic beliefs" (Weis, 1990) that emerge out of inaccuracies and misattributions of accountability or psychosexual conflicts.

From a developmental perspective, we would urge that the concept of "traumatic memory" be placed within the broader concept of "traumatic expectation." In general, childhood traumatic experiences contribute to a schematization of the world, especially of security, safety, risk, injury, loss, protection, and intervention. The importance of traumatic memories lies in their role in shaping expectations of the recurrence of threat, of failure of protective intervention, and/or of helplessness, which govern the child's emotional life and behavior. "Traumatic expectation" provides a more powerful explanatory concept for understanding the long-term consequences of trauma on the child's emerging personality.

DEVELOPMENTAL NEUROBIOLOGY AND TRAUMATIC STRESS

There has been a paucity of neurobiological studies of traumatized children. Despite rapid advances in the characterization of the neurobiology of adult traumatic stress, there has been a tendency to overlook the importance of neurodevelopmental considerations in comparable studies of childhood traumatic stress. These considerations are twofold. First, neurophysiological alterations in traumatized children may disrupt normal biological maturation (Perry, in press). Second, these alterations, along with their effects over time, may have a significant impact on a variety of other aspects of child development.

The startle reaction provides a good example of both of these considerations. The acute impact of traumatic stress may vary according to the relative plasticity or consolidation of the underlying startle mechanism (Ornitz, 1991). Disturbances in the maturation of the startle mechanism may have serious consequences for other developmental spheres. Ornitz and Pynoos (1989) have provided preliminary evidence that consolidation of the inhibitory control of the startle reflex in middle childhood may be interfered with by traumatic exposure, leading to a "neurophysiological regression" to an earlier pattern of startle modulation.

In addition, the central nucleus of the amygdala regulates fear-enhanced startle (Ornitz, 1991) and perhaps the reactivity to novel stimuli of inhibited children (Kagan, 1991). The loss of inhibitory control over the startle reflex may interfere with the acquisition of a number of latency skills—for example, increased control over activity level, and capacity for reflection, academic learning, and focused attention.

Similar developmental considerations may be important to disturbances in other modulatatory mechanisms, such as those governing sleep-related phenomena and aggression. Children appear to be especially prone to non-rapid-eye-movement sleep disturbances after trauma, including increases in the percentage of time in stage 2 and stage 4 sleep, and parasomnia symptoms of somnambulism, vocalization, motor restlessness, and night terrors (Pynoos, 1990). Chronic sleep disturbance can lead to more daytime irritability and difficulties in concentration and attention, which can affect family life, peer relationships, and academic learning. In addition, temporary or chronic difficulty in modulating aggression can make children more irritable and anger-prone. This may result in reduced tolerance of the normal behaviors and slights of peers and family members, followed by unusual acts of aggression or social withdrawal (Pynoos, Nader, & March, 1991). It may alter the emerging balance between hostile and instrumental uses of aggression (Atkins, Stoff, Osborne, & Brown, 1993).

These trauma-induced changes in neuromodulation and physiological reactivity may produce biological analogues of traumatic expectations. These include central nervous system response to trauma-related cues and increased focused attention on external stimuli, in order to detect danger and make appropriate defensive responses (Krystal et al., 1989). These changes may initiate "anticipatory bias," a "state of preparedness" for extremely negative emotions, and "anxiety of premonitions" (Kagan, 1991). These traumatic expectations may be associated with recurrent bouts of fear, thrill seeking, or aggression, which can seriously affect a child's emerging self-concept, including self-attributions of cowardliness, courage, and fearlessness. Rieder and Cicchetti (1989) have suggested that these changes can have a deleterious effect on general information processing.

CHILDHOOD TRAUMA, EMERGING PERSONALITY, AND COMPLEX DISORDERS

Increased knowledge about traumatic stress in childhood, and recent studies implicating childhood trauma in adult personality disorders (e.g., borderline personality disorder; Herman, Perry, & van der Kolk, 1989) and other complex disorders, have generated interest in the long-term implications of childhood trauma for adult personality. Complex, life-trajectory-based, developmental models, similar to those recently proposed for the study of childhood bereavement (Clark, Pynoos, & Goebel, 1994), are needed to guide prospective and retrospective investigations of the long-term impact of childhood traumatic stress. Such a model requires revised thinking about the complex disorders that have been found to be associated with histories of traumatic experiences. Diagnostic symptom criteria need to be conceptualized as reflecting a layering of effects over time. Different symptoms and personality traits may represent the outcome of (1) specific features of traumatic exposures at varying points in development; (2) secondary adversities (including adverse caretaking); (3) disturbances in developmental expectations and in the acquisition and integration of developmental competencies; (4) the disruption of developmental transitions; (5) disturbances in normal biological maturation; and (6) the expression of traumatic expectations and intervention fantasies.

Whereas a general behavioral pattern, such as self-injurious behavior in adults, may be associated with a combination of risk factors, such as childhood trauma, neglect, and deprivation (van der Kolk, Perry, & Herman, 1991), a particular self-injurious or suicidal act may involve reenactment of a specific childhood traumatic experience and its accompanying intervention fantasies. Cooper (1986) has suggested that an unusual, isolated adult symptom may be etiologically related to a specific childhood traumatic experience. Stoller (1989) has commented that the more fixed and compulsive a perverse adult behavior, the more likely it is that traumatic exposures and family forces have contributed to its origin and maintenance.

Symptoms of personality disorders and other complex disorders associated with antecedent childhood trauma also need to be understood from a developmental perspective. For example, a recent study of dissociative identity disorder (formerly multiple personality disorder) in adolescents (Dell & Eisenhower, 1990) suggested that the core "personalities" were found to have originated during preschool years. The three central types described—a fearful, a protective or intervening, and an avenging or aggressive self—were each associated with specific traumatic episodes. Contrary to a state-dependent model of dissociation, a developmental psychopathology approach would reconsider these "selves" as perhaps reflecting a rigidification and persistence of age-related intervention fantasies incorporated into solitary and coordinated role play (Parker & Gottman, 1989).

CONCLUSION

Theoretical, research, and clinical approaches to traumatic stress in children and adolescents are entering a challenging new era. In the next decade, we can look forward to a burgeoning of knowledge in all the areas discussed above. Continued progress in the field requires "reintroducing" development into the discussion of childhood PTSD. An enhanced understanding of the interplay of developmental processes and traumatic stress should guide future research and clinical intervention.

ACKNOWLEDGMENTS

We gratefully acknowledge support for the writing of this chapter from the Bing Fund and the Robert Ellis Simon Foundation.

REFERENCES

American Psychiatric Association. (1994). *Diagnostic and statistical manual of mental diorders* (4th ed.). Washington, DC: Author.
Angelou, M. (1969). *I know why the caged bird sings.* New York: Random House.

Atkins, M., Stoff, D., Osborne, M. L., & Brown, K. (1993). Distinguishing instrumental and hostile aggression: Does it make a difference? *Journal of Abnormal Child Psychology, 21,* 355–365.

Baddeley, A. D. (1976). *The psychology of memory.* New York: Basic Books.

Baddeley, A. D. (1984). Memory theory and memory therapy. In B. Wilson & N. Moffat (Eds.), *Clinical management of memory problems* (pp. 5–27). London: Aspen.

Bat-Zion, N., & Levy-Shiff, R. (1993). Children in war: Stress and coping reactions under the threat of the Scud missile attacks and the effect of proximity. In L. Lewis & N. Fox (Eds.), *The psychological effects of war and violence in children* (pp. 143–161). Hillsdale, NJ: Erlbaum.

Bell, C. C., & Jenkins, E. J. (1993). Community violence and children on Chicago's south side. *Psychiatry, 56,* 46–54

Berkovitz, I. H., Wang, A., Pynoos, R., James, Q., & Wong, M. (Chairs). (1994, October). *Los Angeles earthquake, 1994: School district reduction of trauma effects.* Symposium presented at the annual meeting of the American Academy of Child and Adolescent Psychiatry, New York.

Bernstein, A. E. (1990). The impact of incest trauma on ego development. In H. B. Levine (Ed.), *Adult analysis and childhood sexual abuse* (pp. 65–91). Hillsdale, NJ: Analytic Press.

Bjork, R. A., & Richardson-Klavehn, A. (1989). On the puzzling relationship between environmental context and human memory. In C. Izawa (Ed.), *Current issues in cognitive processes: The Tulane Flowertree Symposium on Cognition* (pp. 313–344). Hillsdale, NJ: Erlbaum.

Bowlby, J. (1973). *Attachment and loss: Vol. 2. Separation: Anxiety and anger.* New York: Basic Books.

Bowlby, J. (1979). *The making and breaking of affectional bonds.* London: Tavistock.

Buck, L., & Axel, R. (1991). A novel multigene family may encode odorant receptors: A molecular basis for odor recognition. *Cell, 65,* 175–187.

Cain, A., & Fast, I. (1972). Children's disturbed reactions to parent suicide: Distortion and guilt, communication and identification. In A. Cain (Ed.), *Survivors of suicide* (pp. 93–111). Springfield, IL: Charles C Thomas.

Cicchetti, D., & Carlson, V. (1989). *Child maltreatment: Theory and research on the causes and consequences of child abuse and neglect.* New York: Cambridge University Press.

Clark, D. C., Pynoos, R. S., & Goebel, A. E. (1994). Mechanisms and processes of adolescent bereavement. In R. J. Haggerty, N. Garmezy, M. Rutter, & L. Sherrod (Eds.), *Stress, risk, and resilience in children and adolescents: Process mechanisms and interventions* (pp. 100–146). Cambridge, England: Cambridge University Press.

Cooper, A. M. (1986). Toward a limited definition of psychic trauma. In A. Rothstein (Ed.), *Clinical Workshop Series of the American Psychoanalytic Association: Monograph 2. The reconstruction of trauma: Its significance* (pp. 41–56). New York: International Universities Press.

De Bellis, M. D., Chrousos, G. P., Dorn, L. D., Burke, L., Helmers, K., Kling, M. A., Trickett, P. K., & Putnam, F. W. (1994). Hypothalamic–pituitary–adrenal axis dysregulation in sexually abused girls. *Journal of Clinical Endocrinology and Metabolism, 78,* 249–255

Dell, P., & Eisenhower, J. W. (1990). Adolescent multiple personality disorder: A preliminary study of eleven cases. *Journal of the American Academy of Child and Adolescent Psychiatry, 29*(3), 359–366.

Dollinger, S. J., O'Donnell, J. P., & Staley, A. A. (1984). Lightning-strike disaster: Effects on children's fears and worries. *Journal of Consulting and Clinical Psychology, 52*(6), 1028–1038.

Emde, R. N. (1991). Positive emotions for psychoanalytic theory: Surprises from infancy research and new directions. *Journal of the American Psychoanalytic Association, 39*, 5–44.

Freedy, J. R., Kilpatrick, D. G., & Resnick, H. S. (1993). Natural disaster and mental health: Theory, assessment, and intervention. *Journal of Social Behavior and Personality, 8*(5), 49–103

Freud, S. (1953). The interpretation of dreams. In J. Strachey (Ed. and Trans.), *The standard edition of the complete psychological works of Sigmund Freud* (Vol. 4, pp. 1–338; Vol. 5, pp. 339–627). London: Hogarth Press. (Original work published 1900)

Freud, S. (1959). Inhibitions, symptoms and anxiety. In J. Strachey (Ed. and Trans.), *The standard edition of the complete psychological works of Sigmund Freud* (Vol. 20, pp. 75–175). London: Hogarth Press. (Original work published 1926)

Garbarino, J., Kostelny, K., & Dubrow, N. (1991). What children can tell us about living in danger. *American Psychologist, 46*(4), 376–383.

Gleser, G., Green, B., & Winget, C. (1981). *Prolonged psychosocial effects of disaster: A study of Buffalo Creek.* New York: Academic Press.

Goenjian, A. (1993). A mental health relief program in Armenia after the 1988 earthquake: Implementation and clinical observations. *British Journal of Psychiatry, 163*, 230–239.

Goenjian, A., Pynoos, R. S., Steinberg, A. M., Najarian, L. M., Asarnow, J. R., Karayan, I., Ghurabi, M., & Fairbanks, L. A. (1995). Psychiatric co-morbidity in children after the 1988 earthquake in Armenia. *Journal of the American Academy of Child and Adolescent Psychiatry, 34*, 1174–1184.

Goenjian, A., Yehuda, R., Pynoos, R. S., Steinberg, A. M., Tashjian, M., Yang, R. K., Najarian, L. M., & Fairbanks, L. A. (in press). Basal cortisol, dexamethasome suppression of cortisol and MHPG among adolescents after the 1988 earthquake in Armenia. *American Journal of Psychiatry.*

Gorky, M. (1965). *My childhood.* (R. Wilks, Trans.). Harmondsworth, England: Penguin Books. (Original work published 1913)

Herman, J. L., Perry, J. C., & van der Kolk, B. A. (1989). Childhood trauma in borderline personality disorder. *American Journal of Psychiatry, 146*, 490–495.

Hendriks, J. H., Black, D., & Kaplan, T. (1993). *When father kills mother: Guiding children through trauma and grief.* London: Routledge.

Hoffman, M. L. (1979). Development of moral thought, feeling, and behavior. *American Psychologist, 34*, 959–966.

Howes, C. (1987). Social competence with peers in young children: Developmental sequences. *Developmental Review, 7*, 252–272.

Johnson, M. K., & Foley, M. A. (1984). Differentiating fact from fantasy: The reliability of children's memory. *Journal of Social Issues, 40*(2), 33–50

Kagan, J. (1991). A conceptual analysis of the affects. *Journal of the American Psychoanalytic Association, 39,* 109–130.

Kestenberg, J. S. (1972). How children remember and parents forget. *International Journal of Psychoanalytic Psychotherapy, 1,* 103–123.

Khan, M. (1963). The concept of cumulative trauma. *Psychoanalytic Study of the Child, 18,* 286–306.

Krystal, H. (1991). Integration and self-healing in post-traumatic states: A ten year retrospective. *American Imago, 48*(1), 93–117

Krystal, J. H., Kosten, T. R., Perry, B. D., Southwick, S., Mason, J. W., & Giller, E. L. (1989). Neurobiological aspects of PTSD: Review of clinical and preclinical studies. *Behavior Therapy, 20,* 177–198.

Kuterovac, G., Dyregrov, A., & Stuvland, R. (1994). Children in war: A silent majority under stress. *British Journal of Medical Psychology, 67,* 363–375.

Lansky, M. R. (1992). *Fathers who fail: Shame and psychopathology in the family system.* Hillsdale, NJ: Analytic Press.

McFarlane, A. C. (1995). Stress and disaster. In S. E. Hobfoll & M. deVries (Eds.), *Extreme stress and communities: Impact and intervention* (pp. 247–265). Dordrecht, The Netherlands: Kluwer.

Macksoud, M. S., Dyregrov, A., & Raundalen, M. (1993). Traumatic war experiences and their effects on children. In, B. Raphael & J. P. Wilson (Eds.), *International handbook of traumatic stress syndromes* (pp. 625–633). New York: Plenum Press.

Marans, S., & Cohen, D. J. (1993). Children and inner-city violence: Strategies for intervention. In L. A. Leavitt & N. A. Fox (Eds.), *The psychological effects of war and violence on children* (pp. 281–301). Hillsdale, NJ: Erlbaum.

Mones, P. (1991). *When a child kills: Abused children who kill their parents.* New York: Pocket Books.

Murray, H. A. (1938). *Explorations in personality.* London: Oxford University Press.

Nader, K., Pynoos, R. S., Fairbanks, L. A., Al-Ajeel, M., & Asfour, A. (1993). Acute posttraumatic reactions among Kuwait children following the Gulf crisis. *British Journal of Clinical Psychology, 32,* 407–416

Osofsky, J. D. (1993). Applied psychoanalysis: How research with infants and adolescents at high psychosocial risk informs psychoanalysis. *Journal of the American Psychoanalytic Association, 41,* 193–207.

Ornitz, E. M. (1991). Developmental aspects of neurophysiology. In M. Lewis (Ed.), *Child and adolescent psychiatry: A comprehensive textbook* (pp. 38–51). Baltimore: Williams & Wilkins.

Ornitz, E. M., & Pynoos, R. S. (1989). Startle modulation in children with post-traumatic stress disorder. *American Journal of Psychiatry, 147,* 866–870.

Parens, H. (1991). A view of the development of hostility in early life. *Journal of the American Psychoanalytic Association, 39,* 75–108.

Parker, J. G., & Gottman, J. M. (1989). Social and emotional development in a relational context. In T. J. Berndt & G. W. Ladd (Eds.), *Peer relationships in child development* (pp. 95–131). New York: Wiley.

Perry, B. D. (1994). Neurobiological sequelae of childhood trauma: Post-traumatic stress disorders in children. In M. Murberg (Ed.), *Catecholamine function in post-*

traumatic stress disorder: Emerging concepts (pp. 233–255). Washington, DC: American Psychiatric Press.

Perry, B. (in press). Incubated in terror: Neurodevelopmental factors in the "cycle of violence." In J. D. Osofsky (Ed.), *Children, youth, and violence: Searching for solutions.* New York: Guilford Press.

Pliny the Younger. (1931). *Letters* (W. Melmoth, Trans., revised by W. M. L. Hutchinson). London: Heinemann. (Original works written 100–113 A.D.)

Prigerson, H. G., Frank, E., Kasl, S. V., Reynolds, C. F., Anderson, B., Zubenko, G. S., Houck, P. R., George, C. J., & Kupfer, D. J. (1995). Complicated grief and bereavement-related depression as distinct disorders: Preliminary empirical validation in elderly bereaved spouses. *American Journal of Psychiatry, 152,* 22–30.

Pynoos, R. S. (1990). Post-traumatic stress disorder in children and adolescents. In B. D. Garfinkel, G. A. Carlson, & E. B. Weller (Eds.), *Psychiatric disorders in children and adolescents* (pp. 48–63). Philadelphia: W.B. Saunders.

Pynoos, R. S. (1992). Grief and trauma in children and adolescents. *Bereavement Care, 11*(1), 2–10.

Pynoos, R. S. (1993). Traumatic stress and developmental psychopathology in children and adolescents. In J. Oldham, M. Riba, & A. Tasman (Eds.), *American Psychiatric Press review of psychiatry* (Vol. 12, pp. 205–238). Washington, DC: American Psychiatric Press.

Pynoos, R. S. (in press). Children exposed to catastrophic violence and disaster. In C. R. Pfeffer (Ed.), *Intense stress and mental disturbance in children.* Washington, DC: American Psychiatric Press.

Pynoos, R. S., Frederick, C., Nader, K., Arroyo, W., Steinberg, A., Eth, S., Nunez, F., & Fairbanks, L. (1987). Life threat and posttraumatic stress in school-age children. *Archives of General Psychiatry, 44,* 1057–1063.

Pynoos, R. S., Goenjian, A., Tashjian, M., Karakashian, M., Manjikian, R., Manoukian, G., Steinberg, A., & Fairbanks, L. (1993a). Posttraumatic stress reactions in children after the 1988 Armenian earthquake. *British Journal of Psychiatry, 163,* 239–247.

Pynoos, R. S., & Nader, K. (1989). Children's memory and proximity to violence. *Journal of the American Academy of Child and Adolescent Psychiatry, 28,* 236–241.

Pynoos, R. S., & Nader, K. (1993). Issues in the treatment of post-traumatic stress in children and adolescents. In J. P. Wilson & B. Raphael (Eds.), *International handbook of traumatic stress syndromes* (pp. 535–549). New York: Plenum Press.

Pynoos, R. S., Nader, K., & March, J. (1991). Post-traumatic stress disorder. In J. Weiner (Ed.), *Textbook of child and adolescent psychiatry* (pp. 339–348). Washington, DC: American Psychiatric Press.

Pynoos, R. S., Sorenson, S. B., & Steinberg, A. M. (1993b). Interpersonal violence and traumatic stress reactions. In L. Goldberger & S. Breznitz (Eds.), *Handbook of stress: Theoretical and clinical aspects* (2nd ed., pp. 573–590). New York: Free Press.

Pynoos, R. S., Steinberg, A. M., & Wraith, R. (1995). A developmental model of childhood traumatic stress. In D. Cicchetti & D. J. Cohen (Eds.), *Manual of developmental psychopathology* (pp. 72–95). New York: Wiley.

Rado, S. (1942). Pathodynamics and treatment of traumatic war neurosis (traumatophobia). *Psychosomatic Medicine, 4,* 362–368.

Rangell, L. (1991). Castration. *Journal of the American Psychoanalytic Association, 39*(1), 3–23.

Rieder, C., & Cicchetti, D. (1989). Organizational perspective on cognitive control functioning and cognitive–affective balance in maltreated children. *Developmental Psychology, 25*(3), 382–393

Richters, J., & Martinez, P. (1993). NIMH Community Violence Project: I. Children as victims of and witnesses to violence. *Psychiatry, 56*, 7–21.

Rolls, E. T. (1989). Functions of neuronal networks in the hippocampus and neocortex in memory. In J. H. Byrne & W. O. Berry (Eds.), *Neural models of plasticity: Experimental and theoretical approaches* (pp. 240–264). New York: Academic Press.

Rose, D. (1991). A model for psychodynamic psychotherapy with the rape victim. *Psychotherapy, 28*(1), 85–95.

Rosenblatt, A. D., & Thickstun, J. T. (1977) *Modern psychoanalytic concepts in a general psychology.* New York: International Universities Press.

Rubin, K. H., LeMare, L. J., & Lollis, S. (1990). Social withdrawal in childhood: Developmental pathways to peer rejection. In S. R. Asher & J. D. Cole (Eds.), *Peer rejection in childhood* (pp. 217–240). Cambridge, England: Cambridge University Press

Saigh, P. A. (1991, November). *Academic variations among traumatized Lebanese adolescents.* Paper presented at the 25th Annual Convention of the Association for Advancement of Behavior Therapy, New York.

Saarni, C., & Harris, P. L. (1991). *Children's understanding of emotion.* Cambridge, England: Cambridge University Press.

Schwarz, E. D., & Kowalski, J. M. (1991). Malignant memories: PTSD in children and adults after a school shooting. *Journal of the American Academy of Child and Adolescent Psychiatry, 30*, 936–944.

Shapiro, T., & Perry, R. (1976). Latency revisited. *Psychoanalytic Study of the Child, 31*, 79–105.

Stoller, R. (1989). Consensual sadomasochistic perversions. In H. Blum, E. Weinshel, & F. Rodman (Eds.), *The psychoanalytic core* (pp. 265–282). Madison, CT: International Universities Press.

Strenz, T. (1982). The Stockholm syndrome. In F. Ochberg & D. Soskis (Eds.), *Victims of terrorism* (pp. 149–164). Boulder, CO: Westview Press.

Stuber, M. L., Nader, K., Yasuda, P., Pynoos, R. S., & Cohen, S. (1991). Stress responses after pediatric bone marrow transplantation: Preliminary results of a prospective longitudinal study. *Journal of the American Academy of Child and Adolescent Psychiatry, 30*(6), 952–957.

Stuvland, R. (1993). *Psychological and educational help to school-children affected by war: Results from a screening of children in Croatia.* Zagreb: Ministry of Education, Government of Croatia, in cooperation with UNICEF Zagreb.

Terr, L. C. (1991). Childhood traumas: An outline and overview. *American Journal of Psychiatry, 148*, 10–20.

Tsui, E., Dagwell, K., & Yule, W. (in press). *Effects of a disaster on children's academic attainment.* Manuscript submitted for publication.

van der Kolk, B. A., Perry, J. C., & Herman, J. L. (1991). Childhood origins of self-destructive behavior. *American Journal of Psychiatry, 148*, 1665–1671.

Weis, R. T. (1990). The centrality of adaptation. *Contemporary Psychoanalysis, 26,* 660–676.

Weisaeth, L. (1993). Disasters: Psychological and psychiatric aspects. In L. Goldberger & S. Breznitz (Eds.), *Handbook of stress: Theoretical and clinical aspects* (2nd ed., pp. 591–616). New York: Free Press.

Wiesel, E. (1960). *Night.* (S. Rodway, Trans.). New York: Hill & Wang. (Original work published 1958)

World Health Organization. (1992). *International classification of diseases* (10th revision). Geneva: Author.

Yule, W. (1991). Resilience and vulnerability in child survivors of disasters. In B. Tizare & V. Varma (Eds.), *Vulnerability and resilience in human development* (pp. 182–197). London: Jessica Kingsley.

Yule, W. (1993). Technology-related disasters. In C. F. Saylor (Ed.), *Children and disasters* (pp. 105–121). New York: Plenum Press.

Yule, W., Bolton, D., & Udwin, O. (1992, June). *Objective and subjective predictors of PTSD in adolescence.* Paper presented at the annual conference of the International Society for Traumatic Stress Studies, Amsterdam.

Yule, W., & Williams, R. M. (1990). Post-traumatic stress reactions in children. *Journal of Traumatic Stress, 3,* 279–295.

CHAPTER 15

Prior Traumatization and the Process of Aging

Theory and Clinical Implications

PETRA G. H. AARTS
WYBRAND OP DEN VELDE

Over the last few decades, it has become commonly known that shocking events or lengthy periods of stress can cause serious damage to individuals' health. Although some trauma survivors display few to no negative responses, in some the damage may be permanent. Several studies have revealed that the course of posttraumatic stress disorder (PTSD) over the individual lifespan is highly variable (Bramsen, 1995; Aarts et al., 1996). There is, however, evidence that a delayed onset or exacerbation of clinical PTSD may emerge during the process of aging.

This chapter offers an explanation of aging as a risk factor for previously traumatized individuals, by means of a comparison between developmental tasks of late life on the one hand and posttraumatic sequelae on the other. Before we describe this explanatory model, however, the thus far prevailing explanations of late-onset PTSD are presented and debated. The chapter begins with a brief overview of clinical and empirical studies on aging World War II survivors. Two clinical vignettes then illustrate the late onset and the intensification of PTSD, respectively, during the later states of the life cycle.

STUDIES ON WORLD WAR II SURVIVORS

Most of what we presently know concerning the long-term effects of trauma is derived from studies on survivors of World War II. In the first few decades after World War II, it became clear that many survivors of Nazi persecution were suffering seriously as a consequence of what they had gone through. Whereas some survivors were able to adjust and to cope fairly adequately, others continued to suffer as a consequence of the horrors they had experienced. Their symptoms have been described by a number of authors (Bastiaans, 1957; Eitinger, 1961; Niederland & Krystal, 1968; Venzlaff, 1964). Although the names that were given to the cluster of symptoms varied from "traumatic neurosis" to "concentration camp syndrome" or "survivor syndrome," the symptomatology recognized in survivors of Nazi persecution was fairly consistent. Anxiety, numbing of affect, depression, dysphoria, cognitive and memory impairment, somatoform complaints, and sleep disturbances were the main symptoms of the survivor syndrome.

Gradually, it became apparent that posttraumatic complaints could be absent or in remission for extended periods of time in individual survivors (Bastiaans, 1957; Hoppe, 1966; Krystal, 1968). The attention of the mental health experts involved was primarily directed toward an explanation of the nature—the why and how—of this so-called "latency period." A strong suppression of symptoms by means of defense mechanisms or reaction formations defined the latency period. The investigators opposed the term "symptom-free interval" for the latency period, because isolated symptoms, in their opinion, were always present. These symptoms, however, did not lead to a clinical survivor syndrome. Only later did researchers contemplate possible causes for the cessation of the latency period (Cath, 1981; Davidson, 1987; Kahana, 1981; Krystal, 1981). Some clinical studies then revealed that during the transition from middle to late life, trauma survivors were at risk of a delayed onset of posttraumatic symptomatology.

To date, very little empirical research has focused specifically on the age of onset or worsening of posttraumatic complaints. Nevertheless, several recent studies have confirmed the clinical impression that survivors of World War II are at risk of a delayed onset or worsening of posttraumatic symptomatology during the later phases of the life cycle, sometimes after decades of adequate coping. This pertains to survivors of Nazi persecution, military veterans, former members of resistance movements, and war sailors (Askevold, 1980; Assael & Givon, 1984; Hartvig, 1977; Randall, Walker, Ross, & Maltbie, 1982; Steinitz, 1992). Op den Velde et al. (1993), for instance, studied former members of the Dutch resistance during World War II ($n = 147$) and found that the time of onset of the first symptoms of PTSD was highly variable. Several resistance veterans reported symptom-free intervals of many years; in 50%, PTSD was first manifested more than 20 years after the end of the war. Tennant, Goulson, and Dent (1993), in a controlled follow-up study with former Australian servicemen who were interned in Japanese prisoner-of-war camps, showed a significant increase of psychiatric disorders when the target group was between 46.5 and 66.5 years of age.

Kuilman and Suttorp (1989) studied 100 World War II survivor patients in The Netherlands. They counted a majority of subjects in which a late onset or worsening of posttraumatic symptomatology during midlife and old age had taken place. In various geriatric institutions in the United States, Honigman-Cooper (1979) observed that elderly survivors of trauma suffered from increased vulnerability to the stresses that go hand in hand with the process of aging. Furthermore, Archibald and Tuddenham (1965) found an increasing incidence of World War II military veterans with "war neuroses." They were among the first investigators to speculate that this late manifestation of posttraumatic symptoms might be age-related.

CASE PRESENTATIONS

The history of Mrs. E. offers an example of late-onset PTSD with a latency period of nearly half a century. Mrs. E., an 83-year-old Dutch Jewish woman, was referred to one of us (Op den Velde) because of suspected dementia. She had escaped the Nazis during World War II by hiding, together with other Jews, in the basement of a farmhouse. On several occasions German troops searched the farm, but she and her companions were able to reach their emergency hiding place in a haystack just in time. She remembers that once the attackers suspected that people were hidden in the haystack, and pierced the hay with bayonets while threatening to set the stack on fire. After the war, she found out that her parents, brother, and three sisters had not survived the Holocaust. The family that had offered her shelter became a kind of foster family to her. Soon after the war, she got married, but her husband fell ill and died only 3 years later.

Mrs. E. was successful and highly respected in her professional career. As a social worker, she was involved with the rehabilitation of convicts. Surprisingly, she stated that she had experienced no emotional problems at all with her work on behalf of convicted collaborators of the German occupiers. Apart from sporadic migraine attacks, she had always been in good health. After her retirement she enjoyed a fairly satisfactory social life with her friends. At the age of 81, however, she moved to a home for the elderly. Gradually she outlived her friends and acquaintances. It was only then that she became preoccupied with the fate of her family members who had perished in Nazi death camps during the war. Frightening dreams about being burned alive interrupted her sleep. She became tense and irritable, lost weight, and isolated herself. Physical examination revealed nothing other than moderate arthrosis of the hips. She was referred to Op den Velde because some organic brain disorder was suspected.

Mrs. E. appeared to have vitality, without conclusive signs of cognitive impairment. After the first interview she was diagnosed as suffering from late-onset PTSD, and treated with weekly counseling. Her insomnia improved considerably with fluvoxamine (50 mg).[1] In the early stages of her psychotherapy, she realized with shock that she had not been able to mourn the loss of the couple who had saved her life. After grief, sorrow, and guilt feelings of her "foster family" and husband had been worked through, she was again astonished to find that she had never mourned for her murdered relatives. She realized that her pain over the loss of her family was so profound that she had not previously been able to feel it. Now, in her efforts to grieve, she wrote an extensive letter to her lost younger sister, to whom she had been particularly close. It was a report on her life during and since the war, and contained a formal apology for her "insensitivity and negligence" with regard to the commemoration of her family. She now also realized that she had suffered from incomprehensible headache attacks at the birthdays of her murdered relatives, and admitted that she had suffered from many other somatoform complaints ever since the war. Her ability to recognize and express her feelings of guilt, grief, and loneliness increased at nearly every session. The incapacity to mourn the immense losses she had suffered had seriously impaired her ability to master her traumatization. She now recognized a deep survivor guilt and identification with the aggressor; the latter was symbolized in her work with convicts, former Nazi sympathizers included. After half a year of treatment, her complaints were significantly diminished.

Losses of family members and friends, and the resulting feelings of loneliness, often seem to play a triggering role in the sudden exacerbation or late onset of posttraumatic symptomatology. Unfortunately, this condition is not always recognized for what it is. Just as in Mrs. E.'s case, the complaints and symptoms of these patients can be easily interpreted as signs of the depression, excessive rumination, or cognitive degeneration commonly associated with old age. The case of Mrs. E. also demonstrates that advanced age is not at all a contraindication for psychotherapy. Finally, Mrs. E.'s case illustrates a typical tardive onset of posttraumatic complaints, after a latency period of nearly five decades.

The second clinical example illustrates the reemergence of PTSD in remission during the process of aging. Mr. K. was a married man, a retired driving instructor. In 1945, at the age of 21, he had joined the Dutch army and

[1]In the treatment of disturbed sleep and dreaming in elderly trauma victims, selective serotonin reuptake inhibitor antidepressants often give better results than benzodiazepine hypnotics (De Boer et al., 1992).

volunteered for duty in the Dutch East Indies, which was at that time still occupied by the Japanese. By the time of his arrival in Asia, the Japanese had surrendered; however, the Dutch troops were ordered to suppress the uprising of the Indonesian nationalists, who demanded independence from the Dutch. For the next 3 years, Mr. K. fought in a guerrilla war. His patrol was ambushed, and once he was separated from his comrades and roamed alone in enemy-controlled territory. He also watched his best friend die before his eyes as they entered a booby-trapped building together. Many years later, he still resented the Dutch government for its decision to negotiate peace with the Indonesian Republic and to withdraw its troops.

For 5 years after his return home, Mr. K. suffered from flashbacks, nightmares, and depression. Gradually these complaints waned. In the 1970s, however, his eldest son was drafted for military duty, and at the same time Dutch newspapers began to report on atrocities committed by Dutch troops during the war in Indonesia. Mr. K. was very angry and upset about the "slander in the newspapers"; he once again became sleepless, tired, and touchy. In his nightmares, he saw his son entering a booby trap and was unable to warn him in time. During this period, his employer threatened Mr. K. with dismissal because of his excessive use of alcohol. His wife and general practitioner tried to refer him to a psychiatrist, but he refused, stating that he certainly "was not insane." After 3 difficult years, he suddenly felt "reborn." His complaints disappeared immediately, and he became very active with his numerous hobbies.

In 1993, while Mr. K. was stopped at a traffic light, his car was hit from behind. He suffered several complicated fractures. After emergency surgery, he was thoroughly confused and mistook the nurses for disguised Indonesian partisans who were trying to kill him. His consciousness cleared, but he remained anxious and was hardly able to sleep. During the night, he warned the other patients to watch for snipers. During 4 months of forced immobilization as a consequence of the fractures, he suffered from full-blown PTSD, with vivid flashbacks and frequent aggressive outbursts. The staff of the surgical ward requested his transfer to the department of psychiatry. Mr. K., however, refused transferral, would not take psychotropic medication, and even declined to see the consulting psychiatrist. The psychiatrist had weekly sessions with both the surgical ward staff and Mr. K.'s wife. Information and explanation about Mr. K.'s history and his related posttraumatic reactions reduced the tension among the surgical staff. After discharge from the hospital, Mr. K.'s posttraumatic complaints worsened, and he finally agreed to psychiatric treatment.

Shame about his "mental weakness" dominated the first five sessions of Mr. K.'s psychotherapy. His youth had been unhappy and hard; he described his father as a tyrant. Because of his rather limited introspective capacities, treatment was mainly supportive. He was brought into contact with a volunteer discussion group of veterans from the war in Indonesia. He was relieved when he discovered that many of the veterans shared his historical views and faced similar health problems. At this writing, he is a volunteer leader of veterans' self-help groups.

In retrospect, one can see that Mr. K. developed PTSD after his return from his combat experiences in Indonesia, and that this first episode lasted for 5 years. After a seemingly symptomless period of 21 years, his PTSD recurred for 3 years, triggered by the newspaper reports on war atrocities and his son's entering the army. Following a second symptomless interval, full-blown PTSD developed after his surgery and lengthy immobilization in the hospital. In our clinical experience, a reemergence of PTSD after illness and hospitalization is not rare. However, this does not invariably occur; some severely traumatized individuals sustain serious illness without intensification of PTSD symptoms (Van Driel & Op den Velde, 1995). Mr. K. found recognition and security in a volunteer organization of veterans. It was obvious that Mr. K.'s self-esteem had suffered a serious blow as a consequence of his being a veteran of a lost and "bad" war. His feelings of humiliation and guilt about this, as well as about his failure to protect his comrade, may well have led to reactive aggressive behavior. His volunteer work with fellow veterans apparently soothed these injuries to his ego, and he regained self-esteem.

THEORIES ON LATE ONSET OR EXACERBATION OF PTSD

In most studies, a decrease in coping capacities and an increase in negative life events are held responsible for the late onset of posttraumatic symptomatology in aging trauma survivors. In order to clarify the delayed onset or sudden exacerbation of PTSD in elderly survivors, it has been assumed that during senescence the individuals' mental and physical resilience gradually diminishes. As a consequence of this assumed general process of "weakening," it has been argued that trauma survivors' ability to ward off or master repressed trauma-related memories and associated affects inevitably decreases during the process of aging. Moreover, it was thought that elderly survivors of trauma are unable to continue to use coping mechanisms that were once available to them (e.g., rigid concentration on external matters and occupational achievements, or defense mechanisms such as denial and repression). Thus, a combination of general lack of resilience and stressful life events, such as retirement, children leaving the parental home, separation, or divorce, was said to lead to decompensation in aging trauma survivors (Cath, 1981; Danieli, 1981; Hertz, 1990; Krystal, 1981; Randal et al., 1981). For instance, Assael and Givon (1984) speculated that aging Israelis in general and Holocaust survivors in particular, as a consequence of previous stress and trauma, "had no strength left to cope with the mental and other difficulties that are a part of old age" (p. 32).

Underlying this point of view was the now obsolete view that senescence is mainly a process of neurophysiological degeneration. In combination with the culturally determined general depreciation of old age, this view may well have colored the clinical and theoretical understanding of the origins of delayed PTSD in aging trauma survivors. In addition, as Schulz (1982) has recognized, professionals tend to attribute a decline in coping capacities to the aged. Yet recent gerontological studies and research indicated that at least some of our perceptions concerning the process of aging are part of a biased belief system and do not necessarily reflect reality (Coleman, 1986; Schmid, 1991). Although, indeed, the elderly often demonstrate an impairment of short-term memory and a decrease in physical and biological functionality, there is no empirical evidence whatsoever that coping mechanisms, cognitive faculties, and affect regulation necessarily deteriorate in the later stages of the life cycle. Moreover, depression is not found to be such a frequent feature in the elderly (Feinson & Thoits, 1986).

Numerous studies now contradict the view that the incidence of depression in the elderly is much higher than in other age groups. Heeren (1992), in a review of recent international empirical research, states that the prevalence of functional disorders in the elderly is equal to that in younger generations. Her own study of 351 Dutch citizens aged 85 or over showed that the prevalence of nonorganic psychiatric disorders (12%), depression (5%) included, did not exceed the prevalence of such disorders in younger generations (Heeren, 1991). In addition, other studies have shown that coping capacities do not necessarily deteriorate as a consequence of old age. Solomon (1991), for example, presented a study with a 1-year follow-up on the effects of contemporary traumatization within different age groups. It appeared that the aged were no more vulnerable to trauma than younger cohorts. Surprisingly, those who suffered most from posttraumatic misery were between 30 and 45 years of age. A comparable longitudinal study (12 years) by Green, Gleser, Lindy, Grace, and Leonard (1996) reached similar conclusions. In a controlled study with aging survivors of Nazi persecution, Shanan and Shahar (1983) found that although the target group showed more cognitive and intellectual impairment and amnesia, they performed better than the controls while facing current stress. Such results should stimulate us to question the assumption that coping capacities and affect regulation necessarily diminish as a consequence of aging.

As we have mentioned above, stressful life events are also considered to be an important reason for a late onset or sudden worsening of posttraumatic complaints in survivors of trauma (Assael & Givon, 1984; Cath, 1981; Davidson, 1987; Hertz, 1990; Krystal, 1981; Ornstein, 1981). Kuilman and Suttorp (1989), for instance, found that the late onset of PTSD was often precipitated by negative life events. Out of 100 patients, 43% reported stressful life events 1 year prior to exacerbation. A study of aging Holocaust survivors by Lomranz, Shmotkin, Zechovoy, and Rosenberg (1985) indicated that the group of survivors was more past-oriented and more pessimistic in their attitudes toward life events than the control group.

The life events that are most commonly reported to precipitate a sudden onset or worsening of posttraumatic symptoms can be classified into two types. First, there are life events that involve personal changes, such as retirement, children leaving the parental home, death of or separation from relatives or friends, physical illness, and hospitalization. A second type of precipitating factor appears to be a confrontation with racism, war, prison camps, or cruelty, whether directly or through the mass media. Survivors of World War II trauma can become deeply desperate when faced with the reality that not much seems to have been learned from that war. To them, their torments and survival appear to have been in vain. There are currently no empirical studies that support this observation; there is, however, some evidence that the Gulf War generated late-onset PTSD in elderly World War II trauma survivors (Musaph, 1991; Robinson, Netanel, & Rapaport, 1992; Shatan, 1991). These two types of life events have the common feature that they somehow resemble or symbolize the original trauma, and this resemblance leads to intrusive reexperiencing of the traumatic past (Davidson, 1987; Musaph, 1991; Krystal, 1968, 1981; Ornstein, 1981). Such life events are therefore often called "retraumatizing events."

Of the first type of life events, retirement is most commonly associated with late-onset PTSD. Given their enforced inactivity, retirees are less able to ward off their emotions through vigorous concentration on external matters (Kahana, 1981; Krystal, 1981; Kuilman & Suttorp, 1989). It is generally assumed that retirement unfavorably affects the physical and mental health of aging workers, as well as their self-esteem and general contentment. The loss of status, productivity, income, and involvement that accompany retirement are considered to be the origins of the adverse effects on mental and physical health. However, in a review of research, Minkler (1981) concludes that there is no distinct confirmation that retirement negatively affects health in the general population. Palmore, Fillenbaum, and George (1984), in a longitudinal study of the consequences of retirement, also conclude that it has no inauspicious effects on health. *Early* retirement, on the other hand, does appear to have adverse effects on health. Palmore et al. have hypothesized that poor health may well be a cause for early retirement and not its consequence; in their article, they refer to several empirical studies that confirm this hypothesis. In a study with former members of the Dutch resistance during World War II (Aarts et al., 1996; Op den Velde et al., 1993), the biographical interviews suggested that severe traumatic experiences did not preclude good or even excellent social and occupational functioning for considerable periods of time. However, most of the 147 veterans retired or were granted a disability pension at the age of 50 to 55 years. At the time of the study, in 1985, only 6 out of 147 veterans (mean age 61.5) were still partially employed. Problems and conflicts with colleagues at work often led the veterans to take early retirement. During the interviews, evidence was collected that, in particular, manifestations of vital exhaustion, chronic fatigue, insomnia, and related irritability forced the subjects to terminate their occupational careers prematurely. A study by Hartvig (1977) with Scandinavian war sailors contains similar findings.

Stressful life events—not only retirement and the subsequent loss of status and activities and reduction in income, but also illness and disease; the deaths of spouses, siblings, and friends; and children leading their own lives away from the parental home—are to some extent inherent to the life cycle. In fact, such events are more or less age-related, since they are more likely to occur and/or to accumulate during the later decades of the lifespan. Therefore, considering such life events to be the causes for posttraumatic decompensation in aging trauma survivors means that "normal" life events are being labeled as pathogenic forces in themselves. Life events may well *trigger* a delayed onset or exacerbation of PTSD in trauma survivors, as has indeed been observed in many instances, but they are certainly not a sufficient *cause* in themselves (see also Miller, 1988).

In conclusion, the two factors commonly assumed to be critical to causing late onset or exacerbation of PTSD—that is, age-related decline of coping capacities and stressful life events—do not adequately explain its occurrence.

In 1981, the *Journal of Geriatric Psychiatry* dedicated a special issue to aging survivors of the Holocaust. In an important contribution, Krystal (1981) utilized Erikson's epigenetic model on identity formation to clarify the late onset of posttraumatic complaints. He recognized that acceptance of loss and ego integrity are not only crucial developmental tasks of aging, but also critical achievements in the process of recovery from trauma (see also Danieli, 1981). A closer scrutiny of the commonalities between the process of aging and posttraumatic reactions has brought us closer to a theoretical understanding of delayed onset or exacerbation of PTSD during the aging process.

TRAUMA AND AGING COMPARED

As we have pointed out earlier in the chapter, modern gerontological theories oppose the formerly dominant "deficiency model" of aging as a process of mainly physical and mental decline (Schmid, 1991). The peculiarities and problems of the presenium and old age are now understood in the light of the individual's life course and the totality of his or her previous experiences. It is increasingly understood that individual reactions to the many challenges of old age differ according to personal life histories. This so-called "lifespan perspective" on aging (Coleman, 1986) is undoubtedly inspired by Erik Erikson's model of identity formation. Like every other phase of the life cycle, senescence holds its own promises and chances. The later phases of the lifespan offer an opportunity to contemplate one's existence and to enjoy its fruits. A reconciliation with the mildness toward one's own and others' trials and errors may emerge; out of this, a new kind of unselfish and rewarding respect and love for others can grow. Erikson (1965) stated that each particular phase in a person's life contains its own challenges and crises to overcome. In addition, the later periods of the life cycle are stages of human identity formation, with their own specific developmental tasks (Erikson, 1965). Erikson understood that human life ideally ends with the completion of these tasks; actual death, by comparison, is a mere fact. Ego integrity and despair are the extreme outcomes on the continuum of this last developmental stage, whereas loss is the main ordeal. Successful adaptation to aging, therefore, is understood as the capacity to cope adequately with the losses and challenges of old age.

Although aging is not necessarily and exclusively a vale of tears, the road toward ego integrity is not neatly paved. If we combine Coleman's (1986) insights with those of Schmid (1991) and Erikson (1965), we see that successful adaptation to aging requires the following:

- Mourning for losses
- Giving meaning to past and present experiences
- Accepting one's past and present states
- (Re)establishing self-coherence and self-continuity
- Achieving ego integration

During the succeeding stages of effective adjustment to aging, memory is a significant vehicle for moving toward ego integrity. An increase of reminiscence during senescence is a well-observed phenomenon. The typical reminiscing of the aged was formerly appraised as a pathological manifestation of neurophysiological degeneration and cognitive passivity. Recently, the awareness has grown that memory helps the individual to give meaning to and accept past experiences and states. The "remembrance of things past," as Proust found, plays a pivotal role in the organization of the individual's identity. Living in the past is a means of coming to terms with the past.

Reminiscence is not only important during the process of aging; it also plays a critical role in posttraumatic symptomatology. The "survivor syndrome" symptoms of intrusive reexperiencing, memory impairment, paroxysmic hypermnesias, and compulsive repetition of nightmares demonstrate the critical significance of memory. On the other hand, posttraumatic reenactment and repetition compulsion are by no means simple pathological manifestations; they also facilitate the mastering of the trauma. Moreover, as Horowitz (1976) pointed out, a more active and controlled remembrance of traumatic events is a prerequisite for a successful recovery from trauma.

Mourning for Losses

Since grief is more or less inherent in old age as a consequence of the many losses that accompany it, mourning is part and parcel of adequate adaptation to aging. Especially in old age, the acceptance and integration of past and present states demand mourning. Among Holocaust survivors, bereavement and loss are crucial themes; at the same time, the capacity to mourn is often impaired as a consequence of traumatization (Danieli, 1981; Krystal, 1981). The mourning for previous, analogous losses is rarely completed, and new losses may well trigger suppressed and postponed grief. Grief was and is hard to bear not only because of the loss and death of loved ones, but also because of the loss of an empathic and positive self-image, of former beliefs, and of basic trust. Krystal (1988) further stresses that posttraumatic states are characterized by affect intolerance. The anxiety-arousing reminiscences of the traumatic past can be serious hindrances in the mourning process. Insomnia, chronic fatigue, and depression can be additional burdens for active mourning in traumatized individuals. Loss and bereavement may be obvious themes for survivors of Nazi persecution, but loss, both real and fantasized, is inherent in any trauma (Herman, 1992). Uncompleted grief, as well as guilt feelings, may be reactivated by the many losses that are part and parcel of the later stages of the life cycle.

Giving Meaning to Experiences and Accepting the Past and Present

To facilitate ego integration during the process of aging, it is important for individuals to be able to accept the course of their lives as inevitably their own (Erikson, 1965). If it is understood that past, present, and possible future events may have some meaning within one's life, both positive and negative experiences gain congruence. To assign meaning to these experiences is a way to comprehend or make sense out of one's life, and advances the acceptance and endurance of the manifold losses of old age. To be able to give a meaning to and accept one's life story is essential for the ability to enjoy the potential pleasures of the last phases of the life cycle. Assigning meaning to and accepting trauma are important means of recovering from trauma as well (Herman, 1992; Krystal, 1988).

In trauma survivors, beliefs in fundamental reason and justice are often severely damaged. The sensation of utter powerlessness during a traumatic event may shatter one's basic trust and feeling of control over one's very existence. A profound mistrust of fellow humans—the impairment of what we could call "social basic trust"—is an important additional phenomenon in survivors of trauma. Horowitz (1976) asserted that in order to recover from the effects of trauma, it is important for an individual to give a meaning to the traumatic experiences. As a consequence of a traumatic event, a person's inner conceptions of the world and life—in Horowitz's vocabulary, "cognitive schemata"—are disrupted. According to Horowitz, it is therefore crucial to match pretraumatic inner schemes or models with the new (posttraumatic) information. To reduce the incongruity of the traumatic information, ideational and cognitive processing is required. Giving meaning to the traumatic experience lessens the distress and restores the sense of self-control in trauma survivors.

We feel, however, that in Horowitz's model of recovery from trauma, cognitive assessment as a way of giving meaning to and accepting traumatic events is overemphasized at the cost of emotional aspects. After all, a rational interpretation of traumatic experiences without emotional association remains meaningless. In particular, the sensations of powerlessness and extreme vulnerability, and the confrontation with ruthless human violence, evoke intense and unendurable emotions. Traumatic events cause not only cognitive confusion but also severe disintegration anxiety. Especially for severely traumatized individuals, such as survivors of Nazi persecution, it is hard to give a meaning to and accept former torments and the murder of many (sometime all) of their loved ones. To find reason or congruity in such horrors seems an impossible task. Furthermore, acceptance of their losses may cause unbearable guilt feelings.

(Re)establishing Self-Coherence and Self-Continuity

Each succeeding phase in human development demands a (re)establishment of psychic coherence and continuity. Self-coherence and self-continuity are closely related concepts. They are essential to feeling that one is a "whole" person. "Self-coherence" refers to integration in the here and now, while "self-continuity" refers to the feeling of integrity in retrospect, over the entire lifespan. The awareness of a discernible association of past, present, and even future states is its vehicle. Each form of loss, however, signifies a rupture in the individual's sense of self-coherence and self-continuity. A temporal deprivation of an emphatic self is likely to accompany any form of loss. The losses that accompany the process of aging and the confrontation with one's future death contain further threats to self-esteem. In some individuals, such narcissistic injuries are serious threats to psychic integrity during the process of aging.

In massive trauma, the split in the life cycle is conclusive. As such, it is a fierce and often successful attack on psychic integrity; as a result, the awareness of the "self" is fragmented. Many World War II survivors, for instance, say that they do not feel themselves to be the same persons as they were before the traumatic events. The trauma of Nazi persecution meant that victims were forced for a long time into a pathological way of dealing with affects. The expression of rage, overwhelming anxiety, anger, or grief was literally life-threatening during the war. Suppression of these emotions was a necessity; survival depended on it. But there were also internal reasons for a stifling of affects. As we have stated earlier, the victims' grief was hard to bear not only because of the loss and death of loved ones, but also as the result of the loss of their empathic and positive self-images. The Nazis treated their prisoners as vermin and as worthless creatures. Sometimes survivor guilt was a consequence of actual antisocial behavior during internment, however necessary it may have been to survive. Also as a result of the loss of the capacity to mourn or feel empathy with other persons, people could fear that they were almost as bad as their persecutors. The sense that they were "bad" and somehow deserving of their harassment infiltrated the minds of some survivors. Shame could be brought forth by the sensation of utter powerlessness and self-accusations (survivor guilt), which are not uncommon phenomena in trauma survivors (Berger, 1977; Lifton, 1980; Niederland & Krystal, 1968). The shame- and guilt-provoking conditions contributed to the massive attack on each person's self-esteem and psychic integrity. There is some agreement among authors that human-inflicted trauma implies a severe narcissistic injury for its victims (Eissler, 1968; Herman, 1992; Krystal, 1968; Ulman & Brothers, 1988). In another context, Kohut (1972) argued that narcissistic injury may disrupt the self-structure and cause intense disintegration anxiety in an individual.

Achieving Ego Integration

At present, trauma experts consider pathology of the self to be the main adverse phenomenon in trauma patients. Inspired by Kohut's self psychology and psychoanalytical object relations theory, Ulman and Brothers (1988) and McCann and Pearlman (1990) postulate a shattering of the self in trauma survivors. A division into so-called "good" and "bad" self-representations is the result. Therefore, the focus of treatment is the integration of the self and thereby restoration of the sense of self-coherence in trauma survivors (Krystal, 1988; McCann & Pearlman, 1990; Ornstein, 1986; Ulman & Brothers, 1988).

With respect to Vietnam veterans, Laufer (1988) has argued that the disintegration of the self is the result of splitting into a pretraumatic, a traumatic, and posttraumatic self. Amnesia for the pretraumatic self or an idealization of that particular period can be understood as an effort to deny the rupture in one's life and to establish a semblance of continuity between the pretraumatic self and the posttraumatic self. The traumatic self is mostly looked upon with awe, shame, and anger. To recover from trauma, integration is a difficult but essential task. It can only be accomplished when these negative affects and memories can be faced, and the loss of the pretraumatic self can be mourned for.

In Figure 15.1, the phases of trauma recovery and the stages of the process of aging are schematized and compared. As the figure indicates, the similarities between these two processes are marked. Mourning for losses, giving

Developmental Tasks of Aging   Trauma Recovery Process

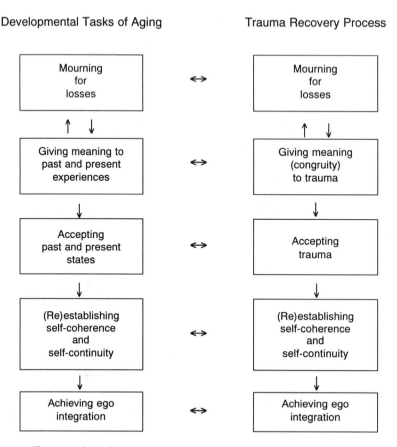

Figure 15.1. Comparative model of aging and trauma recovery.

meaning to and accepting past and present experiences, and (re)creating self-coherence and self-continuity are chores within each process; ego integration is the completion of both. Moreover, memory plays a major role in the process of aging as well as in trauma recovery.

In conclusion, traumatized individuals encounter serious hindrances during and after the transition from middle to late life. In the effort to adapt to aging, traumatic experiences that have not been worked through may surface. Interference between the processes of dealing with the trauma and dealing with old age may well explain a tardive onset or reoccurrence of posttraumatic symptomatology. We therefore argue that prior trauma constitutes a developmental risk during the process of aging.

SUMMARY AND DISCUSSION

There is sufficient evidence that during senescence survivors of trauma are at risk of a worsening or sudden onset of posttraumatic symptomatology, even after decades of adequate coping. An age-related decline of mental and physical resilience that diminishes coping capacities, and/or negative life events, are usually assumed to be responsible for this late onset of posttraumatic symptomatology. However, there appears to be no basis for the assumption that a waning of coping capabilities goes hand in hand with the process of aging. Nor are stressful life events sufficient explanations for a (re)emergence of flourishing PTSD in elderly trauma survivors.

Alternatively, we have argued that posttraumatic states and the specific developmental problems belonging to old age interfere with each other. The observed analogies between the developmental conflicts of aging and trauma responses make the decompensation of elderly trauma survivors more comprehensible, even when the traumatic experiences concerned took place many decades ago. Survivors of trauma have to mourn not only the losses that accompany old age, but also the many losses at the time of their traumatization that have not been worked through. In addition, their capacity to mourn may have been impaired by the trauma. Nevertheless, the disintegrating effects of psychic trauma can only be reduced or undone when sufficient mourning has taken place.

Acceptance of one's past and present states and experiences is another shared prerequisite for an adequate adaptation to aging and for trauma recovery. A further mutual challenge or task is the maintenance or establishment of a sense of self-coherence and feeling of continuity in the self. This is particularly difficult for trauma survivors, because their traumatic experiences may well have caused a serious rupture in their self-perception and sense of continuity. Under these circumstances, ego integrity, as the final goal of identity formation, can only be achieved with tremendous emotional and cognitive efforts. Traumatized subjects encounter various auxiliary hindrances to coping adequately with the process of aging. In fact, they have a double task to perform. It is therefore concluded that prior trauma represents a developmental risk during senescence.

Most of our present state of knowledge concerning delayed and long-term effects of traumatization is derived from treatment of and research with aging survivors of World War II—in particular, those who survived Nazi persecution. A similarity between the particular burdens of old age and the scarring experiences of Holocaust survivors has been recognized before. The losses that accompany senescence have been noted to reactivate not-worked-through traumatic contents. The symbolic likeness of, for instance, death and disease during Nazi persecution and the later phases of the life cycle has been cited to explain the decrease of resilience in elderly Holocaust survivors (Danieli, 1981; Krystal, 1981; Steinitz, 1982). The model presented in this chapter, however, surpasses the idiosyncratic, symbolic association of posttraumatic responses and the process of aging, and described the potentially disintegrative analogies between the two processes in more general and structural terms. Although survivors of World War II are the most thoroughly studied group of elderly trauma survivors, there is no reason to assume that theories concerning this group would not be relevant for trauma survivors in general.

Studies suggest that the immediate and later reactions of elderly people to traumatic events seem to be comparable to those of younger individuals. The literature does not give indications of changed susceptibility or different clinical manifestations and course. Furthermore, no evidence has been found that age or developmental stage at the time of traumatization influences late-life intensification or sudden onset of PTSD. In the empirical research on World War II survivors, military and resistance veterans varied in age at the times of their traumas from adolescents and young adults to mature adults. The ages of survivors of Nazi persecution under study varied widely. Clinical studies reveal that survivors of World War II who were traumatized as children may also suffer from a delayed onset or sudden exacerbation of posttraumatic symptoms during the transition from middle to late life (Bramsen, 1995). All studies, however, refer to long-lasting and severe traumatization. The interference of aging with the late sequelae of a sudden and brief traumatic experience, such as an accident or robbery, has yet to be corroborated.

Unfortunately, in our present society many groups and individuals are, or will be, traumatized. Among those who seemingly adapt fairly well for years or even for decades, some may well suffer from a late onset or aggravation of posttraumatic symptomatology during or after the midlife transition. However, when mental health professionals misconstrue posttraumatic symptoms (e.g., depression, anxiety, intrusive memories, chronic fatigue, and sleep disorders) as part and parcel of the degenerative process of aging, they may well miss the crucial diagnosis and deny aging trauma survivors an empathic understanding of their sufferings and adequate treatment. Probably as a consequence of the formerly dominating "deficiency model" of aging, mental health professionals tend to be pessimistic about the prognosis for psychotherapy in elderly patients (Ford & Sbordone, 1981; Blazer, 1982). For adequate treatment of aging trauma survivors, however, it is important to underscore and explore the psychodynamics that have led to their decompensation.

REFERENCES

Aarts, P. G. H., Op den Velde, W., Falger, P. R. J., Hovens, J. E., De Groen, J. H. M., & Van Duijin, H. (1996). Late onset posttraumatic stress disorder in aging resistance veterans in The Netherlands. In P. E. Ruskin & J. A. Talbott, (Eds.), *Aging and posttraumatic stress disorder* (pp. 53–78). Washington, DC: American Psychiatric Press.

Archibald, H. C., & Tuddenham, R. D. (1965). Persistent stress reaction after combat. *Archives of General Psychiatry, 12,* 475–481.

Askevold, F. (1980). The war sailor syndrome. *Danish Medical Bulletin, 77,* 220–223.

Assael, M., & Givon, M. (1984). The aging process in Holocaust survivors. *American Journal of Social Psychiatry, 4,* 32–36.

Bastiaans, J. (1957). *Psychosomatische gevolgen van onderdrukking en verzet [Psychosomatic consequences of oppression and resistance].* Amsterdam, the Netherlands: Noord-Hollandse Urtgevers Maatsohappij.

Berger, D. M. (1977). The survivor syndrome: A problem of nosology and treatment. *American Journal of Psychotherapy, 31,* 238–251.

Blazer, D. G. (1982). *Depression in late life.* St. Louis: C. V. Mosby.

Bramsen, I. (1995). *Psychological adjustment of World War II survivors.* Delft, The Netherlands: Eburon Press.

Cath, S. H. (1981). The effects of the Holocaust on life cycle experiences: The creation and recreation of families. *Journal of Geriatric Psychiatry, 14*(2), 155–163.

Coleman, P. G. (1986). *Aging and reminiscence processes: Social and clinical implications.* New York: Wiley.

Danieli, Y. (1981). Discussion: On the achievement of integration in aging survivors of the Nazi Holocaust. *Journal of Geriatric Psychiatry, 14*(2), 191–210.

Davidson, S. (1987). Trauma in the life cycle of the individual and the collective consciousness in relation to war and persecution. In H. Dasberg, S. Davidson, G. L. Durlacher, B. C. Filet, & E. de Wind (Eds.), *Society and trauma of war* (Sinaï Series no. 4, pp. 14–32). Assen, The Netherlands: Van Gorcum.

De Boer, M. C., Op den Velde, W., Falger, P. R. J., Hovens, J. E., De Groen, J. H. M., & Van Duijn, H. (1992). Fluvoxamine treatment for chronic PTSD: A pilot study. *Psychotherapy and Psychosomatics, 57,* 158–163.

Eissler, K. R. (1968). Weitere Bemerkungen zur Problem der KZ-Psychologie. *Psyche, 22,* 452–463.

Eitinger, L. (1961). Pathology of the concentration camp syndrome. *Archives of General Psychiatry, 5,* 371–379.

Erikson, E. H. (1965). *Childhood and society* (2nd ed.). Harmondsworth, England: Penguin Books.

Feinson, M. C., & Thoits, P. A. (1968). The distribution of distress among elders. *Journal of Gerontology, 41*(2), 225–233.

Ford, C. V., & Sbordone, R. J. (1981). Attitudes of psychiatrists toward elderly patients. *American Journal of Psychiatry, 137,* 571–575.

Green, B. L., Gleser, G. C., Lindy, J. D., Grace, M. C., & Leonard, A. (1996). Age-related reactions to the Buffalo Creek dam collapse: Second decade effects. In P. E. Ruskin & J. A. Talbott (Eds.), *Aging and posttraumatic stress disorder* (pp. 101–126). Washington, DC: American Psychiatric Press.

Hartvig, P. (1977). Krigsseilerssyndromet [The war-sailor syndrome]. *Nordisk Psykiatrisk Tidsskrift, 29,* 302–312.

Heeren, T. J. (1991). *Psychiatric morbidity in the oldest old: The Leiden 85-plus study.* Unpublished doctoral dissertation, University of Leiden.

Heeren, T. J. (1992). Ouderdom is geen risicofactor [Age is not a risk factor]. *Maandblad Geestelijke Volksgezondheid, 47*, 774–782.

Herman, J. L. (1992). *Trauma and recovery: The aftermath of violence—from domestic abuse to political terror.* New York: Basic Books.

Hertz, D. G. (1990). Trauma and nostalgia: New aspects on the coping of ageing Holocaust survivors. *Israel Journal of Psychiatry and Related Sciences, 27*(4), 189–198.

Honigman-Cooper, R. (1979). Concentration camp survivors: A challenge for geriatric nursing. *Nursing Clinics of North America, 14*(4), 621–628.

Hoppe, K. D. (1966). The psychodynamics of concentration camp victims. *Psychoanalytic Forum, 1*, 76–86.

Horowitz, M. S. (1976). *Stress response syndromes.* New York: Jason Aronson.

Kahana, R. J. (1981). Discussion: Reconciliation between the generations: A last chance. *Journal of Geriatric Psychiatry, 14*(2), 225–289.

Kohut, H. (1972). Thoughts on narcissism and narcissistic rage. *Psychoanalytic Study of the Child, 27*, 360–400.

Krystal, H. (Ed.). (1968). *Massive psychic trauma.* Boston: Little, Brown.

Krystal, H. (1981). Integration and self-healing in posttraumatic states. *Journal of Geriatric Psychiatry, 14*(2), 165–189.

Krystal, H. (1988). *Integration and self-healing: Affect, trauma and alexithymia.* Hillsdale, NJ: Atlantic Press.

Kuilman, M., & Suttorp, O. (1989, October). *Late onset posttraumatic spectrum disorders in survivors of Nazi terror: A retrospective study of 100 patients (1973–1988).* Paper presented at the Psychische Schäden alternder Überlebenden des Nazi-Terrors und ihrer Nachkommen conference, Hannover, West Germany.

Laufer, R. S. (1988). The serial self: War trauma, identity and adult development. In J. P. Wilson, Z. Harel, & B. Kahana (Eds.) *Human adaptation to extreme stress: From the Holocaust to Vietnam* (pp. 33–54). New York: Plenum Press.

Lifton, R. J. (1980). The concept of the survivor. In J. E. Dimsdale (Ed.), *Survivors, victims and perpetrators: Essays on the Nazi Holocaust* (pp. 113–126). New York: Hemisphere.

Lomranz, J., Shmotkin, D., Zechovoy, A., & Rosenberg, E. (1985). Time orientation in Nazi concentration camp survivors: Forty years after. *American Journal of Orthopsychiatry, 55*(2), 230–236.

McCann, J. L., & Pearlman, L. A. (1990). *Psychological trauma and the adult survivor: Theory, therapy and transformation.* New York: Brunner/Mazel.

Miller, T. W. (1988). Advances in understanding the impact of stressful life events on health. *Hospital and Community Psychiatry, 29*(6), 615–622.

Minkler, M. (1981). Research on the health effects of retirement. *Journal of Health and Social Behavior, 22*, 117–130.

Musaph, H. (1991). De Golfoorlog als trigger voor een late post-traumatische stressreactie [The Gulf War as a trigger for late onset PTSD]. *Tijdschrift voor Psychotherapie, 19*(6), 356–361.

Niederland, W. G., & Krystal, H. (1968). Clinical observations on the survivor syndrome. In H. Krystal (Ed.), *Massive psychic trauma* (pp. 327–348). Boston: Little, Brown.

Op den Velde, W., Hovens, J. E., Falger, P. R. J., De Groen, J. H. M., Van Duijn, H., Lasschuit, L. J., & Schouten, E. G. W. (1993). PTSD in Dutch resistance veterans from World War II. In J. P. Wilson & B. Raphael (Eds.), *International handbook of traumatic stress syndromes* (pp. 219–230). New York: Plenum Press.

Ornstein, A. (1981). The effects of the Holocaust on life-cycle experiences: The creation and recreation of families. *Journal of Geriatric Psychiatry, 14*(2), 135–154.

Palmore, E. B., Fillenbaum, G. G., & George, L. K. (1984). Consequences of retirement. *Journal of Gerontology, 39*(1), 109–116.

Randall, M. C., Walker, J. I., Ross, D. R., & Maltbie, A. A. (1981). Reactivation of traumatic conflicts. *American Journal of Psychiatry, 138*(7), 984–985.

Robinson, S., Netanel, R., & Rapaport, J. (1992). Reactions of Holocaust survivors to the Gulf War and Scud missile attacks on Israel. In S. Robinson (Ed.), *Echoes of the Holocaust (Bulletin of the Jerusalem Center for Research into the Late Effects of the Holocaust,* Talbieh Mental Health Center, No. 1, pp. 1–12). Jerusalem: Talbieh Mental Health Center.

Schmid, A. H. (1991). The deficiency model: An exploration of current approaches to late-life disorders. *Psychiatry, 54,* 358–367.

Schulz, R. (1982). Emotionality and aging: A theoretical and empirical analysis. *Journal of Gerontology, 37*(1), 42–51.

Shanan, J., & Shahar, O. (1983). Cognitive and personality functioning of Jewish Holocaust survivors during the midlife transition (46–65) in Israel. *Archiv für Psychologie, 135*(4), 275–294.

Shatan, C. F. (1991, October). *The Gulf—50 year gap in onset of PTSD.* Paper presented at the 7th Annual Conference on the International Society for Traumatic Stress Studies, Washington, DC.

Solomon, S. D. (1991, October). *Effects of aging on response to disaster.* Poster presented at the 7th Annual Conference of the International Society for Traumatic Stress Studies, Washington, DC.

Steinitz, L. Y. (1992). Psycho-social effects on the Holocaust on aging survivors and their families. *Journal of Gerontological Social Work, 4,* 145–152.

Tennant, C. C., Goulson, K., & Dent, O. (1993). Medical and psychiatric consequences of being a prisoner of war of the Japanese: An Australian follow-up study. In J. P. Wilson & B. Raphael (Eds.), *International handbook of traumatic stress syndromes* (pp. 231–240). New York: Plenum Press.

Ulman, R. B., & Brothers, D. (1988). *The shattered self: A psychoanalytic study of trauma.* Hillsdale, NJ: Analytic Press.

Van Driel, R. C., & Op den Velde, W. (1995). Myocardial infarction and posttraumatic stress disorder. *Journal of Traumatic Stress, 8,* 151–159.

Venzlaff, U. (1964). Mental disorders resulting from racial persecution outside of concentration camps. *International Journal of Social Psychiatry, 4,* 177–183.

CHAPTER 16

Legal Issues in Posttraumatic Stress Disorder

ROGER K. PITMAN
LANDY F. SPARR
LINDA S. SAUNDERS
ALEXANDER C. McFARLANE

Perhaps more than any other psychological or medical disorder, posttraumatic stress disorder (PTSD) has influenced, and been influenced by, the law. Nonpsychiatric incentives (e.g., the prospect of financial gain or avoidance of criminal punishment), which are present in all civil and criminal legal systems, have cast a shadow over the validity of the PTSD diagnosis and delayed its acceptance into diagnostic systems in psychiatry. Since this acceptance, however, PTSD has exerted a dramatic impact on forensic psychiatry and the law (Stone, 1993).

In civil law, the PTSD diagnosis represents landmark recognition that an external event can serve as the direct cause of a mental disorder, leading one authority to write, "Accurate assessment of PTSD-specific symptoms forms the basis for defining psychic injury in law" (Raifman, 1983, p.124). In criminal trials, PTSD is unique among mental disorders in its invocation by both prosecution and defense. The dissociative "flashback" experience has opened a new dimension in insanity defenses and related criminal defenses (Appelbaum et al., 1993; Sparr & Atkinson, 1986), insofar as a nonpsychotic defendant with PTSD may be alleged to have briefly lost contact with reality and become "temporarily insane." The presence of PTSD in a victim may be cited by the prosecution as "syndrome evidence" supporting the occurrence of a criminal act such as rape. PTSD is also occasionally invoked as grounds for civil commitment.

This chapter provides an overview and discussion of civil and criminal legal issues in PTSD. It also discusses forensic psychiatric evaluation and testimony in this new and rapidly developing area of forensic psychiatry.

CIVIL ISSUES

Traumatic versus Compensation Neurosis

The concept of mental injury as a compensable entity, of which PTSD represents the culmination, has gradually and incompletely emerged out of the historical context of physical injury. Conditions we would regard as psychiatric today appeared a century ago in physical guises such as "railway spine," "irritable heart," "effort syndrome," "neurocirculatory asthenia," and "shell-shock" (Scrignar, 1988). Even the term "traumatic neurosis" itself denotes physical abnormality (i.e., a pathological condition of the nerves). The recognition of psychological and emotional aspects of the causation and manifestation of injury-related mental disorders has only been accomplished over the past century (Hoffman, Rochon, & Terry, 1992).

Availability of compensation has long created an atmosphere of suspicion about traumatized persons, because of the perceived possibility that their distress is motivated by material gain. This suspicion is exemplified in the oxymoron "compensation neurosis," coined a century ago for the complaints of railway accident victims that were unexplainable on a physical basis. After World War I, the availability of pensions for shell-shock was blamed for the severity of the persisting symptoms. This led to the proposal that in future wars this disorder should not be compensated; in fact,this was the case in Germany after World War II.

It was formerly argued that as soon as the litigation was resolved, the symptoms of so-called "compensation neurosis" would disappear. This simplistic assertion has been largely discredited (for a review, see Resnick, 1994). Mayou, Bryant, and Duthie (1993) examined the effects of motor vehicle accidents in cases where only a portion of the victims were able to sue. Litigation status did not influence the prevalence of psychiatric disorder, course, or chronicity of associated disabilities; severe chronic physical and psychological symptoms were also found in the nonlitigating group. McFarlane (in press) found similar results in groups of litigating and nonlitigating victims of the Ash Wednesday bush fire disaster in Australia, who were followed over an 11-year period. Brooks and McKinlay (1992), using Resnick's criteria, found no evidence of symptom manufacturing in 66 residents of Lockerbie, Scotland, following the crash of a jetliner over that village after a terrorist bomb explosion. In contrast, Frueh, Smith, & Barker (in press) reported more evidence of symptom exaggeration on psychological testing in compensation-seeking Vietnam veterans than in their non-compensation-seeking peers.

Despite the above-described studies, confusion often remains about the difference between PTSD and compensation neurosis. Against this background, a forensic psychiatric claim of PTSD may be expected to be subjected to substantial scrutiny.

Tort Litigation

Roughly speaking, a "tort" is an injury resulting from a wrongful (intentional or negligent) act of omission or commission, which potentially entitles the victim to compensation for damages. Traditionally, legal systems have resisted claims of mental damages. The reasons probably involve a combination of stigmatization of mental illness, belief that mental symptoms are under the individual's voluntary control, suspicion of malingering, dearth of reliable criteria for determining the existence and extent of mental damages, and fear of frivolous litigation.

In order to be successful in a tort action, a claim must pass through a series of "filters" (Spaulding, 1988). First, the defendant must be found to have borne a duty of care to the plaintiff and to have been derelict in that duty. Next, the defendant's act must be shown to have been the proximate cause of the plaintiff's reasonably foreseeable injury. Next, damages must be demonstrated. In many jurisdictions, claims for mental damages must then pass through one or more of several additional filters that reflect the law's distrust of such claims. These may involve, from the most to least restrictive:

1. Requiring a physical impact upon the plaintiff.
2. Requiring the plaintiff to have been in the so-called "zone of danger," and hence exposed to the possibility of physical impact.
3. Requiring a physical injury to have ensued from the mental injury.
4. Requiring the mental injury to have physical manifestations.

PTSD has become the most important diagnosis in the forensic psychiatry of personal injury because of the ways it potentially overcomes traditional legal restrictions on mental damages claims. Psychiatric epidemiological studies have demonstrated that the PTSD syndrome is caused by an external event, thereby supporting proximate causation. Acceptance of the idea that a mental disorder can result from a specific event has had to overcome influential views within psychiatry that mental disorders are caused by either internal conflicts of early childhood origin, inborn genetic abnormalities, or other, unknown factors. Epidemiological studies have shown that the incidence of PTSD resulting from more severe events is substantial, thereby supporting foreseeability (Spaulding, 1988). Although the PTSD diagnosis cannot help a plaintiff pass through the more restrictive "physical impact" or "zone of danger" filters, which are being phased out in most legal jurisdictions, it may help overcome the less restrictive filters arbitrarily applied to mental damages claims. Although courts vary in what they consider to constitute "physical injury" or "physical manifestations," some have held that these concepts require only that that the condition represent a disorder that is susceptible to objective medical determination. Courts generally regard PTSD's inclusion in the official psychiatric nomenclature as grounds for its meeting this standard (Saunders, Pitman, & Orr, 1993). The current diagnostic criteria for PTSD also include potentially measurable physical manifestations (e.g., exaggerated startle response and specific physiological reactivity.)

PTSD is one of only a few disorders for which the cause is considered to be known (American Psychiatric Association, 1994; World Health Organization, 1992). This means that other mental disorders commonly associated with personal injury litigation (e.g., mood disorders, somatoform disorders, and other anxiety disorders) may be expected to encounter more difficulty than PTSD in meeting the legal requirements of proximate causation and foreseeability. As Spaulding (1988) has noted, "The further from the diagnosis of PTSD the evaluator strays, the more speculative the opinion on causation will become" (p. 13). For this reason, Spaulding recommends that the forensic psychiatric "evaluation process should begin with an attempt to sort claims into those that involve a diagnosis of PTSD and those that do not" (p. 12). This illustrates the watershed that PTSD has become in mental tort litigation.

Workers' Compensation

Workers' compensation law shares with tort law a traditional distrust of mental damages claims, reflected in the exclusion in many jurisdictions of "ordinary diseases of life" and so-called "mental–mental" claims (Colbach, 1982; Sersland, 1983–1984). "Mental–mental" claims refer to a psychological problem caused by a psychological stressor, without a physical element in either the cause or the effect. As they do in tort law, the special features of PTSD help it overcome legal barriers under workers' compensation. Whereas mood disorders and other anxiety disorders may be argued to represent "ordinary diseases of life," the recognition that PTSD is caused by a discrete external event (e.g., a workplace accident) removes it from this exclusionary category. PTSD's associated physical manifestations also potentially exempt it from "mental–mental" exclusions. Given the severely traumatic events associated with combat, PTSD logically represents the most compensable of mental disorders under veterans' disability benefits, a form of workers' compensation (Sparr, White, Friedman, & Wiles, 1994).

Private Disability Insurance

Many private insurers offer disability policies that pay when the policy holder becomes unable to perform the specific duties of his or her specific occupation, even though he or she may be able to perform some other occupation. In cases where the disability arises as the result of an occupation-related incident, the presence of PTSD symptoms (e.g., intense psychological distress upon exposure to reminders of the traumatic event and efforts to avoid such reminders) may in some cases be argued to confer on the individual a specific inability to perform his or her own occupation that more general mood and anxiety symptoms may not.

Effect of the Litigation Process on the PTSD Patient

The capacity of the incentive of compensation to reinforce psychiatric symptomatology is embodied in the concept of "secondary gain." However, litigation may also influence primary PTSD symptoms through a process of retraumatization. Requiring the PTSD patient to confront his or her traumatic history during interviews with attorneys and consultants, depositions, and courtroom testimony thwarts characteristic efforts at avoidance and predictably results in the resurgence of intrusive ideation and increased arousal. The wish to avoid the distress caused by retelling the traumatic experience may lead some plaintiffs to accept less than adequate settlements. An adversarial system of justice pits the plaintiff once again against the defendant, whom the patient, through the occurrence of the traumatic event, may already have come to see as an enemy. A patient uneducated as to the workings of such a system, including the purpose of cross-examination, may come to perceive (rightly or wrongly) that the system is protecting the tortfeasor and placing the plaintiff on trial. Such a perception may exacerbate the PTSD patient's sense of vulnerability and victimization. Often a plaintiff will already have sustained major final loss as a result of the traumatic event. Pursuit of litigation involves further financial risk, as well as anxiety, because a positive outcome is not guaranteed. Ironically, many plaintiffs seek understanding more than money; a system that attempts to translate all damages into a financial bottom line may be ill equipped to provide such understanding.

Napier (1991) has argued that delays and failures in public judicial fact-finding procedures regarding the circumstances of disasters may further traumatize victims:

> ... the legal system is poorly designed to cope with disaster aftermath. ... The victims frequently feel that in the legal process their interests come well down in the list of considerations. ... The result is that the medical trauma of the disaster is worsened by further trauma to the victims as they battle with a confusing system that is often slow and ineffective in providing the answers that they and the public reasonably seek. (p. 158)

Civil Commitment

Although the specific legal criteria authorizing involuntary commitment (either emergency or nonemergency) vary across jurisdictions, in principle involuntary civil commitment is justified upon a medical, judicial, or administrative finding of dangerousness to self or others by reason of mental illness. In some jurisdictions, the law may not define requisite mental illness in terms of officially psychiatrically recognized mental disorders. Nevertheless, the presence of one or more such disorders is viewed as significant in assessing the legal mental illness criterion for commitment.

It is not uncommon that a petitioner seeks the involuntary emergency commitment of an allegedly suicidal individual with a past trauma history (e.g., a child abuse victim). Sometimes a PTSD diagnosis in such a person is offered to support the proposition that a suicide attempt or gesture is the product of a mental illness. Self-destructive behavior, however, is not a recognized feature of PTSD. Rather, when present in PTSD individuals, it is almost always the product of one or more comorbid conditions (e.g., depression, substance dependence or abuse, or borderline personality disorder). In such cases, the determination of dangerousness to self properly revolves more around the current status of the comorbid disorder(s) than around that of the PTSD.

Angry outbursts have been formally recognized as manifestations of PTSD arousal disturbance. Such outbursts, however, are usually intermittent. PTSD does not entail the capacity for the kind of sustained disturbance in thinking or affect typically associated with schizophrenia or melancholia, which allows for a confident determination of prospective harmfulness. In summary, reliance on a diagnosis of PTSD alone as a causal basis of harmfulness to self or others sufficient for forcible detention is rarely justified.

Other Civil Issues

In the domestic arena, in jurisdictions retaining fault grounds for divorce, the presence of PTSD in one spouse may be offered as proof of the other's extreme cruelty. Similarly, in child custody determinations, the presence of PTSD in a child may be invoked as proof of parental cruelty and unfitness. Conversely, an adult may occasionally invoke his or her own PTSD condition as a mitigating factor in behavior toward a spouse or child. Indeed, it sometimes seems that there is no end to the creative uses to which the PTSD diagnosis may be put in legal actions, as the following section illustrates further.

CRIMINAL ISSUES

PTSD as a Criminal Defense

In order for a person to be held criminally responsible, two elements are necessary: a criminal act (*actus reus*) and criminal intent (*mens rea*). Criminal defenses in which the presence of a mental illness may be argued to have diminished criminal intent include not guilty by reason of insanity, diminished capacity, and unconsciousness/automatism. The number of defendants seeking either acquittal or sentence reduction because of the alleged effects of PTSD has steadily increased since 1980 (Speir, 1989). Use of PTSD as a basis for reduced criminal intent is difficult, however, because generally persons with PTSD have lost neither their contact with reality nor their appreciation of wrongfulness. For this reason, the dissociative state seems to have become almost the *sine qua non* for the PTSD criminal defense. The PTSD diagnosis is vulnerable to legal challenge on other grounds as well. Stressor identification may be called into question, or symptom assessment or causation may be contested, with prior susceptibility or intervening factors offered in rebuttal.

Insanity Defense

Although the insanity defense has received much public notoriety, its use is uncommon. In most jurisdictions, insanity is an "affirmative" defense; that is, the defendant bears the burden of proving that he or she was insane at the time of the alleged crime. Sometimes this proof must be accomplished by means of "clear and convincing evidence." A recent study of 967,209 felony indictments revealed insanity pleas in only 8,953 instances (0.93%), with an acquittal rate of 26% (Callahan, Steadman, McGreevy, & Robbins, 1991). Of these insanity pleas, only 28 (0.30%) were based on a PTSD diagnosis, with a comparable acquittal rate of 29% (Appelbaum et al., 1993). These data highlight two facts: The PTSD insanity defense is raised infrequently, and, like other insanity pleas, it is usually unsuccessful.

Two types of legal standards for insanity exist, one cognitive and the other volitional. The first and most famous is the "*M'Naghtan* rule," also known as the "right or wrong" test. This standard requires that the defendant did not know the nature and quality of his or her act, or that the act was wrong. It is sufficient to establish insanity in nearly all legal jurisdictions. Many other jurisdictions add an alternative, volitional test of insanity. Typically, the volitional standard requires the individual to have lacked the capacity to conform his or her conduct to the requirements of the law. Another volitional test is that the act was the product of an irresistible impulse. Certain crimes of passion may fit this model. A problem with this rule is immediately apparent, however: how to distinguish an impulse that was truly irresistible from an impulse that was simply, for whatever reason, unresisted (Gutheil, 1989).

Almost the only conceivable way that PTSD can qualify a defendant for insanity under the *M'Naghten* rule is for the disorder to have manifested itself at the time of the act in a full-blown dissociative or flashback state. As a result, the defendant would have to show that he or she lost contact with, and appreciation of, reality. Any evidence of rational behavior at the time of the alleged crime (e.g., trying to conceal it) is highly damaging to such a defense. Under a volitional test of insanity, a PTSD sufferer who was in at least partial contact with reality might still be able to show that extremely powerful impulses deriving from the disorder prevented him or her from adhering to the lawful course of action, even though he or she retained some appreciation of the wrongfulness of the act committed.

To all the above-described insanity tests is added the requirement that the respective cognitive or volitional impairment be caused by a mental disease or defect. Some jurisdictions require that the mental disease or defect be severe, as a means of ensuring that neuroses, nonpsychotic behavior disorders, substance abuse, or antisocial tendencies do not suffice for insanity defenses. A pivotal question is whether PTSD qualifies as a severe mental disorder. As a minimum, a PTSD dissociative state should qualify if it entails a drastic alteration of an individual's cognitive capacity (Davidson, 1988). Nevertheless, the severity restriction tends to work against the effectiveness of PTSD as the basis for an insanity defense.

Diminished Capacity

Evidence of an abnormal mental condition not amounting to insanity is inadmissible in some jurisdictions. In others, however, such evidence is admissible for arguing that the defendant did not possess the requisite mental state pertinent to the crime for which he or she has been charged. This is variably referred to as "diminished responsibility," "partial responsibility," "partial capacity," "diminished capacity," and "partial insanity" (Morris, 1975; Slovenko, 1992). The diminished capacity defense focuses on the question of which crime the defendant may be held responsible for. For example, in a first-degree murder charge, many jurisdictions allow a defendant to introduce evidence that he or she did not have the mental capacity to premeditate the act, and that for this reason, only second-degree murder at most could have been committed. The court may also consider diminished capacity in sentencing.

Since the tightening of insanity defense standards, the use of PTSD in criminal proceedings has more applicability to the question of diminished capacity, and in fact it has been more often used in that role. Several different dynamic aspects of PTSD may potentially reflect diminished capacity in a defendant (Grant & Coons, 1983; Sparr, Reaves, & Atkinson, 1987): (1) sensation seeking or so-called "addiction to trauma"; (2) need for punishment to appease a sense of guilt connected with the traumatic event; and (3) substance abuse in an attempt to numb posttraumatic psychic pain, with resultant disinhibited actions.

Lack of Consciousness/Automatism

Another *mens rea* defense has to do with dissociative states that are beyond conscious control or even conscious awareness. PTSD is on a short list of disorders, mostly organic, that can entail such states. Traumatic experiences in which a person's voluntary will is physically overridden may stimulate dissociation at the time and predispose the individual to subsequent dissociative reactions. Under this defense, the individual charged argues that he or she was not conscious of the act, and therefore cannot be held criminally responsible for it (Higgins, 1991; Thomson, 1991). Courts, however, are traditionally reluctant to excuse wrongdoers from responsibility because of claimed amnesia or subjective nonvolition. Criminals frequently claim amnesia for an illegal act. To separate the malingerers from those persons whose behavior is the result of a true dissociative state is difficult.

A related plea is the little-used defense of "automatism," which arises from the historical legal requirement of a volitional act. This plea may apply to PTSD veterans who performed repeated, sanctioned acts of violence in the combat situation and subsequently find themselves losing control of violent behavior after their return to civilian life (Erlinder, 1984). Perhaps the most commonly encountered clinical example of automatism is that of the combat veteran who awakens in a violent rage after being shaken, prodded, or even only touched while asleep. Another example involves police officers, who may have traumatic backgrounds by virtue of the nature of their work. During shootouts, some police officers report having gone on "automatic pilot," unaware even of the number of bullets they were firing. In such instances, the trier of fact may be called upon to determine whether the preautomatic portion of the violent behavior was lawfully permissible (Kleinman, Martell, & Gioiella, 1993). For example, persons with PTSD, charged with excessive use of force in self-defense, have been exonerated after testimony that they entered a state of automatism after having been assaulted, and subsequently became unable to form requisite intent.

Self-Defense

Feminists and victims' advocates have come to regard the use of PTSD to support a self-defense plea as more politically acceptable than an insanity plea, because it does not stigmatize the victim as irrational. This affirmative defense requires the defendant to demonstrate that self-defensive responses at the time of the act were subjectively reasonable—in other words, that he or she reasonably believed that the use of force was necessary for self-protection. In some case, the existence of PTSD may aid a defendant in showing that a particular type of provocation to which the defendant had become especially sensitive in light of previous traumatization caused him or her to feel physically threatened and evoked a reasonable self-defensive reaction. The most familiar example is use of "battered woman syndrome" (Goodstein & Page, 1981) to explain a female defendant's violent acts toward her spouse or partner. This syndrome may also be evoked to explain why women in such circumstances do not simply leave their abusers. Some courts have held that expert testimony regarding battered woman syndrome is admissible for the purpose of educating the jury as to how a history of abuse at the hands of her spouse or partner may support a woman's claim that she reasonably believed she was in imminent danger. In contrast, other courts have rejected battered woman syndrome evidence by holding that because the defendant was not in imminent danger at the time of the alleged criminal act, such evidence is irrelevant to the question of reasonableness (Lustberg & Jacobi, 1992).

Psychiatric Factors Supporting a PTSD Criminal Defense

The following factors tend to support a PTSD-related criminal defense (Auberry, 1985; Blank, 1985; Marciniak, 1986): (1) the act represents spontaneous, unpremeditated behavior uncharacteristic of the individual; (2) coherent dialogue appropriately related to time and place is lacking; (3) the choice of victim is fortuitous or accidental; (4) the response is disproportionate to the provocation; (5) the act is rationally inexplicable and lacks current motivation; (6) the act recreates in a psychologically meaningful way elements of the original traumatic stressor; (7) the defendant is unaware of the ways in which he or she has reenacted traumatic experiences; (8) the act is precipitated by events or circumstances that realistically or symbolically force the individual to face unresolved conflicts; and (9) there is amnesia for the episode.

PTSD in Criminal Prosecution

The defense has not enjoyed a monopoly on the use of PTSD in criminal trials. The prosecution may attempt to use a PTSD diagnosis in a victim as circumstantial evidence supporting the occurrence of a criminal act. The rationale is clear but potentially circular: Because a traumatic event is required for PTSD, if a victim has the PTSD syndrome, then a traumatic event must have befallen him or her. Such "syndrome evidence" (Slovenko, 1984) has most often arisen in rape trials (Burgess & Holstrom, 1974), although it potentially applies to other violent crimes such as armed robbery and attempted murder. Courts universally allow PTSD testimony in civil rape cases, where the testimony is entered not to show that the rape occurred but to assess damage once it has been proven. In criminal rape trials, however, where testimony is entered to demonstrate that a rape actually occurred, "rape trauma syndrome" has received a mixed legal reception. Such evidence is most often presented in trials where the defendant admits that sexual intercourse occurred but claims that the act was consensual. In this situation, the testimony is offered to corroborate the complainant's version of the facts. Research supports the assumption that jurors are not familiar with the typical reactions of rape victims (Frazier & Borgida, 1988) and may be assisted by expert testimony (e.g., with regard to PTSD).

In the law, determination of witness credibility is traditionally left to the jury. Some courts have excluded expert testimony on rape trauma syndrome, on the grounds that it is prejudicial and invades the jury's fact-finding province. The question of prejudicial impact is closely tied to helpfulness. Rape trauma syndrome evidence is deemed prejudicial when expert testimony improperly bolsters a complainant's credibility by creating an "aura of special reliability and trustworthiness" (Frazier & Borgida, 1985, p. 992). Determination of prejudice is also affected by the way evidence is presented. The testimony is least prejudicial if it merely describes the victim's behavior; more prejudicial if this behavior is causally linked to the alleged rape; and still more prejudicial if the expert testifies that he or she believes the complainant's assertion that a rape actually occurred.

Presentation of PTSD syndrome evidence may be a two-edged sword for the victim, in that it may open the door to cross-examination regarding other details of the victim's personal life (Frazier & Borgida, 1985). The defendant's attorneys may attempt to unearth skeletons from the victim's past in an effort to discredit the notion that the alleged rape, and not some other traumatic life event, caused the PTSD. The defense may insist on having the victim examined by its own psychiatric expert, and this examination may be particularly stressful (Buchele & Buchele, 1985). If the victim does not exhibit sufficient PTSD symptoms to satisfy the defense expert, the defense, by turning the "syndrome evidence" issue on its head, may attempt to use this to contend that no rape occurred (Trosch, 1991).

FORENSIC EVALUATION OF PTSD AND EXPERT TESTIMONY

Forensic Psychiatric Examination

History

History taking poses a dilemma for the forensic evaluator of PTSD. Because of the acknowledged tendency of PTSD patients to avoid painful recollections of the trauma, superficial questioning may fail to elicit all the symptoms that are actually present. On the other hand, direct inquiry regarding the PTSD diagnostic criteria may be treated by motivated respondents as a series of leading questions, evoking answers that lead too readily to a PTSD diagnosis. Since the diagnostic criteria for PTSD are available through publication and word of mouth, there is little to stop a motivated claimant from learning what symptoms must be reported in an attempt to qualify for the diagnosis (Sparr & Pankratz, 1983). The competent psychiatric or clinical psychological evaluator must avoid the Scylla of naive disregard of this reality and the Charybdis of cynical preoccupation with it. These are formidable obstacles to a reliable forensic evaluation of PTSD, but the skilled evaluator is not without tools to overcome them.

The first such tool is nondirective interviewing. The interviewer should begin by asking the claimant to describe the problems he or she has been experiencing, and then should allow the claimant to talk with as little interruption as possible. A claimant who talks for 15 or 30 minutes and hardly mentions a symptom consistent with PTSD, but who answers positively to almost all PTSD symptoms during subsequent direct questioning, should be regarded with justifiable suspicion.

Another tool is insistence on detailed illustration. Knowledgeable or coached claimants may know which PTSD symptoms to report, but being able to illustrate them with convincing, personal life details is another matter. The interviewer should not simply take the claimant's word for it that he or she suffers from nightmares or intrusive recollections, but should require the claimant to describe several of these as fully as possible. Invented symptoms will have a vague and stilted quality. The interviewer must determine whether the history being presented has the quality of a personal autobiography or merely a textbook recitation.

While gathering personal details during the history-taking process, the interviewer should look toward the preparation of the forensic report and ultimately toward the testimony. Just as the evaluator in the forensic (as opposed to therapeutic) setting is unwilling to accept the claimant's word that he or she has a certain symptom without being shown how and why, the evaluator should not expect the jury to accept the evaluator's word that the claimant has or does not have PTSD, without being shown how or why. The evaluator's ultimate goal is to present to the jury a history that speaks for itself.

Use of Structured Interview Instruments

Following the nondirective portion of the interview, the evaluator should conduct a directive interview that inquires into each PTSD diagnostic criterion in turn, as well as into the criteria of every other Axis I and Axis II mental disorder that potentially enters into the differential diagnosis. Psychiatric researchers are now required to determine the presence or absence of diagnostic criteria in a systematic, reliable manner, which is usually accomplished by means of structured interview instruments. Because the need for reliability in the medico-legal setting is equally great, forensic evaluations call for a similar approach. Examples of structured interview instruments include the Clinician-Administered PTSD Scale (CAPS; Blake et al., 1995), the Structured Clinical Interview for DSM-IV Axis I Disorders (SCID-I; First, Spitzer, Gibbon, & Williams, 1994a), and the Structured Clinical Interview for DSM-IV Axis II Personality Disorders (SCID-II; First, Spitzer, Gibbon, & Williams, 1994b). The

CAPS has the additional advantage of incorporating a severity measure as well as a categorical measure of PTSD. An instrument available for the detection of malingering is the Structured Interview for Reported Symptoms (Rogers, Bagby, & Dickens, 1992).

It should be kept in mind that professionally administered instruments such as the CAPS, the SCID-I, and the SCID-II do not require the interviewer to score an item positive just because the interviewee answers affirmatively, or vice versa. It is the interviewer's responsibility through probing to determine whether the detailed historical data satisfy the symptomatic criterion in question.

Mental Status Examination

While eliciting the history, the evaluator should pay close attention to the claimant's behavior. Some PTSD symptoms (e.g., irritability, difficulty concentrating, or exaggerated startle reactions) may be directly observed. Also of relevance is whether the claimant's behavior and affect are consistent with the history he or she is providing. The display of genuine emotion, or the lack of it, during the rendition of the traumatic event and its sequelae can be revealing. Jurors will be looking for the same thing when the plaintiff testifies at trial.

Psychometric Testing

A number of questionnaire instruments yield numerical scores pertinent to the presence or absence, as well as the severity, of PTSD (see Chapter 11, this volume). However, evaluators must be aware that many of these instruments do not incorporate validity scales as checks for symptom exaggeration. Moreover, research has indicated that even the instrument with the best validity scales (viz., the Minnesota Multiphasic Personality Inventory) may fail to detect fabricated PTSD (Lees-Haley, 1990; Perconte & Goreczny, 1990). This consideration makes psychometric tests useful only as screening tools, or as ancillary tests to confirm or call into question the evaluator's total impressions.

Psychophysiological Testing

Laboratory measurement of physiological responsivity during exposure to cues related to a traumatic event has been described as "the best and most specific biological diagnostic test for PTSD" (Friedman, 1991, p. 74). Pitman and Orr (1993) have recently proposed that such measurement "has the potential to redeem the PTSD diagnosis from its current subjectivity and to help separate the wheat from the chaff in the forensic evaluation of PTSD claims" (p. 40). Those proposing the utility of psychophysiological testing emphasize that its results, like the results of psychometric testing, do not stand on their own, but serve as only one component of a comprehensive forensic psychiatric evaluation for PTSD.

Evaluation of Functional Impairment

A PTSD diagnosis by itself is not informative to the legal process. Rather, it is necessary that it be translated into one or more functional impairments (Spaulding, 1988). Prognosis must be made on the basis of the individual case, but should be compatible with research knowledge regarding the course of PTSD (see Chapter 8, this volume). Because the literature indicates that many cases of PTSD improve over time, predictions of total, permanent disability are rarely justified in the immediate aftermath of the traumatic event, although they may on occasion become justified if a chronic course becomes evident. It is generally agreed that the PTSD diagnosis entails an indefinite vulnerability to relapse.

Some functional determinations require delicate clinical judgment. For example, in the case of a work-related traumatic event, the evaluator may be called upon to determine whether the evaluee is capable of returning to the work situation where the traumatic event occurred. Predictably, this will stimulate distressing recollections in a PTSD sufferer. The question will be whether reintroduction will result in eventual desensitization to the work environment and return to employability, with accompanying improvement in the PTSD, or further traumatization and an increase in symptomatology, with accompanying demoralization and loss of self-esteem. In such cases, considerations not immediately related to the PTSD (e.g., the evaluee's motivation or available support system) may be determinative.

Evaluation of functional impairment is also critical in cases of civil commitment, but here the relevant impairment is strictly limited to the individual's ability to refrain from self-harm or harm to others. In criminal insanity defenses, it is not prospective, but retrospective, impairment that is the critical issue.

Use of Collateral Sources

Although psychiatrists and clinical psychologists should not become detectives, there are good reasons to place greater emphasis on outside sources of information in forensic evaluations than in ordinary clinical evaluations. Such sources may either substantiate or cast doubt on the occurrence and severity of the traumatic event, as well as the subsequent emotional disturbance and functional impairment reported by the claimant. In the assessment of combat-related PTSD, military records (including unit activity reports, decorations, and discharge papers) are routinely reviewed by rating boards. Examples of important potential sources of information in nonmilitary PTSD cases include police reports, nurses' notes, and employee proficiency reports. When witnesses to the traumatic event and the claimant's subsequent behavior and functioning are available, they should be interviewed by telephone or in person.

Expert Testimony Regarding PTSD

Scope

Legal advocates seem to have a thirst for expert psychiatric and psychological testimony, and sometimes attempt to push such experts beyond the limits of their knowledge (Sparr & Boehnlein, 1990). This state of affairs emphasizes the need for quality assurance in forensic psychiatric assessments. Mental health professionals who render testimony on either a willing or an unwilling basis can avoid problems if they stick to describing the evaluee's history, signs and symptoms, diagnostic conditions, and mental disabilities, and leave the judge and jury to weigh these in the context of legal standards. The expert should not attempt to resolve questions of damages, competence, or criminal responsibility. In determining the admissibility of an expert's opinion, the judge will weigh its probative value against its possible prejudicial effect. Judges may also evaluate the validity of opinions proffered as scientific (Marwick, 1993; Steinberg, 1993).

Educating Jurors Regarding PTSD

A main task of an expert is to educate jurors on matters beyond their common-sense understanding. PTSD is a good example. Jurors tend projectively to identify with a plaintiff or defendant, and may have trouble understanding how that person could have felt or acted any differently than how they themselves would have (or like to think they would have) felt or acted in the same situation. For example, a juror may fail to understand how a plaintiff could still be bothered by an event that happened many years ago and wonder why the plaintiff just doesn't get on with his or her life, which would be the rational thing to do. The expert must help jurors understand that a mental disorder such as PTSD is an irrational phenomenon.

Misuse of PTSD

Frequently the legal profession is accused of abusing PTSD, but this is a fallacy. Because only a clinician can make a diagnosis, only a clinician can abuse it. Lawyers cannot introduce a PTSD diagnosis into evidence except through the testimony of a clinical expert. Misuse of the PTSD diagnosis by experts may arise out of either ignorance or bias. Some uneducated experts regard virtually any emotional disturbance that follows an untoward event as synonymous with PTSD, and fail to apply the diagnostic criteria or to consider differential possibilities. Other experts never find PTSD because they do not know how to recognize it. Bias regarding PTSD sometimes arises from sympathy with, or antipathy toward, the "sociopolitical ideology of victimization" (Stone, 1993, p. 24). A misapplied PTSD diagnosis at times represents a vehicle for what Szasz (1962) has termed "bootlegging humanistic values through psychiatry." Such misapplication, however well intended, reduces the credibility of the diagnosis and the profession.

Common errors leading to the forensic overdiagnosis of PTSD include the following:

1. Failure to separate expectable emotional distress from mental disorder.
2. Application of fewer criteria than are required for the proper diagnosis.
3. Failure to consider the contribution of earlier, unrelated traumatic events to the evaluee's illness, with resulting false attribution to the traumatic event being litigated.
4. Failure to diagnose preexisting psychopathology.
5. Failure to identify a positive family history of mental disorder that may point to another etiology.
6. Failure to entertain a differential diagnosis.

Common errors leading to the forensic underdiagnosis of PTSD include the following:

1. Characterization of PTSD symptoms as mere understandable, normal reactions to the traumatic event.
2. Basing opinion on superficial, open-ended interviews, without an adequate attempt to explore details of the traumatic event and subsequent symptomatology.
3. Idiosyncratic thresholds for diagnosis.
4. Failure to acknowledge that the diagnosis of PTSD may be made despite the presence of major vulnerability factors.
5. Mistaking predisposition for preexisting psychopathology.
6. False attribution of the evaluee's symptoms to other life events.
7. Espousal of narrow or outdated theories of etiology that may play on popular prejudices (e.g., "All mental illness results from early childhood," or "All mental illness is inherited").
8. Failure to consider relevant, supportive PTSD literature.

Special Considerations in Criminal Cases

For reasons discussed above, experts should be especially wary about rendering testimony that implies that the presence of PTSD proves the factual occurrence of a crime, or even a negligent act, on the part of a defendant. A prominent psychiatric task force has gone so far to declare: "In the absence of a scientific foundation for attributing a person's behavior or mental condition to a single past event, such testimony should be viewed as a misuse of psychiatric expertise" (Halleck, Hoge, Miller, Sadoff, & Halleck, 1992, p. 495). Experts testifying in criminal cases must take care to distinguish between the mere presence of PTSD on the one hand, and a causal connection between the PTSD and the act in question on the other. Often the prosecution will not challenge the diagnosis will but will point to secondary factors, such as financial problems, interpersonal conflicts, or substance abuse, as proximate motivations for the criminal activity. Although some of these factors may reflect PTSD symptoms, they are not generally regarded as sufficient to relieve an individual from criminal responsibility. Experts must be prepared to address these issues.

CONCLUSION

Legal advocates may be expected to continue to turn to psychiatric, psychological, and other mental health professionals familiar with PTSD who can provide opinions they deem helpful to their cases. Professionals responding to such calls, who presumably already possess expertise in PTSD, have the responsibility to educate themselves in the ways the diagnosis can be used and abused in the legal setting, in order that their participation may further rather than hinder the pursuit of justice. Professionals must also remain cognizant of the vulnerability of PTSD patients and their capacity for retraumatization by the legal process. Although forensic clinicians may not bear responsibility for the treatment of their evaluees, they still maintain an ethical obligation to deal with them honestly, objectively, and empathically, and to do them no harm.

REFERENCES

American Psychiatric Association. (1994). *Diagnostic and statistical manual of mental disorders* (4th ed.). Washington, DC: Author.

Appelbaum, P. S., Jick, R. Z., Grisso, T., Givelber, D., Silver, E., & Steadman, H. J. (1993). Use of posttraumatic stress disorder to support an insanity defense. *American Journal of Psychiatry, 150,* 229–234.

Auberry, A. R. (1985). PTSD: Effective representation of a Vietnam veteran in the criminal justice system. *Marquette Law Review, 68,* 648–675.

Blake, D. D., Weathers, F. W., Nagy, L. M., Kaloupek, D. G., Gusman, F. D., Charney, D. S., & Keane, T. M. (1995). The development of a clinician-administered PTSD scale. *Journal of Traumatic Stress, 8,* 75–90.

Blank, A. S. (1985). The unconscious flashback to the war in Viet Nam veterans: Clinical mystery, legal defense, and community problem. In S. M. Sonnenberg, A. S.

Blank, & J. A. Talbott (Eds.), *The trauma of war: Stress and recovery in Viet Nam veterans* (pp. 293–308). Washington, DC: American Psychiatric Press.

Brooks, N., & McKinlay, W. (1992). Mental health consequences of the Lockerbie disaster. *Journal of Traumatic Stress,5,* 527–543.

Buchele, B. J., & Buchele, J. P. (1985). Legal and psychological issues in the use of expert testimony on rape trauma syndrome. *Washburn Law Journal, 25,* 26–42.

Burgess, A., & Holmstrom, L. (1974). Rape trauma syndrome. *American Journal of Psychiatry, 131,* 980–986.

Callahan, L. A., Steadman, H. J., McGreevy, M. A., & Robbins, P. C. (1991). The volume and characteristics of insanity defense pleas: An eight-state study. *Bulletin of the American Academy of Psychiatry and the Law, 19,* 331–338.

Colbach, E. M. (1982). The mental–mental muddle and work comp in Oregon. *Bulletin of the American Academy of Psychiatry and the Law, 10,* 165–169.

Davidson, M. J. (1988). Post-traumatic stress disorder: A controversial defense for veterans of a controversial war. *William and Mary Law Review, 29,* 415–440.

Erlinder, C. P. (1984). Paying the price for Vietnam: Post-traumatic stress disorder and criminal behavior. *Boston College Law Review, 25,* 305–347.

First, M. B., Spitzer, R. L., Gibbon, M., & Williams, J. B. W. (1994a). *Structured Clinical Interview for DSM-IV Axis I Disorders, Version 2.0* (May 1994 draft). New York: New York State Psychiatric Institute.

First, M. B., Spitzer, R. L., Gibbon, M., & Williams, J. B. W. (1994b). *Structured Clinical Interview for DSM-IV Axis II Personality Disorders, Version 2.0* (July 1994 draft). New York: New York State Psychiatric Institute.

Frazier, P., & Borgida, E. (1985). Rape trauma syndrome evidence in court. *American Psychologist, 40,* 984–993.

Frazier, P., & Borgida, E. (1988). Juror common understanding and the admissibility of rape trauma syndrome evidence in court. *Law and Human Behavior, 12,* 101–122.

Friedman, M. J. (1991). Biological approaches to the diagnosis and treatment of post-traumatic stress disorder. *Journal of Traumatic Stress, 4,* 67–91.

Frueh, B. C., Smith, D. W., & Barker, S. E. (in press). Compensation seeking status and psychometric assessment of combat veterans seeking treatment for PTSD. *Journal of Traumatic Stress, 9.*

Goodstein, R. K., & Page, A. W. (1981). Battered wife syndrome: Overview of dynamics and treatment. *American Journal of Psychiatry, 138,* 1036–1044.

Grant, B. L., & Coons, D. J. (1983). Guilty verdict in a murder committed by a veteran with post-traumatic stress disorder. *Bulletin of the American Academy of Psychiatry and the Law, 11,* 355–358.

Gutheil, T. G. (1989). Legal issues in psychiatry. In H. I. Kaplan & B. J. Sadock (Eds.), *Comprehensive textbook of psychiatry* (5th ed., Vol. 2, pp. 2107–2124). Baltimore: Williams & Wilkins.

Halleck, S. L., Hoge, S.K., Miller, R.D., Sadoff, R.L., & Halleck, N.J. (1992). The use of psychiatric diagnoses in the legal process: Task force report of the American Psychiatric Association. *Bulletin of the American Academy of Psychiatry and the Law, 20,* 481–499.

Higgins, S. A. (1991). Post-traumatic stress disorder and its role in the defense of Vietnam veterans. *Law and Psychology Review, 15,* 259–276.

Hoffman, B. F., Rochon, J. P., & Terry, J. A. (1992). *The emotional consequences of personal injury: A handbook for psychiatrists and lawyers.* Toronto: Butterworths.

Kleinman, S. B., Martell, D., & Gioiella, R. (1993). Dissociation and the "mens rea" defense. *American Academy of Psychiatry and the Law Annual Meeting Continuing Medical Education Syllabus, 24,* 21.

Lees-Haley, P. R. (1990). Malingering mental disorder on the Impact of Event (IES) Scale: Toxic exposure and cancerphobia. *Journal of Traumatic Stress, 3,* 315–321.

Lustberg, L. S., & Jacobi, J. V. (1992). The battered woman as reasonable person. *Seton Hall Law Review, 22,* 365–388.

Marciniak, R. D. (1986). Implications to forensic psychiatry of post-traumatic stress disorder: A review. *Military Medicine, 151,* 434–437.

Marwick, C. (1993). Court ruling on "junk science" gives judges more say about what expert witness testimony to allow. *Journal of the American Medical Association, 270,* 423.

Mayou, R., Bryant, B., & Duthie, R. (1993). Psychiatric consequences of road traffic accidents. *British Medical Journal, 307,* 647–651.

McFarlane, A. C. (in press). Attitudes to victims: Issues for medicine, the law and society. In C. Sumner, M. Israel, M. O'Connor, & R. Snare (Eds.), *International victimology: Selected papers from the 8th International Symposium on Victimology.* Canberrra: Australian Institute of Criminology.

Morris, G. H. (1975). *The insanity defense: A blueprint for legislative reform.* Lexington, MA: D. C. Heath.

Napier, M. (1991). The medical and legal trauma of disasters. *Medico-Legal Journal, 59*(3), 157–179.

Perconte, S. T., & Goreczny, A. J. (1990). Failure to detect fabricated posttraumatic stress disorder with the use of the MMPI in a clinical population. *American Journal of Psychiatry, 147,* 1057–1060.

Pitman, R. K., & Orr, S. P. (1993). Psychophysiologic testing for post-traumatic stress disorder: Forensic psychiatric application. *Bulletin of the American Academy of Psychiatry and the Law, 21,* 37–52.

Raifman, L. J. (1983). Problems of diagnosis and legal causation in courtroom use of post-traumatic stress disorder. *Behavioral Sciences and the Law, 1,* 115–131.

Resnick, P. J. (1994). Malingering. In R. Rosner (Ed.), *Principles and practice of forensic psychiatry* (pp. 417–426). New York: Chapman & Hall.

Rogers, R., Bagby, R. M., & Dickens, S. E. (1992). *Structured Interview for Reported Symptoms.* Odessa, FL: Psychological Assessment Resources.

Saunders, L. S., Pitman, R. K., & Orr, S. P. (1993). Providing objective proof of mental harm through psychophysiologic testing for post-traumatic stress disorder. *Trial Bar News, 15,* 72–80.

Scrignar, C. B. (1988). *Post-traumatic stress disorder: Diagnosis, treatment, and legal issues* (2nd ed.). New Orleans: Bruno Press.

Sersland, S. J. (1983–1984). Mental disability caused by mental stress: Standards of proof in workers compensation cases. *Drake Law Review, 4,* 751–816.

Slovenko, R. (1984). Syndrome evidence in establishing a stressor. *Journal of Psychiatry and Law, 12,* 443–467.

Slovenko, R. (1992). Is diminished capacity really dead? *Psychiatric Annals, 22,* 566–570.

Sparr, L. F., & Atkinson, R. M. (1986). Posttraumatic stress disorder as an insanity defense: Medicolegal quicksand. *American Journal of Psychiatry, 143,* 608–613.

Sparr, L. F., & Boehnlein, J. K. (1990). Posttraumatic stress disorder in tort actions: Forensic minefield. *Bulletin of the American Academy of Psychiatry and the Law, 18,* 283–302.

Sparr, L. F., & Pankratz, L. D. (1983). Factitious posttraumatic stress disorder. *American Journal of Psychiatry, 140,* 1016–1019.

Sparr, L. F., Reaves, M. E., & Atkinson, R. M. (1987). Military combat, posttraumatic stress disorder, and criminal behavior in Vietnam veterans. *Bulletin of the American Academy of Psychiatry and the Law, 15,* 141–162.

Sparr, L. F., White, R., Friedman, M. J., & Wiles, D. B. (1994). Veterans psychiatric benefits: Enter courts and attorneys. *Bulletin of the American Academy of Psychiatry and the Law, 22,* 205–222.

Spaulding, W. J. (1988). Compensation for mental disability. In R. Michels (Ed.), *Psychiatry* (Vol. 3, pp. 1–27). Philadelphia: J. B. Lippincott.

Speir, D. E. (1989, June). Application and use of post-traumatic stress disorder as a defense to criminal conduct. *Army Lawyer,* 17–22.

Steinberg, C. E. (1993). The *Daubert* decision: An update on the *Frye* rule. *American Academy of Psychiatry and the Law Newsletter, 18,* 66–69.

Stone, A. A. (1993). Post-traumatic stress disorder and the law: Critical review of the new frontier. *Bulletin of the American Academy of Psychiatry and the Law, 21,* 23–36.

Szasz, T. S. (1962). Bootlegging humanistic values through psychiatry. *Antioch Review, 22,* 341–349.

Thomson, J. (1991). Post traumatic stress disorder and criminal defenses. *University of Western Australia Law Review, 21,* 279–304.

Trosch, L. A. (1991). *State v. Strickland:* Evening the odds in rape trials! North Carolina allows expert testimony on post traumatic stress disorder to disprove victim consent. *North Carolina Law Review, 69,* 1624–1643.

World Health Organization. (1992). *ICD-10 classification of mental and behavioural disorders: Clinical descriptions and diagnostic guidelines.* Geneva: Author.

Trauma in Cultural Perspective

MARTEN W. deVRIES

There is no solution to these problems. One must endure the hardship.

— DINKA REFUGEE, KAKUMA CAMP, KENYA, 1994[1]

Enduring, recovering from, and succumbing to trauma are all aspects of the human condition. The impact of traumatic life events and of the resulting loss and grief on the individual has attracted increasing professional attention over the last 25 years. In the United States, the psychosocial impact of the Vietnam War on the veterans confirmed the psychological suffering of individuals around the world as a result of human-made disasters. The recent exposure of the prevalence of incest within nuclear families has also catapulted the long-term impact of trauma in its various forms into public as well as professional awareness. Today we are bombarded with global information about individual and social problems related to trauma. When a traumatic event, an uprooting, or a social upheaval strikes, the community as well as the individuals within a society are affected (Hobfoll & deVries, 1995).

Although the Third World seems especially prone to catastrophic events, developed countries are in no way immune to them. Europe and Japan were shattered by war just 50 years ago, and today the former Yugoslavia and 48 other countries in the world are involved in violent internal or external strife. Yet traumatized individuals rebuilt both Europe and Japan (with help), and today around the world people are busy reconstructing their devastated countries to provide security for themselves and future generations. This seems a paradox

[1]Cited in Richter (1994).

of devastation and recovery—an ebb and flow of suffering and disintegration, alternating with social unity and hope. Victims as well as heroes seem to pop up everywhere, always demonstrating the effects of a particular cultural and historical context in their reactions to trauma. Questions such as the following arise: Does culture protect against the effects of stress and trauma? And what happens when culture fails? We are very much at the beginning of understanding these processes, but as we puzzle out what lies at the roots of vulnerability or resilience and the process of recovery from traumatic events, the relationship of culture to trauma must be explored.

POSTTRAUMATIC STRESS DISORDER IN CULTURAL PERSPECTIVE

The way in which modern psychological theory has reframed the nature of traumatizing experiences confronts us with some fundamental issues. Historically, the belief that individuals can control their own destinies has only emerged in recent generations. It is likely that the decline of religion is a function of a rise in the illusory hope that human beings can be in charge of their own future. Eastern religions, in particular, do not offer their followers such a promise. For example, both Hinduism and Islam teach that life is entirely determined by fate and that one has to submit oneself to the gods' or Allah's will. Very little scientific work on the relative prevalence of posttraumatic stress disorder (PTSD) has been done in areas of the world where these religions have a large following, so that no information is available on how religious beliefs shape people's responses to trauma. However, the very notion that PTSD occurs as a normal response to an abnormal condition implies that, ordinarily, people can have control over their fate—a decidedly optimistic position.

Psychological trauma and reactions to it have been legitimized in Western diagnostic systems (American Psychiatric Association, 1980, 1994) as PTSD. In contrast to other diagnostic entities, PTSD is defined as having been set in motion by an exogenous event. Whereas other psychopathological disorders are currently aggressively decontextualized and diagnosed only in terms of signs and symptoms, PTSD can occur after a particular event within a particular historical and ontogenic context. PTSD, then, serves as a model for correcting the decontextualized aspects of today's taxonomic systems. It draws our attention away from our overly concrete definition of psychological illness as a thing in itself, bringing us back to the person's experience and the meaning which he or she assigns to it (Nemiah, 1989, p. 1528). PTSD requires us to focus on the life history of the individual interacting with other individuals in the context of society and culture (Brody, 1994). PTSD is thus a description of an illness process based not on the intrinsic nature of the person alone, but rather on the person's sociocultural interaction over time (Bronfenbrenner, 1994).

Research on stress, trauma, and their interaction with health in psychology, physiology, and sociology has demonstrated that the impact of stress and trauma encompasses biological, psychological, social, and cultural phenomena. Recent research has alerted us to the fact that massive disruptions in personal and social life are not the only disturbances that affect health; minor daily events, hassles, and family problems do so as well (Holmes & Rahe, 1967; deVries, 1987; Stone, Neale, & Shiffman, 1993). It is the positive evaluation of the self in the social context, as well as social support, that corrects the negative effects of stressful events (Csikszentmihalyi, 1991; Delongis, Coyne, Dakof, Folkman, & Lazarus, 1982; Kanner,Coyne, Schaefer, & Lazarus, 1981). Culture plays a key role in how individuals cope with potentially traumatizing experiences by providing the context in which social support and other positive and uplifting events can be experienced. The interactions between an individual and his or her environment/community play a significant role in determining whether the person is able to cope with the potentially traumatizing experiences that set the stage for the development of PTSD. Thus, PTSD reflects the sociocultural environment in which it occurs.

Culture is a double-edged sword. Because of human beings' dependence on it, its loss becomes traumatic. The power of culture as a protector, integrator, and security system is evident in studies where the degree of cultural assimilation is a key variable (Brown & Prudo, 1981; Prudo, Brown, Harris, & Dowland, 1981). In these studies, individuals who were strongly identified with cultural values benefited from increased social support; culture buffered them from the impact, and even the occurrence, of traumatic events. For socially less integrated individuals, stress had a strong negative impact on health and psychopathology. However, culture provides protection at a cost. Strong attachments to persons and lifestyles leads to a deeper sense of loss when the life of the culture is disrupted. When people adhere to a system and bond to the other individuals within it, the loss of those persons and the disintegration of the system become traumatic.

CULTURE, STRESS, AND TRAUMA

Culture may in many ways be viewed as a protective and supportive system of values, lifestyles, and knowledge, the disruption of which will have a deleterious effect on its members. During social and cultural upheavals, drastic changes occur in people's expectations, "the meaning of life," and communal values. Cultures, however, are powerfully resilient to the stresses of the environment and resistant to change. Culture thereby buffers its members from the potentially profound impact of stressful experiences. It does so by means of furnishing social support, providing identities in terms of norms and values, and supplying a shared vision of the future. Cultural stories, rituals, and legends highlighting the mastery of communal trauma, the relationship to the spiritual realm, and religion itself are important mechanisms that allow individuals to reorganize their often catastrophic reactions to losses. Culture, as a source of knowledge and information, locates experience in a historical context and forces continuity on discontinuous events.

Materialistically, culture is a health maintenance system whose function is to assure the adequate distribution of goods, as well as physical and social resources for maintaining social relationships and structure. In short, culture's function is the maintenance of an orderly progression through the life cycle (Whiting & Whiting, 1975). Culture provides a complex and flexible set of rules and values, as well as both practical and symbolic means to carry them out. Within the culturally prescribed social and community structure, life cycle roles and the emotional management of transitions from one role or relationship to another are facilitated and ordered (LeVine, 1973). It is in this context that personal life events, trauma, and illness will be mastered or not.

Provided that the individual does not interfere with the group's capacity to reproduce or remain viable in its niche, cultural social roles, shared values, and historical continuity will act as key stress managers. If the individual does not fit, social extrusion and stigmatization may result as a cultural defense reaction to the unwanted information or behavior. Culture is, however, geared toward providing the homeostatic processes that allow the group and the individual to survive under a wide range of stressful conditions. Shalev (Chapter 4, this volume) points out that when trauma strikes, this may not be the case. Trauma may be differentiated from stress at the cultural level in a parallel manner to what Shalev describes for the individual. Trauma, in contrast to stress, profoundly alters the basic structure not just of the individual, but of the cultural system as a whole: Society will never be the same again. Homeostatic mechanisms (e.g., rituals, social organization, and the economic system) no longer suffice to restore a sense of safety and belonging, and other forms of organization or lack of organization need to take their place. In analogy to PTSD at the individual level, a posttraumatic cultural reaction may best be viewed as an abnormal response to an extraordinary event. To understand how culture is disrupted by trauma, we should first look at how cultures work under conditions of relatively normal stress.

WHEN THINGS GO RIGHT: HOW CULTURE PROTECTS INDIVIDUALS

The investigations into traditional societies carried out by anthropologists over the last 100 years constitute a good point of departure for illustrating the working ingredients of culture. Traditional cultural responses to stress are integrated within a frame of belief that holds that problems and illnesses, as well as their causes, do not disappear with time or treatment. Stressful or traumatic events and their consequences are inevitable and unavoidable. Stress, grief and illness must therefore be continually managed and accommodated at both the personal and group levels. Culture in part is adapted to help the community and the individuals to do this. For example, in the medical system of the Digo in East Africa (deVries & deVries, 1977), one never loses a "diagnosis." Diseases and their material or spiritual causes are instead accumulated. They act as parts of the self; they caution against hazards and remind of potential vulnerability. In turn, each disease entity is linked to a mode of continual treatment and supportive social relationships. Society then organizes the process of suffering, rendering it a meaningful mode of action and identity within a larger social framework. A response to stress or danger also operationalizes society's capacity to support its members. In this model, illness and suffering are communications to the group, as well as profound personal experiences.

Indigenous social security systems are the mainstay of the community response. Since in most societies the family/kin group is chiefly responsible for its members, the social security systems are based on filial piety and kin responsibility. After disaster strikes, the indigenous social security or filial (kin) system generally responds to problematic emotional reactions and brings order to an individual's emotional reactions to life events. Depending on the particular culture, they facilitate the provision of help to dependents in various complex ways.

Cultures also create meaning systems that explain the causes of traumatic events. "Fatalistic" cultures believe that traumatic events have external causes that must be continually faced during life; causes and consequences do not disappear. Rituals and symbolic places are necessary to reify and support group members during times of inevitable difficulty (Geertz, 1973). Traditional cultures assign causation either to a god or gods, to others (witchcraft), or to ancestors (breaking of rituals or taboos). Such concepts of external causation have the social function of linking an individual's experience of illness and trauma directly to the larger society. In these settings, filial responsibility and dependence are evoked by the communication of suffering.

Rituals support the individual, repair rents in the social fabric, and reestablish the group. Individuals in traditional societies, then, not only lose their kin support network during social disruptions; they may also lose access to their rituals and symbolic places, and this loss may limit their ability to mobilize healing resources. This stands in contrast to the West, where the prevailing idiom for illness experience is individual responsibility for one's own health. The "duty to be healthy" is a major underpinning of Western medicine, which assesses individual risk and expects compliance, but tolerates the right to refuse. All societies provide rules for emotional expression and illness behavior, ultimately facilitating interpersonal understanding and thereby inviting support or (when these rules, are breached) rejection (deVries, 1995).

If a community remains intact after a traumatic disruption, the culture will make attempts to correct the effects of the traumatic experiences by employing accepted strategies or by developing new ones. Medical practitioners (or traditional healers) are key elements in such a response in most cultures; they are the guardians of the cultural concepts of dependence, family roles, care-seeking behavior, and life cycle expectations. In traditional societies, the work of healers is based on the facts that the body cannot in any way be isolated from the mind, and the mind cannot be removed from its social context. This integration of body, mind, spirit, and culture is a result of the truism that individuals grow up within a particular social context where cultural values and the meaning of health and disease are communicated from birth to death. Individuals, in turn, experience their physical and mental functioning in the context of a larger social and cultural frame of reference (Shweder & LeVine, 1984).

Every culture has its own medical system that embodies ideas of illness and health, as well as hope and the expectation for solutions. The medical system is delicately interwoven with the group's ideas and feelings about the entire range of physical and social events possible or tolerable within the group. The medical system, then, plays a crucial role in shaping individuals' social world and experience (deVries, Lipken, & Berg, 1982). Cultures differ in their religious systems and social organizations; therefore, each provides its own particular interpretation of the causes and the experiences of physical and emotional suffering and trauma. Variations in these interpretations as to whether suffering can be cured, must be endured, or is a means of communicating are functions of cultural differences in the strategies for seeking solutions to suffering (Kleinman, 1988).

During massive upheavals, a culture may be incapable of doing its protective work and cannot adequately fulfill its functions of regulating emotions and of providing identity, support and resources. Such times call forth the best and the worst in men and women. The "up side" of the discontinuity is the possibility for change or the creation of new social forms; the "down side" is the regression to previous historical conditions and to primitive emotions and behaviors. In response to trauma, individuals and groups must help themselves. Glorious altruism and outrageous mendacity can therefore coexist.

CULTURAL ORGANIZATION OF GRIEF: CUSTOMS AND RESTITUTION

Cultures vary in the use of rituals and religion. The functions of rituals during death and loss are to regulate behavior, time, and emotions, and to provide guidance for often fragmented social relationships. Culture organizes emotional expression in a manner appropriate to the established level of "personhood" of the sufferer; such expression may range from stoical perseverance and withdrawal to flamboyant, highly emotional acting out of grief or pain. Key emotions related to bereavement that receive special cultural attention are those related to anger and aggression, with the aims of reducing harm, facilitating restitution, and maintaining cultural production without interruption. Customs and rituals constitute a way of patterning behavior and providing organization during a chaotic period of transition, refining ongoing cultural values, and helping to cut the ties with what may never be again (Rosenblatt, Walsh, & Jackson, 1976).

At the death of an important person in one's life, one generally experiences strong emotions and marked changes in behavior patterns. Among these emotions may be feelings labeled as sadness, anger, fear, anxiety, guilt, loneliness, and numbness. Behavior changes may include loss of appetite and weight loss, disruption of work activities, loss of interest, decrease in sociability, disrupted sleep, and disturbing dreams. These feelings and dispositional changes may result from many things, including uncertainty about what to do, loss of gratification, and disruption of familiar living patterns. The problems are greater when the loss is unexpected, is traumatic, or occurs at times of uncertainty, each of which aggravates the disruption of familiar patterns.

Grief rituals are designed to help bereaved people return to being able to make reasonable contributions in their social and work lives. In the West, we hold that grief should be "worked through." This includes acceptance of the loss; extinction of behaviors that are no longer adaptive; acquisition of new ways of dealing with others; and the amelioration of guilt, anger, and other disruptive emotions. Custom and ritual channel and facilitate the working-through process. Lindemann's (1944) description of the mourning process was helpful in alerting psychiatry to this process. However, today his description seems oversimplified, given the diversity of positive outcomes in response to a range of grief reactions, including denial (Wortman & Silver, 1989). Wortman and Silver point out that loss is very often not worked through—a point made in a different way by the Dinka refugee quoted at the beginning of this chapter: "There is no solution to these problems. One must endure the hardship." Life is real, and trauma, despite the best efforts of cultures or individuals, cannot always be worked through; its effects remain. In traditional societies, however, customs can help by providing structure, a poultice for these sores. They provide a grieving process for people who, if left to their own devices, would not do so, and who thereby might be at risk for developing PTSD. Culture, with its customs and rituals, is thus a key participant in returning a person to normal functioning by moving the person from shock to grief, and ultimately to nonbereavement. In the absence of culturally regulated processes, this reestablishment of normality is less likely to occur.

Custom, by excusing people from social role obligations during the mourning period, decreases the amount of friction grief creates. It also facilitates and integrates dependence on members of a supportive group who help with ceremonies; this obligates the bereaved to those providing the support, with the expectation that the currently traumatized person will reciprocate in the future. Death customs are rites of passage and initiate a change in status for both the dead and the bereaved. As the dead person is ceremonially passed from the realm of the living to that of the dead, the bereaved person is passed from the state of mourner to the state of nonmourner.

Death also empties the roles that have been occupied by the deceased. One thing that must be accomplished following a death is to refill the roles; this requires identifying persons to occupy them, recruiting them, and certifying their new positions. Customs and rituals then attempt to maintain social solidarity by regulating potentially disruptive dispositions. Ceremonies following death will reinforce the remaining social ties, sort out who is in the group and who is not, and reinforce ties through shared work and ceremonially required cooperation. Eulogies are common around the world as one means of promoting solidarity and providing praise for the deceased; they also indirectly serve as a reward for those still living, who could be similarly praised at their own deaths (Rosenblatt et al., 1976).

In summary, cultural customs and rituals help individuals control their emotions, order their behavior, link the sufferers more intimately to the social group, and serve as symbols of continuity. Such processes of restitution, outlined in many ethnographic studies, are disrupted when cultures as a whole are traumatized. Similarly, variations in cultural custom influence individual grief reactions and the types of restitutions after traumatic events that are possible. The reaction to trauma varies a great deal from one place to another (deVries, 1987b). When culture loses important aspects of its ability to function and becomes incapable of guiding grief reactions or to provide support, individuals are left unprotected and left to their own devices.

MEDICALIZATION: LEGITIMIZATION OF SUFFERING DUE TO STRESS AND TRAUMA

One formal social response to overwhelming stress is the expansion of the medical system itself, which legitimizes the reallocation of community resources. Digo medicine provides an example of an increase in the scope of the medical taxonomy to accommodate individual and communal stress (de Vries & deVries, 1977). The Digo live on the East African coast; their territory is bordered to the west by the eastern extension of Masai grazing land. The two cultures, which had previously had little contact, clashed in the 1960–1970s because of drought and the subsequent expanded search by the Masai for grazing land. The Masai began raiding peripheral Digo homesteads for cattle and supplies, creating

406 • DEVELOPMENTAL, SOCIAL, AND CULTURAL ISSUES

panic and generalized anxiety throughout Digo land. The stress experienced by individuals and the group was often expressed in ad hoc "trance dances." In these dissociated states, individuals could experience and relive their anxiety and fear by abreacting and behaving like, or identifying with, the aggressors during the dance. Eventually, the traditional healers gave this specific stress response of anxiety, fear, and behaving like a Masai warrior a label, and incorporated it within the traditional healing rituals. The dances were then formalized and used to alleviate stress, as well as to accumulate resources for the protection of border communities from the Masai threat. Thus, personal fear and anxiety in reaction to community stress were labeled and transformed into an illness and a form of social communication, thereby securing attention and resources. Medicalizing the problem enabled the group not only to protect itself against the Masai, but to provide social support for individuals unable for both personal and social reasons to cope with this threat in their daily lives.

Similar to Digo medicine's taxonomic response to social stress created by the Masai, 20th-century Tibetan medicine has undergone a transformation as a result of the Chinese–Tibetan cultural clash (Janes, 1995). The result of this violent collision of cultures is evident in modern Tibetan medicine's elaboration of the "*rlung*" etiological categories. *Rlung* is a basic tenet of Tibetan medicine related to ordering the life course. During the upheaval, a new class of *rlung* illnesses sprung up, symbolizing the rapid social economic and political changes confronting the Tibetans. The interaction of the Chinese state and Tibetan medicine also provided a new place for Tibetan medicine in the world. This new strength derived from its supportive local role in helping define the traumatic experience of the Tibetan people by means of *rlung*. A solution to this cultural trauma demanded that Tibetan medicine both retain traditional ideas and incorporate the new reality of its changing world. This forced the modernization of Tibetan medicine, and resulted in an internationalization of its practice and ultimately in its acceptance by the Chinese state as a legitimate medical discipline. The current revitalization of Tibetan medicine can be attributed in part to its legitimization of the traumatic experiences of the Tibetans, which grew out of an internal demand by local and exiled Tibetan populations to resist domination (Janes, 1995).

The expansion of taxonomy not only facilitated adjustment to stress but also the management of trauma. For example, it allowed the normalization of war trauma reactions in the United States following the war in Vietnam. Through medical labeling and legal activity centered on the Agent Orange controversy, veterans were able to redress the social problems experienced upon their return to American society. The labeling of PTSD by the American Psychiatric Association (1980) provided a formal place in the taxonomy of Western medicine for their experience and legitimized the suffering of these warriors as they attempted to return to normal life. In all these societies—the Digo culture, Tibet, and the United States—stress experiences, though manifested at the individual level, were intricately tied to larger social issues. A society is constantly challenged and threatened, and it incorporates these group stresses. Its members' experiences and emotions need to be rendered meaningful and legitimated. Medicalization or labeling achieves this by expanding the medical taxonomy (deVries et al., 1982). A medical label justifies and operationalizes social interventions and resource allocation. Culture, then, may cast a net across disruptive human experience by means of its medical system. Human experience thus remains understandable and under control: The individual's suffering is legitimized, and society provides a way of tolerating disability in its members.

WHEN CULTURE FAILS

Culture is supposed to render life predictable. When the cultural defense mechanisms are lost, individuals are left on their own to achieve emotional control. Traumas that occur in the context of social upheavals, such as revolutions, civil wars, and uprootings, create profound discontinuity in the order and predictability that culture has brought to daily life and social situations. When this occurs, traditional systems break down and a conservative element often takes hold. Ethnicity, nationalism, tribalism, and fundamentalism become means of survival; all of these are regressive moves to release individuals behaviorally and ideologically from an intolerable complexity that cannot be managed or used in a more productive way. When culture as the identity giver fails, other models of identity formation and social group formation take its place. The roles and status that had previously organized the system may have no further meaning, as in Turnbull's (1972) classic study of the Ik—a nomadic tribe that, when pushed to the edge of the carrying capacity of its environment in East Africa, relinquished its hold on its traditional values and social structure. Age and family groupings, nurturing of the young, and respect for the old were no longer the underpinnings of the society. In cases such as that of the Ik, the homeostatic mechanisms of culture and behavior adapted to the normal stresses of life break down under the burden of trauma. At such times, new or no social forms take their place. The *de novo* creation of self-help groups is one very positive outcome (see below), but most often negative social forms appear (e.g., warlords, gangs, and brutal usurpations of power). The aims of these are to forge order from emotions through violence and aggression, and in particular to deny anxiety and grief.

Today, we are only at the beginning of our understanding of the process of cultural disintegration, the shock it creates, and the individual and social attempts to correct it. The norm under these traumatized conditions often consists of negative identities derived from the old system (Erikson, 1963). Uprooting has a profound impact on the locus of control of individuals: Where do they belong, and where are they going? (Frankl, 1963). It would be naive to attempt to discuss in precise detail the ramifications of trauma down from culture to the individual. Medicine and anthropology are still too stunned today by having opened their eyes to the reality of the effects of trauma on individuals and communities to make a definitive link.

When cultural protection and security fail, the individual's problems are proportional to the cultural disintegration. The avenues of vulnerability resulting from trauma follow the routes vacated by culture: Paranoia substitutes for trust; aggression replaces nurturance and support; identity confusion or a negative identity substitutes for a positive identity. Social bonding becomes a regression to nationalism and tribalism, thereby permitting individuals to deny the experienced losses or to defend themselves against expected additional losses. Compounding these problems in most areas of the world is that at times of cultural disintegration, the population is often physically depleted and fatigued as well. For example, the citizens of Bosnia, Somalia, and Rwanda are both physically and psychologically traumatized. These psychological and physical consequences will strongly affect their lifestyles and mental states in the future, even if the norms and values of their given cultures are reinstated (Giel, 1994). Yet, paradoxically, the members of a culture will always (or most often) rebuild on a template or remnant of cultural customs and values.

CULTURAL SELF-HELP STRATEGIES

Under a variety of conditions, therefore, culture may be inadequate to maintain individual support and social resources. Individual or group self-help strategies may then be required. Janzen (1982) describes how sufferers have been brought from the isolation of their sickness together with others with the same affliction, and have given one another mutual support to reenter society—indeed, even to become specialized healers of their affliction. Janzen refers to these self-help groups as "drums anonymous"(since drums are frequently employed in African versions of these groups), and describes the striking commonalities among such groups around the world. The gourd dance among the Native Americans of the southern plains is an example. It dates back to before the creation of reservations, when these groups were warrior societies. When the warriors put down their arms in the late 19th century and were placed on reservations, the gourd dance served as a means to work out their frustrations. At the end of the Vietnam War, when Native American veterans came home, they were again warriors who had turned in their weapons. They were sitting around in cities and towns not knowing what to do, drinking, often getting into trouble, and lacking a sense of orientation. The gourd dance, with its unique pulsating circular rhythm and the social activities surrounding it, reemerged as a means of reestablishing orientation. Today, in the cities of the southern plains states and on the reservations, one finds active local gourd dance chapters. In these chapters, veterans counsel one another on alcohol and other problems and dance together (Howard, 1976; Gephardt, 1977).

A common feature that makes a person eligible for belonging to a self-help group is that the affliction comes upon the individual rather suddenly and traumatically, as in a disaster. Despite this initial helplessness, in the group process the "sufferer" is gradually transformed into a healer; in these self-help groups, in striking contrast to orthodox professional medical models, evil is somehow converted into a virtue. Self-help groups emerge when permanent maintenance of help and resources is required and one-time solutions will not do. As in traditional settings (e.g., the Digo medical system), the sufferer never fully loses the illness. The affliction is seen as a permanent characteristic that the sufferer cannot eliminate. Ongoing therapy is therefore necessary. The self-help group is a widespread, if not universal, mode of healing. The examples from the Euroamerican tradition (e.g., Alcoholics Anonymous, Parents Anonymous, cardiac rehabilitation units) demonstrate that it is a viable and specific form of therapy for chronic afflictions,and one that is of particular use when the given social system fails or is irrelevant (Janzen, 1982).

CONCLUSIONS

As I have described in this chapter, culture under normal conditions maintains an arsenal of approaches that can deal quite well with the challenges to its survival. Individuals are provided with identity, predictability, resources, and order. Grieving patterns, as well as the medical and social systems, provide the support required to deal with normal life events and stress. When these fail or do not support the person—as is the case with many displaced Third World residents, as well as with Vietnam veterans and many victims of familial sexual abuse—individuals are thrust back onto themselves. Trauma to some extent may be viewed as the product of a combination of the severity of the stress and the supportive capabilities of the environment. The age at which the trauma occurs, the social context, and the support and resources available will all influence the outcome. Many other chapters in this volume demonstrate that the individual will regress, fixate, or be thrown back to primitive defenses in order to manage trauma. At the group level, a conservative response often takes hold—a historical regression to idealized familiar conditions, to a better and seemingly simpler time. Such a regression holds out the temptation of a new identity and the denial of pain and complexity.

In the other chapters of this volume, psychological and biological explanations form the basis of examining traumatic reactions. To these explorations, this chapter adds cultural aspects. The cultural and the individual levels of explanations are different and may be best understood if applied at different points in time. Neither culture, psychology, nor biology explains the total picture over the period of time relevant for analysis—before, during, and after the trauma. The psychological and cultural explanations fit best at different stages of the trauma response. The psychological level of explanation of the trauma reaction is powerful in explaining immediate reactions to the trauma. The explanations of posttraumatic reactions have more to do with the process of recovery after the event. It is here that culture and social support become important explanatory paradigms. Culture cannot prevent calamity, nor can it blunt the immediate physical power of violence and the emotional shock of betrayal. It can only help with building up resilience before such events, or with providing validation, restitution, and rehabilitation afterward. Cultural processes such as social support and self-help groups are powerful forces for restitution, particularly when combined with formal cultural acceptance of the traumatic experience.

As care providers, we generally appear on the scene after a trauma has occurred. Culture at this point may be fully in place or may have been disrupted by the trauma. Whatever cultural structure remains should be employed to help victims manage the horror. After a traumatic event, rituals and customs that order emotions and create self-help opportunities must be facilitated. This provides individuals with a sense of identity and a locus of control that facilitates their taking adaptive action. The medical system should legitimate suffering by expanding definitions of formally recognized illness categories to encompass the experience of these individuals, such as the Digo, the Tibetans, and the American Psychiatric Association have done. The goal should be to bring order and continuity into the posttraumatic period: to provide help with ordering emotional reactions, social relationships, and resources in response to the initial shock, recoil, denial, and anger. This will help defend against the conservative impulse and the psychopathological processes that may otherwise result in a striving for pathological liberation from trauma and regressive social bonding.

Rituals and the places required to carry them out should be incorporated in rehabilitative programs whenever possible. Following major social disruption, the reestablishment of symbolic places—churches, mosques, trees for gathering under, schoolyards, special places for women and children to gather, and safe places for evening meetings—is an important goal. Symbolic places make visible the normal demographic age distribution of a community, the range from young to old. This helps reestablish previously learned cultural rules and reinstate members of the community in role functions appropriate to their places in the life cycle. Symbolic places and the culturally prescribed behaviors within such places help reinstitute traditional social relationships. These go a long way toward facilitating mature defenses and the potential for altruistic action during times of disorganization and stress, where regressive, primitive defenses such as projection, denial, and narcissistic survival strategies tend to prevail.

Everything should be done to keep the problem from becoming chronic. The "chronic stress" of trauma makes it possible for human beings, singly or in groups, to concretize delusions as reality. This is a well-described process among Russian intelligentsia under the repressive regime in the former Soviet Union (Shalimov, 1980), where the constant pressure of surveillance and mistrust created paranoid delusional states that became the norm for daily life. Such delusions may be necessary for survival and are extremely difficult to give up once they are no longer needed.

Two examples from Uganda are particularly instructive in terms of the continuation of this dissociative, delusional process in response to having become uprooted from one's culture. Giel (1994) reports the story of a girl who, during the war in northern Uganda, was attacked in her local village by soldiers of the national army. Her father and brother, who under threat of death refused to rape her, were killed before her eyes. For 2 years, she was kept and abused by the soldiers as their "guerrilla girl." Every night, as she experienced the lust of another soldier, she would withdraw into her own world. Today she is "free"—wandering around in Uganda, aimlessly searching for her family, detached from all around her, and often wishing she were dead. Another displaced Ugandan described by Giel (1994) is Peter, a somewhat suspicious young fellow who says he's 13 years old, but actually looks like an 8-year-old boy. He laughs and talks very little. For the last 3 years, he has accompanied the freedom fighters in northern Uganda and considers them his only family. He states that he has no memory of his birthplace or school; he doesn't know whether he had friends or whether he ever tended cattle. As the civil war draws to a close, there seems no way that this boy could ever find his way back to his home, nor does he have the social skills to fill a peacetime social role. These young people, uprooted from their cultures, cannot return to their past and seem to have little future: poignant symbols of acculturation.

In summary, when cultural patterns, identities, and relationships are lost, life becomes unpredictable. Under normal stressful conditions, a grieving process with the aim of leaving the old and adjusting to the new takes place. With trauma, however, other patterns are activated—conservative impulses (ethnicity, etc.) at the group level, and psychopathological reactions (depression, paranoia, and aggression) at the individual level. Culture helps protect against these processes. In its absence, loss, regression, and harm occur. The puzzle and paradox of both traumatic reactions and restitution provide a new challenge for understanding and action. The further study of the interplay of culture and trauma will help untangle the web of causal and protective factors that result in trauma's being endured, succumbed to, or recovered from. This provides a major area of study for clinicians and anthropologists alike—one that will help illuminate a dark, worldwide "field site" that sadly appears to be ever-growing and endless.

REFERENCES

American Psychiatric Association. (1980). *Diagnostic and statistical manual of mental disorders* (3rd ed.). Washington, DC: Author.

American Psychiatric Association. (1994). *Diagnostic and statistical manual of mental disorders* (4th ed.). Washington, DC: Author.

Brody, E. B. (1994). Psychiatric diagnosis in sociocultural context. *Journal of Nervous and Mental Disease, 182,* 253–254.

Bronfenbrenner, U. (1994). Nature–nurture reconceptualized in developmental perspective: A bioecological model. *Psychological Review, 10*(4), 568–586.

Brown, G. W., & Prudo, R. (1981). Psychiatric disorders in a rural and an urban population: Vol. 1. Aetiology of depression. *Psychological Medicine, 11,* 581–599.

Csikszentmihalyi, M. (1991). *Flow: The psychology of optimal experience.* New York: Harper.

Delongis, A., Coyne, J. C., Dakof, G., Folkman, S., & Lazarus, R. S. (1982). Relationship of daily hassles, uplifts, and major life events to health status. *Health Psychology, 1,* 119–136.

deVries, M. W. (1987a). Investigating mental disorders in their natural settings. *Journal of Nervous and Mental Disease, 175,* 509–513.

deVries, M. W. (1987b). Cry babies, culture, and catastrophe: Infant temperament among the Masai. In N. Scheper-Hughes (Ed.), *Child survival* (pp. 165–185). Dordrecht, The Netherlands: D. Reidel.

deVries, M. W. (1995). Culture, community, and catastrophe: Issues in understanding communities under difficult conditions. In S. E. Hobfoll & M. W. deVries (Eds.), *Extreme stress and communities: Impact and intervention* (pp. 375–395). Dordrecht, The Netherlands: Kluwer.

deVries, M. W., & deVries, M. R. (1977).The cultural relativity of toilet training readiness: A perspective from East Africa. *Pediatrics, 60,* 170–177.

deVries, M. W., Lipken, M., & Berg, R. (Eds.). (1982). *The use and abuse of medicine.* New York: Praeger.

Eisenbruch, M. (1991). From posttraumatic stress disorder to cultural bereavement: Diagnosis of Southeast Asian refugees. *Social Science and Medicine, 33*(6), 673–680.

Erikson, E. H. (1963). *Childhood and society* (2nd ed.). New York: Norton.

Frankl, V. (1963). *Man's search for meaning.* New York: Washington Square Press.

Geertz, C. (1973). *The interpretation of cultures.* New York: Basic Books.

Gephardt, L. (1977). *The affective structure of the gourd dance.* Unpublished master's thesis, University of Kansas.

Giel, R. (1990). Psychosocial processes in disaster. *International Journal of Mental Health, 19*(1), 7–20.

Giel, R. (1994, December 13). *Afscheidsrede.* Paper presented at the retirement of Professor R. Giel, Rijksuniversiteit Groningen.

Hobfoll, S. E., & deVries, M. W. (Eds.). (1995). *Extreme stress and communities: Impact and intervention.* Dordrecht, The Netherlands: Kluwer.

Holmes, T. H., & Rahe, R. H. (1967). The Social Readjustment Rating Scale. *Journal of Psychosomatic Research, 11,* 213–218.

Howard, J. H. (1976). The plains gourd dance as a revitalization movement. *American Ethnologist, 2,* 243–259.

Janes, C. R. (1995). The transformations of Tibetan medicine. *Medical Anthropology Quarterly, 9*(1), 6–39.

Janzen, J. (1982). Drums anonymous. In M. W. deVries, M. Lipkin, & R. Berg (Eds.), *The use and abuse of medicine* (pp. 154–166). New York: Praeger.

Kanner, A. D., Coyne, J. C., Schaefer, C., & Lazarus, R. S. (1981). Comparison of two modes of stress measurement: Daily hassles and uplifts versus major life events. *Journal of Behavioral Medicine, 4,* 1–39.

Kleinman, A. (1988). *The illness narrative.* New York: Basic Books.

LeVine, R. A. (1973). *Culture, behavior and personality.* Chicago: Aldine.

Lindemann, E. (1944). Symptomatology and management of acute grief. *American Journal of Psychiatry, 101,* 141–148.

Nemiah, J. (1989). Janet redivivus [Editorial]. *American Journal of Psychiatry, 146,* 1527–1529.

Prudo, R., Brown, G. W., Harris, T., & Dowland, J. (1981). Psychiatric disorder in a rural and an urban population: Vol. 2. Sensitivity to loss. *Psychological Medicine, 11,* 601–616.

Richter, A. (1994). *IPSER Internal Report Kakuma Reugee Camp.* Maastricht, the Netherlands: IPSER.

Rosenblatt, P. C., Walsh, R. P., & Jackson, D. A. (1976) *Grief and mourning in cross-cultural perspective.* New Haven, CT: Human Relations Area Files Press.

Schweder, R. A., & LeVine, R. A. (1984). *Culture, theory: Essays on mind, self and emotion.* Cambridge, England: Cambridge University Press.

Shalimov, V. (1980). *Kolyma Tales.* New York: Norton.

Stone, A. A., Neale, J. M., & Shiffman, S. (1993). Daily assessments of stress and coping and their association with mood. *Annals of Behavioral Medicine, 15*(1), 8–16.

Turnbull, C. M. (1972). *The mountain people.* New York: Simon & Schuster.

Whiting, B., & Whiting, J. (1975). *Children of six cultures.* Cambridge, MA: Harvard University Press.

Wortman, C. B., & Silver, R. C. (1989). The myths of coping with loss. *Journal of Consulting and Clinical Psychology, 57,* 349–357.

PART VI

TREATMENT

A General Approach to Treatment of Posttraumatic Stress Disorder

BESSEL A. VAN DER KOLK
ALEXANDER C. McFARLANE
ONNO VAN DER HART

History, despite its wrenching pain, cannot be unlived, but, if faced with courage, need not be lived again.
— MAYA ANGELOU (1993)

Although posttraumatic stress disorder (PTSD) is among the most common psychiatric disorders (e.g., Breslau, Davis, Andreski, & Peterson, 1991; Saxe et al., 1993), systematic investigation of what constitutes effective treatment is still in its infancy. Most of the available published treatment studies have utilized cognitive-behavioral therapy (see Chapter 22, this volume), eye movement desensitization and reprocessing (EMDR; e.g., Wilson, Tinker, & Becker, 1995; Vaughan et al., 1994a; Vaughan, Wiese, Gold, & Tarrier, 1994b), or pharmacotherapy (see Chapter 23, this volume). In contrast with general outcome studies of PTSD, which paint a bleak picture of the long-term prognosis in PTSD (see Chapter 8, this volume), studies utilizing these treatment modalities have shown quite positive results. Few studies have examined the efficacy of psychodynamic therapies; most (e.g., Lindy, 1987) have failed to show robust decreases in PTSD symptoms. Two studies, one of accident victims (Brom & Kleber, 1989) and one of traumatized police officers (Gersons & Carlier, 1994), were notable exceptions.

Despite the fact that most studies with positive results for ameliorating PTSD symptoms have used a cognitive-behavioral framework, most clinicians treating traumatized patients continue to practice psychodynamic therapy (Blake, 1993). This raises these questions: Are most clinicians misguided in their choice of interventions? Or are most patients with PTSD seeking treatment not primarily for their PTSD symptoms, but for the associated features of PTSD (such as affect dysregulation, dissociative problems, somatization, depression, and difficulties with trust and intimacy; see Chapter 9, this volume), which may respond best to dynamic therapies? No treatment studies of PTSD have as yet addressed these questions, because the existing studies have not looked at the effects of treatment both on the core PTSD symptoms and on comorbidity and functional impairment. In addition, there have been no careful studies comparing manualized cognitive-behavioral treatment with a rigorous psychodynamic approach.

Until more comprehensive treatment outcome studies are available, we continue to be critically dependent on clinical wisdom in treating these patients. Thus, we must remain aware of the caveat that there can be significant gaps between clinical impressions and scientific data—a caveat graphically illustrated by the Koach project (Solomon, Bleich, Shoham, Nardi, & Kotler, 1992). This carefully designed treatment study was developed by the Mental Health Department of the Israeli Defense Force to assist a large group of veterans of the 1982 Lebanon War whose chronic PTSD had not responded to treatment. A group of international authorities on traumatic stress organized an innovative treatment program that incorporated the latest understanding of cognitive, behavioral, and social interventions for PTSD. At the end of the study, both therapists and participants were generally positive about its effectiveness and outcome. However, contrary to these subjective impressions, careful psychometric assessment demonstrated both short-term and long-term negative effects. Compared with a control group, treated veterans developed *more* symptoms and disabilities in several areas of functioning.

The reports about this program show that even with a sophisticated knowledge of PTSD, and careful application of the available treatment literature, significant negative outcomes can occur. Moreover, even though both patients and therapists may *feel* good about the treatment process, this does not necessarily mean that patients are actually getting better. The lesson from the Koach project is that health care providers must constantly reevaluate what is being accomplished. This includes a continual need to evaluate what particular interventions are most effective for which trauma-related problems. For example, core PTSD symptoms (intrusions, numbing, and hyperarousal), occupational disabilities, or interpersonal problems and alienation may all need different approaches. Thus, the treatment of PTSD has this in common with other areas of psychotherapy practice: Much of the required research information does not exist. Therefore, the treatment must in large part be derived from clinical judgment and draw from the available knowledge about the etiology and longitudinal course of this condition.

BASIC PRINCIPLES OF TREATMENT

What distinguishes people who develop PTSD from those who are merely temporarily stressed is that they become "stuck" on the trauma; they keep reliving it in thoughts, feelings, actions, or images. This intrusive reliving, rather than the traumatic event itself, is responsible for the complex biobehavioral change that we call PTSD (McFarlane, 1988). Once they become dominated by intrusions of the trauma, traumatized individuals begin organizing their lives around avoiding having these experiences. Avoidance may take many different forms: keeping away from situations, people, or emotions that remind them of the traumatic event; ingesting alcohol or drugs, which numb awareness of distressing emotional states; or utilizing dissociation to keep unpleasant experiences from conscious awareness. A chronic sense of helplessness, physiological hyperarousal, and other trauma-related changes may permanently change how a person deals with stress, alter his or her self-concept, and interfere with his or her view of the world as a manageable place.

A sense of relative safety and predictability is a precondition for effective planning and goal-directed action. Freud (1911/1958) postulated that in order to function properly, people need to be able to define their needs, and to entertain a range of options on how to meet them, without resorting to premature action. He called this capacity "thought as experimental action." Traumatized people have been shown to have trouble tolerating intense emotions and entertaining potentially upsetting cognitions without feeling overwhelmed (van der Kolk & Ducey, 1989). This interferes with their being able to utilize emotions as guides for action. People with PTSD experience their internal world as a danger zone that is filled with trauma-related thoughts and feelings. They seem to spend their energy on *not* thinking and planning. This avoidance of emotional triggers further diminishes the importance of current reality, and, paradoxically, increases their attachment to the past.

The aim of therapy with traumatized patients is to help them move from being haunted by the past and interpreting subsequent emotionally arousing stimuli as a return of the trauma, to being fully engaged in the present and becoming capable of responding to current exigencies. In order to do that, the patients need to regain control over their emotional responses and place the trauma in the larger perspective of their lives—as a historical event (or series of events) that occurred at a particular time and in a particular place, and that can be expected not to recur if the individuals take charge of their lives. The key element of the psychotherapy of people with PTSD is the integration of the alien, the unacceptable, the terrifying, and the incomprehensible into their self-concepts. Life events initially experienced as alien, imposed from outside upon passive victims, must come to be "personalized" as integrated aspects of the individuals' history and life experiences (van der Kolk & Ducey, 1989). The massive defenses, initially established as emergency protective measures, must gradually relax their grip upon the sufferers' psyches, so that dissociated aspects of experience do not continue to intrude into their life experiences, thereby continuing to retraumatize already traumatized victims.

Psychotherapy must address two fundamental aspects of PTSD: (1) deconditioning of anxiety, and (2) altering the way victims views themselves and their world by reestablishing a feeling of personal integrity and control. In only the simplest cases will it be sufficient to decondition the anxiety associated with the trauma; in the vast majority of patients, both aspects need to be treated. This means the use of a combination of procedures for deconditioning anxiety, for reestablishing a personal sense of control (which can range from engaging in physical challenges to reestablishing a sense of spiritual meaning), and for forming meaningful and mutually satisfying relationships with others (often by means of group psychotherapy). Tragically, many traumatized people are involved in ongoing traumatic situations, in which they seem to have little or no personal control over what happens to them. However, even under those circumstances, learning how to assess properly what is going on and to plan responses can still be expected to have significant benefits.

The therapeutic relationship with PTSD patients tends to be extraordinarily complex, particularly since the interpersonal aspects of the trauma, such as mistrust, betrayal, dependency, love, and hate, tend to be replayed within the therapeutic dyad (see Chapters 24 and 25, this volume). Dealing with trauma in therapy confronts all participants with intense emotional experiences ranging from helplessness to intense wishes for revenge, and from vicarious traumatization to vicarious thrills (van der Kolk, 1994). The devastating effects of trauma on affect modulation, attention, perception, and the giving and taking of pleasure bring both patients and therapists face to face with the full range of human emotions—from the desire to love and feel safe, to the wish to dominate, use, and hurt others (Wilson & Lindy, 1994).

DIAGNOSIS AND ASSESSMENT

Prior to the start of treatment, a thorough history needs to be taken. This should include the nature of the traumatic stressor; the patient's role in the traumatic experience; the patient's thoughts and feelings about actions taken and not taken; the effect of the trauma on the patient's life and perceptions of self and others; exposure to prior traumatic experiences; habitual coping styles; level of cognitive functioning; particular personal strengths and capacities; prior psychiatric history; medical, social, family, and occupational history; and cultural and religious explanatory beliefs. During the initial evaluation, particular attention needs to be paid to the issues discussed in detail below.

Intrusive Reexperiencing

Remembrance and intrusions of the trauma are expressed in many different ways: as flashbacks, affective states, somatic sensations, nightmares, interpersonal reenactments (including transference repetitions), character styles, and pervasive life themes. Laub and Auerhahn (1993) have organized the different forms of knowing about trauma along a continuum, according to their emotional distance from the traumatic experience. Each form progressively represents a deeper and more integrated "level of knowing": (1) not knowing; (2) fugue states (in which events are relived in an altered state of consciousness); (3) retention of the traumatic experience as compartmentalized, undigested fragments of perceptions that break into consciousness (with no conscious meaning or relation to oneself); (4) transference phenomena (wherein the traumatic legacy is lived out as one's inevitable fate); (5) partial, hesitant expression of the experience as an overpowering narrative; (6) the expression of compelling, identity-defining, and pervasive life themes (both conscious and unconscious); and (7) organization of the experience as a witnessed narrative. These various forms of knowing are not mutually exclusive.

Autonomic Hyperarousal

Whereas people with PTSD tend to deal with their environment through emotional constriction, their physiological responses are conditioned to react to reminders of the trauma as an emergency. Autonomic arousal, which serves the essential function of alerting the organism to potential danger, loses that function in people with PTSD; the easy triggering of somatic stress reactions causes them to be unable to trust their bodily sensations to warn them against impending threat, and cease to alert them to take appropriate action. Not only does increased autonomic arousal interfere with psychological comfort, but anxiety itself may also trigger memories of previous traumatic experiences. Any arousing situation may trigger memories of long-ago traumatic experiences and precipitate reactions that are irrelevant to present demands (see Chapter 10, this volume).

Numbing of Responsiveness

Aware of their difficulties in controlling their emotions, traumatized people seem to spend their energies on avoiding distressing internal sensations, instead of attending to the demands of the environment. In addition, they take little or no satisfaction in matters that previously gave them a sense of satisfaction, and may feel "dead to the world." This emotional numbing may be expressed as depression, as anhedonia and lack of motivation, as psychosomatic reactions, or as dissociative states. In contrast with the intrusive PTSD symptoms, which occur in response to specific stimuli, numbing is part of these patients' baseline functioning. After being traumatized, many people cease to derive pleasure from exploration and involvement in activities; they feel that they just "go through the motions" of everyday living. Emotional numbness also gets in the way of resolving the trauma in psychotherapy: Many patients can no longer imagine a future for themselves.

Intense Emotional Reactions

The loss of neuromodulation that is at the core of PTSD leads to loss of affect regulation. Traumatized people go immediately from stimulus to response without being able to first figure out what makes them so upset. They tend to experience intense fear, anxiety, anger, and panic in response to even minor stimuli. This makes them either overreact and intimidate others, or shut down and freeze. Both adults and children with such hyperarousal will experience sleep problems, both because they are unable to still themselves sufficiently to go to sleep, and because they are fearful of having traumatic nightmares.

Learning Difficulties

Physiological hyperarousal interferes with the capacity to concentrate and to learn from experience. Aside from amnesias about aspects of the trauma, traumatized people often have trouble remembering ordinary events as well. Easily triggered into hyperarousal by trauma-related stimuli, and beset with difficulties in paying attention, they may display symptoms of attention-deficit/hyperactivity disorder. After a traumatic experience, people often lose some maturational achievements and regress to earlier modes of coping with stress. In children, this may show up as an inability to take care of themselves in such areas as feeding and toilet training; in adults, it is expressed as excessive dependence and in a loss of capacity to make thoughtful, autonomous decisions.

Memory Disturbances and Dissociation

In addition to hypermnesia and intrusive memories, chronically traumatized people, particularly children, may develop amnesic syndromes related to the traumatic event. During the stage of life in which children normally try on different identities in their daily play activities, children who are exposed to prolonged and severe trauma may be capable of organizing whole personality fragments to cope with traumatic experiences (Putnam, 1989). At the far extreme of the spectrum of dissociative responses to traumatic life experiences is the syndrome of dissociative identity disorder (formerly called multiple personality disorder), which occurs in about 4% of psychiatric inpatients in the United States (Saxe et al., 1993).

Patients who have learned to dissociate in response to trauma are likely to continue to utilize dissociative defenses when exposed to new stresses. They develop amnesia for some experiences, and tend to react with fight-or-flight responses to feeling threatened, none of which may be consciously remembered afterwards. People who suffer from dissociative disorders are a clinical challenge, particularly in regard to helping them acquire a sense of personal responsibility for their actions and reactions; forensically, they are a nightmare.

Aggression against Self and Others

Numerous studies have demonstrated that both adults and children who have been traumatized are likely to turn their aggression against others or themselves. Abuse during childhood sharply increases the risk for later delinquency and violent criminal behavior. In one study of 87 psychiatric outpatients, van der Kolk, Perry, and Herman (1991) found that self-mutilators invariably had severe childhood histories of abuse and/or neglect. Problems with aggression against others have been particularly well documented in war veterans, in traumatized children, and in prisoners with histories of early trauma (Lewis, 1990, 1992).

Psychosomatic Reactions

Chronic anxiety and emotional numbing also get in the way of learning to identify and articulate internal states and wishes (Krystal, 1978; Pennebaker, 1993). Many traumatized patients suffer from alexithymia—an inability to translate somatic sensations into basic feelings, such as anger, happiness, or fear. This failure to translate somatic states into words and symbols causes them to experience emotions simply as physical problems. This naturally plays havoc with interpersonal communication. These people experience distress in terms of physical organs, rather than as psychological states (Saxe et al., 1994).

ESTABLISHING A TREATMENT PLAN

The assessment of the relative significance of these various symptom clusters is essential for determining an appropriate treatment plan. For example, flooding therapy may be inappropriate for patients with high levels of avoidance, whereas dissociative patients need to learn to control "spacing out" under stress before actively addressing their memories of their traumatic experiences. Moreover, specific psychological interventions cannot begin until various other issues, often of a very practical nature, have been addressed. For example, victims of a natural disaster may have to secure a place to sleep and a way of protecting their possessions; political prisoners who have been tortured may have to attend to resettlement issues before they can look back at the meaning of their trauma for their further lives. Perhaps one of the greatest challenges is dealing with families in which there is ongoing sexual abuse. The immediate physical protection of the child and legal issues always take precedence over the exploration of the trauma.

Planning for and Dealing with Noncompliance

One serious obstacle to effective treatment is that many traumatized patients will guard against confrontations with reminders of their trauma, including psychotherapeutic interventions. Brom, Kleber, and Defares (1989) found that although 36% of motor accident victims agreed to have their longitudinal course monitored, only 13% were willing to participate in an intervention study, despite the presence of significant levels of distress. High rates of noncompliance in patients who suffer from PTSD make it necessary to spell out explicit treatment agreements and to approach treatment flexibly enough to leave the door open for later contact (Bernstein, 1986). Clinicians need to position themselves as consultants to their patients in continually monitoring what they can tolerate, determining how fast they want to proceed, and collaboratively following the course of various posttraumatic symptoms. A constant reassessment of patients' capacity to face their emotions is essential to prevent high dropout rates and therapeutic failure rates (McFarlane, 1994).

Since interpersonal trauma tends to occur in contexts in which the rules are unclear, under circumstances that are secret, and in conditions where issues of responsibility are often murky, issues of rules, boundaries, contracts, and mutual responsibilities need to be clearly specified and adhered to (Kluft, 1990; Herman, 1992). Failure to attend strictly to these issues is likely to result in a recreation of aspects of the trauma itself in the therapeutic situation.

Taking Different Approaches at Different Stages

Trauma needs to be treated differently at different phases of people's lives following the trauma: Treatments that may be effective at some stages of treatment may not be effective at others. For example, on a pharmacological level, initial management with drugs that decrease autonomic arousal will decrease nightmares and flashbacks, will promote sleep, and may prevent the limbic kindling that is thought to underlie the long-term establishment of PTSD symptomatology (see Chapters 10 and 23, this volume). Once the disorder we call PTSD has been established, these same drugs have at best a palliative function; at this point, serotonin reuptake blockers, which seem to have little immediate benefit, often start being helpful in allowing people to attend to current tasks and to decrease their dwelling upon past fears, interpretations, and fixations.

Similarly, when intrusions of fragmentary memories of the trauma are the predominant symptoms, exposure and desensitization may be what patients most urgently require. At a later stage of the progression of the disorder—when individuals have organized their lives around avoidance of triggers of the trauma, and view other people as potential triggers of traumatic intrusions—helplessness, suspicion, anger, and interpersonal problems may dominate the symptom picture. When this is the case, primary attention needs to be paid to stabilization in the social realm.

TREATMENT OF ACUTE TRAUMA

Immediately after people have been traumatized, the emphasis needs to be on self-regulation and on rebuilding (see Chapters 19, 20, and 21, this volume). This means the reestablishment of security and predictability. It also means active involvement in adaptive action, such as the rebuilding of damaged property, engagement with other victims, and active engagement in the physical care of oneself and other survivors. Only a limited proportion of people who are traumatized develop PTSD; most traumatized people seem to be able to negotiate these initial adaptive phases successfully, without succumbing to the long-term progression of their acute stress reaction into PTSD. For them, the trauma becomes merely a terrible experience in their past.

It is not at all clear whether talking about what has happened is always useful. Some surprising findings have come out of careful research on critical incident stress debriefing. The few controlled studies that have examined the preventive effect of debriefing immediately following exposure to a traumatic event have suggested a *poorer* outcome after debriefing than after no intervention (McFarlane, 1994). Given the paucity of controlled studies, we are left with the clinical impression that the initial response to trauma needs to consist of reconnecting individuals with their ordinary supportive networks, and having them engage in activities that reestablish a sense of mastery. It is obvious that the role of mental health professionals in these initial recuperative efforts is quite limited.

PHASE-ORIENTED TREATMENT OF PTSD

All treatment of traumatized individuals needs to be paced according to the degree of involuntary intrusion of the trauma, as well as the individuals' capacities to deal with intense emotions. Clinicians must identify and respect the different psychic defenses that people use to deal with the memories of traumatic material. Effective treatment needs to proceed in phases, which should include the following (van der Hart, Brown, & van der Kolk, 1989; van der Hart, Steele, Boon, & Brown, 1993; Herman, 1992):

1. Stabilization, including (a) education and (b) identification of feelings through verbalizing somatic states.
2. Deconditioning of traumatic memories and responses.
3. Restructuring of traumatic personal schemes.
4. Reestablishment of secure social connections and interpersonal efficacy.
5. Accumulation of restitutive emotional experiences.

In the treatment of simple cases of PTSD, it is often possible to move quickly from one phase to the next; in more complex cases, the stabilization phase needs to be frequently repeated, as the totality of the personality may react to many aspects of everyday living as a reexperiencing of the trauma (e.g., Brown & Fromm, 1986).

Stabilization: Overcoming the Fear of Trauma-Related Emotions

During the stabilization phase, a patient is taught how to control overwhelming emotions and pathological defensive operations, such as continued dissociation. This includes identifying and labeling emotions; identifying and appropriately utilizing social supports; focusing on content, rather than affects; scheduling, planning, and anticipating daily activities; making judicious use of exercise and food; and engaging in relaxation and stress inoculation exercises (Foa, Rothbaum, Riggs, & Murdock, 1991; Linehan, 1993; van der Hart et al., 1993). Psychopharmacological management is often an integral part of stabilization (see Chapter 23).

Education

Patients are often confused by their symptoms and believe that they are "going crazy." Their families, colleagues, and friends may be equally confused about what to do, and may withdraw in the face of the patients' intense emotionality, anger, grief, and withdrawal. Developing a cognitive frame that helps patients understand their intrusions and avoidance helps them gain some emotional distance from the experience, and begins to put the event into the larger context of their lives. They first need to get a sense of time: This experience had a beginning, now has progressed to the next phase, and eventually will come to an end in some way. The initial encounter with the therapist often provides the first opportunity for making a conscious link between trauma-related thoughts and feelings. A detailed behavioral analysis may explain the range of triggers to memories of the trauma, as well as an individual's autonomic, cognitive, and behavioral responses (Brom et al., 1989; McFarlane, 1994).

Identification of Feelings
through Verbalizing Somatic States

The psychological function of emotions is to alert people to the occurrence, significance, and nature of subjective experience. Thus, emotions function as signals to readjust one's expectations of the world and/or to take adaptive action. Ordinarily, emotions are deactivated when one's conceptions of the world have been brought into line with what is actually happening (Horowitz, 1986). This is done through assimilation (i.e., changing one's concepts of the world to include the new experience) or through accommodation (i.e., taking action that brings the situation back in line with expectations).

Krystal (1978) first noted that in people with PTSD, emotions seem to lose much of their alerting function; a dissociation is set up between emotional arousal and goal-directed action. People with PTSD no longer seem to be able to interpret the meaning of their emotional arousal, which thus becomes irrelevant as a signal for change. Indeed, having feelings in and of itself becomes a negative experience: Because these people can find no release in adaptive action, emotions merely become reminders of their inability to affect the outcome of their lives. Hence, not only do concrete, sensory images of the trauma function as reminders; feelings themselves may come to be experienced as traumatic reminders, and thus need to be avoided (van der Kolk & Ducey, 1989).

Unable to neutralize emotions by taking effective action, traumatized people tend to experience their feelings in their bodies, by way of either their smooth or their striated muscles. Thus, either they somatize (Saxe et al., 1994) or they discharge their emotions with actions that do not match the stimulus precipitating the emotion—often with aggressive actions against self or others (van der Kolk et al., 1991). A critical element in the treatment of traumatized people is to help them find words for emotional states. Naming feelings gives patients a subjective sense of mastery and a mental flexibility that facilitates comparison with other emotions and other situations. As we have noted in Chapters 1, 2, and 13, both children and adults can come to deal effectively with stressful situations by learning to categorize their perceptions.

Again, because in people with PTSD so many roads seem to lead to traumatic associations, much of their efforts are geared toward *not* feeling and thinking. They have given up on believing that they can figure out how to regulate their internal states. Unable to imagine that they are able to master their intense feelings, many people with PTSD cling to caregivers (whom they endow with magical capacities) to do it for them. Like young children, they have problems telling the difference between what something (e.g., a reminder of the trauma) feels like and what is actually happening. PTSD patients with flashbacks cannot distance themselves from what is happening *to* them, and they have difficulty distinguishing between the trigger and their response. Thus, for them, the event seems to be happening over and over again.

Treatment, like human development, consists of learning to master and "own" one's experiences. Traumatized individuals need to learn to detach themselves from being "embedded" in the experience; sensations and perceptions once again need to be placed into personal categories. In order to accomplish this, people need to "know" what these events actually are, and to locate them in space and time. People need to rediscover that what is currently being experienced was preceded by, and will be followed by, other experiences. This knowledge is essential for them to be able to compare what is currently going on with other experiences—a necessary precondition for the development of the critical capacity to imagine playing a role in what is happening, and hence to be able to affect the outcome of events.

2. Deconditioning of Traumatic Memories and Responses

When patients have gained stability, control, and perspective, treatment can be terminated. There is no intrinsic value in dredging up past trauma if a patient's current life provides gratification, and the present is not invaded by emotional, perceptual, or behavioral intrusions from the past. However, if such involuntary emotional, perceptual, or behavioral intrusions continue to interfere with people's current functioning, controlled and predictable exposure to the traumatic memories can help with regaining mastery. The compulsion to repeat the trauma, without any perspective on what is being repeated, does not lead to mastery, but only disrupts people's lives further (van der Kolk, 1989). Merely reexperiencing fragments of the trauma (e.g., in nightmares and flashbacks) cannot lead to resolution, because the incomplete reliving of perceptual or affective elements of the trauma prevents the construction of an integrated memory—one that no longer serves as a trigger for conditioned responses (van der Hart & Op den Velde, 1991).

A therapist's natural proclivity is to help a patient avoid experiencing undue pain; however, learning to tolerate the memories of intense emotional experieces is a critical part of recovery. The psychotherapist who understands the nature of trauma can aid the process of integration by staying with the patient through his or her suffering; by providing a perspective that the suffering is meaningful and bearable; and by helping in the mastery of trauma through putting the experience into symbolic, communicable form (i.e., through putting perception and sensations into words). The patient's "repeating" the trauma in action is the forerunner to his or her "remembering" and symbolizing it in words, which in turn is both a precursor and an accompaniment to "working it through" in emotional experience.

In Chapter 12, we discussed how traumatic memories tend to be stored as perceptual and affective states, with little verbal representation. Many traumatized people continue to be haunted by "them" (unintegrated traumatic memories), without an "I" to put these feelings and perceptions in perspective. Treatment at this stage consists of translating the nonverbal dissociated realm of traumatic memory into secondary mental processes in which words can provide meaning and form, thereby facilitating the transformation of traumatic memory into narrative memory. In other words, what is currently implicit memory needs to be made explicit, autobiographical memory.

The Central Issue of Memory and Dissociation

Pierre Janet (1889) first described how the central issue in trauma is dissociation. Memories of what has happened cannot be integrated into one's general experiential schemes and are split off from the rest of personal experience. Lack of integration on a schematic level causes the experience to be stored as affect states or as somatosensory elements of the trauma, which return into consciousness when reminders activate customary response patterns: physical sensations (such as panic attacks), visual images (such as flashbacks and nightmares), obsessive ruminations, or behavioral reenactments of elements of the trauma. (See Chapters 12 and 13 for fuller discussions.)

Most studies of people who develop PTSD find significant dissociative symptomatology (Bremner et al., 1993; Marmar et al., 1994) The most extreme form of posttraumatic dissociation is seen in patients who suffer from dissociative identity disorder. Janet (1889) first described how traumatized people become "attached" (Freud would later use the term "fixated") to the trauma: "Unable to integrate traumatic memories, they seem to have lost their capacity to assimilate new experiences as well. It is . . . as if their personality definitely stopped at a certain point and cannot enlarge any more by the addition or assimilation of new elements" (Janet, 1919/1925, Vol. 1, p. 532). Clinicians have repeatedly observed that traumatized people tend to revert to earlier modes of cognitive processing of information when faced with new stresses.

Since the core problem in PTSD consists of a failure to integrate an upsetting experience into autobiographical memory, treatment consists of finding ways in which people can acknowledge the reality of what has happened without having to reexperience the trauma all over again. For this to occur, merely uncovering memories is not enough. Traumatic memories need to be become like memories of everyday experience; that is, they need to be modified and transformed by being placed in their proper context and reconstructed into a meaningful narrative. Only if all residual fragments are integrated can full resolution occur. The purpose of full exposure is to make the fragments of the traumatic event lose their power to act as conditioned stimuli that reactivate affects and behaviors relevant to the trauma, but irrelevant to current experience. Thus, in therapy, memory paradoxically becomes an act of creation, rather than the static recording of events that is characteristic of trauma-based memories.

Controlled Exposure and Memory Reactivation

Controlled exposure as a means of reactivating and modifying traumatic memories is a key aspect of the treatment of PTSD and other trauma-induced disorders. Its rationale and practice are described differently by different therapeutic schools; however, all apply Foa, Steketee, and Rothbaum's (1989) rule that some new information incompatible with the rigid traumatic memory must be introduced. According to Foa and Kozak (1985) (see also Chapter 23, this volume), two conditions are required for the reduction of fear, and hence for the treatment of PTSD:

1. The person must attend to trauma-related information in a manner that will activate his or her own traumatic memories. As long as trauma-related affects are not experienced, the traumatic structure cannot be modified. The decrease of fear or anxiety is dependent upon the controlled and coordinated evocation of (a) the stimulus components (environmental cues), (b) the response components (e.g., motoric actions, heart pounding), and (c) the meaning elements (e.g., cues regarding morality and guilt) of the traumatic memory (Keane & Kaloupek, 1982; Foa et al., 1989; Litz & Keane, 1989).

2. In order for the person to form a new, nontraumatic structure, trauma-discrepant information must be provided. The critical issue is to expose the patient to an experience that contains elements that are sufficiently similar to the trauma to activate it, and at the same time contains aspects that are incompatible enough to change it.

The most important new information is probably the fact that the patient is able to confront the traumatic memory with a trusted therapist in a safe environment (van der Hart & Spiegel, 1993). Secure attachment to the therapist is an indispensable element in learning to regulate emotional arousal; the therapeutic alliance is the cornerstone of all treatment. Although behavioral therapists describe exposure procedures extensively, they tend to neglect to write about the intensely personal element in all psychotherapeutic procedures, which is critical to the success of treatment. So, while these clinicians and researchers limit their presentations almost exclusively to data indicating decreases of fear or anxiety through controlled exposure to the stimulus—response components and the meaning elements of the traumatic memories, their results are most likely influenced in a major way by their personal investment in the well-being of their patients, which is communicated and translated into a subjective sense of safety.

Flooding and exposure are by no means risk-free treatment techniques. Exposure to information consistent with a traumatic memory can be expected to increase anxiety (thereby sensitizing and aggravating PTSD symptomatology). Again, in order to overcome the intrusive sensory–motor elements of the trauma, the person must transform the traumatic (nonverbal) memory into a personal narrative; this entails being able to tell the story of the shocking event without totally reliving it. Excessive arousal may make the PTSD patient worse by interfering with the acquisition of new information (Strian & Klicpera, 1978). When that occurs, the traumatic memories will not be corrected, but merely confirmed; instead of promoting habituation, it accidentally fosters sensitization. Another obstacle to effective treatment is that the strong response elements in the PTSD structure may promote avoidance: Strong fear and discomfort may motivate patients to escape confrontation with situations that remind them of the trauma.

Hence, the objective of this part of treatment is for a patient to reexperience a traumatic memory in a safe and controllable environment, and to be able to evoke a traumatic image without feeling overwhelmed by the associated emotions. An increasing body of research demonstrates that once all relevant elements of the total traumatic experience have been identified and thoroughly and deeply examined and experienced in the therapy, successful synthesis will take place (e.g., Resick & Schnicke, 1992).

Restructuring of Trauma-Related Cognitive Schemes: Overcoming the Fear of Life Itself

People are meaning-making creatures. As human beings develop, they organize their world according to a personal theory of reality, some of which may be conscious, but much of which is an unconscious integration of accumulated experience (Harber & Pennebaker, 1992; Janet, 1889). As Horowitz (1986) and Epstein (1991) have pointed out, conceptions of oneself and the world are organized according to relatively stable cognitive schemata (about competence and dependence, power and helplessness, trust and distrust, etc.). These mental schemata organize psychological experience via the processes of assimilation and accommodation, and assure continuity of a person's identity. Although most people cannot clearly articulate the content of their mental schemes, they nonetheless determine what sensory input is selected for further coding and categorization, and what actions they are likely to take in the face of stress. Cognitive schemata allow people to make sense out of emotional and arousing experiences, and thus serve as buffers against their becoming overwhelmed.

Adaptive resolution to a stressful experience consists of a modification of one's view of self and others that permits continued attention to the exigencies of daily life. In order to deal successfully with distressing events, it is necessary not to generalize from that experience to the totality of existence, but to view it merely as one terrible incident that has taken place at a particular place at a particular time (Epstein, 1991; Janoff-Bulman, 1992). Traumatic experiences are not only processed by means of currently existing mental schemes; they may also activate latent self-concepts and views of relationships that were formed earlier in life. This activation of latent schemes is particularly relevant for people with prior histories of trauma, even when they have subsequently been able to make successful adaptations. When trauma activates these earlier self-schemata, these will compete and coexist with more mature schemata in explaining cause-and-effect relationships in regards to the trauma. These different, and often competing, mental schemes will then determine the psychological organization of the traumatic experience.

In many people with PTSD, trauma-related conceptions of themselves and the world come to dominate their everyday existence. When dissociation is a central element of coping with the trauma, there may be a split: Some existing schemes are maintained and come to coexist with trauma-related schemes, which are only activated when the individual is once again exposed to a stressful situation. In many traumatized patients, cognitive schemes include both trauma-based and non-trauma-based schemes. Dissociative patients in some states may believe that "I was not abused," while the dissociated cognitive system may contain beliefs such as "I am weak, helpless, and unworthy" or "I am mean and aggressive." Exposure to subsequent stress tends to reactivate not only traumatic memories, but also trauma-based schemes about self and others.

Often these issues are inadequately assessed in the treatment of PTSD treatment, although studies such as the National Vietnam Veterans Readjustment Study (Kulka et al., 1990) provide rich accounts of the pervasive effects of trauma on the totality of people's functioning. Effective psychotherapy needs to address specifically how the trauma has affected people's sense of self-efficacy, their capacity for trust and intimacy, their ability to negotiate their personal needs, and their ability to feel empathy for other people (McCann & Pearlman, 1990; Herman, 1992). This is often best accomplished in a group psychotherapy setting (see below).

Reestablishment of Secure Social Connections and Interpersonal Efficacy

Emotional attachment is probably the primary protection against being traumatized. People seek close emotional relationships with others in order to help them anticipate, meet, and integrate difficult experiences. Contemporary research (see Chapters 19 and 20, this volume) has shown that as long as the social support network remains intact, people are relatively well protected against even catastrophic stresses. For young children, the family is usually a very effective source of protection against traumatization, and most children are amazingly resilient as long as they have caregivers who are emotionally and physically available (van der Kolk et al., 1991; McFarlane, 1988). Mature people also rely on their families, colleagues, and friends to provide such a "trauma membrane." In recognition of this need for affiliation as a protection against trauma, it has become widely accepted that the central issue in acute crisis intervention is the provision and restoration of social support (Lystad, 1988; Raphael, 1986).

Some form of group therapy is often considered a treatment of choice for both acutely and chronically traumatized individuals. The primary task of group therapy and community interventions is to help victims regain a sense of safety and of mastery. After an acute trauma, fellow victims often provide the most effective short-term bond, because the shared history of trauma can form the nucleus of retrieving a sense of communality. For chronically traumatized individuals, group psychotherapy may provide a sense of mutuality and a forum to explore concerns about safety and trust, which have been affected by earlier interpersonal trauma.

Regardless of the nature of the trauma, or the structure of the group, the aim of group therapy is to help people actively attend to the requirements of the moment, without undue intrusions from past perceptions and experiences. Group therapy has been used for victims of interpersonal violence (Mitchell, 1983), natural disasters (Lystad, 1988; Raphael, 1986), childhood sexual abuse (Herman & Schatzow, 1987; Ganzarian & Buchele, 1987), rape (Yassen & Glass, 1984), spouse battering (Rounsaville, Lifton, & Bieber, 1979), concentration camps (Danieli, 1985), and war trauma (Parson, 1985). In a group of people who have gone through similar experiences, most traumatized people are eventually able to find the appropriate words to express what has happened to them. As was observed over 50 years ago, "by working out their problems in a small group they should be able to face the larger group, i.e., their world, in an easier manner" (Grinker & Spiegel, 1945).

There are many levels of trauma-related group psychotherapies, with different degrees of emphasis on stabilization, memory retrieval, bonding, negotiation of interpersonal differences, and support. However, to varying degrees, the purposes of all trauma-related groups are to help members (1) stabilize psychological and physiological reactions to the trauma, (2) explore and validate perceptions and emotions, (3) understand the effects of past experience on current affects and behaviors, and (4) learn new ways of coping with interpersonal stress (see van der Kolk, 1992).

Accumulation of Restitutive Emotional Experiences

Because the reliving and the warding off of traumatic memories are the central psychological preoccupations of traumatized people, there is little room for new, gratifying experiences that might allow for reparation of past injuries to the self. Patients need to expose themselves actively to experiences that provide them with feelings of mastery and pleasure. Physical activities (such as sports or wilderness ventures), other enjoyable physical experiences (e.g., massages), or artistic accomplishments may be experiences for patients that are not contaminated by the trauma, and that may serve as a source of new gratification.

REVIEW OF AVAILABLE TREATMENT OUTCOME STUDIES

Exposure and Related Treatments

In recent years, a number of treatment outcome studies have roughly supported the essential elements of psychotherapy for PTSD as outlined above. Edna Foa and her colleagues (see Chapter 22, this volume) compared stress inoculation training, prolonged imaginal exposure, supportive counseling, and a waiting-list control in 45 female rape victims with PTSD. Initially, both stress inoculation therapy and imaginal exposure proved to be effective treatments of PTSD symptoms, anxiety, and depression. At a 4-month follow-up, imaginal exposure treatment had better effects than stress inoculation. Foa and her colleagues suggested that this finding might be attributable to the fact that the stress inoculation therapy group did not continue to practice, which is necessary for durable improvement. In contrast, they believed that the lasting effects of prolonged exposure were the results of significant changes in memory representations of the trauma itself, which were translated into long-term symptom relief.

Imaginal flooding has been claimed to be effective in a variety of controlled studies of combat veterans with PTSD. Cooper and Clum (1989) found that imaginal flooding caused reduction in sleep disturbance and anxiety symptoms 3 months after the end of treatment, but had no effect on depression, in comparison to "conventional" PTSD treatment. Keane, Fairbank, Caddell, and Zimering (1989) found that implosion therapy at 6 months was associated with reductions in depression, fear, state anxiety, and intrusive symptoms, but not emotional numbing or avoidance. Boudewyns, Hyer, Woods, Harrison, and McCranie (1990) demonstrated that flooding, but not counseling, led to significant improvement at a 3-month follow-up; symptom scales, as well as heart rate change on exposure to combat stimuli, were used as outcome measures. The effects of implosion therapy seem to be long-lasting, as demonstrated by a 2-year follow-up of eight veterans who were treated with biofeedback-assisted systematic desensitization (Peniston, 1986). These results are bolstered by a variety of single-case studies of other traumatized populations, including some with children (Blake, 1993).

Hence, treatment outcome research strongly supports the idea that exposure to memories of the trauma is an essential element of effective treatment of PTSD. This has been further supported by other forms of treatment that do not involve flooding or implosion techniques. For example, Resick and

Schnicke (1992) found that a combination of education, exposure, and cognitive reprocessing work was significantly superior to a wait-list control group, both immediately after and 6 months following treatment.

It is likely that the particular technique utilized in helping patients confront their traumatic memories is *not* the critical variable. For example, Frank, Kosten, Giller, and Dan (1988) failed to find statistical differences between cognitive therapy and systematic desensitization in the treatment of rape victims. Both led to significant reductions of anxiety, depression, and fear. In another well-conducted study of acutely distressed rape victims, Resick, Jordan, Girelli, Hutter, and Marhoefer-Dvorak (1988) found that assertion training, stress inoculation, and supportive psychotherapy with information and education led to similar significant improvements in anxiety and depression. In one of the few studies that included psychodynamic treatment, in addition to hypnotherapy, desensitization, and wait-list controls, Brom and Kleber (1989) examined 112 patients with PTSD associated with a variety of different traumas. Improvement occurred in all treatment modalities, but not in the wait-list control group. Their study suggests that for many patients flooding may be helpful in controlling intrusions and anxiety, but that dynamic psychotherapy may be most helpful in mastering avoidance (Brom et al., 1989).

It is important to emphasize that exposure may lead to serious complications. Vaughan and Tarrier (1992) reported this technique to be useful in seven subjects; two were not helped, and in one there was an increase in both intrusion and avoidance symptoms. Pitman et al. (1991) stopped a flooding study with Vietnam veterans because a number developed serious adverse reactions.

Eye Movement Desensitization and Reprocessing

EMDR, a new treatment for PTSD using rapid rhythmic eye movements, has been described by Francine Shapiro (1989, 1995). The patient is told to maintain an image of the original traumatic experience, and is encouraged to simultaneously evoke the event and associated feelings while engaging in the eye movements. Although some of the initial studies suffered from serious methodological flaws (Herbert & Mueser, 1992), a steady output of successful case reports has encouraged further investigation of EMDR. While one preliminary report by Lytle (cited by Metter & Michelson, 1993), comparing EMDR with non-eye-movement desensitization and a nondirective counseling session, suggested that EMDR was not significantly different from the controls and possibly less efficacious than having the subjects "stare at a dot on the wall," other studies are very encouraging and indicate that this new form of treatment, despite its incomprehesible technique, seems to be capable of producing powerful therapeutic effects in some patients with PTSD (Wilson et al., 1995; Vaughan et al., 1994a, 1994b).

Psychopharmacological Treatment

Recent years have seen numerous anecdotal reports and five well-controlled studies about the use of pharmacological agents in the treatment of PTSD. These are discussed in Chapter 23.

CONCLUDING REMARKS

After a trauma that fully confronts people with their existential helplessness and vulnerability, things can never be exactly the same; the traumatic experience will somehow become part of their lives. Sorting out exactly what happened and sharing their reactions with others can make a great deal of difference in victims' eventual adaptation. However, putting the feelings and cognitions related to the trauma into words is likely not to be enough: Victims need to find active ways of regaining control over their feelings and actions. After intense efforts to ward off reliving the trauma, therapists cannot expect that their patients' resistances to remembering will suddenly melt away under their empathic efforts. The effects of the the patient's trauma on sense of self and trust in others will inevitably find their way into the therapeutic relationship, in which negotiations about safety, trust, disappointment, and boundaries are likely to yield the greatest therapeutic benefits.

Only when issues of interpersonal security can be safely negotiated can the therapeutic relationship be utilized to hold the patient's psyche together when the threat of physical disintegration is reexperienced. Failure to approach trauma-related material gradually is likely to lead to intensification of posttraumatic symptomatology (i.e., increased somatic, visual, or behavioral reexperiences). Once the traumatic experiences have been located in time and place, the person can start making distinctions between current life stresses and past trauma, and can decrease the impact of the trauma on present experience.

Again, talking about the trauma is rarely if ever enough; trauma survivors need to take some action that symbolizes triumph over helplessness and despair. The Holocaust Memorial (Yad Vashem) in Jerusalem, and the Vietnam War Memorial in Washington, D.C., are good examples of symbols that enable survivors to mourn the dead and establish the historical and cultural meaning of the traumatic events. Most of all, they serve to remind survivors of the ongoing potential for communality and sharing. This also applies to survivors of other types of traumas, who may have to build less visible memorials and common symbols to help them mourn and express their shame about their own vulnerability. This may take the form of writing a book, taking political action, helping other victims, or any of the myriad of creative solutions that human beings can find to defy even the most desperate plight.

REFERENCES

Angelou, M. (1993). *On the pulse of morning.* New York: Random House.

Bernstein, A. (1986). The treatment of non-compliance in patients with posttraumatic stress disorder. *Psychosomatic Medicine, 27,* 37–40.

Blake, D. D. (1993). Treatment outcome research on post traumatic stress disorder. *C P Clinician Newsletter, 3,* 14–17.

Boudewyns, P. A., Hyer, L., Woods, M. G., Harrison, W. R., & McCranie, E. (1990). PTSD among Vietnam veterans: An early look at treatment outcome using direct therapeutic exposure. *Journal of Traumatic Stress, 3,* 359–368.

Bremner, J. D., Scott, T. M., Delaney, R. C., Southwick, S. M., Mason, J. M. (1993). Deficits in short-term memory in posttraumatic stress disorder. *American Journal of Psychiatry, 150*(7), 1015–1019.

Breslau, N., Davis, G. C., Andreski, P., & Peterson, E. (1991). Traumatic events and posttraumatic stress disorder in an urban population of young adults. *Archives of General Psychiatry, 48,* 216–222.

Brom, D., & Kleber, R. J. (1989). Prevention of post-traumatic stress disorders. *Journal of Traumatic Stress, 2*(3), 335–351.

Brom, D., Kleber, R. J., & Defares, P. B. (1989). Brief psychotherapy for posttraumatic stress disorders. *Journal of Consulting and Clinical Psychology, 57*(5), 607–612.

Brown, D. P., & Fromm, E. (1986). *Hypnoanalysis and hypnotherapy.* Hillsdale, NJ: Erlbaum.

Cooper, N. A., & Clum, G. A. (1989). Imaginal flooding as a supplementary treatment for PTSD in combat veterans: A controlled study. *Behavior Therapy, 20*(3), 381–391.

Danieli, Y. (1985). The treatment and prevention of long-term effects and intergenerational transmission of victimization: A lesson from Holocaust survivors and their children. In C. R. Figley (Ed.), *Trauma and its wake* (Vol. 1). New York: Brunner/Mazel.

Epstein, S. (1991). The self-concept, the traumatic neurosis, and the structure of personality. In D. Ozer, J. M. Healy, Jr., & A. J. Stewart (Eds.), *Perspectives in personality* (Vol. 3, Part A, pp. 63–98). London: Jessica Kingsley.

Foa, E. B., & Kozak, M. J. (1985). Treatment of anxiety disorders: Implications for psychopathology. In A. H. Tuma & J. D. Maser (Eds.), *Anxiety and the anxiety disorders.* Hillsdale, NJ: Erlbaum.

Foa, E. B., Rothbaum, B. O., Riggs, D. S., & Murdock, G. B. (1991). Treatment of post-traumatic stress disorder in rape victims: Comparison between cognitive-behavioral procedures and counseling. *Journal of Consulting and Clinical Psychology, 59,* 715–723.

Foa, E. B., Steketee, G., & Rothbaum, B. O. (1989). Behavioral/cognitive conceptualizations of post-traumatic stress disorder. *Behavior Therapy, 20,* 155–176.

Frank, J. B., Kosten, T. R., Giller, E. L., & Dan, E. (1988). A preliminary study of phenelzine and imipramine for post-traumatic stress disorder. *American Journal of Psychiatry, 145,* 1289–1291.

Freud, S. (1958). Formulations on the two principles of mental functioning. In J. Strachey (Ed. and Trans.), *The standard edition of the complete psychological works of Sigmund Freud* (Vol. 12). London: Hogarth Press. (Original work published 1911)

Ganzarian, R., & Buchele, B. (1987). Acting out during group psychotherapy for incest. *International Journal of Group Psychotherapy, 37,* 185–200.

Gersons, B. P. R., & Carlier, I. V. E. (1994). Treatment of work related trauma in police officers: Post-traumatic stress disorder and post-traumatic decline. In M. B. Williams & J. F. Sommer (Eds.), *Handbook of post-trauma therapy* (pp. 325–336). Westport, CT: Greenwood Press.

Grinker, R. R., & Spiegel, J. P. (1945). *Men under stress.* Philadelphia: Blakiston.

Harber, K. D., & Pennebaker, J. W. (1992). Overcoming traumatic memories. In S. A. Christianson (Ed.), *The handbook of emotion and memory: Research and theory* (pp. 359–386). Hillsdale, NJ: Erlbaum.

Herbert, J. D., & Mueser, K. T. (1992). Eye movement desensitization: A critique of the evidence. *Journal of Behavior Therapy and Experimental Psychiatry, 23*(3), 169–174.

Herman, J. L. (1992). *Trauma and recovery.* New York: Basic Books.

Herman, J. L., & Schatzow, E. (1987). Recovery and verification of memories of childhood sexual trauma. *Psychoanalytic Psychology, 4*(1), 1–14.

Horowitz, M. J. (1986). *Stress response syndromes* (2nd ed.). New York: Jason Aronson.

Janet, P. (1889). *L'automatisme psychologique.* Paris: Alcan.

Janet, P. (1925). *Psychological healing* (2 vols.). New York: Macmillan. (Original work published 1919)

Janoff-Bulman, R. (1992). *Shattered assumptions: Towards a new psychology of trauma.* New York: Free Press.

Keane, T. M., Fairbank, J. A., Caddell, J. M., & Zimering, R. T. (1989). Implosive (flooding) therapy reduces symptoms of PTSD in Vietnam combat veterans. *Behavior Therapy, 20*(2), 245–260.

Keane, T. M., & Kaloupek, D. G. (1982). Imaginal flooding in the treatment of post-traumatic stress disorder. *Journal of Consulting and Clinical Psychology, 50,* 138–140.

Kluft, R. (1990). *Incest-related syndromes of adult psychopathology.* Washington, DC: American Psychiatric Press.

Krystal, H. (1978). Trauma and affects. *Psychoanalytic Study of the Child, 33,* 81–116.

Kulka, R. A., Schlenger, W., Fairbank, J., Hough, R. L., Jordan, B. K., Marmar, C. R., & Weiss, D. S. (1990). *Trauma and the Vietnam war generation.* New York: Brunner/Mazel.

Laub, D., & Auerhahn, N. C. (1993). Knowing and not knowing massive psychic trauma: Forms of traumatic memory. *International Journal of Psycho-Analysis, 74,* 287–301.

Lewis, D. O. (1990). Neuropsychiatric and experiential correlates of violent juvenile delinquency. *Neuropsychology Review, 1*(2), 125–136.

Lewis, D. O. (1992). From abuse to violence: Psychophysiological consequences of maltreatment. *Journal of the American Academy of Child and Adolescent Psychiatry, 31,* 383–391.

Litz, B. T., & Keane, T. M. (1989). Information processing in anxiety disorders: Application to the understanding of post-traumatic stress disorder. *Clinical Psychology Review, 9,* 243–257.

Lindy, J. D. (1987). *Vietnam: A casebook.* New York: Brunner/Mazel.

Linehan, M. M. (1993). *Cognitive-behavioral treatment of borderline personality disorder.* New York: Guilford Press.

Lystad, M. (Ed.). (1988). *Mental health response to mass emergencies*. New York: Brunner/ Mazel.

Marmar, C. R., Weiss, D. S., Schlenger, W. E., Fairbank, J. A., Jordan, B. K., Kulka, R. A., & Hough, R. L. (1994). Peritraumatic dissociation and post-traumatic stress in Vietnam theater veterans. *American Journal of Psychiatry, 151*, 902–907.

Metter, J., & Michelson, L. K. (1993). Theoretical clinical research and ethical constraints of the eye movement desensitization reprocessing technique. *Journal of Traumatic Stress, 6*, 413–415.

McCann, I. L., & Pearlman, L. A. (1990). *Psychological trauma and the adult survivor: Theory, therapy, and transformation*. New York: Brunner/Mazel.

McFarlane, A. C. (1988). Recent life events and psychiatric disorder in children: The interaction with preceding extreme adversity. *Journal of Clinical Psychiatry, 29*(5), 677–690.

McFarlane, A. C. (1994). Individual psychotherapy for post-traumatic stress disorder. *Psychiatric Clinics of North America, 17*(2), 393–408.

Mitchell, J. (1983). When disaster strikes: The critical incident stress debriefing process. *Journal of Emergency Medical Services, 8*, 36–39.

Parson, E. R. (1985). Post-traumatic accelerated cohesion: Its recognition and management in group treatment of Vietnam veterans. *Group, 9*(4), 10–23.

Peniston, E. G. (1986). EMG biofeedback-assisted desensitization treatment for Vietnam combat veterans with post-traumatic stress disorder. *Clinical Biofeedback and Health, 9*(1), 35–41.

Pennebaker, J. W. (1993). Putting stress into words: Health, linguistic, and therapeutic implications. *Behaviour Research and Therapy, 31*(6), 539–548.

Pitman, R. K., Altman, B., Greenwald, E., Longpre, R. E., Macklin, M. L., Poire, R. E., & Steketee, G. S. (1991). Psychiatric complications during flooding therapy for posttraumatic stress disorder. *Journal of Clinical Psychiatry, 52*(1), 17–20.

Putnam, F. W. (1989). *Diagnosis and treatment of multiple personality disorder*. New York: Guilford Press.

Raphael, B. (1986). *When disaster strikes: How individuals and communities cope with catastrophe*. New York: Basic Books.

Resick, P. A., Jordan, C. G., Girelli, S. A., Hutter, C. K., & Marhoefer-Dvorak, S. (1988). A Comparative outcome study of behavioral group therapy for sexual assault victims. *Behavior Therapy, 19*, 385–401.

Resick, P. A., & Schnicke, M. K. (1992). Cognitive processing therapy for sexual assault victims. *Journal of Consulting and Clinical Psychology, 60*(5), 748–756.

Rounsaville, B., Lifton, N., & Bieber, M. (1979). The natural history of a psychotherapy group for battered women. *Psychiatry, 42*, 63–78.

Saxe, G. N., Chinman, G., Berkowitz, R., Hall, K., Lieberg, G., Shcwartz, J., & van der Kolk, B. A. (1994). Somatization in patients with dissociative disorders. *American Journal of Psychiatry, 151*, 1329–1335.

Saxe, G. N, van der Kolk, B. A., Hall, K., Schwartz, J., Chinman, G., Hall, M. D., Lieberg, G., & Berkowitz, R. (1993). Dissociative disorders in psychiatric inpatients. *American Journal of Psychiatry, 150*(7), 1037–1042.

Shapiro, F. (1989). Eye movement desensitization: A new treatment for post-traumatic stress disorder. *Journal of Behavior Therapy and Experimental Psychiatry, 20*, 211–217.

Shapiro, F. (1995). *Eye movement desensitization and reprocessing: Basic principles, protocols, and procedures.* New York: Guilford Press.

Solomon, Z., Bleich, A., Shoham, S., Nardi, C., & Kotler, M. (1992). The Koach project for the treatment of combat related PTSD: Rationale, aims and methodology. *Journal of Traumatic Stress, 5,* 175–194.

Strian, F., & Klicpera, C. (1978). Die bedeuting psychoautotonomische reaktionen im entstehung und persistenz von angstzustanden. *Nervenartzt, 49,* 576–583.

van der Hart, O., Brown, P., & van der Kolk, B. A. (1989). Pierre Janet's treatment of posttraumatic stress. *Journal of Traumatic Stress, 2*(4), 379–395.

van der Hart, O., & Op den Velde, W. (1991). Traumatische herinneringen [Traumatic memories]. In O. van der Hart (Ed.), *Trauma, dissociatie en hypnose* [Trauma, dissociation, and hypnosis] (pp. 71–90). Lisse, The Netherlands: Swets & Zeitlinger.

van der Hart, O., & Spiegel, D. (1993). Hypnotic assessment and treatment of trauma-induced psychoses: The early psychotherapy of H. Breukink and modern views. *International Journal of Clinical and Experimental Hypnosis, 41,* 191–209.

van der Hart, O., Steele, K., Boon, S., & Brown, P. (1993). The treatment of traumatic memories: Synthesis, realization, and integration. *Dissociation, 6,* 162–180.

van der Kolk, B. A. (1989). The compulsion to repeat trauma: Revictimization, attachment and masochism. *Psychiatric Clinics of North America, 12,* 389–411.

van der Kolk, B. A. (1992). Group psychotherapy with post traumatic stress disorders. In H. Kaplan & B. Sadock (Eds.), *Comprehensive group psychotherapy* (pp. 550–560). Baltimore: Williams & Wilkins.

van der Kolk, B. A. (1994). Foreword. In J. P. Wilson & D. Lindy (Eds.), *Countertransference in the treatment of PTSD* (pp. vii–xii). New York: Guilford Press.

van der Kolk, B. A., & Ducey, C. P. (1989). The psychological processing of traumatic experience: Rorschach patterns in PTSD. *Journal of Traumatic Stress, 2,* 259–274.

van der Kolk, B. A., Perry, J. C., & Herman, J. L. (1991). Childhood origins of self-destructive behavior. *American Journal of Psychiatry, 148,* 1665–1671.

Vaughan, K., Armstrong, M. S., Gold, R., O'Conner, N., Jenneke, W., & Tarrier, N. (1994a). A trial of eye movement desensitization compared to image habituation training and applied muscle relaxation in post-traumatic stress disorder. *Journal of Behavior Therapy and Experimental Psychiatry, 25,* 283–291.

Vaughan, K., & Tarrier, N. (1992). The use of image habituation training with post-traumatic stress disorders. *British Journal of Psychiatry, 161,* 658–664.

Vaughan, K., Wiese, M., Gold, R., & Tarrier, N. (1994b). Eye movement desensitization: Symptom change in post-traumatic stress disorder. *British Journal of Psychiatry, 164,* 533–541.

Wilson, J. P., & Lindy, J. D. (Eds.). (1994). *Countertransference in the treatment of PTSD.* New York: Guilford Press.

Wilson, S. A., Tinker, R. H., & Becker, L. A. (1995). Eye movement desensitization and reprocessing (EMDR) treatment for psychologically traumatized individuals. *Journal of Clinical and Consulting Psychology, 63,* 928–937.

Yassen, J., & Glass, L. (1984). Sexual assault survivor groups. *Social Work, 37,* 252–257.

CHAPTER 19

Prevention of Posttraumatic Stress

Consultation, Training, and Early Treatment

ROBERT J. URSANO
THOMAS A. GRIEGER
JAMES E. McCARROLL

Disasters and exposures to trauma are much more common aspects of everyday life throughout the world than is often appreciated. The World Health Organization (1988) has estimated that between 1900 and 1988, hurricanes left 1.2 million people without homes and directly affected the lives of 3.5 million people. During this same time, earthquakes, typhoons, and cyclones affected another 26 million people, and 10 million of these were made homeless. Often those without resources are the most affected: Between 1960 and 1987, 41 of the 109 worst natural disasters occurred in developing countries (Berz, 1989). The less developed countries also have higher rates of morbidity and mortality when a disaster strikes than do the more developed countries, even when population density is controlled for (Guha-Sapir, 1989). In general, the less economically developed an area is, the greater the amount of damage and the number of deaths. Those with fewer financial resources often settle in densely populated areas, near natural (e.g., rivers) or human-made (e.g., oil refineries) risk factors, where property values are low, and housing is inexpensive and often poorly constructed. These areas are most likely to sustain heavy damage in a disaster (Lima et al., 1989; Lima, Shaila, Santacruz, & Lozano, 1991; Weisaeth, 1993). In recognition of the human cost of disasters, the United Nations General Assembly designated the 1990s as the decade of natural disaster reduction (World Health Organization, 1988).

Because of the growing knowledge of the predictors of outcome after traumatic events, it is also possible to consider prevention strategies for posttraumatic stress after disaster and traumatic events. The human chaos of disasters is not random. Rather, the behavioral and psychological responses seen in disasters frequently have a predictable structure and time course (Ursano, McCaughey, & Fullerton, 1994). For most individuals, posttraumatic psychiatric symptoms are transitory. However, for some, the effects of a disaster linger long after the traumatic event has passed; new experiences continually remind such persons of the past traumatic event.

In addition, we know that some individuals are predictably exposed to disaster and traumatic stressors (e.g., firefighters, police, disaster workers, soldiers). In other populations, where exposure is unexpected, the opportunity to intervene early after an exposure can provide an opportunity to implement intervention strategies to prevent the development of chronic symptoms and to foster resilience.

How to prevent or at least minimize the psychological ill effects of trauma and disaster, and how to foster resilience, are the topics of this chapter. Prevention can be primary (preparation before the event, sometimes thought of as "inoculation"), secondary (early identification and treatment to limit disability), or tertiary (rehabilitation to prevent chronic social disability). Technically, all forms of treatment reviewed in this volume are attempts to prevent further symptoms and/or disability and chronicity; most would therefore be classified as tertiary prevention. In the rest of this chapter, we will focus on areas of prevention strategies administered prior to the disaster or trauma (primary prevention) and on some aspects of early intervention after trauma exposure (secondary prevention). Review of the chapters on other types of treatment and debriefing will aid the reader in broadening this discussion to all three levels of prevention.

THE GOALS OF PREVENTION: PREVENTING DISEASE AND FOSTERING RESILIENCE

Prevention of posttraumatic stress has as its goal substantially reducing both the human misery and the human cost of trauma and disaster. The prevention of psychiatric disorders often focuses on posttraumatic stress disorder (PTSD). However, PTSD is not the only psychiatric disorder associated with disasters; in fact, it may not even be the most common. PTSD, major depression, substance abuse, generalized anxiety disorder, and adjustment disorder have all been noted following disasters and trauma (Rundell, Ursano, Holloway, & Silberman, 1989), and psychological reactions to physical injury and illness are also important postdisaster responses. (See Table 19.1 for a complete listing.)

The American Psychiatric Association (1994) has added a new disaster-related diagnosis, acute stress disorder (ASD), to its diagnostic manual. ASD, which is applicable soon after a disaster strikes, has only been studied recently. Studies support the idea that ASD (perhaps particularly dissociative symptoms) predicts poorer outcome and later PTSD (Cardeña & Spiegel, 1993; Koopman, Classen, Cardeña, & Spiegel, 1995; Koopman, Classen, & Spiegel, 1994; Staab, Grieger, Fullerton, & Ursano, 1995). Thus, prevention of ASD is an important focus. Depression is often found after disasters and is the most common comorbid disorder with PTSD. The management of loss and death by a community may affect the presence of depression after the disaster (Lundin, 1987; Raphael, 1983, 1986; Wright, Ursano, Bartone, & Ingraham, 1990). Those who (1) have high levels of intrusion and avoidance in the first week after a community disaster, (2) are closest to the dead, (3) have lower levels of social support, and/or (4) have been community members the longest may be at highest risk of depression (Fullerton, Ursano, Kao, & Bhartiya, 1992b, 1992c).

The issues of the acute versus chronic responses to trauma and disaster are particularly important for the prevention of posttraumatic stress. The goal of secondary prevention can be thought of as assuring that early stress symptoms are "digested" or "metabolized," and do not become chronic and crystalized into psychic structure and behavioral patterns.

The prevention of PTSD focuses on both the acute and, importantly, the chronic disorder. Clinically, acute and long-term responses appear to be quite different and are extremely important to distinguish. They may well have

TABLE 19.1. Psychiatric Responses to Disaster

Acute stress disorder
Posttraumatic stress disorder
Major depression
Generalized anxiety disorder
Substance abuse
Psychological factors affecting physical disease (in the injured)
Organic mental disorders secondary to head injury, toxic exposure, infection and dehydration
Adjustment disorder
Bereavement
Family violence
Child and spouse abuse
No psychiatric disorder (normal responses to an abnormal event)

different predictors, and therefore different intervention strategies may well be needed for prevention (Ursano, Fullerton, Kao, & Bhartiya, 1995). Green, Lindy, and Grace (1989) studied survivors of the Buffalo Creek disaster (a dam break and subsequent flooding) and found that the rates of PTSD were 44% at 18–26 months and 28% at 14 years after the disaster. Rates of PTSD in flood victims examined by Steinglass and Gerrity (1990) were 14.5% at 4 months and 4.5% at 16 months after the disaster. At 16 months after a tornado struck one community, Steinglass and Gerrity (1990) found PTSD in 21% of the population.

Similarly, studies of victims of crime and disaster workers indicate the difference between acute and chronic PTSD. In a community sample ($n = 214$), Kilpatrick, Resnick, and Amick (1989) and Kilpatrick, Amick, and Resnick (1990) found that 29% of adult family survivors of criminal homicide experienced PTSD at some point after the death. This dropped to 7% at the time of inquiry (time not specified). In a sample of alcohol-related vehicular homicide survivors, 34.1% reported PTSD at some point after the accident, and 2.2% at the time of inquiry. Kilpatrick and colleagues' findings suggest that in these community samples, only a small percentage of those with acute PTSD develop chronic PTSD (Kilpatrick & Resnick, 1993). Similarly, Ursano et al. (1995) found significant PTSD (11%) shortly after exposure to human remains in disaster workers, but recovery tended to occur by 1 year (2%). Thus, the issues of what may protect people from the onset of PTSD and what may protect them from PTSD's becoming chronic are important and different questions.

Prevention of disease is not, however, the only goal of preventive interventions. Increasing resilience and positive outcomes is an important but often forgotten goal of prevention strategies. In fact, resilience is the most common observation after all disasters. In addition, the effects of traumatic events are not always bad. Although many survivors of the 1974 tornado in Xenia, Ohio, experienced psychological distress, the majority described positive outcomes: They learned that they could handle crises effectively, and felt that they were better off for having met this type of challenge (Quarentelli, 1985; Taylor, 1977). This "benefited response" is also reported in the combat trauma literature. Sledge, Boydstun, and Rahe (1980) found that approximately one-third of U.S. Air Force Vietnam-era prisoners of war (POWs) reported having benefited from their POW experience. These POWs tended to be the ones who had suffered the most traumatic experiences.

For some people, trauma and loss actually facilitate a move toward health (Card, 1983; Sledge et al., 1980; Ursano, 1981). A traumatic experience can become the center around which a victim reorganizes a previously disorganized life, reorienting values and goals (Ursano, 1981, 1987). Traumatic events appear to function as psychic organizers (i.e., "psychic glue"), which link affects, cognitions, and behaviors that are later expressed after symbolic, environmental, or biological stimuli (Holloway & Ursano, 1984).

THEORY OF PREVENTIVE INTERVENTIONS FOR POSTTRAUMATIC STRESS, AND THE ROLE OF CONSULTATION

Knowledge of the responses to disaster and of the interconnected variables that influence outcome is critical to developing effective primary and secondary interventions. Few well-designed empirical studies have directly examined preventive interventions and outcomes. Thus, much of the following relies on clinical observation and implications derived from studies of the mediators of traumatic stress.

Professional groups are some of the few populations in which preventive interventions have been considered, because of their expectable exposure. Groups that are specialized, usually professional, highly trained, and carefully selected—such as firefighters, disaster workers, police, soldiers, and medical personnel—confront trauma on a predictable although episodic basis. Such groups typically have varying degrees of experience and training, but lack specific training in trauma/disaster stress.

One must be careful about generalizing knowledge obtained from any of these groups and uncritically applying it to another professional group. This is even more true when one applies results from highly trained people with special missions to the functioning of a large number of people with varying degrees of training and experience. For example, victims of tornadoes, forest fires, hurricanes, and other natural disasters may require very different interventions than rescue workers, firefighters, and the police may need. Professional groups have various levels of training, selection, and professional supports on the one hand, and often greater exposure, fewer physical supports (sleep, food, etc.), and multiple stressors on the other. With these caveats, however, research on these professional groups is important because of the groups' needs, and because it offers one of the few ways in which to study and learn about expected exposures and possible preventive interventions.

Preventive interventions are targeted to specific exposures, specific types of disability/behavioral disturbance, and specific phases of a disaster. Thus, it is important to distinguish preventive interventions in the following manner (see also Table 19.2): (1) What is the nature of the traumatic experience ("toxin") to which the individuals have been exposed? (2) What symptoms or disabilities are to be prevented? (3) In what stage of the trauma or disaster is the intervention to be administered?

The Toxin

Traumatic events and disasters usually include multiple stressors: threat to life, exposure to death and the dead, bereavement, loss of property, stigmatization, injury, fatigue, and physiological disruption (sleep, food, and water depriva-

TABLE 19.2. Targets of Preventive Interventions

Stressors (toxins)	Symptoms/disabilities	Trauma stage
Threat to life	Intrusive memories	Anticipation of trauma
Exposure to death	Avoidance	Acute trauma exposure
and the dead	Arousal	Early posttrauma phase
Bereavement	Depression	Middle posttrauma phase
Loss of property	Anxiety	Late posttrauma phase
Stigmatization	Dissociation	
Injury	Substance abuse	
Fatigue	Family violence	
Physiological	Social withdrawal	
disruption	Social phobia	
	Responses to injury	
	Hopelessness	
	Expectation of failure	

tion). These toxic elements are elaborated, enhanced, or diminished by their translation into individual meaning and into group responses of support or isolation. These "secondary messengers of the trauma experience"—individual meaning and group responses—can be thought of in the same way in which we think of mediators of exposure to contamination from a poisoned well. They can increase the toxic effects, in the same way that a bacteria can spread more rapidly if it reaches the central water supply versus is contained in a local well; or they can decrease the toxic effects, as when a bacteria must pass a filtration plant before reaching the individuals of the community. Preventive interventions can be designed to affect each of the trauma elements noted above and to affect either the direct toxic exposure or the "secondary messengers."

Symptoms and Disability

The symptoms of posttraumatic stress include the symptoms of the disorders described above and in Table 19.1. These include intrusive memories, avoidance, arousal, depression, anxiety, dissociative symptoms, substance abuse, family violence, social withdrawal, social phobia, and the wide array of responses to physical injury.

The Stages of Disaster Exposure and Response

The stages of disaster and trauma begin before the actual exposure. For groups that are often mobilized for disasters (e.g., police, firefighters, disaster workers, military), as well as for those exposed to disasters for which there may be substantial warning (e.g., hurricanes, toxic clouds, war), there is the anticipatory stage of trauma exposure. This is followed by the impact of the disaster and its aftermath, for which the stages can be summarized as follows: the acute phase of trauma exposure, the early posttrauma phase, the middle posttrauma phase, and the late posttrauma phase. Each stage has its characteristic toxins, responses, and potential interventions.

One important stage of disaster exposure that is often overlooked is the anticipatory stage. The stress of anticipation warrants some review. It is common in professional groups such as firefighters and police, but it also occurs in connection with some natural disasters (hurricanes) and some human-made disasters (airplane crashes). The stress of anticipation has been widely studied in human and animal stress models, and appears to play an important role in many types of stressor events. Czeisler et al. (1976) studied plasma cortisol secretion in patients awaiting elective surgery and in hospitalized controls. The two groups had episodic secretions of cortisol that were indistinguishable, but those awaiting surgery secreted significantly more cortisol during discrete anxiety-provoking experiences such as preoperative preparations. This suggests the need for research to identify the specific stress-producing aspects of predisaster experience. For example, waiting for time to pass during a disaster may not be stressful, whereas receiving instructions or viewing the disaster on television may be.

Anticipated stress of pilots has also been studied during flight preparation for an unaccustomed mission and during the actual mission, using a battery of endocrine measures. A nonspecific stress response occurred during the anticipatory phase. Subsequent stress effects were higher during the first training flight, but decreased on the second leg of the flight, indicating adaptation (Demos, Hale, & Williams, 1969).

Some data suggest that experienced and nonexperienced individuals may differ in anticipatory stress. Studies in parachute jumpers showed that novice and experienced parachute jumpers differed in levels of arousal, as measured by skin conductance, heart rate, and respiration prior to jumping. Both the novices and the experienced jumpers showed an initial activation pattern with elevated levels of arousal. However, in contrast to the novices (who showed continued increased activation up to the time of the jump), the levels of arousal of the experienced jumpers declined as the jump itself came closer. By the time of the jump, their physiological measures were at normal levels (Fenz & Epstein, 1967). Thus, the peak activation of the experienced people occurred earlier than that of the novices. Animal models of stress also support the importance of anticipation as a stressor. Some studies indicate that anticipation of an unavoidable stimulus produces analgesia, perhaps secondary to stimulation of endogenous opioids (Sumova & Jakoubek, 1989).

Anticipation of physical stress has also been examined and is important to disaster work, since disaster environments frequently contain physical threats (Mefferd, Hale, Shannon, Prigmore, & Ellis, 1971; Mefferd & Wieland, 1966). Mefferd and Wieland (1966) compared baseline measures of autonomic, metabolic, and psychological processes of subjects anticipating hypoxia. Upon actual exposure to hypoxia, wide individual differences were noted, but measures generally increased; that is, the rank order of responses was (1) control period, (2) anticipation period, (3) hypoxia exposure.

Specific studies of anticipatory stress in disasters is limited to studies of disaster workers expecting to work with dead bodies (McCarroll et al., 1993b; McCarroll, Ursano, Fullerton, & Lundy, 1993a, 1995; McCarroll, Ursano, Wright, & Fullerton, 1993c). Higher levels of anticipated stress were seen in nonvolunteers, females, those without previous experience, and those with greater mutilation fear. Further study of this stage of disaster exposure is needed.

PREVENTION STRATEGIES

Training

Training can address many of the targets of prevention presented above. Training can be used to limit exposure, alter the type of exposure, decrease surprise and the unexpected, and maximize the sense of mastery and hope (as opposed to hopelessness and defeat). Training can be provided for individuals or groups.

Hytten (1989) interviewed survivors of a helicopter crash to determine which elements of training had been most helpful to survival. The most common advantage reported was that the training allowed the survivors to remain calm and to appraise the situation despite extreme threat; this allowed them to pursue alternate escape routes when the initial routes were found to be blocked. Prior success in a similar training environment provided confidence that the actual experience could be survived.

In studying the cognitive functioning and behaviors of 123 employees involved in an explosion and fire at a paint factory, Weisaeth (1989a, 1989b, 1995) found that 34% in the high-stress group experienced near-total loss of cognitive control, and that 20% had some behavioral response that increased risk to their lives or those of others. Optimal disaster behavior was found in 37%; it was correlated with a high level of prior disaster training/experience and predicted better long-term outcome. The training and experience had been part of military and maritime service and had not been directed to the specific dangers at the factory. It would appear that general disaster and emergency training also offers some advantages—perhaps preparation for the experience of surprise and the unexpected need to act.

Although general disaster training may provide protection from some of the sequelae of trauma, it appears to be less effective when the trauma is of long duration or of an uncontrollable nature. Thus, Weisaeth (1989c) reported the development of PTSD symptoms in 54% of a ship's crew members exposed to torture over a 67-day period. The stress of captivity was dominated by low predictability and control. Because the torture was a terrorist act with little political planning or press coverage, the victims were unable to reappraise the event in terms of either personal or political significance. That is, there was no positive meaning attributable to the experience.

The magnitude of a disaster may exceed that anticipated in training exercises. Ersland, Weisaeth, and Sund (1989) reported the impact of trauma in rescuers at the site of an oil rig collapse. Professional rescue personnel, although trained to respond to disaster situations, found that the severity of the catastrophe was outside the realm of their training experience. There has been no systematic study of the value of including training scenarios in which rescue operations are destined to have limited success, and the workers must manage the feelings of failure as well as success. Such training may aid workers in better managing the common feeling in disasters of not being able to do enough.

Fullerton, McCarroll, Ursano, and Wright (1992a) examined sources of stress and stress mediators among two groups of firefighters involved in disaster work. Four stressful effects of rescue work were found: identification with the victims, feelings of helplessness and guilt, fear of the unknown, and physiological reactions. The investigators also identified four stress mediators: social support, the type of leadership, the level of training, and the use of rituals. They suggested that it may be possible to teach disaster workers to identify less with victims and to enhance their use of social supports in resolving feelings of guilt and helplessness. They suggested that "grief leadership" (Ingraham, 1987)—a group leader's own expression of grief to help others express their feelings—can be a valuable tool in allowing workers to recover as a group. Their examples demonstrated the need for training to develop mastery and optimal performance during actual disasters, and to diminish feelings of guilt and feeling like a victim (see Table 19.3).

Hytten and Hasle (1989) used a questionnaire to assess 58 nonprofessional firefighters who participated in rescue efforts during a hotel blaze. A prominent comment was that "the fire was like an exercise . . . when your exercises are realistic, reality becomes indistinguishable from an exercise" (p. 53). Work-

TABLE 19.3. Interventions to Prevent Traumatic Stress

Training
Experience
Group/organizational leadership
Management of meaning
Management of exposure
Management of fatigue, sleep, and exhaustion
Buddy care
Natural social supports and caretakers
Education in disaster stress and strain
Education of health care providers
Screening

ing in partnership with professionals was also valued. Periods of inactivity, pressure of time, and finding deceased or injured victims caused more anxiety than did concerns about being injured or killed or of being unable to perform according to expectations.

Experience

McCarroll et al. (1993b) studied body handlers and found that the degree of anticipated stress related to the handling of dead bodies was significantly lower in those with prior experience. In comparing groups who handled and those who did not handle the remains of the dead from Operation Desert Storm, McCarroll et al. (1993a, 1995) found that those who were inexperienced in such tasks had significantly higher intrusion, avoidance, and total Impact of Event Scale scores than did those with prior experience.

Solomon, Mikulincer, and Jakob (1987) examined the association of prior combat experience with the development of combat stress reaction (CSR). CSR was lower in soldiers with prior combat experience than in soldiers with no prior combat exposure. Soldiers with prior episodes of CSR were more likely to experience CSR during the Lebanon War than were soldiers with no prior combat experience. Solomon et al. discussed the concept that prior stressful experiences define expectations of subsequent adversities. From a leadership perspective, they suggested that a prior occurrence of CSR may be an indication for assignment to units less likely to experience high-intensity combat. Together, the studies of McCarroll and Solomon support the effects of "inoculation" to the stress of body handling but both inoculation and sensitization to combat.

Other data support the inoculation hypothesis in other trauma exposures. That is, having once survived an experience may protect an individual against the sequelae of subsequent exposures. It has been proposed that when disasters or hazards occur with some frequency, the threat is normalized and can be placed within a framework that makes it meaningful and understandable (Anderson, 1968; Bolin & Kenlow, 1982; Quarantelli, 1985; Warheit, 1985). Norris and Murrell (1988) interviewed 204 adults aged 55 and above who survived floods in rural Kentucky. They found that survival of prior floods and survival of other non-flood-related trauma moderated both trait anxiety and weather-related state anxiety symptoms. In Norris and Murrell's (1988) study, the "inoculating" effect was greater in individuals with similar prior trauma than in those with nonsimilar trauma experiences. The investigators concluded that disaster training should be tied as closely as possible to the anticipated disaster.

Group/Organizational Leadership

Leaders within organizations have responsibility for coordinating and directing the efforts of others to accomplish a common goal or assigned task. Leaders at all levels are responsible for insuring that subordinates are appropriately trained. They also must maintain an environment in which the work tasks can be efficiently performed, and must insure that the organizational structure and operating procedures maximize the delivery of a high-quality product or service. Leaders are also expected to maintain the moral and ethical standards of the societies in which they function, and to foster and direct the meaning and vision of their organizations' efforts.

One task of leaders of groups and organizations is to minimize the occurrence of traumatic events. In individual traumas, such as personal violence, prevention may take place through education about personal safety practices to limit exposure to potentially threatening situations (e.g., teaching children not to walk through the park at night; teaching firefighters not to open hot doors). Such education is also the responsibility of civic and school leaders, as well as employers within the community. In industrial settings, proper training in plant procedures and in adherence to safety standards should minimize disaster stress events. Federal monitoring and regulations play a role in this task of disaster stress prevention, although one must remember that these are not always successful (e.g., Three Mile Island and the Nuclear Regulatory Agency; airline crashes and the National Transportation Board).

In a group of police officers handling the remains of decomposing bodies in a collapsed offshore oil rig, strong organizational and managerial leadership may have decreased the stress involved in the work of body recovery (Alexander & Wells, 1991). Workers reported that their leaders had maintained optimal physical safety and work environments. Required debriefings were held on a daily basis, and the officers were frequently reminded that their task, although unpleasant, was important to the survivors of the disaster victims. Junior officers were paired with more experienced colleagues who demonstrated confidence and competence in their work. Most workers reported a strong sense of group unity and team spirit; they also felt that their tasks were clearly defined and that they were given regular feedback about their performance.

Throughout the disaster, the leaders made sure that consultation by a mental health team was available. Care was taken to insure that workers were not placed in a "patient" role, and that the organizational structure and policies were used to provide the framework for support. Liaison with the mental health team was established prior to the body-handling experience; the consultants were thereby less likely to be perceived as outside of the group. Although some psychological sequelae were reported, such as intrusive images, there was no lost work time or increase of psychiatric symptoms.

The military offers unique opportunities to study the effect of leadership on individuals who have been exposed to trauma. Rundell, Holloway, Ursano, and Jones (1990) reviewed the literature regarding the role of military leadership in preventing combat stress among flyers and ground support personnel within the U.S. Air Force, extending back to World War II. Among flyers, the prevention of combat stress is accomplished by attending to such issues as rest periods, intervals between missions, control of risk, and length of combat tour. Among ground-based personnel, the possibility of chemical and biological warfare places individuals at risk for psychological trauma, as does body handling. General guidance by leaders included providing information to the troops, emphasizing the importance of control of behavior in combat situations, encouraging unit cohesion, providing consistent leadership, and maintaining truthfulness. The importance of various other factors—adequate sleep, "grief leadership," mental health support, chaplain availability, and community support—was also addressed.

An example of effective leadership in the military community occurred in December 1985, after 248 members of one of the U.S. Army's elite combat units were killed in an airplane crash while returning home from a peacekeeping mission in the Middle East. A multidisciplinary mental health team was organized to assist with the grief processes of surviving members of the unit, family members of the deceased, and mortuary workers handling the disfigured bodies of the deceased. Wright (1987) collected and summarized data from the experience, and provided recommendations for those who might be involved in similar future experiences. Although the report was naturalistic in nature and alternative leadership styles were not compared, the findings have strong face validity and were consistent among the 10 contributing authors.

Positive leadership styles were demonstrated at all levels: the president of the United States; division, battalion and brigade commanders; junior officers; and senior noncommissioned officers. Successful leadership qualities included "grief leadership" (Ingraham, 1987), which, again, is the encouragement by group leaders of expression of shared grief to emphasize the normality of and necessity for grieving. Leaders also stressed the role of using social and family support systems to share the pain of loss. Open communication was seen as a means of neutralizing the anxiety and uncertainty arising from rumors. Wright (1987) also noted the need for leaders to reserve time for physical exercise, sleep, and other restorative activities during and after the tragedy to maximize effective functioning. Temporary assignment of a consultant familiar with the operation of the organization proved helpful in terms of information and reassurance. Finally, senior leaders were encouraged to share experiences and feelings with their individual social support networks.

Management of Meaning

As discussed by Alexander and Wells (1991), reinforcing the importance and meaning of gruesome disaster work allowed workers to reframe the experience in a more tolerable fashion. In contrast to the reported good adaptation of the body handlers of the Piper Alpha oil rig disaster, Jones (1985) reported that 32% of rescue workers involved in body recovery after the Jonestown,

Guyana, mass suicides/murders experienced short-term dysphoria. Subjective comments from the participants included anger toward the victims for their participation in the cult, involuntary assignment to the mission, lack of appropriate debriefings, and lack of support from supervisors and the command structure. Jones suggested the value of fostering a sense of meaning, group unity, and recognition by valued authorities as tools for making tolerable an otherwise intolerable situation. The management of meaning is a function of community and group leaders as well as of the mass media (Ursano, Kao, & Fullerton, 1992).

Management of Exposure

The severity of a disaster or traumatic event is perhaps the single best predictor of both the probability and the frequency of postdisaster psychiatric illness. The Epidemiologic Catchment Area study of Vietnam veterans documented a higher rate of PTSD in wounded Vietnam veterans (Helzer, Robins, & McEvoy, 1987). Similar findings were noted in the National Vietnam Veterans Readjustment Study (Kulka et al., 1990, 1991). Greater exposure to combat in Vietnam was also significantly related to higher rates of PTSD, depression, and alcohol abuse (Kulka et al., 1990). In an interesting study, Goldberg, True, Eisen, Henderson, and Robinette (1987) studied monozygotic twins who were discordant for service in Vietnam. Nearly 17% (16.8%) of the twins who had served in Vietnam had PTSD, in contrast to only 5.0% of the twins who had not served. There was a ninefold increase in the prevalence of PTSD in the twins exposed to high levels of combat in Vietnam, compared to their non-combat-exposed siblings. Several studies also found that the intensity of disaster exposure following the Mount St. Helens volcanic eruption predicted psychiatric outcome (Shore, Tatum, & Vollmer, 1986; Shore, Vollmer, & Tatum, 1989). These studies documented higher rates of disaster illnesses in those who lived closer to Mount St. Helens, the illnesses included PTSD, generalized anxiety disorder, and depression.

These most important and consistent findings emphasize the importance of removing individuals from the disaster scene and protecting them from disaster stressors. This can be done for some groups, such as disaster workers, through rotation schedules. For other individuals exposed, providing a sense of safety—through practical provision of housing, food, resources, and assurance of employment (a future)—can greatly decrease the traumatic stress.

Management of Fatigue, Sleep, and Exhaustion

Extreme fatigue and physical exhaustion are often present and seldom measured among disaster workers (Fullerton & Ursano, 1994; Fullerton et al., 1992b, 1992c). Some groups perform their missions in hostile and toxic environments and require extensive protective clothing, which may cause hyperthermia and additional physical demands. Firefighters, as well as chemical spill and radiation contamination cleanup teams, face these additional physical stressors.

Several studies of military personnel in potential chemical and biological warfare (CBW) environments provide some data about these stressors. The 1995 chemical terrorist events in Tokyo make these findings all the more important. Individuals in a CBW environment perform their tasks in uncomfortable protective clothing and are exposed to toxic agents, high workload intensity (possibly alternating with periods of boredom), group stresses, and extensive exposure to the dead and dying (Fullerton & Ursano, 1990). Low prestress anxiety and high social support during the trauma were found to be protective from the psychologically negative effects of the high stress of a CBW environment (Fullerton et al., 1992b, 1992c). A review of the reports of 366 individuals involved in CBW training exercises revealed that 10–20% of participants experienced moderate to severe psychological symptomatology, including anxiety, claustrophobia, and panic (Fullerton & Ursano, 1990). The exercises were terminated prematurely—with reports of hyperventilation, shaking, tremors, confusion, fear of dying, visual distortions, time disorientation, claustrophobia, anxiety, psychophysiological complaints, conversion, and a desire to flee the feared situation—by 4–8% of the participants. Some participants removed their protective clothing, an act that would be fatal in the true toxic environment.

The physical demands of disaster exposure for victims and disaster workers are important to manage, in order to prevent additional stress burdens. Further study is needed to understand the contribution of these stressors to psychological outcomes. Groups expected to be exposed to trauma may benefit from training to limit the physically stressful aspects of their work. Overdedication can be a serious risk factor for the individual, in terms both of psychological outcomes and of performance errors (Fullerton & Ursano, 1994).

Buddy Care

Shalev, Schreiber, and Galai (1993) studied the multiple facets of care and recovery among 16 victims of a terrorist act. They established a two-layer structure for the treatment team, with one layer of case managers involved in direct patient care and a second layer of consultants without direct patient contact. The unexposed consultants were better able to contain the emotional burden of the primary care providers and to help them organize and structure their interventions. A formal debriefing exercise revealed that most primary caretakers failed to take care of themselves (e.g., did not rely on their own social supports and tended to overlook their own symptoms of psychological distress). One conclusion of the study was that unstructured support of primary providers may not be adequate to reducing distress among mental health professionals working in a posttraumatic support role.

Studies of the stress on a medical care team in a simulated CBW environment were also conducted (Fullerton & Ursano, 1994; Fullerton et al., 1992b, 1992c). Higher levels of support provided during the exercise by the members of the health care group to one another predicted better psychological outcomes.

Natural Social Supports and Caretakers

Various types of social support, both instrumental and emotional, are provided by formal and informal networks, family members, friends, and professionals. Professional service providers are often burdened beyond their capacity during large-scale disasters, and families provide the context in which many workers can obtain support when their spouses or significant others can be educated and are able to assist. Studies have shown that the availability and use of naturally occurring social supports are generally associated with lower levels of psychopathology (Fullerton et al., 1992b, 1992c; Fullerton & Ursano, in press; Green, Grace, & Gleser, 1985; Turner, 1981).

One aspect of training for professional disaster aid personnel may be to distribute assistance through training nonprofessionals in providing support. Kiecolt-Glaser et al. (1993) noted that "data from national surveys suggests that marital happiness contributes far more to global happiness than any other variable, including satisfaction with work and friendships" (p. 409). Friends and family are more available to and trusted by persons in need of help than are formally designated helpers (Collins & Pancoast, 1976). Kelly, Kelly, Gauron, and Rawlings (1977) developed a training program for these "natural helpers" in a rural area. Weisenfeld and Weis (1979) trained a group of hairdressers in a form of mental health consultation, to provide them with formal education on how to better meet their customers' emotional needs. Both attempts at training these natural helpers were deemed successful.

Fullerton and Ursano (in press) have also shown that caretaking by spouses of disaster workers is both common and stressful, with disaster workers' wives showing higher levels of intrusive and avoidant symptoms. Education of spouses of disaster workers may facilitate the natural recovery process, and may also protect the spouses from extreme symptoms.

Education in Disaster Stress and Strain

Norris and Uhl (1993) studied the concept that stressors, appraisal of threat, and responses to trauma can be viewed as either chronic or acute, with the implication that a chronic response is most likely when the stressor or appraisal is chronic as well. They considered the stressfulness of any given time interval as influenced both by discrete life events and by less dramatic hassles, pressures, and strains. In studying groups who experienced Hurricane Hugo and comparison groups with similar demographic backgrounds, Norris and Uhl found that chronic stress measures were influenced by acute stress measures, and that chronic stress measures explained 18–32% of the variance in psychological distress scales. Chronic physical stress had the strongest independent effect on distress, followed by financial stress and marital stress. The effects of injury on depression and hostility were completely explained by the indirect effects of injury through chronic stress. The study was limited in its retrospective nature, and Norris and Uhl acknowledged that acute stressors might have influenced perceptions of chronic stressors. For example, hypervigilance resulting from perception of danger in the storm might have led to subsequent perceptions of crowding, noise, and fear of crime following the disaster.

All in all, relief workers and victims should be educated in the expected stressors of disasters and trauma—including the role of daily hassles and strain. Relief begins with restoring basic human needs, but includes assistance with marital strain, filial burden, financial problems, ecological stress, and physical disability. Since relief workers may also be "victims," they should also be well aware of their own day-to-day hassles.

Education of Health Care Providers

Often the victims of disasters will present to primary care health providers. It is important that these "gatekeepers" be alert to the normal responses to trauma, in order not to "pathologize" normal recovery. In addition, it is important that they recognize cases in which traumatic stress may become chronic, and also recognize that somatic symptoms may be the first presentation of PTSD. Outreach education programs to health care providers can decrease long-term illness and chronicity.

Screening

Preexisting psychiatric illnesses or symptoms are neither necessary nor sufficient to the diagnosis of psychiatric morbidity after a traumatic event (Goldberg, True, Eisen, & Henderson, 1990; Ursano, 1981; Ursano, Boydstun, & Wheatley, 1981). For this reason, as well as the financial costs (as shown in the United States during World War II), screening programs may have limited utility except in selected high-risk and high-cost occupations. Most studies show that performance criteria (e.g., training) may offer the best screening, rather than traditional mental health measures, which are usually too gross and create too many false positives when used in large community samples. The less severe the disaster or traumatic event, the more important predisaster psychopathology appears to be (McFarlane, 1986a, 1986b, 1988a, 1988b). In contrast to screening, findings on risk factors do help in identifying high-risk groups for early intervention programs. Women, nonvolunteers, and those with higher mutilation fears may be at greater risk when exposed to body recovery tasks (McCarroll et al., 1995). McFarlane (1988a, 1988b), in his study of 469 firefighters exposed to a bush fire disaster, found that a pattern of persistently chronic morbidity could be predicted when individuals displayed a pattern of adversity before the event, neuroticism, treated past psychiatric disorder, and a tendency to avoid thinking about problems. He found that individuals without PTSD symptoms had a greater tendency to forget about injuries sustained during the trauma than did individuals who developed PTSD symptoms. His study suggests that screening individuals for certain personality and cognitive styles may decrease the likelihood of development of PTSD; this is perhaps more likely in less serious trauma exposures, where personality appears to be more of a predictor than the degree of trauma. Bartone, Ursano, Saczynski, and Ingraham (1989) found that individuals high in "hardiness," a personality construct related to feelings of control, mastery, and challenge, had better outcomes after exposure to disaster stress. These studies are important for our increasing understanding of the mechanisms of traumatic stress. However, at present, screening as a prevention strategy does not have a sufficient scientific base to be implemented.

CONCLUSION

The prevention of negative psychological, behavioral, and health outcomes from disasters and traumatic events requires further empirical study. Many intriguing possibilities are suggested in the literature, but few have been well investigated. The opportunities for prevention highlight the important role of consultation following disasters. The consultant can organize the community leaders in implementing interventions directed to limit disability and to restore individual community structure and function. PTSD and other post-traumatic psychiatric illnesses and reactions are important targets for preventive interventions. Future research should address the types of toxic exposure and the specific symptoms and disabilities expected, and these must be conceptualized across time in the various stages of disaster, including the anticipatory stage prior to disaster impact.

REFERENCES

Alexander, D. A., & Wells, A. (1991). Reactions of police officers to body-handling after a major disaster: A before-and-after comparison. *British Journal of Psychiatry, 159*, 547–555.

American Psychiatric Association. (1994). *Diagnostic and statistical manual of mental disorders* (4th ed.). Washington, DC: Author.

Anderson, J. W. (1968). Cultural adaptation to threatened disaster. *Human Organization*, *27*, 298–307.

Bartone, P., Ursano, R. J., Saczynski, K., & Ingraham, L. H. (1989). The impact of a military air disaster on the health of assistance workers: A prospective study. *Journal of Nervous and Mental Disease*, *177*, 317–327.

Berz, G. (1989). List of major natural disasters, 1960–87. *Earthquakes and Volcanoes*, *20*, 226–228.

Bolin, R., & Kenlow, D. (1982). Response of the elderly to disaster: An age-stratified analysis. *International Journal of Aging and Human Development*, *16*, 283–296.

Card, J. J. (1983). *Lives after Viet Nam*. Lexington, MA: Lexington Books.

Cardeña, E., & Spiegel, D. (1993). Dissociative reactions to the San Francisco Bay Area earthquake of 1989. *American Journal of Psychiatry*, *150*, 474–478.

Collins, A. G., & Pancoast, D. L. (1976). *Natural helping networks: A strategy for prevention*. Washington, DC: National Association of Social Workers.

Czeisler, C. A., Ede, M. C. M., Regestein, Q. R., Kish, E. S., Fang, V. S., & Ehrlich, E. N. (1976). Episodic 24-hour cortisol secretory patterns in patients awaiting elective cardiac surgery. *Journal of Clinical Endocrinology and Metabolism*, *42*, 273–283.

Demos, G. T., Hale, H. B., & Williams, E. W. (1969). Anticipatory stress and flight stress in F-102 pilots. *Aerospace Medicine*, *40*, 385–388.

Ersland, S., Weisaeth, L., & Sund, A. (1989). The stress upon rescuers involved in an oil rig disaster: "Alexander L. Kielland" 1980. *Acta Psychiatrica Scandinavica*, *80*(Suppl. 355), 38–49.

Fenz, W. D., & Epstein, S. E. (1967). Gradients of physiological arousal in parachutists as a function of an approaching jump. *Psychosomatic Medicine*, *29*, 33–51.

Fullerton, C. S., McCarroll, J. E., Ursano, R. J., & Wright, K. M. (1992a). Psychological responses of rescue workers: Fire fighters and trauma. *American Journal of Orthopsychiatry*, *62*, 371–378.

Fullerton, C. S., & Ursano, R. J. (1990). Behavioral and psychological responses to chemical and biological warfare. *Military Medicine*, *155*(2), 54–59.

Fullerton, C. S., & Ursano, R. J. (1994). Health care delivery in the high-stress environment of chemical and biological warfare. *Military Medicine*, *159*(7), 524–528.

Fullerton, C. S., & Ursano, R. J. (in press). Post-traumatic response in spouse/significant others of disaster workers. In C. S. Fullerton & R. J. Ursano (Eds.), *Posttraumatic stress disorder: Acute and long-term responses to trauma and disaster*. Washington, DC: American Psychiatric Press.

Fullerton, C. S., Ursano, R. J., Kao, T., & Bhartiya, V. (1992b). The chemical and biological warfare environment: Psychological responses and social support in a high stress environment. *Journal of Applied Social Psychology*, *22*, 1608–1623.

Fullerton, C. S., Ursano, R. J., Kao, T., & Bhartiya, V. (1992c). *Community bereavement following an airplane crash*. Paper presented at the annual conference of the International Society of Traumatic Stress Studies, Amsterdam.

Goldberg, J., True, W. R., Eisen, S. A., & Henderson, W. G. (1990). A twin study of the effects of the Vietnam War on posttraumatic stress disorder. *Journal of the American Medical Association*, *263*(9), 1227–1232.

Goldberg, J., True, W., Eisen, S., Henderson, W., & Robinette, C. D. (1987). The Vietnam Era Twin (VET) Registry: Ascertainment bias. *Acta Geneticae Medicae Gemellologiae* (Roma), *36*, 67–78.

Green, B. L., Grace, M. C., & Gleser, G. C. (1985). Identifying survivors at risk: Long term impairment following the Beverly Hills supper club fire. *Journal of Consulting and Clinical Psychology, 53*(5), 672–678.

Green, B. L., Lindy, J. D., & Grace, M. C. (1989). Posttraumatic stress disorder. *Journal of Nervous and Mental Disease, 173,* 406–411.

Guha-Sapir, D. (1989). Rapid assessment of health needs in mass emergencies: Review of current concepts and methods. *World Health Statistics Annual, 43,* 171–181.

Helzer, J. E., Robins, L. N., & McEvoy, L. (1987). Post-traumatic stress disorder in the general population. *New England Journal of Medicine, 317,* 1630–1634.

Holloway, H. C., & Ursano, R. J. (1984). The Vietnam veteran: Memory, social context, and metaphor. *Psychiatry, 47,* 103–108.

Hytten, K. (1989). Helicopter crash in water: Effects of simulator escape training. *Acta Psychiatrica Scandinavica, 80*(Suppl. 355), 73–78.

Hytten, K., & Hasle, A. (1989). Fire fighters: A study of stress and coping. *Acta Psychiatrica Scandinavica, 80*(Suppl. 355), 50–55.

Ingraham, L. H. (1987). Grief leadership. In K. Wright (Ed.), *The human response to the Gander military air disaster: A summary report* (Division of Neuropsychiatry Report No. 88-12, pp. 10–13). Washington, DC: Walter Reed Army Institute of Research.

Jones, D. R. (1985). Secondary disaster victims: The emotional effects of recovering and identifying human remains. *American Journal of Psychiatry, 142,* 303–307.

Kelly, V. R., Kelly, P. L., Gauron, E. F., & Rawlings, E. I. (1977). Training helpers in rural mental health delivery. *Social Work, 22,* 229–232.

Kiecolt-Glaser, J. K., Mararkey, W. B., Chee, M. A., Newton, T., Cacioppo, J. T., Mao, H. Y., & Glaser, R. (1993). Negative behavior during marital conflict is associated with immunological down-regulation. *Psychosomatic Medicine, 55,* 395–409.

Kilpatrick, D. G., Amick, A., & Resnick, H. S. (1990). *The impact of homicide on surviving family members.* Bethesda, MD: National Institute of Justice. (Grant No. 87-IJ-CX-0017, Final Report).

Kilpatrick, D. G., & Resnick, H. S. (1993). Posttraumatic stress disorder associated with exposure to criminal victimization in clinical and community populations. In J. R. T. Davidson & E. B. Foa (Eds.), *Posttraumatic stress disorder: DSM-IV and beyond* (pp. 113–143). Washington, DC: American Psychiatric Press.

Kilpatrick, D. G., Resnick, H. S., & Amick, A. (1989, August). *Family members of homicide victims: Search for meaning and post-traumatic stress disorder.* Paper presented at 97th Annual Convention of the American Psychological Association, New Orleans.

Koopman, C., Classen C., Cardeña, E., & Spiegel, D. (1995). When disaster strikes, acute stress disorder may follow. *Journal of Traumatic Stress, 8,* 29–46.

Koopman, C., Classen, C., & Spiegel, D. (1994). Predictors of posttraumatic stress symptoms among survivors of the Oakland/Berkeley, California firestorms. *American Journal of Psychiatry, 151,* 888–894.

Kulka, R. A., Schlenger, W. E., Fairbank, J. A. Hough, R. L., Jordan, B. K., Marmar, C. R., & Weiss, D. S. (1990). *Trauma and the Vietnam War generation.* New York: Brunner/Mazel.

Kulka, R. A., Schlenger, W. E., Fairbank, J. A., Jordan, B. K., Hough, R. L., Marmar, C. R., & Weiss, D. S. (1991). Assessment of posttraumatic stress disorder in the community: Prospects and pitfalls from recent studies of Vietnam veterans. *Psychological Assessment: A Journal of Consulting and Clinical Psychology, 3*(4), 547–560.

Lima, B. R., Chavez, H., Samaniego, N., Pompei, S., Pai, S., Santacruz, H., & Lozano, J. (1989). Disaster severity and emotional response: Implications for primary mental health care in developing countries. *Acta Psychiatrica Scandinavica, 79,* 74–82.

Lima, B. R., Shaila, P., Santacruz, H., & Lozano, J. (1991). Psychiatric disorders among poor victims following a major disaster: Armero, Colombia. *Journal of Nervous and Mental Disease, 179,* 420–427.

Lundin, T. (1987). The stress of unexpected bereavement. *Stress Medicine, 4,* 109–114.

McCarroll, J. E., Ursano, R. J., Fullerton, C. S., & Lundy, A. C. (1993a). Traumatic stress of a wartime mortuary: Anticipation of exposure to mass death. *Journal of Nervous and Mental Disease, 181,* 545–551.

McCarroll, J. E., Ursano, R. J., Fullerton, C. S., & Lundy, A. C. (1995). Anticipatory stress of handling human remains from the Persian Gulf War: Predictors of intrusion and avoidance. *Journal of Nervous and Mental Disease, 183,* 700–705.

McCarroll, J. E., Ursano, R. J., Ventis, W. L., Fullerton, C. S., Oates, G. L., Friedman, H., Shean, G. L., & Wright, K. M. (1993b). Anticipation of handling the dead: Effects of gender and experience. *British Journal of Clinical Psychology, 32,* 466–468.

McCarroll, J. E., Ursano, R. J., Wright, K. M., & Fullerton, C. S. (1993c). Handling of bodies after violent death: Strategies for coping. *American Journal of Orthopsychiatry, 63,* 209–214.

McFarlane, A. C. (1986a). Long-term psychiatric morbidity after a natural disaster. *Medical Journal of Australia, 145,* 561–563.

McFarlane, A. C. (1986b). Posttraumatic morbidity of a disaster: A study of cases presenting for psychiatric treatment. *Journal of Nervous and Mental Disease, 174,* 4–14.

McFarlane, A. C. (1988a). The phenomenology of post-traumatic stress disorders following a natural disaster. *Journal of Nervous and Mental Disease, 176,* 22–29.

McFarlane, A. C. (1988b). The longitudinal course of posttraumatic morbidity: The range of outcomes and their predictors. *Journal of Nervous and Mental Disease, 176,* 30–39.

Mefferd, R. B., Hale, H. B., Shannon, I. L., Prigmore, J. R., & Ellis, J. P. (1971). Stress responses as criteria for personnel selection: Baseline study. *Aerospace Medicine, 42,* 42–51.

Mefferd, R. B., & Wieland, B. A. (1966). Comparison of responses to anticipated stress and stress. *Psychosomatic Medicine, 28,* 795–807.

Norris, F. H., & Murrell, S. A. (1988). Prior experience as a moderator of disaster impact on anxiety symptoms in older adults. *American Journal of Community Psychology, 16*(5), 665–683.

Norris, F. H., & Uhl, G. A. (1993). Chronic stress as a mediator of acute stress: The case of Hurricane Hugo. *Journal of Applied Social Psychology, 23*(16), 1263–1284.

Quarentelli, E. L. (1985). An assessment of conflicting views on mental health: The consequences of traumatic events. In C. R. Figley (Ed.), *Trauma and its wake.* New York: Brunner/Mazel.

Raphael, B. (1983). *The anatomy of bereavement.* New York: Basic Books.

Raphael, B. (1986). *When disaster strikes: How individuals and communities cope with catastrophe.* New York: Basic Books.

Rundell, J. R., Holloway, H. C., Ursano, R. J., & Jones, D. R. (1990). Combat stress disorders and the U.S. Air Force. *Military Medicine, 155*(11), 515–518.

Rundell, J. R., Ursano, R. J., Holloway, H. C., & Silberman, E. K. (1989). Psychiatric responses to trauma. *Hospital and Community Psychiatry, 40*(1), 68–74.

Shalev, A. Y., Schreiber, S., & Galai, T. (1993). Early psychological responses to traumatic injury. *Journal of Traumatic Stress, 6*(4), 441–450.

Shore, J. H., Tatum, E. L., & Vollmer, W. M. (1986). Psychiatric reactions to disaster: The Mount St. Helens experience. *American Journal of Psychiatry, 143*, 590–595.

Shore, J. H., Vollmer, W. M., & Tatum, E. L. (1989). Community pattern of posttraumatic stress disorders. *Journal of Nervous and Mental Disease, 177*, 681–685.

Sledge, W. H., Boydstun, J. A., & Rahe, A. J. (1980). Self-concept changes related to war captivity. *Archives of General Psychiatry, 37*, 430–443.

Solomon, A., Mikulincer, M., & Jakob, B. R. (1987). Exposure to recurrent combat stress: Combat stress reactions among Israeli soldiers in the Lebanon War. *Psychological Medicine, 17*, 433–440.

Staab, J., Grieger, T. A., Fullerton, C. S., & Ursano, R. J. (1995). *Acute stress disorder and PTSD after Typhoon Omar.* Paper presented to the Braceland Seminar, conducted at the annual meeting of the American Psychiatric Association, Miami, FL.

Steinglass, P., & Gerrity, E. (1990). Natural disasters and post-traumatic stress disorder: Short-term versus long-term recovery in two disaster-affected communities. *Journal of Applied Psychology, 20*, 1746–1765.

Sumova, A., & Jakoubek, B. (1989). Analgesia and impact induced by anticipation stress: Involvement of the endogenous opioid peptide system. *Brain Research, 503*, 273–280.

Taylor, V. (1977). Good news about disaster. *Psychology Today*, pp. 93–94, 124–126.

Turner, R. J. (1981). Social support as a contingency in psychological well being. *Journal of Health and Social Behavior, 22*, 357–367.

Ursano, R. J. (1981). The Vietnam era prisoner of war: Precaptivity personality and development of psychiatric illness. *American Journal of Psychiatry, 138*(3), 315–318.

Ursano, R. J. (1987). Comments on "Posttraumatic stress disorder: The stressor criterion." *Journal of Nervous and Mental Disease, 175*, 273–275.

Ursano, R. J., Boydstun, J. A., & Wheatley, R. D. (1981). Psychiatric illness in U.S. Air Force Vietnam prisoners of war: A five-year follow-up. *American Journal of Psychiatry, 138*, 310–314.

Ursano, R. J., Fullerton, C. S., Kao, T. C., & Bhartiya, V. R. (1995). Longitudinal assessment of posttraumatic stress disorder and depression after exposure to traumatic death. *Journal of Nervous and Mental Disease, 183*, 36–43.

Ursano, R. J., Kao, T., & Fullerton, C. S. (1992). PTSD and meaning: Structuring human chaos. *Journal of Nervous and Mental Disease, 180*, 756–759.

Ursano R. J., McCaughey, B. C., & Fullerton, C. S. (1994). *Individual and community responses to trauma and disaster: The structure of human chaos.* Cambridge, England: Cambridge University Press.

Warheit, G. T. (1985). A propositional paradigm for estimating the effects of disasters on mental health. In B. J. Sowder (Ed.), *Disasters and mental health: Selected contemporary perspectives* (pp. 196–214). Rockville, MD: National Institutes of Mental Health.

Weisaeth, L. (1989a). The stressors and the post-traumatic stress syndrome after an industrial disaster. *Acta Psychiatrica Scandinavica, 80*(Suppl. 355), 25–37.

Weisaeth, L. (1989b). A study of behavioral responses to an industrial disaster. *Acta Psychiatrica Scandinavica, 80*(Suppl. 355), 13–24.

Weisaeth, L. (1989c). Torture of a Norwegian ship's crew. *Acta Psychiatrica Scandinavica, 80*(Suppl. 355), 63–72.

Weisaeth, L. (1993). Disaster: Psychological and psychiatric aspects. In L. Goldberger & S. Breznitz (Eds.), *Handbook of stress* (pp. 591–616). New York: Free Press.

Weisaeth, L. (1995). Risk and preventive intervention. In B. Raphael & E. Burrows (Eds.), *Handbook of preventive psychiatry* (pp. 301–322). Amsterdam: Elsevier.

Weisenfeld, A. R., & Weis, H. M. (1979). Hairdressers and helping: Influencing the behavior of informal caregivers. *Professional Psychology, 10*, 786–792.

World Health Organization. (1988). *Resolution on the International Decade for Natural Disaster Reduction.* Geneva: Author.

Wright, K. (Ed.). (1987). *The human response to the Gander military air disaster: A summary report* (Division of Neuropsychiatry Report No. 88-12). Washington, DC: Walter Reed Army Institute of Research.

Wright, K., Ursano, R. J., Bartone, P., & Ingraham, L. H. (1990). The shared experience of catastrophe: An expanded classification of the disaster community. *American Journal of Orthopsychiatry, 60*, 35–42.

CHAPTER 20

Acute Preventive Interventions

BEVERLEY RAPHAEL
JOHN WILSON
LENORE MELDRUM
ALEXANDER C. McFARLANE

A powerful motivation for clinicians working in the field of trauma is the wish to prevent or minimize chronic posttraumatic reactions. Traumatic events offer an unusual opportunity in mental health work generally, where prevention is a much-desired but elusive goal. Is the possibility of prevention a realistic hope or a forlorn attempt to create a world of safety in settings of overwhelming danger and suffering? Can the wounds of the horror, the confrontation with death, and the vulnerability arising out of the loss of control be quickly sealed over?

The question of what acute preventive interventions are possible, and the evidence about their effectiveness, need to be considered from several perspectives. Interest in the field has often developed ahead of empirical knowledge, because of the compelling imperative to intervene with what are seen to be highly vulnerable groups of victims. For mental health workers, this type of intervention has a substantial appeal, because it enables them to get involved in very different work from their typical day-to-day roles. Traumatic situations provide opportunities for them to feel helpful and to deal with the general population, rather than the chronically mentally ill groups that constitute their typical clientele. The explosion of interest and knowledge about posttraumatic stress disorder (PTSD) since 1980 has facilitated an increasing focus in the mass media on these issues in the immediate aftermath of disasters; this encourages disaster authorities to take the necessary actions to provide debriefing.

However, what to do is a difficult question. First, there has been little systematic examination of the critical features of effective interventions. Our

knowledge is largely derived from clinical wisdom. Adequate outcome evaluation is difficult in the face of the immediate trauma and chaos that disasters
and wars bring. There is also a need to define the value of preventive interventions for victims who are at particularly high risk, in contrast to victims with a
normative stress response, for whom no benefit or even negative effects may
be apparent (Raphael, 1980). Furthermore, knowledge of likely course and
etiological factors in the case of posttraumatic outcomes is only currently developing, and many questions remain about what interventions may be useful
at what time for which group. The choice of intervention is also not just a matter
of scientific evidence; secular influences have a powerful impact as well. Support groups for victims and similiar social movements, actively advocate debriefing programs that are allegedly preventive. The widespread existence of these
programs complicates the assessment of natural course and etiology of disorders following many disasters, and the acceptability to a community of any systematic evaluation of outcome.

The use of interventions following traumatic events builds on the model
by Gerald Caplan (1964), who proposed crisis intervention as a preventive technique to lessen the likelihood of unfavorable outcomes after stressful life events.
There are studies that demonstrate beneficial effects of such interventions with
the crises of conjugal bereavement (e.g., Raphael, 1977; Parkes, 1980) and
accidents (Bordow & Porritt, 1979), and others that show substantial negative
effects (e.g., Polak, Egan, Vandebergh, & Williams, 1975). The mechanism as
to how crisis intervention works to prevent psychological disorder is unclear;
it may be either a means of preventing development of a disorder (primary
prevention), or a way of dealing with heightened distress that represents an
early stage in the onset of a disorder. These arguments are of less significance
than the need to evaluate the effectiveness of this type of intervention in improving short- and longer-term outcomes, among the morass of other influences that may operate (including the "secular processes" identified above).
Furthermore, the recognition of the public health impact of mental disorders
in general and of posttraumatic morbidity in particular has highlighted the
need for brief, efficient, and broadly applicable approaches that may mitigate
the likelihood of adverse outcomes. It is in this context that acute preventive
interventions in the field of psychological trauma should be considered.

SOCIAL CONTEXT
OF TRAUMATIC EXPERIENCE

The provision of any preventive intervention needs to take account of the
atmosphere and social processes that emerge following traumatic events.
Trauma in the context of a major natural or human-made disaster will be likely
to evoke a significant positive and sympathetic response to those affected and

to the "heroic" rescuers. The "therapeutic community" response of the social system in the postdisaster period may support and facilitate acute preventive interventions—or, alternatively, may present barriers to these interventions. Often there is a delay before the full impact of a trauma is felt, and this impact begins to emerge once the initial outpouring of community support begins to wane. This period of "disillusionment" can be characterized by negativism, scapegoating, disorganization, withdrawal of support, and a full realization of the extent of the trauma and loss. These factors may complicate the outcome, bringing additional stressors beyond the period when acute preventive interventions are likely to be applied; therefore, such interventions may miss the period of greatest need.

Ultimately, preventive interventions may have little effect in the face of these and other enduring social forces. Often traumas do not provoke widespread interest, particularly if only one or a few people are involved in each trauma, as is generally the case with motor vehicle accidents, rapes, or assaults (Green, McFarlane, Hunter, & Griggs, 1993). Such experiences can be very isolating, and mental health workers may not take the same interest in providing preventive interventions for them, despite the fact that the total number of people exposed to these events is greater than the number exposed to large-scale disasters. For these reasons, individual traumas present a greater public health challenge than disasters do (Norris, 1992). The degree of public acknowledgment and support for a traumatic event may be a significant positive factor, or its absence may be an additional vulnerability or stressor factor—indeed, a second trauma.

Some social contexts are particularly negative (e.g., those of murder and suicide). Moreover, certain groups are already traumatized and marginalized (e.g., refugees, indigenous minority groups), and their needs may not be identified with additional trauma experience. Thus, societal frameworks both at the point of the trauma and over time need to be taken into account in the provision of acute preventive interventions.

Cultural prescriptions, beliefs, and values are also important and should be understood and respected. Social processes within particular cultures that may be seen as rituals for posttrauma healing (e.g., the Native American sweat lodge; Wilson, 1989), should be acknowledged respectfully, and any prevention approach should take these into account. The acceptance of fate or "karma" may also be dictated. Cultural processes may be more subtle—for instance, the organizational culture of expected behavior following a traumatic experience—and these may or may not be adaptive. For example, heavy alcohol intake may be "prescribed" to deal with trauma reactions, and this may set in motion patterns of substance abuse that are seen as the norm. Any intervention program must be sensitive to both positive and negative processes of this kind. Of particular significance are issues of disclosure and privacy; shame and "face"; affect expression and restraint; gender role behaviors; and individual as opposed to interactive processes or solutions.

ACUTE ASSESSMENT, TRIAGE, AND PSYCHOLOGICAL FIRST AID

The initial contact and assessment must encompass a compassionate and human response; the insuring of safety and survival; and the assessment and management of any physical injury or threat to life. Solomon (Chapter 5, this volume) describes the range of acute traumatic reactions that may be observed. Experience suggests that following most traumatic events, very few individuals require immediate treatment because of the severity of their behavioral decompensation. An individual may or may not be in a state in which he or she wishes, or is prepared, to discuss what has happened. Nevertheless, some gentle querying may be an essential component of a "therapeutic assessment" to identify whether a traumatized person needs emergency mental health care, the various dimensions of the trauma experienced (see Chapter 7, this volume), the person's reaction to it, and the degree of his or her risk for the development of a chronic posttraumatic disorder.

This querying provides the basis for triage, and, if done gently and supportively at the person's own pace, may facilitate the commencement of an integrative working-through process (Raphael, 1986). Nevertheless, it must take into account the traumatized person's state; the need to "dose" affective release (Lindy, 1993); the potentially adaptive purposes of dissociation, denial, numbing, and forgetting at some stages and for some people; and the "trauma membrane" that may be developed protectively at this stage, to protect an individual from overwhelming affect.

In times of disaster, mental health professionals providing acute assessment and intervention may need to do so alongside emergency support and assistance in the recovery process and in the provision of other roles (Raphael, 1986; Valent, 1984). The provision of practical help may ultimately be seen as more helpful and positive than the specific psychological care offered (Singh & Raphael, 1981). Giving accurate information and insuring the reunion of primary attachment figures may be essential to acute recovery and longer-term adaptation. It has been shown that separations of children from parents at this time may have unwanted long-term effects, even when such separations are ostensibly provided in the best interests of the children (McFarlane, 1987).

The principles of psychological first aid should be taught alongside other first aid, so that they can be applied by all those responding to traumatized individuals in an acute emergency period. The components of psychological first aid include the following: the basic human responses of comforting and consoling a distressed person; protecting the person from further threat or distress, as far as is possible; furnishing immediate care for physical necessities, including shelter; providing goal orientation and support for specific reality-based tasks ("reinforcing the concrete world"); facilitating reunion with loved ones from whom the individual has been separated; facilitating some telling of the "trauma story" and ventilation of feelings as appropriate for the particular individual; linking the person to systems of support and sources of help that will be ongoing; facilitating the beginning of some sense of mastery; and identifying needs for further counseling or intervention (Raphael, 1986).

The immediate assessment of trauma victims and the provision of acute preventive interventions need to be considered in terms of how they may fit in a range of preventive responses to a traumatic stressor experience. First, Ursano, Grieger, and McCarroll (Chapter 19, this volume) highlight the importance of training in protecting military and rescue workers from the effects of trauma: It enables them to develop a repertoire of behaviors and strategies to mitigate the impact of trauma (see also Weisaeth, 1983). It is important that any preventive intervention not disrupt the adaptive coping of well-trained groups unless there is evidence of a clear benefit.

Second, following major disasters, there may be insufficient resources to provide an intervention for all those exposed; this will necessitate the definition of groups or individuals at particular risk. The intervention approach used may also be modified according to the characteristics defined, and the benefits of prevention may thus be maximized. Risk factors requiring particular attention include the following: major organizational change (e.g., threat to job security); other recent traumatic experiences (e.g., repeated emergencies); transitional factors (e.g., recent immigration or refugee status); threat to significant others (e.g., disaster workers' own families' lives at risk); breakup of usual support systems (e.g., devastation of a community by a hurricane); and traumatic childhood experience for individuals (e.g., past history of abuse). The presence of one or more of these factors may mean that a preventive approach is more necessary. But it also suggests that an understanding of the potentially complex societal, group, and individual dynamics existing in a high-risk situation will be required, as will the skills to take these factors into account in providing acute preventive interventions.

TYPES OF ACUTE PREVENTIVE INTERVENTIONS AND THEIR RATIONALES

Various types of acute interventions have been developed and implemented, according to the circumstances. The management of acute combat stress reactions in military psychiatry (see Chapter 21, this volume), using the principles of "proximity, immediacy, and expectancy," highlights the confusion as to whether such intervention is a treatment of the early stages of a disorder or a primary prevention strategy. Studies have suggested that although this intervention is effective in lessening immediate distress and in its purpose of returning soldiers to combat with its associated risk of further traumatization, it is not effective in preventing PTSD (Solomon, 1993). Recent interventions of this kind in the Gulf War showed positive outcomes at follow-up (not in a controlled trial), but longer-term benefits in terms of prevention remain to be established (Johnson, Cline, Marcum, & Intress, 1992). At present there is little support for the view that there are substantial long-term benefits for the soldiers who are managed in this way, as many still run a high risk of developing chronic and severe PTSD.

Many emergency or rescue team leaders have long recognized the value of a "wake" after a traumatic episode, with talking through, emotional release, and "winding down," perhaps in a relaxed social setting that includes alcohol use. Thus, well before the current processes of stress debriefing became popular, formalized, and widely utilized, informal social processes may have partly fulfilled some of the same functions. More recently, various forms of psychological debriefing have evolved alongside the model of operational debriefing utilized by emergency/rescue personnel in regard to view of tasks, procedures, roles, equipment, and so forth.

The military principles of proximity, immediacy, and expectancy have been transferred into the model of, "critical incident stress debriefing" (CISD) as developed by Mitchell (1983), to serve similar purposes in emergency services workers exposed to critical stress (e.g., disasters, traumatic incidents). These organizations are often militaristic in their frameworks, and military-style debriefing represents an organized format to deal with distress and return workers to effective front-line functioning. CISD is widely utilized and is formalized in terms of specific processes and stages. Initially Mitchell insisted that it must take place in the first 24–72 hours, follow a specific format, and be limited to one specific intervention. More recently, however, he has broadened his approach, recognizing that follow-up debriefing and individual counseling may be necessary, and that time frames may need to be more flexible.

The stages proposed by Mitchell and utilized to varying degrees by mental health workers following the CISD model include the following: an introduction, which spells out confidentiality, process, and proposed benefits; a fact phase, where group members are asked to describe their roles and tasks during the incident, and to provide some facts about what happened from their own perspective; the thought phase, where members of the group are asked to tap their first thoughts during the stressful incident, leading to a more personal perspective; the reaction phase, which seeks to explore the worst part of the experience and hence to encourage people to acknowledge their emotional reactions and express their feelings; the symptom phase, which asks respondents to review their own symptoms of cognitive, physical, emotional, and behavioral distress at the scene and subsequently, up to and including the time of the debriefing; the teaching phase, which emphasizes the normality of these distress signals and gives information about the management of them and about general health issues; and the relating phase, which wraps up the meeting and summarizes it plus any plans. The debriefing is supposed to be run by at least one and preferably two specially trained mental health professionals, and to be supported by peer support personnel who have been previously trained in CISD and who are part of this work force. The aim of this process is to support people through a "normal" reaction to an abnormal event. Sessions may last 1 to 3 hours.

Dunning (1988) has reviewed intervention strategies for emergency workers and identified three distinct debriefing protocols: one that is "didactic" or "teaching," and two that are "psychological" or "therapeutic." These are not mutually exclusive in terms of content, but they do differ in their emphasis and goals. The didactic debriefing is an informational model: Participants are educated about stress, ways to recognize it, and techniques of self-management. The psychological debriefing is based on the conception that ventilation or catharsis facilitates the healing process. Mitchell's CISD is one version of this, and Bergmann and Queen's (1988a, 1988b) "continuum of care" approach is another. This latter places emphasis on coping skills and cognitive restructuring, with less emphasis on disclosure. Training, peer support, and ongoing stress management are emphasized as part of the overall context in Bergmann and Queen's approach, but Mitchell's recent work also emphasizes an overall comprehensive and integrated approach: psychologically based components, including support services at the scene of the incident/disaster; "defusing," which is a much shorter (30–45 minutes) and less structured form of debriefing, offered perhaps as workers come off shift; and follow-up counseling and other services (Mitchell & Dyregrov, 1993).

A "multiple stressor debriefing" model (Armstrong, O'Callahan, & Marmar, 1991) was developed after the 1989 San Francisco Bay Area earthquake for emergency service personnel and is a modification of Mitchell's model. In the immediate aftermath of the earthquake, a number of stress areas were identified: multiple contacts with trauma victims; long hours and poor work environment; administrative/organizational stressors; other recent stressors; being away from home; inexperience and volunteer status; and specific disaster and situation characteristics. This model was carried out in groups of fewer than 20 and involved four stages: (1) disclosure of events covering all stressor events (aspects); (2) feelings and reactions; (3) coping strategies; and (4) termination, which included goodbyes and transition to home and regular roles. In discussing this model, Armstrong et al. (1991) contextualize it with five other intervention models: crisis intervention (Cohen & Ahern, 1980); National Organization of Victim Assistance debriefing (Young, 1988); didactic debriefing (Dunning, 1988); CISD (Mitchell, 1983, 1986), and psychological debriefing (Raphael, 1977, 1986).

Although physiological arousal is a central component of PTSD and may respond to techniques such as those described above, there is little evidence to support their specific effectiveness for arousal (see below). Whether early use of pharmacological agents may be relevant as an acute preventive intervention is simply not established, but it may warrant consideration in some acute and severe situations. This modality would have to be examined in a carefully controlled methodology evaluating shorter- and longer-term outcomes, as with other acute preventive interventions. A. Y. Shalev (personal communication) has examined the use of benzodiazepines in this setting and found that they have no effect on the long-term course, although they do provide acute symptomatic relief.

Social system interventions involve community action, organization, and mobilization; education and consultation with advice for leaders; mobilization of action plans and recovery processes; facilitation of adaptation and mastery in social change; development of community networks; development of a positive recovery organization; communication; and community theater and art geared to working through and recovering from the trauma (Raphael, 1986). The implementation of a public health perspective is extremely difficult to evaluate, but it is often likely to be significant in the recovery of individuals and communities.

The confusion as to whether an acute intervention is treatment of the early stages of a disorder or a primary prevention strategy is reflected in the proposal that eye movement desensitization and reprocessing (EMDR) and cognitive-behavioral techniques should be used in the setting of the acute distress following traumatic events. These methods are described in Chapter 21 of this volume.

STUDIES AND EVALUATIONS
OF PREVENTIVE INTERVENTIONS

To date, there have been no systematic, controlled trials of the effectiveness of the various models of stress debriefing. Mitchell and Bray (1990) claim from anecdotal evidence that CISD has significantly diminished the problems experienced by emergency personnel, including job turnover, early retirement, and mental and other health problems. They suggest that following a critical incident, 3–10% of emergency personnel will have no adverse effects; 80–85% will have acute or delayed effects; and there will be a small group of 3–10%, out of which 3–4% (of the original total) will go on to develop chronic severe PTSD. The sources of these estimates are not quoted.

Subjective anecdotal evaluations report positive outcomes, but an attempt at systematic appraisal of CISD has only recently been made (Robinson & Mitchell, 1993). In an Australian sample of emergency personnel (male) and welfare and hospital personnel, the majority of respondents perceived the debriefing as valuable. The 60% of participants who experienced "stress symptoms" reported reduced symptoms after CISD, and they attributed this reduction to the debriefing. The debriefing was reported as helpful by another

34% of the respondents because it (1) facilitated talking with others about the incident; (2) encouraged talking about the incident; (3) improved their self-understanding; and (4) improved between-agency cohesion. The authors acknowledge the need for more in-depth evaluations to follow this exploratory study, and also note that such debriefing is just one component of a support program. These results are of interest; however, further objective and long-term outcome assessments are also needed, for (as R. Robinson herself reports; personal communication, 1990), there have been a number of longer-term problems appearing.

These findings should be seen in the context of other studies, which have used objective symptom measures (usually in naturalistic experimental frameworks) and have compared debriefed and nondebriefed personnel who have passed through a particular traumatic experience and have been assessed some time subsequently (Watts, 1994; Deahl, Gillham, Thomas, Searle, & Srinivasan, 1994). The positive effects of the short-term CISD intervention outlined above suggest that the disclosure component may be very helpful, and this is reinforced by the emphasis on disclosure in most focal and crisis therapy models, including behavioral models. Research conducted after the fire at King's Cross Station in London found that those victims who had discussed their difficulties with others appeared to have better outcomes (Turner, Thompson, & Rosser, 1993).

On the other hand, there are circumstances where opportunities for disclosure have resulted in no demonstrable benefit. Weisaeth (1989) reports his detailed interviewing of disaster victims after a factory fire/explosion, which covered every aspect of the disaster experience and reaction to it, and commenced within 2 days of the disaster. The intervention did not appear to prevent PTSD from developing to substantial levels in the affected population, although the levels might have been higher without it. However, it was also suggested by Weisaeth's Norwegian group (Ersland, Weisaeth, & Sund, 1989) that after the North Sea oil rig disaster, one group of workers who were rescued were all provided with opportunities for talking through their experience and none had long-term morbidity, whereas a second group of rescued workers who did not have this provision subsequently developed significant problems. Many variables could account for such differences, so that again these findings do not provide adequate support for debriefing's effectiveness.

Tyrer (1989) adds a further positive report, but his interventions were more specific and involved the rotation and support of personnel rather than specific debriefing. It is also clear that even when debriefing has been provided, significant levels of posttraumatic morbidity still occur. This is evidenced by the rate of 33% in a study by Creamer, Burgess, Buckingham, and Pattison (1989), despite extensive mental health outreach, support, and debriefing programs.

Hytten and Hasle (1989) report specifically on the effects of debriefing and rescue action on firefighters who had dealt with a hotel fire. Of the 39 men who participated in the debriefing sessions, 38 stated that the debriefing had been helpful. Two-thirds said that it had been professionally helpful, increasing their self-confidence. Nevertheless, there was no significant difference in Impact of Event Scale (IES) scores between those who received formal debriefing and those who only talked with their colleagues in more informal settings. Morbidity levels were not high for the total sample, but nevertheless were present, so these talking-through processes did not prevent them.

Griffiths and Watts (1992), following up emergency personnel involved in bus crashes, found that those who attended debriefing had significantly higher levels of symptoms at 12 months (both intrusive and avoidance symptoms as measured by the IES) than those who did not. They also found no relationship between the perceived helpfulness of debriefing and such symptoms. It should be noted, however, that those experiencing the greatest distress were more likely to have attended debriefing and found it helpful.

After the Hillsborough football stadium disaster in Sheffield, England, two hospitals dealt with 159 casualties, including 95 deaths. Thirty-two psychological debriefing groups took place from 4 days after the trauma until 13 days after the incident at the first receiving hospital, which dealt with most of the dead. At the second hospital involved, only three requests for individual support and two for group debriefing were received by the psychologists. During the 6 months following the disaster, support services were also provided for staff members at both hospitals. It was found that those who had the highest levels of exposure to the disaster were those seeking prolonged psychological help. In the evaluation of the support services, staff members indicated that both they themselves and their families could have benefited from "preincident" training in knowledge of stress responses to be expected after exposure to trauma. Combined data from both hospitals indicated that 68% of respondents found the counseling and psychological debriefing sessions helpful, although some found them unhelpful. Respondents suggested that more than one method of providing support to those exposed to trauma should be available (Shapiro & Kunkler, 1990a, 1990b).

Effective management and careful planning were utilized in the operation to recover bodies from the accommodation modules of the Piper Alpha oil rig. All those participating in the operation were provided with detailed induction into their specific assignments, which reinforced the importance of their task. The group members were also educated about the need to identify and care for their own possible emotional, physical, and social reactions. Each younger officer was paired with an older, more experienced officer, and each team was debriefed each day by a senior officer, with backup support provided informally by a psychiatrist supporting the team. It was found that officers showed no higher levels of anxiety than were determined in a health study conducted before the task began. This was attributed to the planning and support services provided (Alexander & Wells, 1991).

Kenardy et al. (1996) have reported the most detailed follow-up studies to date in their assessment of outcomes for persons debriefed following the Newcastle earthquake (New South Wales, Australia), as part of their overall assessment of the effects of the earthquake on that community over a 2-year period. The researchers assessed subjects who completed all four phases of the impact study (6 months after the quake and then at intervals of 6–8 months) and who reported that they had acted in the roles of helpers (e.g., police, ambulance officers, counselors) or volunteers (e.g., state, emergency services, welfare roles). Those who were debriefed (via traditional CISD; $n = 56$) were compared with those who were not ($n = 117$). The two groups showed no differences in terms of key demographic variables such as age, sex, and socioeconomic status, or in terms of disaster variables (exposure to threat, exposure to disruption, helping in threat situations). The debriefed group did have a higher educational level, were more likely to have been helping in nonthreat situations, and were more likely to be counselors or coordinators of services. These latter points may be relevant to the outcomes identified below, because they may in general indicate a group more like the one identified in Raphael, Singh, Bradbury, and Lambert (1983–1984)—a group with more ill-defined, less targeted roles and a different type of stressor experience complicating their disaster outcomes, as well as with more depressive symptoms.

Outcomes were measured by General Health Questionnaire (GHQ; Goldberg & Hiller, 1979) and IES (Horowitz, Wilner, & Alvarez, 1979) symptom scores, and perceived helpfulness of debriefing was also assessed. Kenardy et al. (1996) found that there was a significant reduction in IES scores over time, with little change between phases 1 and 2, then a reduction between phases 2 and 3, and little overall change between phases 3 and 4. Higher exposure to threat and disruption were associated with higher scores on the IES and GHQ. However, those who were *not* debriefed showed a more rapid reduction in GHQ scores over time. The researchers conclude from their findings that there was no evidence of enhanced rate or extent of recovery in those who were debriefed, compared to those who were not. Personality, sensitivity, and neuroticism may actually increase reactivity with debriefing. Clearly, these results are of interest, although this was not a controlled study and the groups may have in some way been self-selected (i.e., the most vulnerable may have been debriefed). If this latter was the case, the more vulnerable may have been protected to some degree from even more pronounced morbidity. The differences in the nature of the stressor experience of this group, and the fact that traditional CISD was developed more in relation to single-incident life threat stressors and may not have been appropriate here, should also be noted.

Thus, although debriefing in one form or another is widely used, strongly supported, and generally valued as a helpful preventive intervention, there is no evidence to date of its effectiveness as a preventive intervention in terms of posttraumatic morbidity. In fact, some findings raise questions about the negative effects of these interventions.

A number of studies have investigated the effectiveness of crisis intervention in forms other than a debriefing format, such as a focal or individual approach. Although these approaches have been applied to populations who might have been at risk for posttraumatic stress reactions, most studies have not identified this component or specifically aimed at preventing it. The effectiveness of crisis intervention as a preventive intervention for high-risk bereaved widows has been established (Raphael, 1977). This preventive approach did not encompass specific investigation of PTSD phenomenology, although it should be noted that one risk factor was traumatic circumstances of the death, which may have contributed to the development of PTSD in relation to that stressor rather than to the bereavement. The phenomenology of bereavement and PTSD are different, although they may overlap in traumatic bereavements.

Studies of crisis intervention with accident victims (e.g., Bordow & Porritt, 1979) have shown beneficial outcomes. More recently, Brom, Kleber, and Hofman (1993) assessed motor vehicle accident victims at 1 month with follow-up at 6 months, using the IES, the Trauma Symptom Inventory, and other measures. The intervention was counseling for three to six sessions, carried out by experienced psychotherapists according to a preestablished protocol. The majority were satisfied with the intervention, and the intervention group showed a statistically significant decrease over time; unfortunately, however, this group was more symptomatic to begin with and could not be shown to have benefited.

Models of crisis intervention that have been tested have usually involved a similar number of focused counselling sessions in the early weeks or months after an incident. They have operated generally on the basis of some psychodynamic understanding. And in those instances and in other studies of both bereavement (e.g., Parkes, 1980) and other crises (Viney, Clark, Bunn, & Benjamin, 1985), counseling has been shown to be effective. Whether this timing has better suited situations of loss, or been appropriate for situations of trauma or stressors such as traumatic encounters with death, has not been established. However, despite the differences between the two sets of phenomena, it is interesting to note that one very early, acute, brief preventive intervention with bereaved people (Polak et al., 1975) was also not shown to be effective. This too took place within the first few days (similar to debriefing), as opposed to more targeted crisis intervention formats, which are usually commenced after a few weeks.

In summary, the evidence that acute preventive interventions have a substantial positive benefit for victims of trauma is disappointingly scarce. The possibility that these interventions may actually have negative effects is a cause for concern and caution. These are settings where a sense of imperative to act may undermine the propensity for reflection—a possibility that may account for these disappointing findings. Given the resources and training being devoted to debriefing, there is an obvious need to improve the standards of the evaluation literature.

POSTTRAUMATIC STRESS REACTIONS AND ACUTE PREVENTIVE INTERVENTIONS

Little is known about the exact processes of evolution of acute posttraumatic reactive processes and morbidity that could provide a firm basis for a specific preventive approach, other than the general issues outlined above (see Chapter 4). Although, many of the approaches described in this chapter rely on catharsis, disclosure, reconfronting the trauma, and group and social support, the relative appropriateness of these factors to posttraumatic processes and their resolution remains to be established. For instance, the reviewing of the incident or trauma may inhibit natural processes of "forgetting" or letting memories fade for some people; arousal may be increased; or avoidance may be reinforced.

Furthermore, because past traumatization (e.g., childhood sexual abuse) may be a risk factor for later disorder, the reawakening of such repressed experiences may inevitably create further problems for recovery, yet possibly may also provide opportunities for "working through." The role of underlying personality styles and coping has not been either adequately assessed or taken into account with the current methods of intervention. Although active problem solving is usually endorsed as the most effective means of coping, it may be for others that at this stage or this time that denial is appropriate, and techniques that diminish it are counterproductive.

Dangers also lie in the apparent simplicity of many of the approaches, any effects of which may be empirical. The dangers may arise either from false expectations of providers and recipients, or from potential negative consequences that are not acknowledged or recognized. For example, unrealistic expectations may mean that inadequate attention and resources are given to the planning of services to treat PTSD and other disorders that emerge in the aftermath of the event. This is a particular concern, because interventions provided during the first 6 months after a disaster or accident may have more pronounced and enduring benefits (R. S. Pynoos, personal communication). Many supporters of the acute interventions that are currently in vogue contend that they are sufficient to prevent adverse consequences, although this contention has been somewhat softened in recent years. It is essential that any acute preventive interventions are linked to the concept of a "safety net" of other follow-up services—individual treatment, referral to specialist services, and monitoring over time—so that opportunities exist for interventions or support in cases of delayed reactions or of more chronic and severe problems that may arise.

Evaluation and monitoring of effectiveness are key aspects of such overall management. The evaluation of acute preventive interventions must include both shorter and longer time frames and must take into account potential positive and negative outcomes. A stress reaction that was apparently resolving may evolve into disorder through complex effects related to preexisting vulnerability, new stressor effects, secondary traumatization, failure of support, and many other factors (see Chapter 8, this volume). The timing of the provision of preventive intervention is a related issue. No one would suggest that bereavement counseling should be provided on the day following the death of a spouse; there are many reasons why this would be seen to be inappropriate. These issues could equally apply to the provision of acute interventions immediatly following traumatic events.

QUALITY CONTROL AND TRAINING

The high levels of distress and the enormity of trauma create an environment of intense need, evoking powerful feelings in those who hear and share the story, as well as in those who experience the trauma directly. The transference issues that may arise for a distressed person may involve intense expectations and idealization of help initially given, and subsequent disillusionment or dependency. On the other hand, the nature of the acute crisis, the lowered defensiveness, the empathic identification, the intensity of an acute caseload in a major traumatic incident, the lack of traditional professional boundaries, and the enormity of the incident may all contribute particular stresses for the worker. Lindy and Wilson (1994) suggest that there is a balance between empathic enmeshment on the one hand, and cold distancing and nonresponsiveness to the needs of the traumatized person on the other. Failure to address these issues may well contribute to "burnout," detachment, and withdrawal from service provision (Raphael, Meldrum, & O'Toole, 1991); these possibilities necessitate, debriefing, supervision, and support for workers in the field.

Individuals responsible for the provision of services to a traumatized population must consider issues of evaluation and quality control when planning interventions. Critical issues include what was delivered, when, by whom, to which populations. The plethora of approaches currently presented, the enthusiastic marketing of stress debriefing, and the wide range of professionals (and others) offering acute interventions all indicate a need for close scrutiny. Not only is there the risk that unreal expectations will be created in recipients and payees: there is the risk that in fact negative consequences may result, either from an intervention itself or from a failure to acknowledge that further care may be necessary.

Furthermore, as will be obvious from the present discussion, the tasks of acute preventive intervention are far from simple; they require a sensitive, skilled approach and a knowledge of complex personal and social dynamics. As in major disasters, there may be a need to "protect" victims from the convergence of those who would offer help. There is a firm need for quality control, training, and accreditation for those who offer such services, as well as for systematic evaluation of outcomes. The mental health professionals who do this work need to have extensive skills and training, to have a specific understanding of the complexity of psychological trauma, and at the same time to maintain a human and compassionate approach.

REFERENCES

Alexander, D., & Wells, A.(1991). Reactions of police officers to body handling after a major disaster: A before-and-after comparison. *British Journal of Psychiatry, 159,* 547–555.

Armstrong, K., O'Callahan, W., & Marmar, C. R. (1991). Debriefing Red Cross disaster personnel: The multiple stressor debriefing model. *Journal of Traumatic Stress, 4*(4), 581–594.

Bergmann, L. H., & Queen, T. (1988a, October). Maintaining posttrauma programs. *Fire Engineering,* pp. 73–75.

Bergmann, L. H., & Queen, T. (1988b, August). Posttrauma response programs. *Fire Engineering,* pp. 89–91.

Bordow, S., & Porrit, D. (1979). An experimental evaluation of crisis intervention. *Social Science and Medicine, 13a,* 251–256.

Brom, D., Kleber, R. J. & Hofman, M. (1993). Victims of traffic accidents: Incidence and prevention of post-traumatic stress disorder. *Journal of Clinical Psychology, 49*(2), 131–140.

Caplan, G. (1964). *Principles of preventive psychiatry.* New York: Basic Books.

Cohen, R. E., & Ahern, F. L. (1980). *Handbook for mental health care of disaster victims.* Baltimore: Johns Hopkins University Press.

Creamer, M., Burgess, P., Buckingham, W., & Pattison, P. (1989). *The psychological aftermath of the Queen Street shootings.* Melbourne: Department of Psychology, University of Melbourne.

Deahl, M. P., Gillham, A. B., Thomas, J., Searle, M. M., & Srinivasan, M. (1994). Psychological sequelae following the Gulf War: Factors associated with subsequent morbidity and the effectiveness of psychological debriefing. *British Journal of Psychiatry, 165,* 60–65.

Dunning, C. (1988). Intervention strategies for emergency workers. In M. Lystad (Ed.), *Mental health response to mass emergencies* (pp. 284–307). New York: Brunner/ Mazel.

Ersland, S., Weisaeth, L., & Sund, A. (1989). The stress upon rescuers involved in an oil rig disaster: "Alexander L. Kielland" 1980. *Acta Psychiatrica Scandinavica, 80* (Suppl. 355), 38–49.

Goldberg, D. P., & Hillier, V. F. (1979). A scaled version of the General Health Questionnaire. *Psychological Medicine, 9,* 139–145.

Green, M. M., McFarlane, A. C., Hunter, C. E., & Griggs, W. M. (1993). Undiagnosed post-traumatic stress disorder following motor vehicle accidents. *Medical Journal of Australia, 159*(8), 529–534.

Griffiths, J., & Watts, R. (1992). *The Kempsey and Grafton bus crashes: The aftermath.* East Lismore, Australia: Instructional Design Solutions.

Horowitz, M., Wilner, M. E., & Alvarez, W. (1979). Impact of event scale: A measure of subjective stress. *Psychosomatic Medicine, 41,* 209–215.

Hytten, L., & Hasle, A. (1989). Firefighters: A study of stress and coping. *Acta Psychiatrica Scandinavica, 80* (Suppl. 355), 50–55.

Johnson, L. B., Cline, D. W., Marcum, J. M., & Intress, J. L. (1992). Effectiveness of a stress recovery unit during the Persian Gulf War. *Hospital and Community Psychiatry, 43*(8), 829–830.

Kenardy, J. A., Webster, R. A., Lewin, T. J., Carr, V. J., Hazell, P. L., & Carter, G. L. (1996). Stress debriefing and patterns of recovery following a natural disaster. *Journal of Traumatic Stress, 9*(1), 37–49.

Lindy, J. D. (1993). Focal psychoanalytic psychotherapy of posttraumatic stress disorder. In J. P. Wilson & B. Raphael (Eds.), *International handbook of traumatic stress syndromes* (pp. 803–809). New York: Plenum Press.

Lindy, J. D., & Wilson, J. P. (1994). Beyond empathy: New directions for the future. In J. P. Wilson & J. D. Lindy (Eds.), *Countertransference in the treatment of PTSD* (pp. 389–394). New York: Guilford Press.

McFarlane, A. C. (1987). Post-traumatic phenomena in a longitudinal study of children following a natural disaster. *Journal of the American Academy of Child and Adolescent Psychiatry, 26,* 764–769.

Mitchell, J. (1983). When disaster strikes: The critical incident stress debriefing process. *Journal of Emergency Medical Services, 8,* 36–39.

Mitchell, J. (1986, September–October). Critical incident stress management: Response! *The Magazine of Rescue and Emergency Management,* pp. 24–25.

Mitchell, J., & Bray, G. (1990). *Emergency services stress.* Englewood Cliffs, NJ: Prentice-Hall.

Mitchell, J., & Dyregrov, A. (1993). Traumatic stress in disaster workers and emergency personnel: Prevention and intervention. In J. P. Wilson & B. Raphael (Eds.), *International handbook of traumatic stress syndromes* (pp. 905–914). New York: Plenum Press.

Norris, F. H. (1992). Epidemiology of trauma: Frequency and impact of different potentially traumatic events on different demographic groups. *Journal of Consulting and Clinical Psychology, 60*(3), 409–418.

Parkes, C. M. (1980). Bereavement counselling: Does it work? *British Medical Journal, 281,* 3–6.

Polak, P. R., Egan, D., Vandebergh, R., & Williams, W. V. (1975). Prevention in mental health: A controlled study. *American Journal of Psychiatry, 132,* 146–149.

Raphael, B. (1977). Preventive intervention with the recently bereaved. *Archives of General Psychiatry, 34*(12), 1450–1454.

Raphael, B. (1980). Primary prevention: Fact or fiction? *Australian and New Zealand of Psychiatry, 14,* 163–174.

Raphael, B. (1986). *When disaster strikes.* New York: Basic Books.

Raphael, B., Meldrum, L., & O'Toole, B. (1991). Rescuers' psychological responses to disasters. *British Medical Journal, 303,* 1346–1347.

Raphael, B., Singh, B., Bradbury, L., & Lambert, F. (1983–1984). Who helps the helpers? The effects of disaster on rescue workers. *Omega, 14*(1), 9–20.

Robinson, R., & Mitchell, J. (1993). Evaluation of psychological debriefings. *Journal of Traumatic Stress, 6*(3), 367–382.

Shapiro, D., & Kunkler, J. (1990a). *Psychological support for hospital staff initiated by clinical psychologists in the aftermath of the Hillsborough disaster.* Sheffield, England: Sheffield Health Authority Mental Health Services Unit.

Shapiro, D., & Kunkler, J. (1990b). *Summary of a report on psychological support for hospital staff initiated by clinical psychologists in the aftermath of the Hillsborough disaster.* Sheffield, England: Sheffield Health Authority Mental Health Services Unit.

Singh, B., & Raphael, B. (1981). Postdisaster morbidity of the bereaved: A possible role for preventive psychiatry? *Journal of Nervous and Mental Disease, 169*(4), 203–212.

Solomon, Z. (1993). Immediate and long-term effects of traumatic combat stress among Israeli veterans of the Lebanon War. In J. P. Wilson & B. Raphael (Eds.), *International handbook of traumatic stress syndromes* (pp. 321–332). New York: Plenum Press.

Turner, S. W., Thompson, J., & Rosser, R. M. (1993). The King's Cross fire: Early psychological response and implications for organizing a "phase-two" response. In J. P. Wilson & B. Raphael (Eds.), *International handbook of traumatic stress syndromes* (pp. 451–459). New York: Plenum Press.

Tyrer, P. (1989). Community psychiatry: Are we coping? [Letter]. *British Journal of Hospital Medicine, 42*(5), 426.

Valent, P. (1984). The Ash Wednesday bushfires in Victoria. *Medical Journal of Australia, 141*, 291–300.

Viney, L. L., Clark, A. M., Bunn, T. A., & Benjamin, Y. N. (1985). Crisis intervention counselling: An evaluation of long and short term effects. *Journal of Counselling Psychology, 32*(1), 29–39.

Watts, R. (1994). The efficacy of critical incident stress debriefing for personnel. *Bulletin of the Australian Psychological Society, 16*(3), 6–7.

Weisaeth, L. (1983). *The study of a factory fire.* Unpublished doctoral dissertation, University of Oslo.

Weisaeth, L. (1989). The stressors and the post-traumatic stress syndrome after an industrial disaster. *Acta Psychiatrica Scandinavica, 80* (Suppl. 355), 25–37.

Wilson, J. P. (1989). *Trauma, transformation and healing.* New York: Brunner/Mazel.

Young, M. A. (1988). Support services for victims. In F. M. Ochberg (Ed.), *Posttraumatic therapy and victims of violence* (pp. 330–351). New York: Brunner/Mazel.

CHAPTER 21

Acute Treatments

GORDON J. TURNBULL
ALEXANDER C. McFARLANE

The treatment of victims with acute traumatic reactions presents a particular challenge to the field of traumatic stress. To date, most of the treatment literature has examined the use of a range of techniques in sufferers with established diagnoses of posttraumatic stress disorder (PTSD) (see Chapter 18, this volume). There is very little empirical information from outcome studies to guide the clinician as to how best to treat acute traumatic reactions. The treatment of acute combat stress reactions in the military setting is the one area of collective clinical knowledge. However, as indicated in Chapter 5 of this volume, although this treatment may be effective in ameliorating the acute symptoms, these individuals are still at major risk of going on to develop PTSD in the longer term. The experience of the military has done more to show what does *not* work than to prove which interventions *are* effective. However, the military treatment principles of "immediacy, proximity, and expectancy" have been shown to result in better acute and long-term outcomes for military casualties (Sargant & Slater, 1972).

This chapter therefore highlights some of the key strategies and principles that can assist clinicians in an approach to patients who have recently been exposed to a traumatic event and require more than a preventive intervention. In most disaster situations or civilian accidents, there will be relatively few people who require acute treatment because their behavior or distress is disruptive or unmanageable. The assessment and containment of distress are major components of early treatment, and our current knowledge of these is drawn to a significant degree from the crisis intervention literature. The presence of severe dissociative reactions is probably the most common challenge for the clinician dealing with victims of acute trauma. The presence of prior psychiatric disorder as an important modifying factor in acute presentations should always be assessed. Moreover, various treatment strategies need to be systematically assessed for their relative effectiveness in minimizing secondary morbidity. Treatments that are effective in the latter stages of PTSD may not be effective in the immediate postdisaster period, and vice versa. In particular, our knowledge of the neurobiology of the acute disorder versus chronic PTSD is in a state of evolution.

The acute disorder should be conceived of as a combination of biological, psychological, and social dimensions. Treatment of one domain may help to unravel other dimensional strands. For example, a victim's level of anxiety may be so severe as to interfere with useful cognitive processing or prevent it altogether. The judicious use of anxiolytic medication may allow the individual's distress to decrease to a level at which the psychological work of addressing the meaning of the experience can begin. Given the range of treatment strategies used by therapists, a staged approach to treatment that involves a careful integration of such strategies is of critical importance. The techniques currently used represent an amalgamation of psychological treatments already widely used in other clinical settings.

The increasing recognition of PTSD as a clinical entity with the potential for successful treatment has led patients to present earlier than before, often in the first weeks following exposure. The absence of established patterns of disability, and survivors' greater degree of reactivity at this stage, mean that certain specific issues may be addressed in this acute period with some confidence of success. However, there is no single recognized method for the effective treatment of acute traumatic reactions. Given that many acutely distressed individuals have the potential for recovery in the absence of treatment, the nature of the recovery process should be considered in the acute treatment setting. In part, acute interventions should be conceived of as catalysts to recovery—means of assisting individuals in moving toward restitution. Traditional concepts of psychopathology and treatment therefore have their limitations in this setting. Several themes and principles have emerged in treatment programs used in the early management of individuals with acute traumatic reaction.

THE SETTING OF SERVICES

Among psychiatric service providers, there has been a general recognition of the need to break down the normal models of office-based service delivery if effective outreach is to be achieved. This need is particularly great in the acute trauma field. One of the major issues for any clinician is that those most in need of treatment will often avoid initiating contact with a treatment service or will turn down offers for intervention. Brom, Kleber, and Hofman (1993) found that although 36% of motor accident victims agreed to have their longitudinal course monitored, only 13% agreed to participate in an intervention study, despite the presence of significant levels of distress in this population. This indicates that many sufferers may avoid or reject the idea of psychological treatments for PTSD. Thus, although such treatments may be highly effective in the small subgroup of victims who do seek treatment, it is important to consider the issue of their general acceptability.

Service providers must also actively consider the issues of outreach and service structure. After disasters, the practical demands of rebuilding shattered communities, especially isolated areas, may prevent victims from seeking specialist treatment services (which are often located at a distance). In addition, motor accident victims and burn victims require active contact during their hospitalization. This should occur not only with those who are actively symptomatic during their inpatient stay, but with all such victims. Roca, Spence, and Munster (1992) found that only 7% of adult burn patients had PTSD at discharge, but that this increased to over 22% at follow-up. Finally, it is important for emergency services to include the provision of peer support programs in a variety of high-risk professions. These can act as extended systems of care, and in cases where specialist referral may be needed, they can help individuals to overcome their apprehension about seeking treatment. Such programs are described in greater detail in Chapter 19, this volume.

EDUCATION

Victims of acute trauma are often confused by their symptoms and are uncertain about the best ways of adapting their current distress. Information giving is an essential part of the treatment process. This allows individuals to develop a cognitive structure in order to begin to pursue the issues of meaning, as well as to gain a greater sense of control over their intrusive and avoidant symptoms. The initial assessment is part of the information-giving process. Education needs to center on explaining how the physiological accompaniments of arousal can lead to a somatic focus on the trauma, particularly in conjunction with the residual effects of an injury sustained at the time of the trauma. These residual symptoms can act as subtle symbolic triggers of traumatic images.

ISSUES TO BE ADDRESSED
BEFORE TREATMENT BEGINS

More specific psychological interventions cannot begin until a range of other issues have been addressed. For example, the victims of a natural disaster may have to secure their physical safety and protect their possessions. Refugees and other victims of political upheaval may have a variety of resettlement issues that are paramount in their minds. Perhaps one of the greatest challenges is dealing with a family in which child sexual abuse is ongoing. The immediate physical protection of the child(ren) and legal issues may take precedence over treatment; when treatment does begin, its initial aim must be to restore a modicum of safety and control. Similarly, with rape victims, assisting them with the criminal prosecution and addressing the immediate concerns about their safety will be essential.

The direct or indirect impact of trauma on other family members besides the index sufferer is another issue that requires ongoing assessment. Trauma does not occur in a vacuum, and often a number of family members may be similarly traumatized (e.g., by a natural disaster, sexual abuse, or torture). Even when family members are not directly victimized, the indirect effects on them (e.g., spouses of emergency service workers or rape victims) may be severe. The success of any treatment intervention may be influenced by whether other family members are affected, and treatment may well need to be extended to include all such members.

NONSPECIFIC FACTORS AND COMMON ELEMENTS IN TREATMENT

Much of what is written in the PTSD area emphasizes the specific ingredients of each treatment approach. To date, however, no study has independently assessed the therapeutic process to insure that the specific ingredients of treatment are as "specific" as claimed. Indeed, the most frequently used treatment approaches have a number of common goals. The provisions of hope and of a sense of control is particularly important for victims of trauma. Another primary aim is to help victims develop a realistic appraisal of the threat experienced during the trauma and their actual opportunities for response. On the one hand, this may involve confronting an individual's denial of realistic danger; on the other hand, it may involve providing reassurance about the actions taken (or not taken) and the impossibility of the apparent choices. A related central issue is to overcome the cognitive and behavioral avoidance of both internal cues and external reminders of trauma by assisting the individuals to work through the meaning of their traumatic exposure and to gain a sense of mastery over their intrusive recollections.

It is also necessary to focus on the development of affective modulation, because the victims of trauma often fluctuate between numbing/withdrawal and hypervigilance/overarousal. This can be done both through focused activity and through specific anxiety management strategies. One way of confronting ongoing hypervigilance is to identify the point at which the victims first felt out of danger following the trauma; this should encourage them to focus on their current safety and to begin dealing with their traumatic memories. Of course, therapists will need to insure that the individuals are not retraumatized by the process of treatment if they feel unable or unready to confront their traumatic memories. Helping traumatized individuals progress from the sense of being helpless victims to a sense of being survivors involves helping them shift from a feeling of being persecuted by the trauma to one of being able to look to the present and to develop a sense of future goals. A central dimension of this reengagement is slowly initiating attempts at intimate and rewarding social relationships, instead of progressive withdrawal and social detachment. This often involves dealing with the sense of irritability and preoccupation associated with traumatic reminders.

CRISIS INTERVENTION

There is a long tradition of crisis intervention as an approach to acute trauma. Crisis theory (Lindemann, 1944; Caplan, 1961; Greenstone & Leviton, 1981; Burgess & Baldwin, 1981) describes a balance or "homeostasis" in individuals as a "reasonably consistent balance between affective and cognitive experience" (Caplan, 1961), which, if disrupted, leads inevitably to distortions in affect and cognitive effectiveness. Traumatic stress leads to the deployment of conscious and unconscious coping strategies and behaviors, whose failure is followed by maladaptive behavioral manifestations. The point of crisis intervention therapy is to deal with the situation as soon as possible. As PTSD becomes more entrenched and chronic, the prognosis becomes more guarded, and the therapeutic strategies become more difficult and rigorous. Various aspects of crisis intervention, particularly "psychological debriefing," are discussed in detail in Chapter 20, this volume.

BRIEF INTERVENTIONS

The current literature focuses on the importance of brevity in the treatment of acute traumatic reactions. Symonds (1980) has summarized the essential ingredients of brief intervention:

1. Beginning to restore a sense of power (control) to the survivors by asking permission to interview them. For example, (a) "Is this a good time to talk to you?" (b) "Do you mind if I ask you some questions?"
2. Reducing isolation through nurturing behavior, which diminishes the experience of the hostile environment to which the survivors were subjected.
3. Diminishing feelings of helplessness and hopelessness of the survivors by helping them to build a plan for coping for the present and future.
4. In the case of hostage situations, using various strategies to reduce the survivors' feelings of having been subjected to the dominant behavior of their captors (e.g., the therapist identifies himself or herself to the survivors' satisfaction, asks for permission even to sit down in the survivors' presence, allows the survivors to smoke if they wish, etc.).

These interventions are designed specifically to restore the survivors' sense of personal importance, integrity, and dignity, and to assist them in the process of regaining control. The goal of brief interventions in the treatment of acute traumatic stress reactions should not be directed at complete resolution. The traumatized individuals are seeking help, not therapy in the established sense of the word, and they need a sense of freedom, guidance, and responsibility to be able to undertake the work successfully.

Although Figley (1988) and Horowitz (1976) describe the aim of working with traumatically stressed patients as helping them return to their level of functioning prior to the traumatizing experience, therapists should also not ignore the very real potential for personal "growth" afforded by the disruption to the patients' preexisting schematic model of the world and the need to build a new one. The emphasis should be on construction rather than restoration. Meichenbaum and Cameron (1983) have described the process of development of more flexible affective, cognitive, and behavioral responses—ones that are adaptive for the current traumatic adjustment and, ideally, also for the future. However, the possibility that the adjustment reaction to the impact of the trauma will become maladaptive cannot be ignored, and longer-term therapy may be required.

THE USE OF MEDICATIONS

Drugs may be used in the treatment of acute PTSD. These have been used with the following purposes in mind: (1) sedation if there is extreme agitation or disorganization; or (2) uncovering, confrontation, and abreaction of the dissociated traumatic fragments. Historically, intravenous barbiturates or benzodiazepines have been used for the purposes of abreaction (Sargent & Slater, 1940, 1972). However, symptoms of startle reaction and hypervigilance were noted to persist even following successful abreaction (Sargent & Slater, 1940). These techniques are now regarded as being of historical interest only.

The traditional reason for the use of drugs in acute PTSD has been to reduce or ablate the symptoms of acute, severe stress/anxiety reactions. Most drug treatment interventions in both acute and chronic PTSD attempt to relieve symptoms rather than to effect a cure (Schwartz, 1990). Psychopharmacological treatment often occurs in conjunction with and as an adjunct to psychotherapeutic approaches (Solomon, Gerrity, & Muff, 1992; Peterson, Prout, & Schwartz, 1991). As the understanding of the underlying psychopathology has improved, other medications have been employed in acute states. The current rationale for drug treatment appears twofold: first, to reduce troublesome symptoms and thus to facilitate response to psychotherapeutic intervention and new adaptive coping (Peterson et al., 1991); and second, to influence the biological systems that are thought to be involved in the disorder (van der Kolk, 1988).

The results of controlled drug trials in the literature suggest that tricyclic antidepressants and monoamine oxidase inhibitors may have clinically useful roles to play (Davidson, 1992). There is also increasing research evidence that other classes of drugs, such as the selective serotonin reuptake inhibitors (SSRIs), beta-adrenergic blockers, alpha$_2$-adrenergic agonists, and benzodiazepines, may be of benefit; however, the relative advantage of each class remains to be more fully elucidated (Davidson, 1992; Davidson, Roth, & Newman, 1991; Schwartz, 1990; McFarlane, 1989; Friedman, 1988; van der Kolk, 1987; Lipper, Davidson, & Grady, 1986). The SSRI group (including fluoxetine, peroxetine, sertraline) has found increasing favor in recent years (van der Kolk et al., 1995). The value of these drugs in the acute stage of the disorder remains to be demonstrated in systematic studies. One clinical report (Famularo, Kinscherff, & Fenton, 1988) described positive results after propranolol was administered to children with acute PTSD; the drug reduced symptoms of hyperarousal and hypervigilance.

SPECIFIC NOVEL TECHNIQUES

Apart from the general techniques employed in reduction of anxiety levels—medications (as discussed above and in Chapter 23, this volume) and cognitive and behavioral techniques (see Chapter 22, this volume)—two specific techniques are described here. These have been found to be useful during the phase of assimilation and integration of the memory material that has been brought to the surface as a result of the debriefing process. The techniques are known as the "lines" and "ladders" exercises (Busuttil et al., 1995). To date, their efficacy has not been systematically examined.

The "lines" exercise involves the plotting of a chronological map of survivors' lives. Significant high and low points are noted, with positive and negative events plotted on the vertical axis (including a neutral midway point representing zero). On the horizontal axis, age in years is represented. Survivors are asked to include the whole of their lifetime experiences, in addition to the period of time when they were exposed to the traumatic experience; this brings into perspective positive and negative coping mechanisms used both in the past and during the trauma itself. The "lines" exercise may be used in either an individual or a group setting, but the latter has several advantages. Within a group, the level of intimacy may be enhanced when the map of each participant's life becomes a subject for group discussion. The participants often develop a sense of cooperation and focus on the task, which enhances their sense of purpose and control in the rehabilitation process. Insight is gained not only into personal coping styles, but also into those of the others involved in the exercise. Peer criticism and review help the process along.

Two main benefits are thought to be derived from the "lines" exercise. First, the current stressor is put into the perspective of the whole of a survivor's life experience and is compared with other high and low points. This may promote a new sense of perspective, and permits the survivor to view the traumatic experience and his or her reaction to it with a sense of continuity; the task of recovery thus becomes less formidable. Second, adaptive and maladaptive coping styles can be more readily identified from the previous life challenges, and positive choices can more readily be made for the reentry process. The first of these advantages brings the past and the current experiences together, and the second provides a more solid platform from which initial (often hesitant) steps may be made away from the impact of the traumatic experience and into the future.

The second exercise involves assimilating the lessons learned from a close, focused examination of personal past life challenges (the "lines" exercise) and moving on into the future. This is a stepwise strategy known as the "ladders" exercise. The aim is to encourage survivors to make plans for the future by identifying short- and long-term goals; in a group setting, these are then presented to the survivor group for discussion and reality testing. Plans must be realistic and feasible, and in keeping with each survivor's coping styles as identified in the "lines" exercise. In addition, emphasis is placed on utilizing positive coping strategies and on diminishing the use of maladaptive strategies. Each member of the survivor group is instructed to draw a ladder with several rungs on a large sheet of paper or on a board. Survivors are asked to place a long-term goal on the top rung, and the lowest point in their lives on the bottom rung. (This lowest point is often, but not always, occupied by the experiences surrounding the current trauma.) The intervening rungs are then filled in as steps that should be taken in order for the ultimate goal to be achieved. The "ladders" exercise has intrinsic multidimensional significance, and possible dimensions include personal, marital, family, social, occupational, and financial issues. Each member of the survivor group presents a structured plan to the other members, and peer review takes place. This strategy has been found to be a valuable instrument in the restoration of control and dignity, and to enhance survivors' powers of positive self-criticism, self-awareness, and self-esteem.

CONCLUSIONS

Burgess-Watson, Hoffman, and Wilson (1988) have observed that PTSD may indeed provide the best example—for the process of study—of a disorder that can only be properly understood by a bio/psycho/social approach. We hope that this brief review of acute treatment methods employed in PTSD has demonstrated that effective treatment also requires a multidimensional approach. The future probably promises the development of support mobilized at different levels in the acute management of posttraumatic stress reactions. These levels may include the following (Weisaeth, 1992):

1. Survivors themselves (who must be provided with advice about intra-psychic, interpersonal, and activity-related coping techniques).
2. Survivors' social networks (family, friends, workmates, and neighbors).
3. Helpers outside the health care and social services (community leaders, clergy, police, rescuers, firefighters, volunteer organizations, etc.).
4. Providers of general and specialized physical health care services.
5. Mental health professionals.
6. Specialist psychiatric teams.

If acute treatments of traumatic stress reactions are demonstrated to resolve immediate issues and prevent secondary, long-term morbidity, then it will become necessary for considerable resources to be made available for them. Acute treatments, therefore, must be properly evaluated before they are provided as routine services. Psychological debriefing represents a special case, which needs to be undertaken by professionals especially trained in this technique (see Chapter 20, this volume). In-depth evaluation should indicate whether the acute interventions described should be routinely offered to all survivors of traumatic events, restricted to those at high risk of development of secondary morbidity, or abandoned altogether. This last possibility appears to be unlikely in the light of current research findings (Hiley-Young & Gerrity, 1994; Raphael, McFarlane, & Meldrum, 1994). Meticulous research, longitudinal studies of exposed populations, and standardized methodologies (at the national and international levels) are essential if these questions are to be answered. Because of the promising research data already available from uncontrolled studies, prospective controlled studies of intervention and nonintervention groups are sorely needed, but these require difficult decisions about the ethics of withholding treatment to be made.

REFERENCES

Brom, D., Kleber, R. J., & Hofman, M. C. (1993). Victims of traffic accidents: Incidence and prevention of post-traumatic stress disorder. *Journal of Clinical Psychology*, *49*(2), 131–140.
Burgess, A. W., & Baldwin, B. A. (1981). *Crisis intervention theory and practice: A clinical handbook*. Englewood Cliff, NJ: Prentice-Hall.
Burgess-Watson, I. P., Hofmann, L., & Wilson, G. V. (1988). The neuropsychiatry of post-traumatic stress disorder. *British Journal of Psychiatry*, *152*, 164–173.
Busuttil, W., Turnbull, G. J., Neal, L. A., Rollins, J., West, A. G., Blanch, N., & Herepath, R. (1995). Incorporating psychological debriefing techniques within a brief group psychotherapy programme for the treatment of post-traumatic stress disorder. *British Journal of Psychiatry*, *167*, 495–502.
Caplan, G. (1961). *An approach to community mental health*. London: Tavistock.

Davidson, J. R. T. (1992). Drug therapy of post-traumatic stress disorder. *British Journal of Psychiatry, 160,* 309–314.

Davidson, J. R. T., Roth, S., & Newman, E. (1991). Treatment of post-traumatic stress disorder with fluoxetine. *Journal of Traumatic Stress, 4,* 419–423.

Famularo, R., Kinscherff, R., & Fenton, T. (1988). Propranolol treatment for childhood post-traumatic stress disorder, acute type. *American Journal of Diseases of Children, 142,* 1244–1247.

Figley, C. R. (1988). Post-traumatic family therapy. In F. Ochberg (Ed.), *Post-traumatic therapy and victims of violence.* New York: Brunner/Mazel.

Friedman, M. J. (1988). Towards rational pharmacotherapy for post-traumatic stress disorder: An interim report. *American Journal of Psychiatry, 145,* 281–285.

Greenstone, J. L., & Leviton, S. C. (1981). Crisis management. In R. J. Corsini (Ed.), *Handbook of innovative psychotherapies* (pp. 216–228). New York: Wiley.

Hiley-Young, B., & Gerrity, E. T. (1994). Critical incident stress debriefing (CISD): Value and limitations in disaster response. *National Center for PTSD Clinical Quarterly, 4,* 17–19.

Horowitz, M. J. (1976). *Stress response syndromes.* New York: Jason Aronson.

Lindemann, E. (1944). Symptomatology and management of acute grief. *American Journal of Psychiatry, 101,* 141–148.

Lipper, S., Davidson, J. R. T., & Grady, T. A. (1986). Preliminary study of carbamazepine in post-traumatic stress disorder. *Psychosomatics, 27,* 849–854.

McFarlane, A. C. (1989). The treatment of post-traumatic stress disorder. *British Journal of Psychiatry, 62,* 81–90.

Meichenbaum, D., & Cameron, R. (1983). Stress inoculation training: Toward a general paradigm for training in coping skills. In D. Meichenbaum & M. Jaremko (Eds.), *Stress reduction and prevention.* New York: Plenum Press.

Peterson, K. C., Prout, M. F., & Schwartz, R. A. (1991). *Post-traumatic stress disorder: A clinician's guide.* New York: Plenum Press.

Raphael, B., McFarlane, A. C., & Meldrum, L. (1994). *Acute interventions after traumatic events.* Unpublished manuscript, Department of Psychiatry, Royal Brisbane Hospital, University of Queensland, Australia.

Roca, R. P., Spence, R. J., & Munster, A. M. (1992). Posttraumatic adaptation and distress among adult burn survivors. *American Journal of Psychiatry, 149*(9), 1234–1238.

Sargant, W. W., & Slater, E. (1940). Acute war neuroses. *Lancet, 140,* 1–2.

Sargant, W. W., & Slater, E. (1972). The use of drugs in psychotherapy. In W. W. Sargant & E. Slater (Eds.), *An introduction to physical methods of treatment in psychiatry* (pp. 142–162). New York: Science House.

Schwartz, L. S. (1990). A biopsychosocial treatment approach for post-traumatic stress disorder. *Journal of Traumatic Stress, 3,* 221–238.

Solomon, S. D., Gerrity, E. T., & Muff, A. M. (1992). Efficacy of treatments for post-traumatic stress disorder. *Journal of the American Medical Association, 265,* 633–637.

Symonds, M. (1980). Victim responses to terror. *Annals of the New York Academy of Sciences, 347,* 129–136.

van der Kolk, B. A. (Ed.). (1987). *Psychological trauma.* Washington, DC: American Psychiatric Press.

van der Kolk, B. A. (1988). The trauma spectrum: The interaction of biological and social events in genesis of the trauma response. *Journal of Traumatic Stress, 1*(3), 273–290.

van der Kolk, B. A., Dreyfuss, D., Michaels, M., Shera, D., Berkowitz, R., Fisler, R., & Saxe, G. (1994). Fluoxetine in posttraumatic stress disorder. *Journal of Clinical Psychiatry, 55*(12), 517–522.

Weisaeth, L. (1992). Prepare and repair: Some principles in prevention of psychiatric consequences of traumatic stress. *Psychiatria Fennica, 23*(Suppl.), 11–18.

Cognitive-Behavioral Therapy for Posttraumatic Stress Disorder

BARBARA OLASOV ROTHBAUM
EDNA B. FOA

If one considers the sheer masses of individuals exposed to assault, natural disasters, accidents, war, and other major stressors, traumatic experiences are extremely common. The disturbance most frequently observed following such experiences is posttraumatic stress disorder (PTSD). This disorder has been estimated to affect 9% of the U.S. population (Breslau, Davis, Andreski, & Peterson, 1991), and if one adds subthreshold cases, then the combined prevalence increases to approximately 14–15% (Davidson, Hughes, Blazer, & George, 1991). Epidemiological studies thus suggest that PTSD has become a serious problem in the Western world.

The increasing attention now given by the professional community to PTSD reflects the magnitude of this disorder as a worldwide problem, and serves as a constant reminder that one of the top priorities is to develop treatments that are effective, efficient, and enduring. Given the scope of PTSD, its chronicity, and its often severe disruption of daily functioning, it is of utmost importance to have effective and efficient therapies. This constitutes one of the biggest challenges for health care providers.

Over the past decade, psychosocial treatments for PTSD, including group psychotherapy, individual psychodynamic therapy, and cognitive-behavioral therapy, have been discussed in numerous papers (for a comprehensive review, see Solomon, Gerrity, & Muff, 1992). Within psychosocial treatments, cognitive-behavioral therapy in its various forms has been the most studied treatment modality, and several well-controlled investigations have been conducted to ascertain its efficacy. However, the information about these programs has not been widely disseminated among the mental health professionals who are the front-line helpers for trauma victims. In this chapter, we summarize only cognitive-behavioral interventions examined in well-controlled studies or in case reports that included at least semistructured assessments for evaluating treatment outcome. We begin with a brief review of the theory underlying the cognitive-behavioral treatment of PTSD.

THEORETICAL CONSIDERATIONS

It has been proposed that PTSD occurs because of a person's inability to process a traumatic experience adequately (Foa, Steketee, & Rothbaum, 1989b). If PTSD symptoms are the result of inadequate emotional processing, then therapy, aiming at the reduction of these symptoms, can be perceived as facilitating such processing. In an attempt to explain why exposure therapy is effective in reducing pathological anxiety, Foa and Kozak (1986) adopted Lang's (1977) theory of fear as a cognitive structure containing representations of feared stimuli, fear responses, and the meaning associated with these stimuli and responses. They suggested that the fear structures of anxiety-disordered individuals include pathological elements, and that treatment should be construed as modifying these elements.

According to this theory, two conditions are required for the reduction of fear. First, the fear memory must be activated. Second, new information must be provided—information including elements that are incompatible with existing pathological elements in the structure, so that a new memory can be formed. Exposure procedures activate the structure (i.e., elicit fear) and constitute an opportunity for corrective information to be integrated, and thus to modify the fear structure. The result of such modification should be the reduction of symptomatology. Repeated exposure to the memory of the trauma is expected to result in habituation, so that a survivor can remember it without intense fear responses. Via exposure, situations that had aroused intense fear cease to do so. When the fear elements in the structure are attenuated, many stimuli that were associated with fear through generalization no longer elicit fear. Foa and Kozak (1986) suggested that habituation within and across exposure sessions, and changes in threat appraisals, are indicators that changes in the fear structure have taken place. Several studies lend support to these hypotheses (for details, see Foa & Kozak, 1986; Kozak, Foa, & Steketee, 1988). Of particular relevance to PTSD are two studies demonstrating that fear activation during treatment promotes successful outcome (Brom, Kleber, & Defares, 1989; Foa, Riggs, Massie, & Yarczower, 1993).

Expanding on the Foa et al. (1989b) work, Foa and Riggs (1993) suggested that the trauma memory of a PTSD sufferer is distinguished by representations of the world as indiscriminately dangerous and of the self as an inadequate coper. The observation that victims with PTSD engage in this dichotomous type of thinking was also discussed by Alford, Mahone, and Fielstein (1988). Foa and Riggs further suggested that the fear structures of traumatic memories are more disorganized than other memories and that a disorganized memory is more difficult to modify. If true, then treatment should be directed toward both organizing the memory and correcting the maladaptive beliefs.

On the basis of their work with rape victims, Foa and Riggs (1993) suggested that prolonged exposure (PE), because it brings about a decrease in the anxiety associated with a traumatic memory, permits a reevaluation of the meaning representations in the memory. The repeated reliving in PE, they proposed, generates a more organized memory record that can be more readily integrated with existing schemata. Support for this contention comes from a study analyzing victims' narratives of trauma during exposure (DiSavino et al., 1993). Expressions of disorganization (e.g., unfinished thoughts and repetitions) decreased from the first to the last descriptions of the trauma, and this decrease was correlated with improvement. Treatment by reliving of the trauma does not directly address the victim's schemata about the world and the self. However, once the trauma memory is emotionally processed, the victim is able to view the trauma as a distinct event rather than a representation of the world as a whole, and thus to discriminate between danger and safety. Moreover, the successful processing of the traumatic memories leads to a reduction in PTSD symptoms, especially intrusion and avoidance. This symptom reduction helps change the victim's self-perception as an adequate, rather than inadequate, coper. Indirectly, exposure treatments may also foster positive social interactions: If the victim no longer perceives the world as indiscriminately dangerous and the self as an inadequate coper, then he or she will more readily seek social support.

Stress inoculation training (SIT) techniques seem to have a more direct impact on the self-schemata of the victim, but do not directly address the organization of the trauma memory. Teaching the victim techniques for coping with stress and anxiety, such as relaxation and cognitive restructuring, fosters a self-image of a successful coper. SIT may indirectly affect the victim's perception of the world in two ways. First, the increased perception of control may allow the victim to tolerate the trauma memories for longer periods of time, which may serve as self-directed PE. Second, the perception of oneself as able to cope with stress reduces the negative valence of potential future threats: A victim who perceives himself or herself as an "adequate coper" will expect to be better able to avert potential dangers. Again, these schematic changes are likely to facilitate positive social interactions, which in turn will strengthen the functional schemata.

In summary, Foa and Riggs (1993) suggested that repeated reliving of the trauma directly addresses the organization of the trauma memory and the resulting change in the world schema. SIT has a direct impact on the self-schema. It is therefore not surprising that a combination of the two treatments should prove more effective than either procedure alone in reducing PTSD symptoms, by altering the victim's schemata of the self and the world. Indeed, the effectiveness of treatments such as counseling that focus on problem solving (Foa, Rothbaum, Riggs, & Murdock, 1991; Resick, Jordan, Girelli, Hutter, & Marhoefer-Dvorak, 1988) may be attributable to changes they produce in the victim's self-schema.

The identification of the specific impairments underlying panic disorder has led to very powerful treatments (Margraf, Barlow, Clark, & Telch, 1993). We hope that the elucidation of the specific cognitive impairments underlying PTSD will result in the development of programs that directly address these impairments, and that thus should be more effective and efficient in reducing PTSD and related psychopathology.

DEFINITION OF TREATMENT MODALITIES

Cognitive-behavioral treatment for anxiety disorders can be divided into two categories: exposure therapy and anxiety management training (AMT). Exposure therapy is a set of techniques whose common denominator is helping the client confront feared situations. AMT involves teaching the client how to control intense anxiety by using specific skills. Exposure therapy is the most effective intervention with phobic fears; AMT is the treatment of choice for chronic anxiety, such as is evident in generalized anxiety disorder. Both specific fears and general chronic arousal are among the defining characteristics of PTSD, and therefore both treatment categories are applicable to this disorder.

Exposure therapy techniques are designed to activate the trauma memories in order to modify pathological associations in these memories to generate new, nonpathological associations. AMT is designed to manage anxiety when it occurs; in this case, the emphasis is not on fear activation as much as on furnishing the client with tools to manage it. First, we consider the literature on the success of exposure therapy, followed by a summary of the literature on the efficacy of AMT. Studies employing both exposure and AMT are examined next, and we conclude with some clinical considerations.

EXPOSURE THERAPY

The efficacy of exposure treatment for PTSD was first demonstrated with several case reports on war veterans (Fairbank, Gross, & Keane, 1983; Fairbank & Keane, 1982; Johnson, Gilmore, & Shenoy, 1982; Keane & Kaloupek, 1982; Schindler, 1980). Both flooding in imagination (e.g., Fairbank & Keane, 1982;

Keane, Fairbank, Caddell, & Zimering, 1989) and flooding *in vivo* to trauma-related events (Johnson et al., 1982) appeared to be therapeutic. Most of these treatments, however, included additional techniques, such as anger control or relaxation training; thus, the contribution of exposure to the overall improvement is unclear.

The successful outcome of systematic desensitization (SD), in which clients are exposed to fearful imagery in a state of relaxation, has been reported in two studies with war veterans (Peniston, 1986; Bowen & Lambert, 1986). The treatment was effective compared to a no-treatment control condition, but required a large number of sessions over an extended period of time. The magnitude of the effects of this treatment on the PTSD symptom patterns and on general functioning cannot be ascertained, however, because the severity of PTSD and related pathology was not assessed. *systematic desen.*

Several uncontrolled studies demonstrated that SD is also effective with rape victims in reducing fear, anxiety, depression, and social maladjustment (Frank & Stewart, 1983, 1984; Turner, 1979). In contrast to the work with war veterans, these treatments involved fewer sessions; again, though, it is impossible to judge how successful the treatment was in ameliorating PTSD symptoms, because these symptoms were not assessed. Moreover, in the absence of a control group, the positive effects of the treatment on anxiety and depression are difficult to interpret. Also, because many of the clients were recent victims, some of the observed improvement at the posttreatment assessment may have been attributable to the natural recovery of symptoms over the first several months following assault (see Kilpatrick & Calhoun, 1988). Support for this interpretation comes from a report on the failure of SD to decrease disturbance in women who suffered from chronic assault-related anxiety (Becker & Abel, 1981). *Muse 1986*

Direct evidence for the success of SD in reducing PTSD symptoms comes from two reports that included victims of various traumas. SD (13–18 sessions, with the last 2 sessions devoted to *in vivo* exposure) was used successfully with three automobile accident victims, according to the therapists' and clients' reports (Muse, 1986). A controlled study compared the efficacy of 15 sessions of SD, hypnotherapy, and brief psychodynamic therapy to a waiting-list condition (Brom et al., 1989). Most of the clients suffered from bereavement, often as a result of crime, accident, or sudden illness. All treatments were more effective in reducing symptoms of PTSD and general psychopathology than was the control condition.

In summary, several studies examined the effects of SD with a variety of trauma victims, and most showed some beneficial results. However, the lack of methodological rigor and the absence of PTSD diagnosis and measures in most of the studies limit the conclusions that can be drawn from them.

With the realization that relaxation during confrontation with feared material is not necessary (Foa, Rothbaum, & Kozak, 1989a), and with evidence for the inferiority of SD to flooding in complex anxiety disorders such as ago-raphobia (Marks, Boulougouris, & Marset, 1971), the use of SD for PTSD was abandoned. In its place, researchers have employed a variety of imaginal and *in vivo* exposure procedures involving confrontation with moderate to high levels of anxiety. With PTSD, exposure involves repeated reliving of the trauma in imagination; as noted earlier, the aim is to promote the processing of the traumatic memory, which is thought to be impaired in victims with chronic PTSD (Foa et al., 1989b; Foa, Rothbaum, & Molnar, 1995b).

Five controlled studies have examined the utility of imaginal exposure for reducing PTSD and related pathology; three of these involved male Vietnam veterans, and two involved female assault victims. In the studies of veterans, treatment by imaginal exposure to trauma-related material was conducted over 6 to 16 sessions. In one study, all clients received the "standard" PTSD treat-ment (weekly individual and group therapies) in addition to exposure (Coo-per & Clum, 1989). In the second study, imaginal exposure was compared to a no-treatment waiting-list condition (Keane et al., 1989). During each session, clients were initially instructed to relax. The clients subsequently received 45 minutes of imaginal flooding, followed by relaxation. In the third study, all clients received a group treatment; one-half received additional imaginal ex-posure, and the remaining clients received weekly individual traditional psy-chotherapy (Boudewyns & Hyer, 1990; Boudewyns, Hyer, Woods, Harrison, & McCranie, 1990).

All three studies found that imaginal exposure yielded some benefit as compared to the control conditions, but the effect sizes were small. In the Cooper and Clum (1989) study, imaginal exposure improved the PTSD symp-toms, but had little effect on depression or trait anxiety. In the Keane et al. (1989) study, a mixed picture emerged: Therapists rated exposure clients as more improved on PTSD symptoms than control subjects, but no group differ-ences emerged on self-report measures of these symptoms. Exposure clients did rate themselves as more improved on general psychopathology measures than did those in the waiting-list control condition. The use of relaxation be-fore and after exposure is not customary, and it would be important to exam-ine the separate effects of exposure and relaxation training in order to ascer-tain the separate contribution of each modality.

Boudewyns and Hyer (1990) found no group differences on psychophysi-ological measures, but at the 3-month follow-up, the exposure group showed more improvement on the Veterans Adjustment Scale. Interestingly, regard-less of treatment, a positive relationship was found between psychophysiologi-cal reduction to combat-related stimuli following treatment and improvement on the Veterans Adjustment Scale. In a further analysis of the data with some additional clients, a slight superiority emerged for the exposure group. A higher percentage of the clients treated with exposure than of those receiving tradi-tional therapy were classified as "successes" (Boudewyns et al., 1990).

Prolonged exposure

In two studies, PE treatment for PTSD in female assault victims was compared to other treatment modalities and to waiting-list controls. To control for the natural decline in symptoms that occurs following an assault (Rothbaum, Foa, Riggs, Murdock, & Walsh, 1992), postassault time for all victims was at least 3 months (mean time since assault was 6.7 years in one study and 4.2 years in the other). Treatment efficacy was evaluated by independent assessors who were unaware of the treatment assignment. Assessment included a measure of PTSD severity as defined by the American Psychiatric Association (1980), as well as other standard measures of trauma-related pathology. PE treatment consisted of nine biweekly individual sessions. The first two sessions were devoted to information gathering, presentation of treatment rationale, and treatment planning, including the construction of a hierarchy of feared situations for *in vivo* exposure. During the remaining seven sessions, victims were instructed to relive in imagery their traumatic experiences and to describe the trauma aloud "as if it were happening now." Exposure continued for about 60 minutes and was tape-recorded, so that victims could practice imaginal exposure as homework by listening to the tape. Also for homework, victims were instructed to approach feared situations or objects that were realistically safe. More details on administering PE are presented in the "Clinical Considerations" section at the end of this chapter.

In the first study (Foa et al., 1991), PE was compared to SIT (which is described in the next section), to supportive counseling, and to a waiting-list control. All treatments were delivered in the same nine-session biweekly individual format. Supportive counseling focused on assisting clients to solve daily problems, which may or may not have been assault-related. Discussion of the assault itself was largely avoided, and when clients recounted their trauma they were redirected to "here-and-now" issues. Clients were taught problem solving, and therapists engaged in active listening and support. Victims in the waiting-list condition were assessed at the same 5-week intervals as the treated victims and were contacted by phone in between to maintain contact.

Immediately after treatment, victims who received PE treatment improved on all three clusters of PTSD symptoms. Victims in the supportive counseling and waiting-list conditions evidenced improvement on arousal symptoms, but not on avoidance and reexperiencing symptoms. At 3.5 months following treatment, PE appeared to be the superior treatment; however, the superiority of PE was evidenced only on measures of PTSD symptoms and not on other measures of psychopathology. At follow-up, 50% of the clients who received SIT and 55% of those receiving PE did not meet criteria for PTSD.

A second study (still in progress) is comparing PE, SIT, a combination of SIT and PE, and a waiting-list control condition. Preliminary analyses indicated that PE was more effective than the waiting-list control. At posttreatment, only 29% of victims who received PE retained their PTSD diagnosis, versus 100% of victims in the waiting-list control group. Moreover, 68% of victims in the PE group evidenced at least 50% improvement in PTSD symptoms, as opposed to 7% of the control victims. The superiority of PE over the waiting list was also evidenced on measures of depression (Foa et al., 1994).

A new technique, eye movement desensitization and reprocessing (EMDR; Shapiro, 1989) is a form of exposure (desensitization) with a strong cognitive component accompanied by saccadic eye movements. Briefly, the technique involves the client's imagining a scene from the trauma, focusing on the accompanying thoughts and physiological arousal, and tracking the therapist's rapidly moving finger. The sequence is repeated until the client no longer reports anxiety, at which point the client is instructed to adopt a more positive thought while imagining the trauma and continuing the eye movements. The efficacy of EMDR is equivocal. Proponents of this treatment have interpreted the reported anxiety reduction within a treatment session as indicative of its success (e.g., Lipke & Botkin, 1993; Shapiro, 1989). However, they did not include standardized outcome measures such as PTSD symptom ratings or depression inventories, so that the efficacy of EMDR cannot be ascertained.

Two controlled studies have compared EMDR to an exposure control (eyes-fixed) treatment (Boudewyns, Stwertka, Hyer, Albrecht, & Sperr, 1993; Pitman et al., 1993) and inpatient milieu treatment (Boudewyns et al., 1993). It appears that in both studies, within-session reported anxiety decreased more in the EMDR group than in the exposure control group. However, neither study detected differences between the groups on outcome as assessed by standardized self-report measures or psychophysiological reactivity to taped accounts of the trauma (Boudewyns et al., 1993). When one considers these two studies on the usefulness of EMDR, it is also important to remember that both utilized Vietnam veterans—a population that may be resistant to treatment in general.

In summary, exposure techniques have received strong support for their ability to alleviate posttraumatic suffering. It appears, however, that the effects of this treatment on PTSD symptoms in the studies of female assault victims are more impressive than those found in the studies of Vietnam veterans. As noted above, the latter are resistant to psychosocial as well as pharmacological treatments (Foa, Davidson, & Rothbaum, 1995a). Perhaps the higher comorbidity in veterans accounts in part for their inferior response to treatment in comparison to the assault victims. In addition, many of the traumatic memories in Vietnam veterans are associated with guilt concerning atrocities they perpetrated or witnessed, whereas the traumatic memories of assault survivors involve anxiety associated with having been the victims of violence. There is ample evidence to suggest that anxiety habituates with repeated exposure, but no studies have explored whether repeated exposure to guilt-evoking experiences reduces guilt. Clinical wisdom suggests that repeatedly exposing clients to guilt and depressive thoughts may actually exacerbate rather than ameliorate the discomfort associated with these thoughts. This may account for the fact that some researchers have found adverse effects of exposure (Pitman et al., 1991). Given the prominent role of guilt in PTSD sufferers, it is imperative to develop and evaluate techniques for guilt reduction. In the meantime, we would advocate the use of exposure techniques for anxiety-provoking stimuli and possibly cognitive techniques for guilt issues.

biofeedback
relaxation
ANXIETY MANAGEMENT TRAINING *cog restruct*

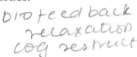

AMT typically includes a variety of procedures, including biofeedback, relaxation, and cognitive restructuring, among others. Therefore, it is impossible to ascertain the contribution of any specific procedure to overall outcome. Several treatment programs are discussed below.

Frank and her colleagues have studied the effects of cognitive therapy targeted at depression and anxiety following rape (Frank et al., 1988; Frank & Stewart, 1984; Turner & Frank, 1981). Some of the clients in these studies entered treatment soon after the rape (mean of 20 days), whereas others were seen several months after the assault (mean of 129 days). No diagnostic criteria were incorporated into the studies. The therapy produced positive changes on ratings of fear, anxiety, depression, and social adjustment. When compared with SD, cognitive therapy produced equivalent outcomes. The absence of a control group and the lack of a PTSD diagnosis limit the conclusions that can be drawn from this study. Interestingly, the time elapsed since rape did not influence the treatment outcome. The improvement evidenced by delayed treatment seekers, who were initially more symptomatic than the immediate treatment seekers suggests that both cognitive therapy and SD had active therapeutic ingredients. *Stress inoculation training*

Of the various AMT programs, SIT (Kilpatrick, Veronen, & Resick, 1982), developed for victims with chronic disturbances, has received the most attention. The original SIT program included 20 therapy hours and homework assignments. Treatment began with a 2-hour educational phase in which the treatment program rationale and theoretical basis for the treatment were explained. The second phase of SIT focused on the acquisition and application of coping skills. This included training in deep muscle relaxation, breathing control, role playing, covert modeling, thought stopping, and guided self-dialogue following Meichenbaum's (1974) stress inoculation training.

In investigating the efficacy of this program, Veronen and Kilpatrick (1982) selected female rape victims who showed elevated fear and avoidance to specific phobic stimuli 3 months after the rape. A clear treatment effect emerged on rape-related fear, anxiety, phobic anxiety, tension, and depression. No control group was included, and therefore the interpretation of the data is limited. In a subsequent study, Veronen and Kilpatrick (1983) incorporated 10 sessions each of SIT, peer counseling, and SD. Victims were permitted to select their treatment, and more than one-half of the potential subject pool rejected therapy. Of those who opted for treatment, the majority selected SIT, few chose peer counseling, and none selected SD. Although no formal statistical analyses were conducted on the clients who completed SIT, the authors reported noticeable pre- to posttreatment improvement on most measures.

In a controlled investigation, also with rape victims (Resick et al., 1988), six 2-hour group sessions of SIT were compared to the same format of assertion training and supportive psychotherapy. The three treatments were compared to a naturally occurring waiting-list control group. Cognitive restructuring, assertiveness training, and role play were excluded from the program described by Kilpatrick et al. (1982), since they were used in the comparative treatment, and exposure *in vivo* was added to the application phase. All three treatments were equally effective in reducing symptoms. Improvement was maintained at 6-month follow-up on rape-related fear measures, but not on depression, self-esteem, and social fears. No improvements were found in the waiting-list control group.

Two studies, described earlier, examined the efficacy of SIT with female victims of rape and nonsexual assault who met criteria for PTSD. In the first study, this treatment was compared to PE, supportive counseling, and a waiting-list control (Foa et al., 1991). The design of the study and the results for PE and counseling have been described earlier. In the second study, SIT was compared to PE, the combination of SIT and PE, and a waiting-list control (Foa, 1993).

The SIT program in both of these studies was adapted from Kilpatrick et al.'s (1982) program described above. In the first session, data regarding the assault and the victim's history were gathered, followed by brief breathing retraining to alleviate anxiety aroused by the discussion of the assault. The rationale for treatment was explained in session 2, and coping skills were taught in sessions 3–9. Coping skills included deep muscle relaxation and differential relaxation, thought stopping, cognitive restructuring, preparing for a stressor, covert modeling, and role play. Each skill was applied first to a non-assault-related example and then to an assault-related example. The sessions began with a review of the previous session's activity and an update on the utilization of coping skills in the client's natural environment and review of the client's homework assignments. Practice of skills taught in that and previous sessions was assigned for homework.

In the first study, SIT produced significantly more improvement on PTSD symptoms than did the waiting-list control immediately following treatment. At follow-up, PE produced superior outcome on PTSD symptoms but not on other measures. Clients who received PE continued to improve after treatment termination, whereas clients in the SIT and supportive counseling conditions evidenced no change between posttreatment and follow-up (Foa et al., 1991).

In the continuation study, preliminary analyses indicated that in clients who received SIT, 60% no longer had PTSD when assessed immediately after treatment (Foa et al., 1994). The results of the combined treatment are described in the next section.

In summary, with the exception of the Foa (1993) study that included female nonsexual assault victims, the AMT studies reviewed above all employed female rape victims and indicated that these techniques produced positive changes on measures of fear and depression. With the exception of the Foa et al. (1991) and Foa et al. (1994) studies, none incorporated either the presence of PTSD diagnosis as an inclusion criterion or measures of PTSD severity. This was partly because postrape sequelae were not conceived of as PTSD until the introduction of the disorder into the nosological system (American Psychiatric Association, 1980). However, with the exception of the Frank et al. studies, clients were all assaulted at least 3 months before entering treatment, indicating that they had suffered chronic disturbances and thus were likely to have had PTSD.

EXPOSURE THERAPY AND AMT

The successes of PE for PTSD and SIT for chronically fearful rape victims led to the supposition that a program including confrontations with feared stimuli in combination with anxiety management skills would enhance the treatment benefit. This idea has led to the development of such combined treatments. It was thought that these treatments would offer sufferers ways to manage the extreme stress and anxiety while learning to confront the feared memories and cues. Two such programs have been studied with female assault victims who manifested chronic PTSD.

One program consisted of the combination of SIT and PE (SIT/PE). This program was compared to PE alone, SIT alone, and a waiting-list control. Details of the individual SIT and PE programs have been described in the previous sections. In SIT/PE, information was gathered in session 1, followed by breathing retraining; treatment was explained in session 2. Deep muscle relaxation was taught in session 3, and imaginal exposure was conducted in session 4. In sessions 5–9, both SIT skills and exposure were presented within the same session. Preliminary analysis indicated that all three treatments were equally effective in reducing PTSD symptoms, but PE tended to be more effective in reducing related psychopathology (Foa et al., 1994).

The second program for rape victims with PTSD was tested in a quasi-experimental design (Resick & Schnicke, 1992). Female sexual assault survivors received cognitive processing therapy over 12 weekly sessions in a group format. This therapy included education, exposure, and cognitive restructuring, and was based on an information-processing theory of PTSD. Exposure consisted of writing a detailed account of the assault and reading it aloud in the treatment group. Cognitive restructuring was based on Beck, Rush, Shaw, and Emery's (1979) cognitive therapy for depression. It focused on areas of functioning thought to be disrupted by victimization, according to the theory of McCann, Sakheim, and Abrahamson (1988); these issues include safety, trust, power, esteem, and intimacy.

Treated clients were compared to a naturally occurring waiting-list control group, but clients were not randomly assigned, and all control subjects did not receive all of the same measures as treated clients. In addition, therapists performed many of the assessments, although apparently therapists did not show bias in ratings. Cognitive processing clients improved significantly from pre- to posttreatment on PTSD and depression ratings, and maintained their improvement throughout the 6-month follow-up period. In fact, at posttreatment none of the treated clients met PTSD criteria, although 12.5% did so at follow-up. The waiting-list subjects evidenced no change during a comparable 12-week period.

DISCUSSION OF THE RESEARCH

In this chapter thus far, we have attempted to provide a critical review of what is known about the success of cognitive-behavioral treatment for PTSD. The vast majority of the knowledge in this area comes from studies and case reports that included either Vietnam veterans or rape victims. Early applications of cognitive-behavioral therapy consisted of flooding, SD, and AMT. By the beginning of the 1980s, PE, in which clients experience moderate to high levels of anxiety, replaced SD as the most common treatment for anxiety disorders and was employed with PTSD veterans. There was hesitation, however, to submit rape victims to this treatment; it was because of this hesitation that treatment studies with rape victims utilized either AMT or SD. Theoretical consideration led to the hypothesis that rape victims with PTSD, like war veterans, should benefit from treatment that activates their rape-related anxiety and modifies it. Indeed, the two studies that employed PE with female assault victims confirmed this hypothesis.

The few well-controlled studies are consistent with case reports in indicating that both exposure therapy and AMT are effective in reducing PTSD symptoms, as well as related symptoms such as depression. There is preliminary evidence to indicate that the combination of PE and AMT may constitute the treatment of choice for chronic PTSD.

CLINICAL CONSIDERATIONS

As is apparent from the literature review, cognitive-behavioral techniques are quite effective in reducing PTSD severity, although some clients do not benefit from treatment and others remain somewhat symptomatic. Although both

PE and AMT are helpful, it should be noted that all of the studies cited were conducted by experts who recognize pitfalls and are apt in overcoming them. Some of these pitfalls and remedies are discussed below.

An important point regarding exposure is that PTSD sufferers are naturally reluctant to engage in reliving their trauma. After all, two cardinal features of this disorder are effortful avoidance and numbing—that is, tendencies to evade engagement with the traumatic memory. In our experience, clients who are randomly assigned to PE do not drop out of treatment more than those assigned to AMT, perhaps because we provide them with an elaborate rationale for why they should submit themselves to this temporary increase in suffering. A summary of this rationale is as follows:

> It is not easy to digest painful experiences. If you think about the trauma or are reminded of it, you may experience extreme fear and other negative feelings associated with it. It is unpleasant to feel this way, so most people tend to push away fearful, painful memories or ignore them. Other people may influence you not to talk or think about it. Unfortunately, ignoring a traumatic event does not make it go away. Often the experience comes back to haunt you through nightmares, flashbacks, phobias, and other ways because it is "unfinished business." What we are going to do in this treatment is the opposite of our tendency to avoid. We will help you to process the experience by having you remember what happened and stay with it long enough to get more used to it. The goal is to be able to have these thoughts, talk about the trauma, or see cues associated with it without experiencing the intense anxiety that is disrupting your life.

Often, therapists themselves are uncomfortable using a treatment method that elicits intense emotional pain. It is important for such therapists to be convinced that short-term suffering will lead to long-term benefit, and to relay this conviction to their clients. It is also imperative that the therapists be willing to hear the horrible stories that the clients will relay while recounting their traumatic experiences. Sometimes debriefing with other health care professionals is helpful for therapists to process this information.

Some clients are reluctant to emotionally engage in reliving their trauma even after they are convinced that it is necessary. This may be especially true if dissociation is a problem. Several sessions of AMT may assist in overcoming this reluctance. In this respect, a treatment that combines PE and AMT offers sufferers ways to manage the extreme stress and anxiety while learning to confront the feared memories and cues. It may also be necessary for a therapist to use exposure techniques creatively. Some examples include asking a client to recount the incident as if it were happening in slow motion, or to attend just to internal sensations and thoughts.

In conducting PE, a therapist should allow a client to approach the trauma memory gradually in his or her first attempt to relive it. It is important for the client to feel in control of the process of remembering the feelings associated with the trauma. During the first imaginal exposure, the client should be allowed to determine the level of detail with which he or she recounts the narrative of the incident. In subsequent imaginal exposures, the therapist should encourage the client to describe the event in more detail by probing for the emotional and physiological reactions that accompanied the trauma.

The therapist should not discontinue the session immediately after the imaginal exposure portion if the client is experiencing high anxiety. Treatment sessions should be planned so that there will be sufficient time at the end to evaluate the client's level of distress. It is very important to encourage the client to talk about his or her reactions to reliving the trauma and to discuss new details and associations that emerge. Breathing retraining after the imaginal exposure may be helpful to reduce distress, if necessary. The therapist may need to be available to talk to the client on the telephone between sessions, in the event that the imaginal or *in vivo* exposure exercises cause extreme distress. Clients should be informed that it is normal to feel initially as if they are getting worse; they may find themselves thinking about the trauma more and experiencing more symptoms. We give the following explanation to clients before imaginal exposure:

> I'm going to ask you to recall the memories of the trauma. It is best for you to close your eyes so you won't be distracted and so that you can envision these events in your mind's eye. I will ask you to recall these painful memories as vividly as possible. We call this "reliving." I don't want you to tell a story about the trauma in the past tense. What I would like you to do is describe the trauma in the present tense, as if it were happening now, right here. I'd like you to close your eyes and tell me what happened during the trauma in as much detail as you remember. We will work on this together. If you start to feel too uncomfortable and want to run away or avoid it by leaving the image, I will help you to stay with it. We will audiotape the narrative so you can take the tape home and listen to it for homework. From time to time while you are reliving the trauma, I will ask you for your anxiety level on a scale from 0 to 100, in which 0 indicates no anxiety or discomfort and 100 indicates panic-level anxiety. Please answer quickly and don't leave the image. Do you have any questions before we start?

We recommend using the entire 60 minutes for the imaginal exposure. If it takes 15 minutes for the client to recount the trauma, then the therapist should ask him or her to start from the beginning and go through it again, repeating it four times. If it takes 20 minutes, the client should repeat it three times, and so on. The following statements are helpful to encourage the client during the exposure: "You are doing fine; stay with the image." "You've done very well. It took some courage to stick it out, even though you were quite afraid." "I know this is difficult. You are doing a good job." "Stay with the image; you are safe here." "Let yourself feel safe and let go of the feelings." The following questions may facilitate confrontation with fear-evoking cues during imaginal exposure: "What are you feeling?" "What are you thinking?" "Are you experiencing any physical reactions? Describe them." "What is your body feeling?" "What are you seeing/smelling/doing now?" "Where do you feel that in your body?" After about 60 minutes of imaginal exposure, the therapist should terminate the exercise by asking the client to open his or her eyes and take several breaths. The therapist and client should then talk about the experience of reliving the trauma. Did the client remember things he or she had not previously recalled? Was it easier or more difficult than the client thought it would be? Was there something the therapist could have done to help?

The therapist needs to express confidence that he or she will be able to handle, and help the client handle, whatever comes up. Sometimes clients are frightened of what they may remember during imaginal exposure and need reassurance. It helps to remind them that whatever they remember, it does not change what happened, or the fact that they survived and therefore obviously did the right thing for survival. We have not yet encountered a client who remembered details during imaginal exposure that he or she could not cope with. One of our patients described each session of exposure therapy as "peeling a layer off of an onion, and after a few sessions, you get to the stinky part in the middle, and then it doesn't stink any more."

Most of the studies that examined the efficacy of cognitive-behavioral therapy included victims with posttrauma times of at least 3 months. This was done to insure that changes after treatment were attributable to the intervention rather than to natural recovery with the passage of time. In the clinical arena, treatment does not have to be delayed. It is natural for trauma victims to show severe disturbances in the first few weeks after trauma. Sometimes, merely normalizing these reactions has therapeutic benefit, and one or two therapy sessions may suffice. In a pilot study (Hearst, Foa, & Riggs, 1993), three to four sessions that included education regarding posttrauma reactions, relaxation, recounting the trauma, and cognitive restructuring were of great benefit in averting chronic PTSD and depression, compared to an assessment control.

Traumatic experiences are extremely prevalent throughout the world, and as mental health professionals we have the responsibility of providing services to those victimized. Because of the vast number of victims, it is incumbent upon us to deliver efficient and effective interventions that are readily available and easy to implement. As experts in cognitive-behavioral therapy, we have come a long way in achieving this goal. The task now is to disseminate the available knowledge while continuing to improve upon the existing techniques.

REFERENCES

Alford, J. D., Mahone, C., & Fielstein, E. M. (1988). Cognitive and behavioral sequelae of combat: Conceptualization and implication for treatment. *Journal of Traumatic Stress, 1,* 489–501.

American Psychiatric Association (1980). *Diagnostic and statistical manual of mental disorders* (3rd ed.). Washington, DC: Author.

Beck, A. T., Rush, A. J., Shaw, B. F., & Emery, G. (1979). *Cognitive therapy of depression.* New York: Guilford Press.

Becker, J. V., & Abel, G. G. (1981). Behavioral treatment of victims of sexual assault. In S. M. Turner, K. S. Calhoun, & H. E. Adams (Eds.), *Handbook of clinical behavior therapy* (pp. 347–379). New York: Wiley.

Boudewyns, P. A., & Hyer, L. (1990). Physiological response to combat memories and preliminary treatment outcome in Vietnam veteran PTSD patients treated with direct therapeutic exposure. *Behavior Therapy, 21,* 63–87.

Boudewyns, P. A., Hyer, L., Woods, M. G., Harrison, W. R., & McCranie, E. (1990). PTSD among Vietnam veterans: An early look at treatment outcome using direct therapeutic exposure. *Journal of Traumatic Stress, 3,* 359–368.

Boudewyns, P. A., Stwertka, S. A., Hyer, L. A., Albrecht, J. W., & Sperr, E. V. (1993). Eye movement desensitization for PTSD of combat: A treatment outcome pilot study. *The Behavior Therapist, 16,* 29–33.

Bowen, G. R., & Lambert, J. A. (1986). Systematic desensitization therapy with posttraumatic stress disorder cases. In C. R. Figley (Ed.), *Trauma and its wake* (Vol. 2, pp. 280–291). New York: Brunner/Mazel.

Breslau, N., Davis, G. C., Andreski, P., & Peterson, E. (1991). Traumatic events and posttraumatic stress disorder in an urban population of young adults. *Archives of General Psychiatry, 48,* 216–222.

Brom, D., Kleber, R. J., & Defares, P. B. (1989). Brief psychotherapy for post-traumatic stress disorder. *Journal of Consulting and Clinical Psychology, 57,* 607–612.

Cooper, N. A., & Clum, G. A. (1989). Imaginal flooding as a supplementary treatment for PTSD in combat veterans: A controlled study. *Behavior Therapy, 20,* 381–391.

Davidson, J. R. T., Hughes, D., Blazer, D. G., & George, L. K. (1991). Post-traumatic stress disorder in the community: An epidemiological study. *Psychological Medicine, 21,* 713–721.

DiSavino, P., Turk, E., Massie, E. D., Riggs, D. S., Penkower, D. S., Molnar, C., & Foa, E. B. (1993, November). *The content of traumatic memories: Evaluating treatment efficacy by analysis of verbatim descriptions of the rape scene.* Paper presented at the 27th Annual Meeting of the Association for Advancement of Behavior Therapy, Atlanta, GA.

Fairbank, J. A., Gross, R. T., & Keane, T. M. (1983). Treatment of posttraumatic stress disorder: Evaluation of outcome with a behavioral code. *Behavior Modification, 7,* 557–568.

Fairbank, J. A., & Keane, T. M. (1982). Flooding for combat-related stress disorders: Assessment of anxiety reduction across traumatic memories. *Behavior Therapy, 13,* 499–510.

Foa, E. B., Davidson, J., & Rothbaum, B. O. (1995a). Treatment of posttraumatic stress disorder. In G. O. Gabbard (Ed.), *Treatments of psychiatric disorders: The DSM-IV edition* (pp. 1499–1519). Washington, DC: American Psychiatric Press.

Foa, E. B., Freund, B. F., Hembree, E., Dancu, C. V., Franklin, M. E., Perry, K. J., Riggs, D. S., & Molnar, C. (1994, November). *Efficacy of short term behavioral treatments of PTSD in sexual and nonsexual assault victims.* Paper presented at the annual meeting of the Association for Advancement of Behavior Therapy, San Diego, CA.

Foa, E. B., & Kozak, M. J. (1986). Emotional processing of fear: Exposure to corrective information. *Psychological Bulletin, 99*, 20–35.

Foa, E. B., & Riggs, D. S. (1993). Post-traumatic stress disorder in rape victims. In J. Oldham, M. B. Riba, & A. Tasman (Eds.) *American psychiatric press review of psychiatry* (Vol. 12, pp. 273–303). Washington, DC: American Psychiatric Press.

Foa, E. B., Riggs, D. S., Massie, E. D., & Yarczower, M. (1993). *The impact of fear activation and anger on the efficacy of exposure treatment for PTSD.* Unpublished manuscript.

Foa, E. B., Rothbaum, B. O., & Kozak, M. J. (1989a). Behavioral treatments of anxiety and depression. In P. Kendall & D. Watson (Eds.), *Anxiety and depression: Distinctive and overlapping features.* New York: Academic Press.

Foa, E. B., Rothbaum, B. O., & Molnar, C. (1995b). Cognitive-behavioral treatment of post-traumatic stress disorder. In M. J. Friedman, D. S. Charney, & A. Y. Deutch (Eds.), *Neurobiological and clinical consequences of stress: From normal adaptation to post-traumatic stress disorder* (pp. 483–494). New York: Raven Press.

Foa, E. B., Rothbaum, B. O., Riggs, D. S., & Murdock, T. (1991). Treatment of post-traumatic stress disorder in rape victims: A comparison between cognitive-behavioral procedures and counseling. *Journal of Consulting and Clinical Psychology, 59*, 715–723.

Foa, E. B., Steketee, G., & Rothbaum, B. O. (1989b). Behavioral/cognitive conceptualizations of post-traumatic stress disorder. *Behavior Therapy, 20*, 155–176.

Frank, E., Anderson, B., Stewart, B. D., Dancu, C., Hughes, C., & West, D. (1988). Efficacy of cognitive behavior therapy and systematic desensitization in the treatment of rape trauma. *Behavior Therapy, 19*, 403–420.

Frank, E., & Stewart, B. D. (1983). Physical aggression: Treating the victims. In E. A. Blechman (Ed.), *Behavior modification with women* (pp. 245–272). New York: Guilford Press.

Frank, E., & Stewart, B. D. (1984). Depressive symptoms in rape victims. *Journal of Affective Disorders, 1*, 269–277.

Hearst, D. E., Foa, E. B., & Riggs, D. S. (1993, November). *Brief cognitive-behavioral program to prevent the development of chronic post-trauma reactions in assault survivors.* Paper presented at the 27th Annual Meeting of the Association for Advancement of Behavior Therapy, Atlanta, GA.

Johnson, C. H., Gilmore, J. D., & Shenoy, R. Z. (1982). Use of a feeding procedure in the treatment of a stress-related anxiety disorder. *Journal of Behavior Therapy and Experimental Psychiatry, 13*, 235–237.

Keane, T. M., Fairbank, J. A., Caddell, J. M., & Zimering, R. T. (1989). Implosive (flooding) therapy reduces symptoms of PTSD in Vietnam combat veterans. *Behavior Therapy, 20*, 245–260.

Keane, T. M., & Kaloupek, D. G. (1982). Imaginal flooding in the treatment of post-traumatic stress disorder. *Journal of Consulting and Clinical Psychology, 50*, 138–140.

Kilpatrick, D. G., & Calhoun, K. S. (1988). Early behavioral treatment for rape trauma: Efficacy or artifact? *Behavior Therapy, 19*, 421–427.

Kilpatrick, D. G., Veronen, L. J., & Resick, P. A. (1982). Psychological sequelae to rape: Assessment and treatment strategies. In D. M. Dolays & R. L. Meredith (Eds.), *Behavioral medicine: Assessment and treatment strategies* (pp. 473–497). New York: Plenum Press.

Kozak, M. J., Foa, E. B., & Steketee, G. (1988). Process and outcome of exposure treatment with obsessive–compulsives: Psychophysiological indicators of emotional processing. *Behavior Therapy, 19,* 157–169.

Lang, P. J. (1977). Imagery in therapy: An information processing analysis of fear. *Behavior Therapy, 8,* 862–886.

Lipke, H. J., & Botkin, A. L. (1993). Case studies of eye movement desensitization and reprocessing (EMD/R) with chronic post-traumatic stress disorder. *Psychotherapy, 29,* 591–595.

Margraf, J., Barlow, D. H., Clark, D., & Telch, M. (1993). Psychological treatment of panic: Work in progress on outcome, active ingredients, and follow-up. *Behaviour Research and Therapy, 31,* 1–8.

Marks, I. M., Boulougouris, J., & Marset, P. (1971). Flooding versus desensitization in the treatment of phobic disorders. *British Journal of Psychiatry, 119,* 353–375.

McCann, I. L., Sakheim, D. K., & Abrahamson, D. J. (1988). Trauma and victimization: A model of psychological adaptation. *The Counseling Psychologist, 16,* 531–594.

Meichenbaum, D. (1974). *Cognitive behavior modification.* Morristown, NJ: General Learning Press.

Muse, M. (1986). Stress-related, posttraumatic chronic pain syndrome: Behavioral treatment approach. *Pain, 25,* 389–394.

Peniston, E. G. (1986). EMG biofeedback-assisted desensitization treatment for Vietnam combat veterans with post-traumatic stress disorder. *Clinical Biofeedback and Health, 9,* 35–41.

Pitman, R. K., Altman, B., Greenwald, E., Longpre, R. E., Macklin, M. L., Poire, R. E., & Steketee, G. (1991). Psychiatric complications during flooding therapy for posttraumatic stress disorder. *Journal of Clinical Psychiatry, 52,* 17–20.

Pitman, R., Orr, S. P., Altman, B., Longpre, R. E., Poire, R. E., & Lasko, N. B. (1993, October). *A controlled study of eye movement desensitization/reprocessing (EMDR) treatment for post-traumatic stress disorder.* Paper presented at the annual meeting of the International Society for Traumatic Stress Studies, San Antonio, TX.

Resick, P. A., Jordan, C. G., Girelli, S. A., Hutter, C. K., & Marhoefer-Dvorak, S. (1988). A comparative outcome study of behavioral group therapy for sexual assault victims. *Behavior Therapy, 19,* 385–401.

Resick, P. A., & Schnicke, M. K. (1992). Cognitive processing therapy for sexual assault victims. *Journal of Consulting and Clinical Psychology, 60,* 748–756.

Rothbaum, B. O., Foa, E. B., Riggs, D. S., Murdock, T., & Walsh, W. (1992). A prospective examination of post-traumatic stress disorder in rape victims. *Journal of Traumatic Stress, 5,* 455–475.

Schindler, F. E. (1980). Treatment of systematic desensitization of a recurring nightmare of a real life trauma. *Journal of Behavior Therapy and Experimental Psychiatry, 11,* 53–54.

Shapiro, F. (1989). Efficacy of the eye movement desensitization procedure in the treatment of traumatic memories. *Journal of Traumatic Stress, 2,* 199–223.

Solomon, S. D., Gerrity, E. T., & Muff, A. M. (1992). Efficacy of treatments for posttraumatic stress disorder: An empirical review. *Journal of the American Medical Association, 268,* 633–638.

Turner, S. M. (1979). *Systematic desensitization of fears and anxiety in rape victims.* Paper presented at the 13th Annual Meeting of the Association for Advancement of Behavior Therapy, San Francisco.

Turner, S. M., & Frank, E. (1981). Behavior therapy in the treatment of rape victims. In L. Michelson, M. Hersen, & S. M. Turner (Eds.), *Future perspectives in behavior therapy* (pp. 269–291). New York: Plenum Press.

Veronen, L. J., & Kilpatrick, D. G. (1982, November). *Stress inoculation training for victims of rape: Efficacy and differential findings.* Paper presented at the 16th Annual Meeting of the Association for Advancement of Behavior Therapy, Los Angeles.

Veronen, L. J., & Kilpatrick, D. G. (1983). Stress management for rape victims. In D. Meichenbaum & M. E. Jaremko (Eds.), *Stress reduction and prevention* (pp. 341–374). New York: Plenum Press.

CHAPTER 23

The Psychopharmacological Treatment of Posttraumatic Stress Disorder

JONATHAN R. T. DAVIDSON
BESSEL A. VAN DER KOLK

When Abram Kardiner (1941) first defined what is now called posttraumatic stress disorder (PTSD), he called it a "physioneurosis," claiming that these patients' bodies are on constant alert for return of the trauma. Although several studies have found psychotherapy to be an effective treatment (see Chapters 18 and 22, this volume), numerous patients with PTSD take medications in the hope of ameliorating their symptomatology. What can drugs do for these patients? There is a long history attesting to the use of medications and substances, both prescribed and self-administered, to reduce distress in victims of trauma (Davidson & Nemeroff, 1989). In an apparent effort to regulate their own excessive arousal and other PTSD-related problems, these patients have high rates of self-medication: Among treatment-seeking patients, from 60% to 80% suffer from alcohol or drug abuse or dependence (Branchey, Davis, & Lieber, 1984; Keane, Gerardi, Lyons, & Wolfe, 1988). Opioids, alcohol, and benzodiazepines are the self-medications most frequently chosen (Bremner, 1994).

Although just about every group of psychotropic agents has been claimed to be effective for the treatment of some aspect of PTSD symptomatology, very few such agents have been systematically studied. Most studies have been done with male combat veterans suffering from chronic PTSD, which they first developed as adults. A recent study (van der Kolk et al., 1994; see below) showed a marked difference in responsiveness to fluoxetine between a combat veteran population and a sample of nonveterans with PTSD. This study has thus confirmed clinical concerns that the studies of the effects of medications in combat veterans may not be generalizable to nonveteran populations.

Since double-blind studies are enormously expensive in terms of time and money, only a few drugs have been exhaustively studied. Which drug is selected is a function of not only clinical promise, but also availability of funding and interest of the investigators. The fact that a particular drug has been proven to be effective in a double-blind study means only that it has been shown to be more effective than placebo in a particular patient population, within which some patients are likely to have responded better than others (van der Kolk et al., 1994). It does *not* mean that this drug is necessarily more effective than the ones that have not been tested. Clinicians should rely both on the body of published research and on their own clinical experience when trying to decide which particular drug to perscribe for any particular patient. Although it is important to stay abreast of research findings, clinicians are encouraged to explore new medications for their patients as well, and to collect data that can be shared with colleagues, in the hope that this can contribute to more systematic explorations.

RATIONALE

Drug therapy for PTSD can be understood in the context of several biological models, which have been advanced as mechanistic explanations of PTSD, and/or as explanations of how drugs may work. The major biological models are briefly described here.

1. *Noradrenergic dysregulation.* There is cumulative evidence to suggest dysregulation of the catecholaminergic system in PTSD, as reviewed elsewhere (Davidson, 1992). The locus coeruleus may serve as an alarm center, which is poorly regulated and perhaps overresponsive in people with chronic PTSD. Kolb (1987) has hypothesized that treatments that reduce locus coeruleus activity are likely to be effective in PTSD. These treatments include the monoamine oxidase (MAO) inhibitors and tricyclic antidepressants, as well as other drugs (e.g., clonidine, benzodiazepines, and beta-adrenergic blockers).

2. *Serotonergic dysfunction.* More recent data point to the likelihood that serotonin activity is disturbed in PTSD, and it is possible that individuals differ selectively as to whether they show a serotonergic or catecholaminergic dysfunction (Krystal, 1990; see Chapter 10, this volume). Conditioned avoidance,

stress resilience, sleep regulation, and impulse control are all strongly influenced by serotonergic activity, and all four of these variables are crucial aspects of PTSD. We have reviewed the possible importance of serotonin in PTSD elsewhere (van der Kolk, 1994; Vargas & Davidson, 1993). Recent clinical trials, as described below, support the efficacy of serotonergic drugs in PTSD.

3. *Kindling.* "Kindling" refers to a lowering of seizure threshold after repeated electrical stimulation of the brain at a level that is initially insufficient to produce a seizure. By analogy, some intrusive PTSD symptoms may develop through a kindling-like process in which long-term changes in excitability occur, rendering the victim increasingly likely to develop certain symptoms; that is, the excitability threshold has been lowered (van der Kolk, 1987). Antikindling drugs (e.g., carbamazepine) can be useful in PTSD and offer partial support for this notion.

4. *Increased startle responsiveness.* PTSD is in some ways a disorder of heightened startle and arousal, for which there may be a genetic vulnerability, since the startle phenomenon has been associated with a gene locus in the long arm of chromosome 5. Startle remains one of the more persistent symptoms of PTSD, often enduring even after successful abreaction at the time of acute PTSD (Kardiner, 1941; Sargant and Slater, 1940, 1941). Some antidepressants have no impact upon animal models of startle, and fluoxetine actually increases startle in people with PTSD (Fisler, Orr, & van der Kolk, 1995), even when the fluoxetine is clinically helpful. In contrast, animal models of startle suggest that anxiolytic drugs such as clonazepam and buspirone can be effective (Ryan et al., 1992; Shalev, 1993).

THE PURPOSES OF MEDICATIONS IN PTSD

The principal goals of using medications in PTSD are as follows:

1. Reduction of frequency and/or severity of intrusive symptoms.
2. Reduction in the tendency to interpret incoming stimuli as recurrences of the trauma.
3. Reduction in conditioned hyperarousal to stimuli reminiscent of the trauma, as well as in generalized hyperarousal.
4. Reduction in avoidance behavior.
5. Improvement in depressed mood and numbing.
6. Reduction in psychotic or dissociative symptoms.
7. Reduction of impulsive aggression against self and others.

Reduction of Intrusive Reexperiencing

Intrusion of the trauma is expressed on many different levels: flashbacks, affective states, somatic sensations, nightmares, and interpersonal reenactments. Autonomic arousal has the capacity to precipitate flashback phenomena, seemingly in state-dependent fashion (Rainey et al., 1987; Southwick et al., 1993). Drugs that decrease autonomic arousal, including the benzodiazepines, beta-adrenergic blockers, and clonidine, are generally thought to be effective for these symptoms. Since intrusive reexperiencing is the single most important predictor for the development of PTSD (see Chapters 4 and 7, this volume), it is reasonable to think that aggressive treatment of intrusions shortly after the trauma will have beneficial effects on the long-term development of PTSD. However, in the only empirical study of this proposition, the effects were negative. Shalev and his colleagues recently gave alprazolam to a group of acutely traumatized patients and compared them with an unmedicated control group; the alprazolam group had more PTSD symptomatology at a 6-month follow-up (A. Y. Shalev, personal communication, 1995). Obviously, this study needs to be replicated before firm conclusions can be drawn from its findings.

Reduction in the Tendency to Interpret Incoming Stimuli as Recurrences of the Trauma

Clinical experience and psychological testing show that traumatized individuals tend to overinterpret incoming stimuli as reminders of the trauma. It is as if their trauma-related associative networks are extraordinarily susceptible to activation by even the slightest trigger that matches an element of the trauma. Fluoxetine has been shown to be able to significantly decrease people's propensity to interpret sensory stimuli as a recurrence of the trauma and to increase their capacity to use cognitive functions to interpret affectively laden issues (van der Kolk et al., 1994).

Reduction in Conditioned and Generalized Hyperarousal

Reminders of the trauma may activate autonomic arousal; conversely, arousal itself may trigger memories of traumatic experiences (see van der Kolk, Chapter 10). Excessive reactions that are irrelevant to present demands probably play a major role in making PTSD patients avoid reminders of the trauma and consequently constrict their involvement in their surroundings. Both generalized hyperarousal and conditioned physiological reactivity to reminders of the trauma contribute to "all-or-none" emotional reactions.

The physiological responses of people with PTSD are conditioned to react to reminders of the trauma as emergencies. Autonomic arousal, which serves the essential function of alerting the organism to potential danger, loses that function in people with PTSD; the easy triggering of somatic stress reactions causes them to be unable to trust their bodily sensations to warn them against impending threat and to alert them to take appropriate action. This loss of neuromodulation, which is at the core of PTSD, leads to loss of affect regulation. Traumatized people are prone to go immediately from stimulus to response without being able to figure out first what makes them so upset. They tend to experience intense fear, anxiety, anger, and panic in response to even minor stimuli. These negative emotions make them either overreact and intimidate others, or shut down and freeze. Both adults and children with such hyperarousal are vulnerable to sleep problems, both because they are unable to calm themselves sufficiently to go to sleep, and because they may be fearful of having traumatic nightmares.

Since people with PTSD tend to move immediately from stimulus to response, they often have difficulty making use of psychotherapy to help them reflect on the meaning of their experience and to plan for restorative action. As long as they are so vulnerable to hyperarousal, they are prevented both from reestablishing stable occupational and interpersonal relationships, and from being able to address the impact of the trauma in their lives without getting more upset. The emotional and cognitive constriction seen in PTSD cuts off these individuals' access to an inner world of fantasy and symbols (see Chapters 13 and 18, this volume). Hyperarousal interferes with the capacity to put experience into words, and is likely to result in the discharge of emotional tensions in actions, and/or in self-medication with drugs of alcohol. Benzodiazepines, as well as alcohol, have been shown to decrease conditioned and generalized arousal in both animals and people.

Reduction in Avoidance Behavior

Aware of their difficulties in controlling their emotions, traumatized people seem to spend their energy on avoiding distressing internal sensations, instead of attending to the demands of the environment. Avoidance behavior is likely to lift once people with PTSD become aware that they are less sensitive to environmental triggers. After effective treatment for generalized and specific hyperarousal, the focus of treatment may require shifting to any remaining phobic avoidance.

Improvement in Depression and Numbing

Comorbidity between depression and PTSD is extremely high (Davidson, Swartz, Storck, Hammett, & Krishnan, 1985; Davidson et al., 1990). When depression occurs together with PTSD in war veterans, it has been shown to be psychologically and biologically distinct from major depression occurring without PTSD, and to be more resistant to standard antidepressant agents (Southwick, Yehuda, & Giller, 1991). A recent study (van der Kolk et al., 1994; see below) found that depression and numbing showed a differential treatment response in a combat veteran population: Even when depression was effectively treated, numbing persisted.

Numbing is one of the most intractable PTSD symptoms; many people who stop suffering from intrusions of the trauma continue to feel unmotivated and "dead to the world." In contrast with the intrusive PTSD symptoms, which occur in response to outside stimuli, numbing is part of these patients' baseline functioning. Emotional numbness also gets in the way of resolving the trauma in psychotherapy, since the inability to imagine a future for oneself kills the capacity to look for new solutions. The recent study by van der Kolk et al. (1994; see below) found that fluoxetine produced an improvement in numbing in a civilian population.

Reduction in Psychotic or Dissociative Symptoms

Intrusive reexperiences, particularly in patients who are victims of childhood trauma and who continue to dissociate, may be so vivid that patients are unable to distinguish them from reality. By definition, these experiences are psychotic; however, they are different from psychotic symptoms seen in other disorders because these patients seem to be reexperiencing actual events, which may or may not have been distorted. The hallucinations and delusions seen in flashbacks may be better conceptualized as dissociative phenomena. Clinical experience has shown that these often respond well to very low doses of antipsychotic medications (Saporta & Case, 1991).

Patients who have learned to dissociate in response to trauma are likely to continue to utilize dissociative defenses when exposed to new stresses. They develop amnesia for some experiences, and tend to react with fight-or-flight responses to feeling threatened, none of which may be consciously remembered afterwards. People who suffer from dissociative disorders are both a clinical and a research challenge. Evaluating the efficacy of a particular medication on the basis of statements such as "The monster does not scream so loud any more" and "The 2-year-old has stopped crying" may give the clinician a sense that something actually works, but is difficult to translate into a language that is useful for scientific investigation. Patients with multiple personality disorder (now dissociative identity disorder) often complain of auditory hallucinations (usually heard inside the head) and can experience thought withdrawal, delusions of passive influence, and other symptoms suggestive of schizophrenia (Kluft, 1987). However, these symptoms are thought to respond only rarely to antipsychotic medications (Loewenstein, Hornstein, & Farber, 1988; Putnam, 1989).

Reduction of Impulsive Aggression against Self and Others

Numerous studies have demonstrated that both adults and children who have been traumatized are likely to turn their aggression against others or themselves (see Chapter 9, this volume). Problems with aggression against others have been particularly well documented in war veterans, traumatized children, and prisoners with histories of early trauma (Lewis, 1990, 1992). Because self-destructive behavior is associated with decreased serotonin function (Brown, Goodwin, Ballenger, Goyes, & Major, 1979; Coccaro et al., 1989), fluoxetine and other serotonergic agonists should theoretically be effective. This has not as yet been documented. Carbamazepine has been shown to be effective for treatment of self-destructive behaviors in patients with borderline personality disorder (Cowdry & Gardner, 1988). One study showed that lithium carbonate can be helpful (Wickman & Reed, 1987), whereas opiate receptor blockers have been found to decrease self-destructive behaviors in other populations (Herman et al., 1987).

Aggressive patients with PTSD frequently meet diagnostic criteria for other Axis I psychiatric syndromes as well. Those other disorders have generally been studied more thoroughly than the PTSD component. For example, there is a good treatment literature on atypical depression/hysteroid dysphoria, which has demonstrated the effectiveness of MAO inhibitors (Liebowitz et al., 1988; Quitkin et al., 1989), and "unstable" or "impulsive" character disorders, which have been shown to respond well to lithium carbonate (Rifkin, Quitkin, Carillo, Blumberg, & Klein, 1972; Wickman & Reed, 1987). Although in those studies the prevalence of PTSD was left unexamined, our clinical experience suggests that many patients with PTSD can also be characterized as suffering from atypical depression and/or from impulsive disorders.

EFFICACY OF DRUG GROUPS

Several different psychotropic drug categories have been systematically evaluated in PTSD, most particularly the MAO inhibitors, tricyclics, and selective serotonin reuptake inhibitors (SSRIs), and to a lesser extent anticonvulsants, beta-adrenergic blockers and alpha$_2$-adrenergic agonists.

MAO Inhibitors

The category of MAO inhibitors is discussed first, primarily because these drugs were historically the first to be studied in detail, and also because phenelzine is the most thoroughly studied drug in the pharmacotherapy of PTSD at this time. However, few clinicians will elect to use a traditional MAO inhibitor until several other treatments have first been tried and found to be ineffective.

Two double-blind trials have been completed by Kosten(1992) and Shestatzky, Greenberg, and Lerer (1988). The study by Kosten showed impressive effects for phenelzine, which were already apparent relative to the effects for placebo at week 3. Overall, the drug induced an approximately 50% reduction in intrusive and avoidance symptoms, with a slightly greater effect on the former. These results suggest that phenelzine not only can suppress the obsessive, recurrent, and intrusive images/thoughts of combat trauma, but also may have direct antiphobic effects. By contrast, the Shestatzky et al. (1988) study of phenelzine, in Israeli combat veterans, produced negative results. In this study, however, the short duration of treatment, the suboptimal dose, and the crossover design may all have militated against the chance of finding a positive outcome.

The side effects of phenelzine can be problematic in PTSD, most notably sleep cycle disruption, sexual dysfunction, and dizziness (Davidson, Walker, & Kilts, 1987). Overall, phenelzine may be more effective than imipramine (Kosten, 1992), but it would be premature to draw firm conclusions in this regard. Given the seeming superiority of phenelzine, we await with eagerness the development and testing of safer, better-tolerated, selective, reversible MAO inhibitors. Brofaramine appeared promising in this regard until its development was unfortunately halted by the manufacturer.

Tricyclic Antidepressants

There have now been double-blind trials of three tricyclic antidepressants: amitriptyline (Davidson et al., 1990, 1993), imipramine (Kosten, 1992), and desipramine (Reist et al., 1989). All these studies were conducted with male combat veterans; the amitriptyline study was conducted with a mixed inpatient and outpatient population. Amitriptyline was found to be more effective than placebo on a variety of measures, including measures of PTSD, depression, and anxiety. Both observed and self-rated PTSD symptoms were responsive to the drug, although its effect was modest. Subsequent analysis (Davidson et al., 1993) revealed that the drug–placebo difference was greatest in patients who were less severely symptomatic, had lower intensity of combat exposure, had more stable personalities, and were less likely to have frequent panic attacks. Specific symptoms of impaired concentration, somatic anxiety, and guilt feelings, and several symptoms of trauma avoidance, were all predictive of poorer response to amitriptyline. Similar findings have been reported for direct therapeutic exposure in combat veterans (Litz, Blake, Gerardi, & Keane, 1990).

Imipramine also proved to be more effective than placebo in outpatients with combat-induced PTSD; this effect took approximately 5 weeks to emerge (Kosten, 1992).

The study of desipramine (Reist et al., 1989) produced no evidence for drug superiority in effects on PTSD symptoms, and its failure to support the results obtained in the studies of amitriptyline and imipramine raises some questions. One possible explanation is that lower maximum doses of desipramine were used, the length of treatment was no greater than 4 weeks, and the crossover study design (which confounded time effects and treatment effects) may also have limited the likelihood of detecting drug–placebo differences. A second possible explanation lies in the fact that desipramine is a purely noradrenergic drug, whereas imipramine, phenelzine, and amitriptyline have marked serotonergic effects as well. A suitable test of this possibility would be to compare bupropion (a selective catecholaminergic drug) with an SSRI.

Fluoxetine and Other SSRIs

Fluoxetine has been reported to reduce symptoms of PTSD in a number of open studies (Davidson, Roth, & Newman, 1991; Nagy, Morgan, Southwick, & Charney, 1993). van der Kolk et al. (1994) have published a double-blind fluoxetine versus placebo study of subjects drawn both from a Department of Veterans Affairs (VA) clinic and a civilian outpatient trauma clinic. This was a 5-week trial, using maximum doses of 60 mg fluoxetine, although this dose was only needed in some instances. A total of 12 males and 21 females were recruited through the trauma clinic, while 30 male war veterans and one 1 female war veteran came from the VA clinic. Fluoxetine significantly decreased overall PTSD symptomatology, though site (trauma clinic vs. VA clinic) made a more significant difference than did administration of the drug. Basically, the fluoxetine had few effects in the VA group, whereas the trauma clinic group proved to be very responsive to being in the study, with both the placebo and the fluoxetine group improving significantly. However, fluoxetine was significantly more effective in the trauma clinic population than was placebo. The PTSD symptoms of numbing and arousal were most affected by fluoxetine.

Interestingly, while fluoxetine was a very effective antidepressant, improvement in the depression score did not predict improvement in the PTSD score (not even in numbing). Although there was substantial improvement in depression in the VA sample, there was no meaningful change in numbing symptoms. Conversely, whereas the trauma clinic sample had a more modest improvement in depression, it showed a substantial improvement in numbing symptoms. When numbing symptoms were separated from the avoidance, fluoxetine turned out to affect only numbing. It is likely that 5 weeks' worth of improvement in PTSD symptomatology is insufficient for people to realize that exposure to stimuli reminiscent of the trauma will not lead to overwhelming distress. A longer trial might demonstrate whether, over time, patients feel better able to face trauma-related stressors and thus develop a decrease in avoidant symptoms as well.

Because most previous controlled studies were carried out with veterans, it is difficult to draw conclusions from this study about the overall superiority of one drug over another. The civilian trauma clinic sample improved more in 5 weeks on fluoxetine than any of the veteran groups in other studies who were given any of the other drugs over a longer period of time. However, the VA sample, after 5 weeks of fluoxetine, did not nearly have the same beneficial effects as the veterans in other studies who had been maintained on imipramine, amitriptyline, or phenelzine over longer periods of time. Whether a longer trial on fluoxetine would have allowed the veterans to catch up with the trauma clinic civilians, or with the veterans in other studies, clearly would be an important issue to investigate further.

The van der Kolk et al. (1994) study also showed that numbing and depression are not overlapping psychological categories. Although the VA sample became much less depressed on fluoxetine, there was no meaningful change in numbing symptoms. In contrast, the trauma clinic sample showed substantial improvement in both numbing and depression. Thus, the beneficial effect of fluoxetine on PTSD is not necessarily a function of its antidepressant effects.

A recent study by Kline (1994) suggests that sertraline is also of benefit in PTSD.

Anticonvulsants

Studies by Lipper et al. (1986) and Wolf, Alavi, and Mosnaim (1988) both suggest that carbamazepine may have beneficial effects in chronic PTSD. A study of valproic acid by Fesler (1991) also gives support to the idea that valproate may have a role in treatment of this disorder. At this time, no double-blind trials of anticonvulsants in PTSD have been conducted. These drugs, including the new anticonvulsant gabapentin, deserve further close attention for the treatment of chronic PTSD and dissociative disorders.

Beta-Adrenergic Blockers

Two open studies have found effectiveness for propranolol in PTSD. Kolb, Burris, and Griffiths (1984) reported positive effects of the drug at doses of 120–160 mg per day in 12 Vietnam combat veterans. General symptom improvement occurred; the most notable specific effects were those on explosiveness, nightmares, intrusive recollections, sleep impairment, hyperalertness, and startle symptoms. It was also noted that self-esteem and psychosocial functioning improved. Problems with the drug included depression, tiredness, poor memory, impaired sexual functioning, bradycardia, lowering of blood pressure, and confusion at higher doses. Beta-adrenergic blockers may have salutary antiaggressive effects in some cases of PTSD. Famularo, Kinscherff, and Fenton (1988) reported a study of children with acute PTSD who responded to propranolol. All children had been victims of physical or sexual abuse, and the drug improved hypervigilance and hyperarousal, as in the study by Kolb et al. (1984).

Alpha₂-Adrenergic Agonists

Clonidine suppresses alpha$_2$-noradrenergic receptor activity in the locus coeruleus and thereby reduces adrenergic tone. Kolb et al. (1984) noted positive findings with the drug at doses of 0.2–0.4 mg per day in Vietnam veterans. van der Kolk (1987) has found that clonidine can reduce self-mutilative behavior in patients with PTSD. A third report, by Kinzie and Leung (1989), found that combined treatment of nine Cambodian refugees with imipramine and clonidine led to improved sleep and fewer nightmares, and some improvement in startle, but no benefit for avoidant behavior.

Other Drugs

Benzodiazepines have clear theoretical appeal for treating PTSD and are widely used in clinical practice. There is concern about the use of short-acting benzo-diazepines such as alprazolam, which are more likely to produce clinical complications, including rebound anxiety and withdrawal symptoms (Friedman, 1991; Higgitt, Lader, & Fonagy, 1985). From a theoretical point of view, the kindling model of PTSD offers a neurobiological justification for prescribing benzodiazepines for appropriate patients, since limbic kindling is associated with increased benzodiazepine receptor binding (Friedman, 1991; McNamara et al., 1985). Vargas, Bissette, Owens, Ehlers, and Nemeroff (1992) reported that acute administration of adinazolam and alprazolam led to a decrease in corticotropin-releasing factor (CRF) concentrations in the locus coeruleus. On the other hand, concentrations of CRF increased in the hypothalamus. These effects are opposite to those normally observed following exposure of rats to acute or chronic stress. Vargas et al. also found that chronic administration of alprazolam led to a sustained reduction in CRF concentrations in the locus coeruleus. These would support the use of benzodiazepines in PTSD, and two open studies suggest positive effects for alprazolam (Dunner, Edwards, & Copeland, 1985) and clonazepam (Loewenstein et al., 1988). However, the process of withdrawal from alprazolam in combat veterans with PTSD may give rise to some very disturbing withdrawal and relapse symptoms (Risse et al., 1990). The antistartle effects of benzodiazepines have already been referred to, and it is not inconceivable that some patients may be optimally managed by a combination of psychotropic drugs: an antidepressant or anticonvulsant for regulation of intrusive and/or avoidance symptoms and poor impulse control, and possibly a high-potency benzodiazepine for management of startle and hyperarousal symptoms.

The literature on lithium, neuroleptics, and cyproheptadine is sparse and at this point is of little assistance (see van der Kolk, 1987; Brophy, 1991).

Lastly, Vargas and Davidson (1993) have speculated that electroconvulsive therapy, which is a nondrug, somatic treatment, may have a limited role in treating PTSD when there is attendant major depression.

CONCLUSIONS

Over the last 10 years, there has been growing interest in the neurobiology and psychopharmacological treatment of PTSD. The different models that have been advanced to explain PTSD mechanistically also lend themselves to an understanding of how certain medications may work, as well as serving to guide treatment selection according to symptomatology. At the present time, it appears that acute trauma is best treated with any of the drugs that decrease autonomic arousal, such as benzodiazepines or clonidine. In this population it is probably critical to provide a way to avoid nightmares and other intrusive symptoms, in order to prevent kindling of the trauma. Theoretically, anticonvulsants may also be of use, but these have not been tried.

Once a person has developed PTSD, a clinician should initially select either an SSRI or a tricyclic antidepressant, with willingness to introduce a second drug (either an anticonvulsant, a mood stabilizer, or a benzodiazepine) after a few weeks if response is only partial. Choice of the second drug should be guided largely by the symptom profile. In chronic PTSD, in which comorbid psychopathology may be prominent, clinicians can start relying on the studies that have shown different drugs to be effective for such problems as self-destructive behavior, impulsivity, and depression. Unfortunately, at this point there is no evidence that any drug is particularly effective in the treatment of dissociative phenomena.

Although pharmacotherapy is no more likely to induce cure of PTSD than of any other major psychiatric disorder, the symptom relief that results from effective drug therapy enables patients to move ahead toward more productive lives and to participate more effectively in other forms of therapy. Effective pharmacotherapy may also be expected to cut down on some of the attendant morbidity (and possibly mortality) of PTSD.

REFERENCES

Branchey, L., Davis, W., & Lieber, C. S. (1984). Alcoholism in Vietnam and Korean veterans: A long term follow-up. *Alcoholism: Clinical and Experimental Research, 8*, 572–575.

Bremner, J. D. (1994). Neurobiology of post-traumatic stress disorder. In R. S. Pynoos (Ed.), *Posttraumatic stress disorder: A critical review* (pp. 43–64). Lutherville, MD: Sidran Press.

Brophy, M. H. (1991). Cyproheptadine for combat nightmares in posttraumatic stress disorder and dream anxiety disorder. *Military Medicine, 156*, 100–101.

Brown, G. L., Goodwin, F. K., Ballenger, J. C., Goyer, P. F., & Major, L. F. (1979). Aggression in humans correlates with cerebrospinal fluid metabolites. *Psychiatry Research, 1*, 131–139.

Coccaro, E. F., Siever, L. J., Klar, H. M., Maurer, G., Cochrane, K., Cooper, T. B., Mohs, R. C., & Davis, K. L. (1989). Serotonergic studies in patients with affective and personality disorders: Correlates with suicidal and impulsive aggressive behavior. *Archives of General Psychiatry, 46*, 587–599.

Cowdry, R. W., & Gardner, D. L. (1988). Pharmacotherapy of borderline personality disorder with alprazolam, carbamazepine, trifluoperazine, and tranylcypromine. *Archives of General Psychiatry, 45*, 111–119.

Davidson, J. R. T. (1992). Drug therapy of post-traumatic stress disorder. *British Journal of Psychiatry, 160*, 309–314.

Davidson, J. R. T., Kudler, H. S., Saunders, W. B., Erickson, L., Smith, R. D., Stein, R. M., Lipper, S., Hammett, E. B., Mahorney, S. L., & Cavenar, J. O. (1993). Predicting response to amitriptyline in posttraumatic stress disorder. *American Journal of Psychiatry, 150*(7), 1024–1029.

Davidson, J. R. T., Kudler, H., Smith, R., Mahoney, S. L., Lipper, S. Hammett, E., Saunders, W. B., & Cavenar, J. (1990). Treatment of post-traumatic stress disorder with amitriptyline and placebo. *Archives of General Psychiatry, 47*, 259–266.

Davidson, J. R. T., & Nemeroff, C. M. (1989). Pharmacotherapy in PTSD: Historical and clinical considerations and future directions. *Psychopharmacology Bulletin, 25*, 422–425.

Davidson, J. R. T., Roth, S., & Newman, E. (1991). Fluoxetine in post-traumatic stress disorder. *Journal of Traumatic Stress, 4*, 419–423.

Davidson, J. R. T., Swartz, M., Storck, M., Hammett, E. B., & Krishnan, K. R. R. (1985). A family and diagnostic study of PTSD. *American Journal of Psychiatry, 142*, 90–93.

Davidson, J. R. T., Walker, J. I., & Kilts, C. D. (1987). A pilot study of phenelzine in the treatment of post-traumatic stress disorder. *British Journal of Psychiatry, 150*, 252–255.

Dunner, F. J., Edwards, W. P., & Copeland, P. C. (1985). *Clinical efficacy of alprazolam in PTSD patients* [Abstract]. New Research, American Psychiatric Association, 138th Annual Meeting, Los Angeles.

Famularo, R., Kinscherff, R., & Fenton, T. (1988). Propranolol treatment for childhood posttraumatic stress disorder, acute type. *American Journal of Diseases of Children, 142*, 1244–1247.

Fesler, F. A. (1991). Valproate in combat-related posttraumatic stress disorder. *Journal of Clinical Psychiatry, 52*, 361–364.

Fisler, R., Orr, S., & van der Kolk, B. A. (1995). *Fluoxetine increases the startle response in successfully treated PTSD.* Manuscript submitted for publication.

Friedman, M. J. (1991). Biological approaches to the diagnosis and treatment of post-traumatic stress disorder. *Journal of Traumatic Stress, 4*, 67–91.

Herman, B. H., Hammock, M. K., Arthur-Smith, M. A., Egan, J., Chatoor, I., Werner, A., & Zelnick, N. (1987). Naltrexone decreases self-injurious behavior. *Annals of Neurology, 22*, 550–552.

Higgitt, A. C., Lader, M. H., & Fonagy, P. (1985). Clinical management of benzodiazepine dependence. *British Medical Journal, 291*, 688–690.

Kardiner, A. (1941). *The traumatic neuroses of war.* New York: Hoeber.

Keane, T. M., Gerardi, R. J., Lyons, J. A., & Wolfe, J. (1988). The interrelationship of substance abuse and posttraumatic stress disorder in Vietnam veterans. *The Behavior Therapist, 8*, 9–12.

Kinzie, J. D., & Leung, P. (1989). Clonidine in Cambodian patients with posttraumatic stress disorder. *Journal of Nervous and Mental Disease, 177*, 546–550.

Kline, N. A. (1994). Sertraline efficacy in depressed combat veterans with posttraumatic stress disorder. *American Journal of Psychiatry, 151*(4), 621.

Kluft, R. P. (1987). First rank symptoms as a diagnostic clue to multiple personality disorder. *American Journal of Psychiatry, 144*(3), 293–298.

Kolb, L. C. (1987). Neuropsychological hypothesis explaining posttraumatic stress disorder. *American Journal of Psychiatry, 144*(8), 989–995.

Kolb, L. C., Burris, B., & Griffiths, S. (1984). Propranolol and clonidine in the treatment of chronic posttraumatic stress of war. In B. A. van der Kolk (Ed.), *Posttraumatic stress disorder: Psychological and biological sequelae* (pp. 97–107). Washington, DC: American Psychiatric Press.

Kosten, T. R. (1992). Alexithymia as a predictor of treatment response in PTSD. *Journal of Traumatic Stress, 5*(4), 563–573.

Krystal, J. H. (1990). Animal models for post traumatic stress disorder. In E. L. Giller (Ed.), *Biological assessment and treatment of post-traumatic stress disorder* (pp. 1–26). Washington, DC: American Psychiatric Press.

Lewis, D. O. (1990). Neuropsychiatric and experiential correlates of violent juvenile delinquency. *Neuropsychology Review, 1*(2), 125–136.

Lewis, D. O. (1992). From abuse to violence: Psychophysiological consequences of maltreatment. *Journal of the American Academy of Child and Adolescent Psychiatry, 31*, 383–391.

Liebowitz, M. R., Quitkin, F. M., Stewart, J. W., McGrath, P. J., Harrison, W. M., Markowitz, J. S., Rabkin, J. G., Tricamo, E., Goetz, D. M., & Klein, D. F. (1988). Antidepressant specificity in atypical depression. *Archives of General Psychiatry, 45*, 129–137.

Lipper, S., Davidson, J. R. T., Grady, T. A., Edinger, J. D., Hammett, E. B., Mahorney, S. L., & Cavenar, J. O., Jr. (1986). Preliminary study of carbamazepine in posttraumatic stress disorder. *Psychosomatics, 27*, 849–854.

Litz, B. T., Blake, D. D., Gerardi, R. J., & Keane, T. M. (1990). Decision-making guidelines for the use of direct therapeutic exposure in the treatment of post-traumatic stress disorder. *The Behavior Therapist, 13*, 91–93.

Lowenstein, R. J., Hornstein, N., & Farber, B. (1988). Open trial of clonazepam in the treatment of post traumatic stress symptoms in multiple personality disorder. *Dissociation, 1*, 3–12.

McNamara, J. O., Bonhaus, D. W., Shin, C., Crain, B. J., Gellman, R. L., & Giacchino, J. L. (1985). The kindling model of epilepsy: A critical review. *CRC Critical Reviews of Clinical Neurobiology, 1*, 341–391.

Nagy, L. M., Morgan, C. A., Southwick, S. M., & Charney, D. S. (1993). Open prospective trial of fluoxetine for posttraumatic stress disorder. *Journal of Clinical Psychopharmacology, 13*, 107–114.

Putnam, F. W. (1989). *Diagnosis and treatment of multiple personality disorder.* New York: Guilford Press.

Quitkin, F. M., McGrath, P. J., Stewart, J. W., Harrison, W., Wager, S. G., Nunes, E., Rabkin, J. G., Tricamo, E., Markowitz, J., & Klein, D. F. (1989). Phenelzine and imipramine in mood reactive depressives: Further delineation of the syndrome of atypical depression. *Archives of General Psychiatry, 46*, 787–793.

Rainey, J. M., Aleem, A., Ortiz, A., Yeragani, V., Pohl, R., & Berchou, R. (1987). Laboratory procedures for the inducement of flashbacks. *American Journal of Psychiatry, 144*, 1317–1319.

Reist, C., Kauffmann, C. D., Haier, R. J., Sangdahl, C., De Mer, E. M., Chicz-DeMet, A., & Nelson, J. M. (1989). A controlled trial of desipramine in 18 men with posttraumatic stress disorder. *American Journal of Psychiatry, 146*, 513–516.

Rifkin, A., Quitkin, F., Carillo, C., Blumberg, A. G., & Klein, D. F. (1972). Lithium carbonate in emotionally unstable character disorder. *Archives of General Psychiatry*, 27, 519–523.

Risse, S. C., Whitters, A., Burke, J., Chen, S., Scurfield, R. M., & Raskind, M. A. (1990). Severe withdrawal symptoms after discontinuation of alprazolam in eight patients with combat-induced posttraumatic stress disorder. *Journal of Clinical Psychiatry*, 51, 206–209.

Ryan, S. G., Sherman, S. L., Terry, J. C., Sparkes, R. S., Torres, M. C., & Mackey, R. W. (1992). Startle disease or hyperekplexia: Response to clonazepam and assignment of the gene (STHE) to chromosome 5q by image analysis. *Annals of Neurology*, 3(6), 663–668.

Saporta, J. A., Jr., & Case, J. (1991). The role of medication in treating adult survivors of childhood trauma. In P. Paddison (Ed.), *Treating adult survivors of incest* (pp. 101–134). Washington, DC: American Psychiatric Press.

Sargant, W. W., & Slater, E. (1940). Acute war neuroses. *Lancet*, 140, 1–2.

Sargant, W. W., & Slater, E. (1941). Amnesic syndromes in war. *Proceedings of the Royal Society of Medicine*, 34, 757–764.

Shalev, A. Y. (1993). Posttraumatic stress disorder: A biopsychological perspective. *Israel Journal of Psychiatry*, 30(2), 102–109.

Shestatzky, M., Greenberg, D., & Lerer, B. (1988). A controlled trial of phenelzine in posttraumatic stress disorder. *Psychiatry Research*, 24, 149–155.

Southwick, S. M., Krystal, J. H., Morgan, A., Johnson, D., Nagy, L., Nicolaou, A., Heninger, G. R., & Charney, D. S. (1993). Abnormal noradrenergic function in post-traumatic stress disorder. *Archives of General Psychiatry*, 50, 266–274.

Southwick, S. M., Yehuda, R., & Giller, E. L. (1991). Characterization of depression in war related posttraumatic stress disorder. *American Journal of Psychiatry*, 148, 179–183.

van der Kolk, B. A. (1987). The drug treatment of post-traumatic stress disorder. *Journal of Affective Disorders*, 13, 203–213.

van der Kolk, B. A. (1994). The body keeps the score: Memory and the evolving psychobiology of posttraumatic stress. *Harvard Review of Psychiatry*, 1, 253–265.

van der Kolk, B. A., Dreyfuss, D., Michaels, M., Shera, D., Berkowitz, B., Fisler, R., & Saxe, G. (1994). Fluoxetine in posttraumatic stress disorder. *Journal of Clinical Psychiatry*, 55(12), 517–522.

Vargas, M. A., & Davidson, J. R. T. (1993). Post-traumatic stress disorder. *Psychiatric Clinics of North America*, 16(4), 737–748.

Vargas, M. A., Bissette, G., Owens, M. J., Ehlers, C. L., & Nemeroff, C. B. (1992). Effects of chronic ethanol and benzodiazepine treatment and withdrawal on corticotropin-releasing factor neural systems. *Annals of the New York Academy of Sciences*, 654, 145–152.

Wickman, E. A., & Reed, J. V. (1987). Lithium for the control of aggressive and self-mutilating behavior. *International Clinical Psychopharmacology*, 2, 181–190.

Wolf, M. E., Alavi, A., & Mosnaim, A. D. (1988). Posttraumatic stress disorder in Vietnam veterans: Clinical and EEG findings. Possible therapeutic effects of carbamazepine. *Biological Psychiatry*, 23, 642–644.

CHAPTER 24

Psychoanalytic Psychotherapy of Posttraumatic Stress Disorder

The Nature of the Therapeutic Relationship

JACOB D. LINDY

The tendency toward repetition of trauma within the treatment situation holds a central place in the psychoanalytic psychotherapy of posttraumatic stress disorder (PTSD) (Lindy, 1989). Indeed, for this form of psychotherapy these repetitions are not primarily interferences in the therapeutic plan, as they may be for other forms of therapy; rather, they are expectable and essential elements in the therapeutic process (Lindy, Spitz, & Moss, 1995). Consistent with the findings of Janet and the neurobiologists, sensory–motor long-term traumatic memory stores intrude themselves in the present, in special configurations or schemata (Janet, 1889). It is in these same schemata in which the trauma survivor unwittingly places the therapist's behaviors and person, as well as the therapist's spatial and temporal environment.

The treatment situation thus offers many opportunities to provide the backdrop or day residue onto which the traumatic events of the past play themselves out in the present. Otherwise indifferent components of the therapist's space may serve to set off intrusive sensory recollections, symptoms of anxiety, somatic reenactment, and affective states such as terror or shame. Such intrusions can also remind the patient of moments of fantasied safety within the trauma. For example, one patient, in complying with her therapist's wish that she describe elements of her trauma, proceeded while wishing she could remove herself from the pain. She found herself taking solace in looking at a high window in her doctor's office. It became the reminder of the skylight on which she would fix her eyes when she, as a child, was forced to perform fellatio on her uncle in the upstairs bathroom as the rest of the family enjoyed Thanksgiving dinner downstairs. For another patient, however, the sound of water running from a faucet to the sink in the doctor's office served to set off anxiety and somatic reenactment. In one session, for example, as the patient became increasingly anxious, the doctor, in an effort to help his patient compose herself, decided to get her a glass of water. However, the sound of the faucet running triggered a reenactment in which the patient writhed on the floor in uncontrollable terror, lest the water be filling the enema bag that her mother would soon be using to torture her.

While observing such reenactments in the transference from the outset, the psychoanalytically oriented psychotherapist, following the dictum "Above all do no harm," must remain judicious in choosing when and how to use these observations in clinical interventions. On the one hand, the therapist may appreciate the survivor's intense need to fend off the recall of the trauma; in other circumstances, the therapist may recognize an imperative to explore or reconstruct the content of previously split-off traumatic material. But usually it is only gradually that reenactment becomes amenable to the therapeutic process, as a therapeutic alliance develops and as the treatment becomes a secure enough holding environment for the trauma to be expressed and worked on within the alliance. During this complex dyadic process, traumatic memory for the survivor gradually becomes narrative memory; inchoate sensations and dysphoric affect, complete with the emergency defenses used at the time (e.g., dissociation, splitting, or disavowal), come to be personal stories of tragedy, trauma, and loss. These stories come to have enormous significance, for understanding not only the survivor's truncated past, but his or her present and future. For both the survivor and the therapist, unconscious reenactments that place both participants back in the affective, defensive, and adaptive world of the trauma itself become compelling elements in understanding how the traumatic assault has marked the survivor's inner sense of self. It is precisely in this arena that the psychoanalytic psychotherapist must monitor personal subjective responses while finding sufficient neutral ego resources to carry out sound clinical work, and especially to help the survivor find words to express nuances of subjective meaning in an empathic context. Moreover, insofar as schemata not only set off specific posttraumatic reactions but act as organizers of everyday experience for traumatized individuals, the management of traumatic repetitions within the therapeutic context—that is, within the transference and countertransference—becomes crucial for the entire recovery process.

One should keep in mind that the schemata repeating themselves are not simple ones, composed of unidimensional cardboard constructs captured simply by such words as "perpetrator" and "victim," for example. They are more likely to be complex ones in which "victim" and "perpetrator" are imbedded in numerous affect states, defenses, object relations, and meaning configurations. Pertinent to these are subjective decision points in which critical self-judgments are embedded, such as insufficient anticipation of danger, naive trust, impossible choices, guilt and shame, and terror at revealing the content of the traumatic experience to someone new. Other elements of the schemata include temporally contiguous ego states (e.g., splitting, denial, dissociation) and temporally contiguous fantasy states (e.g., murderous vengeance and wishes to die).

The perspective represented in this chapter grows from 20 years of clinical and research studies at the University of Cincinnati and at the Cincinnati Psychoanalytic Institute (Lindy, with MacLeod, Spitz, Green, & Grace, 1988; Honig, Grace, Lindy, Newman, & Titchener, 1993; Lindy, Green, Grace, & Titchener, 1983). In this chapter I wish to demonstrate the uniqueness, texture, and depth of traumatic responses as they appear within the clinical engagement. I wish to emphasize the subtleties that are present from moment to moment within the clinical session, as the therapist tries to determine how and when to help the patient discover more, or, alternatively, how and when to encapsulate trauma so that it intrudes less harmfully into the survivor's life. I examine uniqueness by looking at several pairs of trauma survivors; I examine texture by looking at ego states near, but not necessarily identical with, the trauma itself; I examine depth by looking at patients whose trauma symptoms have multiple origins; and I look at technique by examining the issue of timing (when do clinical situations call for reconstructive interpretation, and when do they call for support of distancing defenses?). I conclude the chapter with a brief discussion of transference and countertransference issues, and a summary of technical principles. Whenever possible, I draw this material from clinical situations arising within a research context and in which additional empirical evidence is available to approach some of the variables through research design.

UNIQUENESS OF THE TRAUMA RESPONSE

The specific ways in which schemata are organized vary enormously from person to person and from circumstance to circumstance. All natural disaster survivors, all rape survivors, and all combat survivors do not share the same traumatic schemata; and their symptoms, if present, do not repeat themselves in quite the same manner. We therapists cannot assume that because a person has endured a specific traumatic event, we have *a priori* knowledge of the person's internal subjective state at the time or access to the specific form that the person's traumatic configuration may take in the present. We cannot assume that the trauma we are aware of is the only one that affects a current symptom (often the person has experienced earlier traumas that are not so readily available for understanding). We cannot assume that we know the affects of the survivor because they fit with what we have been told of the survivor's experience. Finally, we cannot assume that a traumatic situation is amenable to interpretive reconstructive or insight-promoting work at the time we may feel ready to dispense it. However, keeping a watchful eye out for the complex ways in which the trauma may be repeating itself in the present, both in the transference and in the countertransference, may be useful in each of the situations described above.

Two pairs of survivors illustrate how different people can experience almost the same external event with massive differences in long-term clinical presentation. In March 1972, Pam and her younger sister Louise were children aged 10 and 4 living in a small house near Buffalo Creek in West Virginia. A slag dam burst, releasing millions of gallons of water; the water swept down the creek hollow, lifting houses off their foundations, killing hundreds of people, and displacing thousands more. My colleagues and I had occasion to interview survivors 2 years after the flood in 1974, and 20 years after, in 1992. As the water was rising in the creek, Louise remembered herself being whisked off by her older siblings; she was told to take her blanket, run up the nearby hill, and wait for the older children and her mother. She did as she was told. She felt frightened and excited by the adventure; however, she fell asleep once the family made it to the shelter on high ground. Twenty years later, Louise had experienced her share of hardships, as many young women in Appalachia do. But she had no particularly traumatic dreams or memories of the terrible day of the flood. She saw the psychiatric interviewer as a friendly person who (like the lawyers working with the survivors) widened her usual frame of reference by asking interesting questions, and opened broader horizons for her life.

Pam had been in charge of her younger sisters as they were watching television the morning of the flood. Their mother had just been screaming at her for not keeping them quiet enough when Pam looked out the window and saw the creek rising rapidly. She pointed this out to her mother, who became panicky. (Louise tried to look out, but the window was too high up for her.) Although the younger kids got out of the house safely and quickly, managing the mother's exit was no easy matter. The mother couldn't decide what to take; in the end, there were not enough heavy clothes or blankets; the mother became trapped in the door as the foundations were unhinged. Pam was terrified. Caught between the impossible choice of saving herself or her mother, she headed up the hill not knowing whether her mother would make it. Once in the shelter, Pam became fixated with the sight of a dead baby caked with mud—a sight from which Louise was shielded and of which she had no memory in 1992.

Twenty years later, Pam sat in her rocking chair looking out of the window in the direction from which the flood had come in 1972. She hovered over her two children, frightened lest something dreadful should happen to them if they were to get out of her sight. The present seemed to have no meaning. When she spoke of the flood, there was a far-off look in her eyes; the moments of the distant past seemed as though they had happened yesterday. She had frequent nightmares of the flood, especially of the dead mud-caked baby. Her PTSD was omnipresent, as she had arranged her furniture to face the window so that she could continually watch for a return of that terrible day. Pam's and Louise's experiences of the same flood from within the same household were different in a number of important ways. Pam's age and sibling order put greater responsibility on her shoulders. Pam experienced guilt on leaving the house. Pam saw both the terrifying sight of the rising water and the grotesque image of the dead baby. Louise was spared all these elements in the trauma experience. Empirically, we now know that these qualitative differences in the experience (role, guilt, exposure to the grotesque) predict greater long-term pathology (Green, Grace, & Geser, 1985; Green, Grace, Lindy, Glazer, & Leonard, 1990a; Green et al., 1990b). They also help define a different subjective experience to the same disaster.

In the second example, a husband and wife sat across from each other at the same table as fire broke out in a large supper club (the fire soon killed 165 people). Turning toward the main exit, the husband saw dangerous crowding, leaped across table tops, and was among the last to exit safely. Six months later he had lost two jobs, was agitated and depressed, and was suffering from severe intrusions of his trauma at the fire. In his psychotherapy, he reenacted the fire as the wall of his doctor's office suddenly felt hot. He escaped the building in panic; later, he sobbed that the issue was not that he misperceived danger, but that he once more ran to safety before insuring that the other person was out of danger. His wife's experience couldn't have been more different. Noting that a side exit was located immediately behind her, she joined others from the group and exited quickly. Six months later she was suffering no significant signs of PTSD. The marriage did not survive the fire's aftermath.

A *priori* assumptions about these two pairs of survivors, based on their exposure to what seemed like the same disaster in each case, would have been quite misleading. Rather, it is in the details of their separate experiences and subjective states that we get a more accurate picture. Furthermore, reenactments within the therapeutic or diagnostic setting provide many details about the differences.

TEXTURE OF THE TRAUMA RESPONSE

The components in the trauma experience that are eventually reenacted in the therapeutic situation are often near, but not congruent with, what is generally assumed to be the central objective danger point of a given traumatic experience. The trauma becomes imbedded in the victim's schemata of self and others, and rarely remains as an isolated fragment. For instance, on the second anniversary of a traumatizing accident in which Ms. A. nearly died by forcing open and then falling through a glass door, lacerating her radial artery, her sister called her therapist to report that Ms. A. was terrified and mute. On arrival for an emergency session, Ms. A. was not plagued primarily with intrusions (such as the sound of crashing glass and the sensation of warm blood pouring over her), which had become familiar flashbacks to the trauma and which her therapist expected to see. Rather, she spoke haltingly and incomprehensibly, finally clarifying that a letter from her attorney was what had set a horrifyingly helpless affect state in motion. The letter referred to a legal action against her landlord that day, which was the source of the current disabling crisis. She was unable to utter a complete sentence; she looked terrified and enraged.

Fortunately, the therapist was able to remember that shortly after Ms. A.'s admission to the hospital at the time of her severed artery, while she was barely able to maintain consciousness, a miscommunication had led the staff to think that her accident had been a suicide attempt. Soon thereafter, staff members were taking over all "judgment calls" regarding her care, including certain steps that violated her deeply held and highly valued religious convictions. She was terrified and near death, but mostly focused on how these people who should be helping her were taking over her most precious possession—her autonomy and right to have her views heard and respected. It was this affect state and object configuration—having her voice ignored in the presence of personal crisis—that was the centerpiece of her reaction, rather than the more expectable terror of near-death. The poignant part of the trauma that was reenacted was close to, but not synchronous with, the point of maximum danger to her life. On this occasion, helping the patient to understand the meaning of her anniversary reaction (i.e., the fear of having her voice taken away), together with the knowledge that now in the present she did have options, was sufficient to remedy the emergency regression. Later in the chapter, I discuss an initially hidden transference component to this affective reenactment.

Similarly, Mrs. C. did not present with an affect state easily recognizable as a delayed grief reaction, but rather an overactive, overcontrolling coping mode of watching out for the needs of others. Mrs. C., a health care worker and mother of four, was suffering from extreme depression (suicidal) and PTSD; however, she refused to give up her many overcommitments to caring for bereaved children and parents, as well as her own family. Mrs. C. had lost her youngest child, a neurologically damaged 5-year-old, in a pulmonary-related sudden death 2 years earlier. She had failed, she believed, to pay enough attention to the child's pulmonary distress, and chose instead to listen to her pediatrician, whom she heard telling her not to worry so much. At the time that her child stopped breathing, she chose to complete the laundry—a task that seemed more pressing. In the years following this tragedy, it was not so much the affect of loss and grief that became fixed in Mrs. C.'s psychological state; rather, it was the hypervigilant coping state that she put in place following the death.

It was in this state that Mrs. C. confronted her doctor. Although she seemed desperate to begin her treatment experience, she canceled appointments and even signed out of the emergency room in order to tend to apparently minor illnesses of her children. Because she unconsciously thought that remaining busy in the act of bringing help to others or watching for their safety would atone for her misdeed and prevent a recurrence of her tragic loss, Mrs. C. could not attend to her own needs; it was safer for her to overextend herself by watching out for others. Thus she was trapped in the task of meeting ever-increasing demands to take care of more and more needy people. Piecing together and making explicit to the patient the nature of this coping response through unconscious reenactment helped get the treatment started. Once again, transference and countertransference were important: Mrs. C. ran from the doctor even before she saw him, and the doctor felt angry with Mrs. C. even before the treatment began. And, again, I return to these elements in this case later in the chapter.

DEPTH OF THE TRAUMA RESPONSE

Persistent points of condensation of affect in the traumatic narrative may suggest traumas in addition to the one of which the therapist is aware. Ms. K., a quite competent middle management executive who had been raped 15 years previously, was panic-stricken when a senior member of her firm forced himself on her while intoxicated at a company party. The incident involved his thrusting himself against her pelvis as she stood against the wall in a crowded room. Her reaction was severe. Knowing that her PTSD from the rape had been activated, she made an appointment to see a trauma specialist. But after a safe and promising beginning, as Ms. K. started to describe her rape, she was both terrified and unable to speak. The silence was a horrifying one. Ms. K. appeared in agony, with her mouth and face contorted; there was a pleading mixed with horror in that expression. But she could form no words. This state lasted several minutes. Later in the therapy, she was able to relate that the rape had occurred near an amusement park, where she had been pulled into an alley and told she would be killed with a knife if she made any sound that might arouse suspision. She attempted to scream nonetheless, but the rapists stuffed cloth in her mouth and throat and attacked her more brutally. Her effort to bring help through words had not only failed; it had caused greater suffering.

At a subsequent interview, the phenomenon repeated itself: The patient was terrified, grimacing, and (at first) silent, but this time the silence was broken with gutteral efforts to verbalize that were not comprehensible. As her trust in her doctor increased over time, she was able to say that this episode reflected an even more terrifying rape/torture that occurred about 2 years after the first experience. Her captors, taking her to a remote site, had insisted that she cry aloud to meet their sadistic urges. Caught in the double bind of the previous trauma, Ms. K. could neither cry nor not cry—a circumstance she repeated with her therapist. Of course, much work in the therapeutic relationship was necessary to allow this narrative to take form. In her repeated efforts to tell and reenact the trauma, the therapist had initially been seen as a cold and unresponsive police officer, an ineffective administrator, and a persecutor. But gradually she came to see the therapist in the same way she saw the sister of childhood with whom she had gone through so much, and the friends in the present who were of such support. Ms. K. continued to be hopeful in her courageous effort to share her trauma with someone who might understand, and to perceive the therapist as a rational and humane presence with whom to bear witness to her trauma.

Ms. J., a single laboratory specialist at an industrial plant, suffered from severe PTSD following an explosion in her plant that killed several people and badly injured several of her friends. In contrast to others badly affected by the explosion, who sought help early, Ms. J. denied that she was having difficulty; she finally agreed to see someone only after reports of episodes of isolating herself from others at work and crying while she was alone reached her supervisors. These reports warranted attention from the company medical officer. During the delay, she had avoided any contact with the others who were terrified by the explosion, feeling that she was quite alone in her suffering. Her crying spells finally interrupted her efforts to pretend that nothing had happened. In recounting the traumatic experience and the circumstances surrounding it to her therapist, Ms. J. focused frequently on her great shame that attention should come to her, her feeling that she had not behaved courageously, and her fear that somehow she had done something wrong; she even irrationally worried that she had made some mistake in the lab to bring on the explosion itself.

A little later, Ms. J. reported a specific symptom of dropping a test tube with her right hand. The symptom repeated itself, especially when she was expecting a chemical reaction to take place. After a neurological evaluation was negative, her doctor suggested that the symptom might condense an earlier trauma. The warm exploding cylinder in her hand became then an inroad to multiple childhood incest experiences, which most often involved her being forced to masturbate her stepfather. The incest history had left Ms. J. with trauma, which then superimposed itself upon the trauma in adulthood at the chemical plant. In particular, her shame, her feeling isolated in her suffering, her feelings of complicity in terrible happenings, and her feeling guilty for casting blame on those at fault all came from the earlier trauma, without which she and her therapist could not understand the special configuration of her reaction to the adult trauma. The dominant transference configuration in this treatment was one of testing the therapist as to her convictions in the case versus her possible meekness; Ms. J. equated weakness with her mother, who understood the incest but was too frightened to live with the consequences of its exposure.

The discovery of earlier childhood trauma in an individual with multiple adult traumas sometimes also gives important clues as to why the adult trauma seems to be precipitating its particular pathological picture. In the following case of a Vietnam veteran, it was unclear why the trauma of the war (which had occurred during the patient's late adolescence) was also taking the form of a dissociative identity disorder. Mr. F., a creative toolmaker and father of one, had a most refractory form of PTSD following his experiences as a demolition expert in Vietnam. For many months, his treatment uncovered one layer after another of previously repressed memories of his Vietnam experience. Usually the work began with a dream fragment or a recurrent intrusive sound, sensation, or fragment of an image. Gradually the missing pieces formed more comprehensive memories including examining dead bodies (American especially) on which the Vietcong might have set booby traps; exploding a live bomb inside a soldier who was still alive (it was impossible to dislodge it without setting it off); plowing a field full of bodies; and designing devices that would explode in enemy hands. Yet certain dissociative tendencies that continued in the present remained puzzling.

It was actually an event in the transference that set off an early childhood memory of trauma, which was evidently a precursor of the later ones. As Mr. F. began his session on this day, the doctor, aware that he was running late in his schedule, noted that the patient's usually friendly demeanor was rough and sullen. The doctor also remembered that at the preceding appointment Mr. F. had been late, and so he had taken another patient early. The doctor explored with Mr. F. his reaction to this situation of being "sandwiched in." Did it make him feel roughed up and sullen? "Yes, like the times my older brothers would sandwich me between them and bugger me. It was so painful and I felt so humiliated and helpless. But they wouldn't get to me; no, I would turn into someone else, a fierce fighter." In retrospect this was the beginning of the patient's tendency to develop several split-off ego states, which returned in Vietnam. It helped account for the dissociated memories, in that different ones were stored in different ego states.

TIMING OF TRAUMA INTERPRETATIONS

The art of trauma therapy often lies in knowing when to search for missing pieces, in the hope that their inclusion and understanding will build a comprehensible picture for the survivor that makes sense of the memory; when to respect the need to keep traumatic details of memories away from consciousness; and how to accomplish this differentiation while providing hope that meaning and mastery are goals worth the pain of pursuing. Are there any guidelines regarding when and to what degree we as therapists should make our understanding of trauma survivors' experience explicit to them?

In the cases described above, long periods of work took place in which the therapists remained silent with regard to their understanding of the details of trauma experiences. Ms. J., the laboratory specialist, required a lengthy period to build trust in regard to her acknowledged adult trauma. This was especially true when she felt alone, alienated, and numb. The symptom of dropping the test tube actually occurred in a period of relative psychological recovery, with an improvement in her relationships and energy. She was curious about the symptom and was conscientious about getting a neurological workup. In short, during this period of consolidation, a single symptom seemed to have intrusive qualities that, if understood correctly, would help considerably in understanding the larger clinical picture.

Mrs. C., the health care worker whose young son had died, was in an acute crisis of suicidal proportions and seemed unable to get a handle on it. Her reenactments were occurring so rapidly and in such a disguised form that she felt there was no understanding the torrent around her. Interpretation of a trauma-related coping pattern was made, along with a prescription for antidepressant medication, simply to settle down a clinical situation that was spiraling out of control. The interpretation here became necessary because the patient's unconscious reenactments were preventing the possibility of developing a working alliance.

Ms. A., in the midst of her disorganization at the second anniversary of the severing of her artery, combined a number of the features of the preceding two cases. A long period of alliance building was already present. The presence of sudden intrusive phenomena against this background of a good alliance indicated that interpretation would probably be useful.

Mr. F., on the other hand, was the person to make his own revelation of childhood trauma. Here, the therapist was simply following the intensely negative affect being directed at him in the transference.

TRANSFERENCE AND COUNTERTRANSFERENCE

Finally, I should comment on some of the transference and countertransference aspects of cases in which dramatic reenactments occur well into the treatment. In other words, is there some aspect of the here-and-now situation with the therapist that is unwittingly precipitating the configuration of the traumatic event, and which, if understood, would aid in the working through of the trauma? Let us first return to Ms. A., the woman who nearly died from a lacerated artery and became terrified and nearly mute during a reenactment in the course of therapy. From a transference perspective, Ms. A. was tense not only because of the letter from her attorney about her landlord, but because she had been unable to pay her bill to the doctor. She felt guilty about this, but had no way of raising the funds without pressing her attorney for a settlement on the case. Forcefulness (she had forced open the glass door that nearly killed her) was a dangerous state of mind. Now, she believed, her doctor was requiring her to be too forceful; the result would be catastrophic, as with the accident. Deciphering the here-and-now configuration of the trauma, in which the therapist was unwittingly participating in a negative role, provided an opportunity for a new solution and potential mastery.

Mrs. C. immediately placed her doctor in the transference role of the harsh, judgmental mother of childhood, who (although she was dead at the time of Mrs. C.'s son's death) would certainly have criticized her mercilessly for failing to attend to her neurologically impaired child. Thus the initial efforts to make any intervention in the case, particularly her former therapist's effort to get her hospitalized, backfired. On the other hand, the patient's dismissal of advice while persevering in a self-destructive manner, and her missing appointments while in such terrible need, tended to provoke a rejecting countertransference. The therapist found himself angry when he hardly even knew the patient. When the therapist was able to identify his countertransference anger within the trauma context, as a split-off and projected superego punishing the patient for not saving her child, he was able to see her cancellations as related to a traumatic reenactment in which she was to be punished. Given this understanding within the trauma context, her hostility could be seen more centrally not as an attack on the therapist, but as a plaintive cry for help.

SUMMARY OF TECHNICAL PRINCIPLES

The cases described in this chapter serve to provide some guidelines with regard to the indications of when to reconstruct trauma narratives in the treatment. The following points appear important:

1. Trauma reconstructions should occur when intrusive rather than numbing aspects of the PTSD are present.
2. Under ideal circumstances, the alliance should be strong and the general transference positive; the intrusion should be limited and should be occurring in the context of a generally improving clinical condition.
3. However, when the therapist is faced with a rapidly deteriorating clinical situation in which there is a significant negative component to the trans-

ference, reconstruction of trauma can provide a new temporary structure around which ego functions can be consolidated rather than fragmented and an alliance has the opportunity to develop.

These cases also provide some guidelines in regard to the question of how to reconstruct trauma. The following points are central:

1. It is the therapist's task to keep as empathically in contact with the patient in the here and now as possible, including strong feelings directed toward the place or person of the therapist.
2. The therapist, through introspection, should use words to describe feelings in the here and now that can also be applied to the there and then of the trauma. However, it is the patient who should make the reconstruction of the memory, not the doctor.
3. Repetitions in the present, in which the therapist has struggled internally to find words that express anguished meaning, provide an open door for the survivor to find better words to describe his or her uniquely traumatizing events of the past.

REFERENCES

Green, B. L., Grace, M. C., & Geser, C. G. (1985). Identifying survivors at risk: Long-term impairment following the Beverly Hills Supper Club fire. *Journal of Consulting and Clinical Psychology, 53*, 672–678.

Green, B. L., Grace, M. C., Lindy, J. D., Glazer, G., & Leonard, A. (1990a). Risk factors for PTSD and other diagnoses in a general sample of Vietnam veterans. *American Journal of Psychiatry, 147*, 729–733.

Green, B. L., Lindy, J. D., Grace, M. C., Glazer, G., Leonard, A., Korol, M., & Windget, C. (1990b). Buffalo Creek survivors in the second decade: Stability of stress symptoms. *American Journal of Psychiatry, 60*, 45–54.

Honig, R., Grace, M. C., Lindy, J. D., Newman, J., & Titchener, J. (1993). Portraits of survival: A twenty-year follow-up of the children of Buffalo Creek. *Psychoanalytic Study of the Child, 48*, 327–355.

Janet, P. (1889). *L'automatisme psychologique.* Paris: Ballière.

Lindy, J. D. (1989). Transference and posttraumatic stress disorder. *Journal of the American Academy of Psychoanalysis, 17*(3), 415–426.

Lindy, J. D., Green, B. L., Grace, M., & Titchener, J. (1983, October). Psychotherapy with survivors of Beverly Hills fire. *American Journal of Psychotherapy, 37*(4), 593–610.

Lindy, J. D., with MacLeod, J., Spitz, L., Green, B., & Grace, M. (1989). *Vietnam: A casebook.* New York: Brunner/Mazel.

Lindy, J. D., Spitz, L., & Moss, F. (1995). The posttraumatic patient. In E. Schwartz, E. Bleiberg, & S. Weissman (Eds.), *Psychodynamic concepts in general psychiatry* (pp. 263–278). Washington, DC: American Psychiatric Press.

CHAPTER 25

The Therapeutic Environment and New Explorations in the Treatment of Posttraumatic Stress Disorder

STUART W. TURNER
ALEXANDER C. McFARLANE
BESSEL A. VAN DER KOLK

Helping people who develop posttraumatic stress disorder (PTSD) in the aftermath of a traumatic experience is a complex process that cannot simply be described like a cookbook recipe. This chapter explores elements of treatment not discussed in the other chapters in this section, which focus on specific treatment approaches and techniques. Central to the process of treatment are the ways in which an individual comes to engage in therapy and is held within the subsequent therapeutic relationship. Prospective patients may have to struggle with their need for help; this entails acknowledging their dependence and overcoming their fear of confronting their shame and pain, as well as their fears of being humiliated as they acknowledge their grief and helplessness. Therapists have to cope with the challenge of being constantly confronted with the horrendous experiences that can befall people, and with the sense of disinte-

The section on countertransference in this chapter is adapted from van der Kolk (1994). Copyright 1994 by The Guilford Press. Adapted by permission.

gration and despair that these experiences can bring. In this chapter we explore the steps involved in the treatment-seeking process, as well as the feelings invoked in the therapist who tries to manage dealing with traumatized individuals. Finally, the desire to help traumatized individuals has motivated the exploration of several approaches that have not yet been subjected to systematic scientific scrutiny. These methods are based either on common sense or on novel ways of approaching the process of treatment. This chapter aims to examine these approaches and the ways in which they interrelate with, or supplement, conventional treatments.

Traumatic experiences present victims with the inescapable truth that reality can damage their sense of safety and trust. In order to sustain a sense of hope in the face of such an external onslaught, a person has to have a sufficiently enduring sense of identity and interpersonal connectedness. The ability to tolerate the truth of the traumatic experience involves a capacity to bear pain in the presence of another human being; this constitutes the core of mature intimacy.

THE TOLERANCE OF INTIMACY: A CRITICAL DETERMINANT OF ADAPTATION AND TREATMENT OUTCOME

Reestablishing a sense of personal safety and equilibrium is a primary goal of all treatment. This is generally grounded on the perceived safety of the patient–therapist relationship, which is the cornerstone of the therapeutic alliance. The success of treatment depends on the patient's ability to tolerate intimacy—in other words, on the patients capacity to trust another person with his or her helplessness and pain. Independent of the trauma that brings an individual to treatment, different people have different capacities to tolerate such intimacy. This ability is an important determinant not only of the success of treatment, but also of the individual's initial reaction to the trauma.

Intimacy involves a capacity to relate to oneself and others in a modulated and open manner. This potential for intimacy is primarily an ability to tolerate one's inner world and the contradictions it presents. Withdrawal from intimacy in personal relationships is one of the more enduring effects of trauma. This makes it particularly important to understand the role of intimacy in the therapeutic relationship. Many relationships are built on patterns of intimacy that are based on the partners' unspoken promise to validate each other by sharing a set of common assumptions and beliefs. This type of intimacy is based on asserting the similarities in the partners' concepts of each other and the world, rather than exploring the differences. This lack of differentiation depends on avoiding points of conflict and incompatibility. The lack of exploration of significant differences between the partners in a relationship imposes a pseudomutuality. More mature relationships depend on the partners' ability to focus on and explore differences between them; this involves a tolerance of differentiation and conflict. Thus, mature relationships, including therapeutic relationships, do not merely validate the partners. They also confront individual differences and points of conflict, and this confrontation keeps in motion a continual process of growth and exploration.

People's personal realities are to a large degree defined by the accumulation of their interpersonal connections. The ability to tolerate closeness with another person is largely defined by the capacity to negotiate the coexistence of the other's diverse realities. There are significant similarities between a person's ability to tolerate interpersonal intimacy and the capacity to tolerate the challenges to cherished beliefs that follow a traumatic event. Maturity involves people's capacity to withstand challenges to their most cherished beliefs and aspirations. If a traumatized individual is to integrate the trauma successfully, the internal dialogue following the experience requires the same types of adjustments that occur in mature relationships. Reiker and Carmen (1986) have pointed out that "confrontations with violence challenge one's most basic assumptions about the self as invulnerable and intrinsically worthy, and about the world as orderly and just. After abuse, the victim's view of self and world can never be the same again: it must be reconstructed to incorporate the abuse experience" (p. 367).

FACTORS INFLUENCING THE CHOICE AND DEVELOPMENT OF TREATMENT APPROACHES

Whereas the previous chapters on treatment have discussed either treatment outcome research results or well-established clinical wisdom, the daily practice of treating patients who suffer from trauma-related disorders entails many elements that cannot be captured by either randomized clinical trials or systematic treatment protocols. Much of the treatment of victims of trauma is intuitive; it depends on both a sensitive understanding of the unique issues that make every individual different from all others, and clinical knowledge about the accurate timing of appropriate interventions. What occurs between a patient and a therapist is a function not only of the particular diagnosis of the patient, but also of the unique and personal relationship between patient and therapist. Despite the fact that the nature of the therapeutic relationship and the appropriate timing of interventions form the backbone of all treatment, these factors cannot be easily quantified, and probably can never be satisfactorily studied with acceptable scientific methodology.

Because so many elements of the treatment of a traumatized individual are a function of the individual peculiarities of both patient and therapist, and because a traumatized patient is so vulnerable to being revictimized in the therapeutic relationship, it is critical for the therapist continually to take stock of the safety of the relationship and the patient's progress in accomplishing the goals he or she has set out to accomplish. Because there are no clear guidelines about the best way to approach each individual patient, therapists often find themselves faced with a desire to act without having a firmly established canon of knowledge to tell them what to do. This sometimes leads to an uneasy conflict between the desire to know and the desire to help.

Traditionally, most psychotherapeutic approaches have developed as the result of the teachings of particular individuals who have set up schools of theoretical and therapeutic approaches. These individuals and their pupils have generally become partisan advocates of particular treatment approaches, for which there has rarely been much empirical support. In studies where various treatment modalities have been compared for their efficacy (e.g., Strupp & Hadley, 1979), effective therapies have been those in which patients are encouraged to make meaning of their life experiences and in which they feel personally supported by their therapists. The field of traumatic stress has been fortunate to have had a number of thorough investigations into treatment efficacy, which have been discussed in previous chapters. When treating patients with PTSD, clinicians are faced with unique problems regarding physiological stabilization and processing of traumatic memories; various approaches to these problems have been proposed, but only pharmacological approaches, cognitive-behavioral treatment, and eye movement desensitization and reprocessing (EMDR) have been subjected to careful clinical trials. In recent years a number of innovative therapies have been proposed, which, like most new therapies, have been accompanied by unqualified claims of success. Over time, it is critical for these new therapies to be subjected to scientific scrutiny, and some efforts to do so are currently underway (e.g., Figley, 1996). Lewis Thomas said about research: "You either have science, or you don't, and if you have it you are obliged to accept the surprising and disturbing pieces of information, even the overwhelming and upsetting ones, along with the neat and useful bits. It is like that" (quoted in Andrews, 1991). Thus, clinicians always need to be open to examining the results of their therapeutic interventions, and to adjusting their methods, without becoming paralyzed by therapeutic nihilism.

As we have discussed throughout this volume, traumatized individuals, with their histories of helplessness and confusion, are vulnerable to being retraumatized, particularly at the hands of people who are intended to be their caregivers. This includes revictimization by unscrupulous or poorly trained therapists. Historically, societies have always recognized the need to protect the infirm from the exploitation of hope and the rash promises of charlatans: The oldest known written laws, which were inscribed in Babylon, enshrined at length the need to protect patients from medical malpractice. Today, professional boards of registration and restrictions on the advertising of treatments are testaments to the need to safeguard the vulnerability and suggestibility of the sick.

The expectation in medicine is that any new pharmacological treatment should be examined in placebo-controlled trials before the agent can be marketed. The same criterion cannot necessarily be applied to psychosocial interventions, in which the nature of the relationship and the establishment of therapeutic rapport are vital but often elusive therapeutic elements. Yet measuring treatment outcome is critical. The history of psychiatry is littered with treatments that were advocated with great enthusiasm by their inventors, but that ultimately were found to have little or no enduring value beyond their nonspecific effects of instilling hope and providing nonjudgmental support. In the current environment of increasing scrutiny of the health care budget, novel and unconventional treatments are barred from reimbursement.

The power of the placebo effect is one of the ironies that have to be dealt with in the desire to prove the effectiveness of new treatments. In drug studies, up to 40% of subjects may be placebo responders. This means that there has to be a powerful therapeutic effect before a treatment is of proven benefit (Jackson, 1992), and that the placebo effect is actually one of the most powerful treatments in the therapeutic arsenal. It is important not to scoff at the placebo response, but rather to maximize its potential and usefulness. It is possible that the strength of the placebo response accounts for the power of some of the less conventional forms of psychotherapy. The conviction with which these forms are practiced may maximize people's natural capacity for healing. The problem lies with the equally natural propensity of helpless humans to ascribe extraordinary powers to other humans. This promotes loyalty to people (gurus), the advocates of a particular form of treatment, rather than to the facts. This may be the basis of the historical tendency of psychiatry to be organized around theoretical schools named after particular individuals, rather than based on empirical observations.

THE TRANSITION FROM "VICTIM" TO "PATIENT"

The process of entering and maintaining a treatment relationship is always extraordinarily complex. However, it becomes even more so when a patient has been humiliated, hurt, and betrayed, often by people on whom the patient counted to provide safety and protection. When the treatment outcome literature discusses the differences in outcome between groups of patients, it rarely addresses the complexity of the therapeutic interaction, and hence seldom fully deals with the issue of why a particular approach works with one patient and not with the next.

Many of the issues that influence the patient–therapist relationship are played out in the struggle a patient goes through in making the decision to seek treatment. Reiker and Carmen (1986) describe this struggle as the "victim-to-patient process." Two stages exist in this process: In order for a patient to enter treatment, he or she must first come to consider himself or herself as "sick," and then make the decision to seek treatment and enter the patient role (see Chapter 5, this volume). The first step is for the individual to accept and acknowledge his or her distress as both something that is highly unpleasant and something that can be helped. Even in cases when victims' distress dominates their daily lives, disrupts their relationships, and interferes with their capacity to attend to what needs to be done, they are likely to put up with it as long as they see their distress as a natural reaction of their exposure to an abnormal situation. The setting in which a trauma occurs may play an important role in whether people will tolerate their suffering. In wars, and in disasters where many people are killed and there is extensive property loss, the threshold for suffering is especially high. Complaint tends to be less restrained following individual accidents, particularly if financial compensation is involved.

To complain is a threat to oneself and to others. It sets an individual apart from those who are undamaged, and it can undermine the person's sense of self-control; thus, becoming a complainer may reinforce the sense of feeling sick and damaged. Willingness to accept an illness role is influenced by a variety of individual, situational, social, and cultural factors. When professionals plan a treatment service for a group of victims, these factors need to be taken into account. For example, the point at which individuals are most willing to acknowledge their suffering will depend on the type of traumatic event they have experienced. In one study of a brief trauma (Weisaeth, 1989), the worst time for the majority of victims was the first night after exposure and the following day. On the other hand, the first reaction after a prolonged trauma may consist of euphoria (a "honeymoon" period), with a sense of lessening or even absence of distress.

The second hurdle is for the traumatized person to admit that he or she cannot resolve the problem alone and needs help. Again, various social and cultural factors will influence whether and how it is acceptable to seek treatment. Ultimately, the individual's decision will be determined by whether the distress and despair outweigh the fear of being misunderstood, humiliated, or retraumatized. Often information about these questions is obtained from other victims who have sought treatment. Informal networks have a powerful influence on treatment seeking.

BARRIERS TO SUCCESSFUL TREATMENT

Avoidance

The suffering caused by recurrent intrusive memories, combined with hyperarousal symptoms, tends to be a powerful motivation to seek treatment. Paradoxically, numbing and withdrawal cause major disruptions in a traumatized individual's lifestyle, but also act as significant deterrents to acknowledging a need for treatment. Most traumatic experiences are associated with feelings of shame and guilt, which are important barriers to seeking treatment. The importance of shame is illustrated by a study showing that asylum seekers who had been sexually tortured had more pronounced avoidance reactions than victims of other forms of organized state violence, such as physical torture (Ramsay, Gorst-Unsworth, & Turner, 1993). When shame dominates, victims are likely to disclose the most traumatic experience only late in the course of treatment.

Weisaeth's (1989) study of a factory explosion and fire tracked down an entire group of exposed victims. Those with the most severe posttraumatic reactions were the most reluctant to become involved in treatment. This avoidance of exploring their reactions to the disaster extended to a reluctance to present for routine health checks. In a large study of psychiatric outpatients, Sparr, Moffitt, and Ward (1993) found that people with PTSD and/or substance misuse were the most likely to miss appointments.

Alienation

Many victims experience a sense of alienation from others who have not shared the traumatic experience. This may be a powerful motivation to avoid professional help, and instead to seek out self-help groups. For example, 51% of a group of U.K. civilian Gulf War hostages reported feeling misunderstood by others (Easton & Turner, 1991). The same issue emerged more strongly in a study of a group of survivors of torture, where 86% reported described feeling misunderstood and 89% reported feeling different from other people (Gorst-Unsworth, Van Velsen, & Turner, 1993). Specialist health and legal professionals are not exempted from this pervasive feeling of distrust.

Personal Constructions

Although the acceptance of the definition of PTSD has led to legal and therapeutic validation for many victims, it has also been a source of confusion. The notion that an experience of trauma produces an illness that requires a medical diagnosis is an affront to many bystanders, as well as many survivors. The words "victim," "survivor," "patient," and "client" all have significant connotations about the relationship between the traumatized individual and the professionals he or she encounters. Who defines whether the person with a trauma experience is a victim or a survivor? Is this something that professionals do, or is it something that reflects the mental attitude and personal choice of the individual who has been traumatized?

There is an understandable desire to keep the trauma concept at the center of any understanding of the subsequent psychological reaction, and hence to regard a victim's response as entirely understandable within the framework of the *Diagnostic and Statistical Manual of Mental Disorders,* fourth edition (DSM-IV; American Psychiatric Association, 1994) and *International Classification of Diseases,* 10th revision (ICD-10; World Health Organization, 1992) criteria for PTSD. These criteria are unique in including a tightly defined psychological event as a requirement for the emergence of the disorder. However, scientific evidence suggests that there are significant person–event interactions (e.g., McFarlane, 1987), such as the issue of personal responsibility for what has happened. Any suggestion that part of the problem may be attributable to factors intrinsic to the victim becomes a problem in settings that advocate the rights and needs of victims. Many practitioners have found their own simplified ways of explaining posttraumatic reactions. Concepts such as a normal reaction to an abnormal event, or (probably better) a notion of a psychological "injury" rather than a disorder, are easy to explain—however inadequate they may be from a scientific point of view (see Chapter 18, this volume). So, in some circumstances, the conflict between advocacy and science may act as a barrier to engagement and treatment.

Political considerations may even result in a total rejection of an individual psychological model. For example, there is a strongly argued position that diagnosis may depoliticize issues such as state violence, and hence may devalue the fundamental issues of causation, impunity, and prevention (e.g., Martin-Baro, 1988). Similar arguments have been raised by the survivors of other forms of malicious violence, such as child sexual abuse and adult rape. These political conceptualizations present a challenge in medically oriented treatment settings. Following political violence, a therapist may be asked to demonstrate political beliefs compatible with those of a survivor; following sexual assault of a woman, treatment by a male therapist may be unacceptable. With the introduction in both DSM-IV and ICD-10 of acute stress syndromes, these difficulties may emerge earlier than before, and people with short-lived emotional reactions now are at risk of being labeled as "disordered." This may increase the likelihood of stigmatization.

Cultural Factors

Cultural factors (see Chapters 2 and 17, this volume) can have profound effects on the way in which trauma manifests itself. For example, one stereotype of an Englishman is that he possesses a "stiff upper lip," by which it is meant that he does not (or at least should not) show emotion, especially distress. Traditionally, this may be related to learning how to survive in private boarding schools (Cooper, 1993). Such stereotypes and cultural values have an impact on how both victims themselves, and the cultures within which they live, approach trauma. One Far East prisoner of war (during World War II) returned to the United Kingdom after the war; in the face of perceived rejection by his family, he threw himself into work and a relationship (marriage to a stranger within 3 weeks of his return). He only presented for treatment over 40 years later, following his retirement. Similar cultural reactions may be a significant factor elsewhere, especially in predominantly male communities from non-Western cultural and ethnic backgrounds. For example, a therapist working with a male survivor of torture from a Middle Eastern country found it impossible to utilize an interpreter, because the patient expected that he would cry. The treatment proceeded at a snail's pace, with a limited vocabulary, a dictionary, and much tolerance for ambiguity.

Working through interpreters can present many difficulties, especially with victims of torture. It may be hard to know whether the emotional inhibition shown by patients is the result of their reluctance to disclose their experience, their concern about the political content leaking back to their community through an interpreter, or their difficulty with raising distressing subjects in the presence of another person from their own community. These issues must be explored with both patients and interpreters (Turner, 1992). Operating in a cross-cultural setting also helps to illuminate the issue of cultural diversity. The field of traumatic stress is in dire need of studies that will elucidate cultural conceptualizations of PTSD and culturally based variations in the patterns of psychological reaction (e.g., Kinzie, 1985; Penk et al., 1989).

COMMON-SENSE AND NOVEL TREATMENT APPROACHES

Therapists who treat traumatized individuals need to have a range of therapeutic options at their disposal, and to be able to tailor these to the needs of individual patients. These therapists must specifically take into account such issues as avoidance and outreach, acceptance and tolerance, cultural appropriateness, safety and security, and instillation of hope. A trauma survivor may initially only disclose part of the story, or disclose none of what has happened at all. Accessibility, timing, and length of treatment are therefore important. Often it is not enough to wait passively for people to show up. Community agencies may have to use a variety of interventions to involve potential patients in treatment, such as critical incident stress debriefing, active outreach, a well-planned use of the mass media, and the distribution of leaflets.

Any approach designed to achieve maximal benefit must be both credible to the traumatized individual and flexible. Avoidance should be understood as a legitimate choice of the survivor, but also as a form of adaptation with potentially long-term negative consequences. Each individual has the right to balance treatment between arousal reduction and exposure-based approaches. Arousal reduction may be accomplished both by providing secure conditions and by prescribing medications that can help with sleep, startle, and generalized arousal (see Chapter 23).

The role of treatment should be considered in three domains (see Chapter 18). First, treatment needs to focus on stabilization—controlling and mastering physiological and biological stress reactions. The second focus of treatment is on helping the individual to process and come to terms with the horrifying, overwhelming experience. The importance of capturing the experience in its full range of representations goes beyond the person's simply remembering and reporting the verbal schemata. Treatment must address the somatosensory, emotional, and biological, as well as the cognitive, dimensions of experience.

The final focus of treatment is on helping the individual to reengage in his or her current life; this includes reestablishing personal efficacy and secure social connections. Group treatments may be of particular benefit in this. However, the actual value of these treatments has seldom been subjected to close scrutiny; furthermore, if they were to be examined for efficacy, there would be many methodological challenges to overcome in designing treatment trials.

Approaches to Establishing Safety and Stability

When the threat of recurrence of a trauma persists, the first step is to negotiate how the patient can achieve a state of greater safety. When it appears that the risk of further traumatization is ended, there may still be residual vulnerability if the traumatic circumstances should return. A supportive approach, including personal validation through acknowledging the reality of symptoms, is often of considerable help; the mere opportunity to disclose to another human being some part of one's experience can be enormously comforting.

As we have seen in Chapter 18, the first condition for effective treatment of patients with PTSD consists of establishing personal safety and stability (Herman, 1992). When they first come to the attention of mental health professionals, traumatized patients can be quite disorganized and suffer from irregular sleeping and eating habits. They may habitually dissociate under stress, engage in substance abuse, and exhibit various dangerous reenactment behaviors. The cognitive-behavioral treatment of patients with borderline personality disorder, as described by Marsha Linehan (1993), can be particularly helpful at this stage. Stabilization may need to include the following: attention to the patient's safety; the establishment of regular day and night rhythms, appropriate self-care (including adequate food and rest), and structuring of daily activities; the establishment of an "emotional emergency line" (people or institutions that the patient can reliably turn to in times of extreme distress); and the prescription of appropriate medications.

In addition, although many patients who suffer from PTSD may be competent in many areas of functioning, they sometimes exhibit poor judgment—particularly in unstructured situations that are reminiscent of their original traumas, and/or in which trust, aggression, or sexuality plays a significant role. Confronted with such situations, they may rely on dissociation as an ongoing way of coping with stress. It is therefore important to establish the triggers of any particular patient's irrational behaviors. Over time, the patient and therapist may come to understand these as representing fragmented traumatic re-experiences. These reliving experiences may or may not have visual flashback components; without these it is difficult to make a direct connection between the flashback and a particular traumatic event in the patient's life. In all this, it is critical for the therapist to help focus the patient on the facts of what is happening, and to bolster the patient's capacity to attend to the details of living while developing adequate problem-solving strategies.

Many therapists of patients with dissociative problems have found hypnotic techniques that use the metaphoric imagery of placing traumatic memories inside some imaginary "safe," "vault," or "box" helpful in fostering the containment of such memories. Additional hypnotic suggestions may be given for creating an imaginary "safe place," which may serve as a base from which the dissociated memories may be eventually approached (Brown & Fromm, 1986; Spiegel, 1989; van der Hart, van der Kolk, & Boon, 1996).

Approaches to Uncovering and Processing Traumatic Experiences

Direct Therapeutic Exposure

After relative stabilization has been achieved, patients with PTSD need to process their helplessness and dissociation through some form of direct therapeutic exposure. This is a critical element of posttraumatic therapy, since avoidance of traumatic triggers can lead to considerable impairment and to possible recurrence of posttraumatic helpless states. Direct therapeutic exposure is necessary to overcome learned helplessness, to integrate the traumatic experience as a personal event that belongs to the past, and to confer a sense of mastery. Direct therapeutic exposure may take many different forms, ranging from "helicopter ride therapy" for inpatient Vietnam veterans with war-related PTSD (Scurfield, Wong, & Zeerocah, 1992) to Outward Bound programs and "model mugging," to merely reimagining and learning to tolerate the memories of the trauma. What all these therapies have in common is the exposure of traumatized individuals to feared conditions in contexts where the individuals experience social bonding and some degree of personal control.

Hypnosis

Hypnosis is no longer a novel approach, but it represents one of the oldest and possibly one of the most effective ways of helping people revisit past trauma without becoming overwhelmed. Unfortunately, in the context of the "false memory" controversy (see Chapter 2), and of the confusion between what constitutes a valid therapeutic and a valid forensic approach, hypnosis has recently fallen into disrepute as an effective treatment of PTSD and related disorders. First systematically applied in World War I, abreaction (the dramatic reliving of traumatic events under hypnosis), coupled with psychotherapeutic processing of the recovered material, has been used with victims of child abuse and chronic PTSD (Putnam, 1992).

Hypnosis can serve several functions: (1) recovering dissociated or repressed traumatic material; (2) reconnecting missing affect with recalled material; and (3) transforming traumatic memories. It may provide a means of direct therapeutic exposure that allows the traumatic memory to become reasonably accessible. It may also be helpful in the psychogenic amnesia of PTSD (Spiegel & Cardeña, 1990; van der Hart, Brown, & Turco, 1990; Brown & Fromm, 1986). In addition, hypnosis can be used to help patients face and bear a traumatic experience by embedding it in a new context—for example, by dealing with issues such as guilt arising from false sense of personal responsibility at the time of the event. It is important for clinicians to have utter respect for the notion that traumatic memories are dissociated and "forgotten" because of the overwhelming emotions associated with them. Even when the excellent treatment techniques prescribed by Spiegel (1989) and Brown and Fromm (1986) are used, evoking traumatic memories under hypnosis may precipitate the unmodified reliving of traumatic experiences. Such "abreactions" are unlikely to produce any significant therapeutic benefit, and indeed may retraumatize patients. It is also important to be aware of the fact that memories that are recovered under hypnosis cannot be used as forensic evidence.

Alternating Movements and Completing the Story

In recent years several unusual and novel techniques have been proposed to assist in the integration of traumatic memories, including EMDR. We have already discussed EMDR in Chapter 18, but other forms of rhythmic alternating movements have recently been proposed for the treatment of intrusive recollections of traumatic events.

After an initial flurry of single-case reports and open studies, a number of systematic studies of EMDR have been conducted in recent years. Positive results have been found in at least four controlled studies (Shapiro, 1989; Wilson, Covi, Foster, & Silver, 1993; Wilson, Tinker, & Becker, in press; Vaughan, Wiese, Gold, & Tarrier, 1994), equivocal results in two studies (Boudewyns, Stwertka, Hyer, Albrecht, & Speer, 1993; Pitman et al., 1996a), and negative outcomes in two studies (Jensen, 1994; Sanderson & Carpenter, 1992). The equivocal and negative studies were conducted on very chronic populations; such patients have also proven resistant to pharmacological (e.g., van der Kolk et al., 1994) and cognitive-behavioral (Pitman et al., 1996b) interventions. In the EMDR studies with positive treatment outcomes, beneficial effects have particularly been demonstrated in the frequency and intensity of intrusive recollections, such as nightmares and flashbacks (e.g., Vaughan et al., 1994; Shapiro, 1995; Wilson et al., in press).

In a recent open treatment outcome comparison of novel techniques at Florida State University's Psychosocial Stress Research Program (Figley & Carbonell, 1995), EMDR was but one of several novel techniques that showed promise in helping people reduce the frequency and intensity of intrusive traumatic recollections. What is interesting about all these techniques is that patients are not required to spell out the entirety of their traumatic experiences in words in order to achieve a reduction in their PTSD scores. Thought Field Therapy (TFT; Callahan & Callahan, in press) is a procedure that claims to assist patients in reversing their disinclination to reach a certain clinical goal, and in accessing the sensations related to their traumatic stress not only cognitively, but also kinesthetically, emotionally, and physiologically. Similar claims have been made for visual/kinesthetic dissociation (V/KD; Koziey & McLeod, 1987), which is adapted from neurolinguistic programming and the methods of Milton Erickson. Erickson was a master at helping his clients recover lost memories, reframe (develop an alternate view of) their more troubling traumatic experiences, and thus achieve at least a significant reduction in traumatic stress (if not complete elimination of it). Like EMDR and TFT, V/KD is claimed to work in a very brief span of time to reduce subjective distress. The originators of these methods claim that the principal active ingredient in these new therapies involves enabling patients to experience their memories in a way that distances them from their original experiences. By doing so, the clients can view the experience from at least one additional vantage point, and as a result can change their current perspective and begin to make peace with the past (Figley, 1996).

The rationales provided for these treatments at this point tend to be largely untested post hoc hypotheses constructed to justify the methods. Figley (personal communication, 1996) argues that there are particular benefits because these novel treatments provide patients with a treatment setting where they have more control over the pace and process of treatment and do not have to verbalize the totality of their pain.

Group Psychotherapy Approaches

In the aftermath of traumatic stress, there is a primary need to affiliate and to repair damaged attachments. The principles of group treatment approaches to PTSD are discussed in Chapter 18; group treatment has been a primary vehicle for repair in many settings. Group psychotherapy as a form of treatment was born during World War II as a consequence of a shortage of clinicians and an overabundance of traumatized veterans. In the post-Vietnam era, "rap groups" were among the first formally acknowledged treatments for veterans, and provided much of the political impetus for the addition of PTSD to the DSM-III. Groups are also the core of many programs for survivors of abuse, because they provide opportunities for validation and reframing, which overcome the intense legacy of isolation left by many forms of abuse. Finally, groups provide a vehicle for the acknowledgment and sharing of the life challenges and stresses that often come to dominate the lives of PTSD sufferers as consequences of their symptoms and disability.

There are two general categories of group therapies for people who have been exposed to catastrophic trauma. The first category consists of trauma-focused groups, which encompass a variety of short-term and long-term approaches. Groups that fall into this category include (1) acute crisis intervention groups for people affected by the same traumatic experience, such as a natural disaster, the witnessing of a homicide, or a kidnapping; (2) homogeneous groups for people with a similar history of past trauma, such as childhood incest, Holocaust survival, war trauma, or hostage experiences; and (3) a large variety of self-help groups that define themselves according to the past traumas or symptoms of their members. In the second category of trauma groups—that is, long-term heterogeneous groups—the emphasis is less on the trauma itself, and more on the exploration of interpersonal reenactments and the personality changes that have occurred secondary to the traumatization (van der Kolk, 1993a).

What all these group modalities have in common is the provision of a "safe place" in which the keeping of secrets is possible, and further physical or sexual assaults are unacceptable. These groups provide a space in which members can give voice to their traumatic memories and create narratives of their trauma and its effects on them. Once the traumatic experiences have been located in time and place, people can begin to make distinctions between further life stresses and past trauma, and become able to decrease the impact of the trauma on current experience (van der Kolk, 1993b).

In recent years there has been a dramatic increase in self-help organizations for people with adult or childhood trauma. Their models of treatment and containment seem to address a spectrum of real psychological needs related to the long-term effects of repetitive traumatization. They provide people with a predictable structure for being in the company of like-minded individuals who share a meaningful cognitive frame for dealing with the residual sense of helplessness, shame, and secrecy. Many of these self-help groups focus on the development of "serenity," which can be understood both as a state of autonomic stability and as a sense of being at peace with one's surroundings. They teach that the way to gain this serenity is by developing "spiritual values"— in other words, new meaning systems that transcend daily concerns. They promote interdependence through (re)learning to trust, and through making contact and developing interpersonal commitments. By insuring the anonymity of their members, self-help groups provide a support network that attempts to circumvent the barriers people create to bolster their individual differences. This structure also helps to diminish the shame attached to traumatization and helplessness, which would otherwise perpetuate social isolation (van der Kolk, 1993a, 1993b). In these circles, it is said that "No pain is so devastating as the pain a person refuses to face and no suffering is so lasting as suffering left unacknowledged" (Cermak & Brown, 1982).

Spiritual and Religious Ceremonies

The search for meaning is a critical aspect of traumatized people's efforts to master their helplessness and sense of vulnerability. Professionals in the mental health area can take a constricted view of how people rebuild a sense of purpose and meaning when their assumptive world has been shattered and reconstructed around the images of the traumatic experience. Concepts such as fragmentation of awareness and conditioning, which are central to psychotherapy, do not address the spiritual and philosophical beliefs that are central to individual identity and motivation. These beliefs are also sustained by the cultural context and social fabric, which bind individuals in their social groups. These beliefs can be damaged in many traumas, but perhaps most destructively in interpersonal violence. For example, victims of torture suffer not only the ignominy of the destruction of the spirit, but also often the loss of their countries and cultures when they are forced to flee.

The role of religious leaders in the provision of religious ceremonies that address issues of forgiveness and create a rationale for suffering can provide a critical vehicle for recovery. Religion provides a historical lineage of human suffering and capacity for regeneration. Prayers, music, and icons provide a powerful sense of endurance, despite the repeated onslaughts of disaster and war; prayer and identification with the suffering of others can also provide a way forward. The importance of ceremony is important to capture in civilian memorials and rituals as well. The memorials for fallen soldiers and public acknowledgment of gratitude for people who gave their lives in war all create a sense of purpose for the bereaved and traumatized. The importance of the lack of such remembering as part of the healing process was all too clearly demonstrated by the often hostile or indifferent reception given to returning Vietnam veterans.

In multicultural societies, the importance of drawing on the healing customs of the past from various cultures can all too readily be forgotten. Reestablishing enduring links with the past can rebuild shattered assumptions. Wilson (1989) used these principles in designing a recovery program for Native Americans who were Vietnam veterans. Building social links with ethnic groups is critical in the stabilization of refugees. Including the leaders of such groups in the design and support of treatment programs often gives them an authority that can facilitate the involvement of individuals whose suspiciousness is a major barrier to care. The involvement of self-help group representatives and religious leaders in treatment programs is also important to creating a social and treatment environment that encourages integration.

Testimony

Finally, in working with survivors of state persecution and torture, a technique called "testimony" has been used and adapted widely (Cienfuegos & Monelli, 1983; Jensen & Agger, 1988; Agger, 1992/1994). Originally applied within a country with a strong Roman Catholic tradition of confession and trust in the confessor, under a regime in which systematic torture was widespread, it includes a strong political as well as a psychological component. It typically starts with one or two familiarization sessions, then continues with a detailed reconstruction of the events during torture. A tape recorder may be used to record the detailed history, and the typed transcript of the tape provides the starting point for the discussion in the subsequent session. A long document (possibly over 100 pages) is produced and worked through for accuracy. This is the property of the client and may be used for its political value as much as for its psychological meaning. The process appears to have two key beneficial effects. First, there is detailed exposure to memories and triggers related to the torture experience; thus, the criterion of direct therapeutic exposure is met. Second, there is inevitably a process of perceptual change, with the survivor coming to regard the events and his or her role within them in a different light. Going into the details of the event allows the survivor to confront not just the emotion but also the meaning of what happened. The therapist actively encourages a reframing of the trauma, especially in regard to such issues as apparent choice and subsequent guilt reactions. This cognitive element is likely to be at least as important as direct exposure in overall symptom reduction.

COUNTERTRANSFERENCE IN PTSD

Working with people who have been traumatized confronts therapists as well as patients with intense emotional experiences; it forces them to explore the darkest corners of the mind, and to face the entire spectrum of human glory and degradation. Sooner or later, those experiences have the potential to overwhelm therapists. The repeated exposure to their own vulnerability becomes too intense, the display of the infinite human capacity for cruelty too unbearable, the enactment of the trauma within the therapeutic relationship too terrifying.

The recognition of the wide variety of adaptations to traumatic life experiences makes it all too easy to resort to facile constructs. Facing trauma tempts therapists to split the world into uncomplicated realms of good and evil. But such simple distinctions can only be maintained at the cost of ignoring the complex issues of attachment, dominance, and competition—of the universal tendency to split the world into dichotomies of "us" versus "them," good versus evil. These issues are even more complicated with people who have been traumatized: Bizarre attachments may have developed between victims and perpetrators, victims and their helpers, and victims and the people they are supposed to care for, all of whom may get to play roles in a compulsive repetition of the trauma. There is a constant pressure on the people in victims' lives to help the victims reenact rather than remember the trauma; to give in to the frustration of being unable to help them engage and experiment with new challenges; and to get fed up with continually having to earn their fragile trust. How does a therapist help someone deal with the issue of taking responsibility for his or her life after the person has experienced that it is futile to take action? How does the therapist persuade such a person to agree to abide by the rules when the rules were made solely to gratify the whims of others?

The therapist must become the figure who personifies predictability and safety for the patient, as well as the person with whom the dimensions of control and ambivalence can be worked through. Idealization is a necessary component of this transaction, but so is the space to experience and explore disappointment, autonomy, and disagreement. This is the real challenge of intimacy. As Kohut (1977) has pointed out, idealization of a caregiver is necessary as long as a person is not capable of restoring internal homeostasis after being upset. Ideally, children gradually gain a feeling of control and autonomy as they gain mastery over their internal and external world. An increased sense of mastery allows for an increasingly realistic assessment of caregivers, and thus for the development of ambivalence. Trauma destroys this sense of mastery and throws a person back into a state where external sources are vitally needed to regulate internal emotional states. The need for deep attachments is proportional to the intensity of the victim's terror: When the trauma was inflicted by a human agent, particularly by a familiar person, the conflict between the need for external reassurance and the fear of revictimization becomes the central issue in the transference.

It is important for therapists to accept the fact that this need for idealization is not founded on their real attributes (which, in the anxiety to stay in control, patients often barely perceive), and that patients idealize them in order to replace the sources of security that were destroyed by the trauma. This need for security in patients is echoed in therapists' own needs—to be effective, to be good caregivers in contrast with evil perpetrators, and to have their help accepted and appreciated. Patients' passive dependence or stubborn inability to trust is mirrored in therapists' feelings of being powerless and incompetent. Patients' fragility and vulnerability is reflected in therapists' attempts to be perfect and in control. It is a tremendous strain on therapists to maintain an honest appraisal of their own capacities while tolerating their patients' intense need for rescue and constant scanning for imperfections. Only when both a patient and a therapist understand the etiology of these interactions—the traumatic past—can ambivalence and humor enter the therapeutic relationship. If the origins of this tenacious clinging and intolerance of flaws remain unaddressed, the therapy is likely to evolve into what Kohut (1977) called "transference bondage," in which the patient trades autonomy for safety.

Thus, idealization is a double-edged sword: It provides an illusory sense of safety, while preventing a person from taking autonomous action. Treatment must reach a stage where it provides more than validation by the therapist, and comes to include a tolerance of the conflicts and ambivalence that safety brings. If this does not happen, the patient will focus his or her energies on watching the therapist like a hawk and keeping the situation under control. PTSD patients' inability to establish an autonomous sense of security without resorting to withdrawal, sensation seeking, or substance abuse places tremendous demands on the therapists who become the patients' lifelines. As early as possible, each therapist and patient need to gain an understanding of how trauma-induced vulnerability sets the stage for the patient's exquisite sensitivity to specific actions and aspects of the therapist. Setting limits and establishing clear therapeutic contracts are essential to insure the safety of the therapeutic dyad. The therapeutic challenge is simultaneously to set limits and to keep open the exploration of aggressive feelings.

While therapists need to feel safe as well, they need to beware of their own needs to be comforted by their patients. After all, abusers often attempt to find solace in their victims as well, and find it at the victims' expense (see Chapter 9). Safety also does not consist of providing answers to the incomprehensible. Nor does the therapy of traumatized people consist of giving patients sage advice about how to live their lives; they are the survivors and often have skills that therapists can only marvel at. There is no way for therapists to guess how they themselves would have reacted to their patients' traumatic experiences. They can only help the patients recall the ways in which they once coped, help them understand how the trauma continues to get in their way, and assist them in exploring new options.

When the safety of relationships is threatened, people resort to the emergency responses of fight or flight. In traumatized patients it often does not take much to trigger these reactions, which may have been appropriate to being helpless children or traumatized adults, but which are not very helpful in the context of current reality (see Chapter 1). The threatened loss of a powerful protector will activate very primitive responses. At times, traumatized patients may see death as their only means of escaping an intolerable threat. In a study of traumatized borderline patients (Herman, Perry, & van der Kolk, 1989), many subjects specifically identified their therapists' reaction to suicide attempts and other self-destructive actions as critical in helping them gain a sense of autonomy: "Good therapists were the ones who helped me figure out how to control my behavior, rather than attempting to control me." Crises centering around issues of control are common and often inevitable in the treatment of trauma, and provoke shame, powerlessness, and longing for revenge in therapists. Yet often these crises will provide new building blocks for the capacity to tolerate ambivalence, which is essential for the restoration of a sense of autonomy. Only when patients and therapists learn to tolerate ambivalence will the patients become less clinging, and will their self-esteem (long sapped in the service of self-protection) be liberated and mobilized for action.

Clinicians have long noticed that before a patient can achieve autonomy, the safety of the therapeutic relationship first needs to be internalized. Research has confirmed that when a patient has not previously idealized another person, as occurs in cases of chronic neglect, it is virtually impossible to mobilize the trust necessary for eventual internalization and growth (van der Kolk, Perry, & Herman, 1991). Psychotherapy is a business that tries its practitioners' patience. The psychotherapy of frightened, paralyzed, angry, and secretive survivors of trauma requires the patience of saints. Since the schooling of psychotherapists rarely includes religious training, they may be personally ill prepared for this enterprise. Patience is quite incompatible with the intense feelings of helplessness, rage, rescue, and sadness that these patients evoke. Victims invite their therapists to violate some of the most basic tenets of psychotherapy, which are to suspend value judgments, to avoid moralizing, and to eschew therapeutic activism. The need to take a moral stance—to side actively with positive action, interpersonal connectedness, and empowerment—puts a great strain on the capacity to reflect and to help patients figure out how the trauma has affected their inner world and their ways of dealing with the world. The less therapists are in a position to address and explore the effects of trauma on perceptions and decision-making processes, the more they may be tempted to do something to take over control or to pass control on to outside parties. Therapeutic activism involves the danger of accepting the patients' helplessness as inevitable, and of taking over control where patients need to learn to establish control themselves. When this tack fails, as it usually does, the price for trying to run the patients' lives is abandonment.

Whether therapists prefer a behavioral or a psychodynamic approach, the work of therapy is an intensely intimate process. The goal of making thought rather than action the currency of the therapeutic process is extremely difficult to accomplish, in view of the fact that trauma-related thoughts and feelings bring back the intolerable affects that patients so carefully avoid—affects that, if countenanced to their full extent, may prove to be well-nigh unbearable for therapists as well.

REFERENCES

Agger, I. (1994). *The blue room: Trauma and testimony among refugee women. A psycho-social exploration* (M. Bille, Trans.). London: Zed Books. (Original work published 1992)

American Psychiatric Association. (1994). *Diagnostic and statistical manual of mental disorders* (4th ed.). Washington, DC: Author.

Andrews, G. (1991). The evaluation of psychotherapy. *Current Opinions in Psychiatry, 4,* 379–383.

Boudewyns, P. A., Stwertka, S. A., Hyer, L. E., Albrecht, J. W., & Speer, E. V. (1993). Eye movement desensitization and reprocessing: A pilot study. *The Behavior Therapist, 16,* 30–33.

Brown, D., & Fromm, E. (1986). *Hypnotherapy and hypnoanalysis.* Hillsdale, NJ: Erlbaum.

Callahan, R., & Callahan, J. (in press). Thought field therapy: An algorithm for eliminating the suffering of grief trauma. In C. R. Figley, B. Bride, & N. Mazza (Eds.), *Death and trauma.* London: Taylor & Francis.

Cermak, T. L., & Brown, S. (1982). Interactional group psychotherapy with adult children of alcoholics. *International Journal of Group Psychotherapy, 32,* 375–389.

Cienfuegos, A. J., & Monelli, C. (1983). The testimony of political repression as a therapeutic instrument. *American Journal of Orthopsychiatry, 53,* 43–51.

Cooper, R. (1993). *Death plus ten years.* London: HarperCollins.

Easton, J. A., & Turner, S. W. (1991). Detention of British citizens as hostages in the Gulf: Health, psychological, and family consequences. *British Medical Journal, 303,* 1231–1234.

Figley C. R. (1996). The death was traumatic to say the least! In K. Doka (Ed.), *Living with grief after sudden loss.* London: Taylor & Francis.

Figley, C. R., & Carbonell, J. (1995, March). *Treating PTSD: What works and what does not.* Paper presented at the Family Therapy Networker Symposium, Washington, DC.

Gorst-Unsworth, C., Van Velsen, C., & Turner, S. W. (1993). Prospective study of survivors of torture and organised violence: Examining the existential dilemma. *Journal of Nervous and Mental Disease, 181,* 263–264.

Herman, J. L. (1992) *Trauma and recovery.* New York: Basic Books.

Herman, J. L., Perry, J. C., & van der Kolk, B. A. (1989). Childhood trauma in borderline personality disorder. *American Journal of Psychiatry, 146,* 490–495.

Jackson, S. W. (1992). The listening healer in the history of psychological healing. *American Journal of Psychiatry, 149*(12), 1623–1632.

Jensen, J. A. (1994). An investigation of eye movement desensitization and reprocessing (EMDR) as a treatment for posttraumatic stress disorder (PTSD) symptoms of Vietnam combat veterans. *Behavior Therapy, 25,* 311–325.

Jensen, S. B., & Agger, I. (1988). The testimony method: The use of testimony as a psychotherapeutic tool in the treatment of traumatized refugees in Denmark. *Refugee Participation Network, 3,* 14–18.

Kinzie, J. D. (1985). Cultural aspects of psychiatric treatment with Indo-Chinese refugees. *American Journal of Social Psychiatry, 5,* 47–53.

Kohut, H. (1977). *The restoration of the self.* New York: International Universities Press.

Koziey, P. W., & McLeod, G. L. (1987). Visual–kinesthetic dissociation in treatment of victims of rape. *Professional Psychology: Research and Practice, 18*(3), 276–282.

Linehan, M. M. (1993). *Cognitive-behavioral treatment of borderline personality disorder.* New York: Guilford Press.

Martin-Baro, I. (1988). From dirty war to psychological war: The case of El Salvador. In A. Aron (Ed.), *Flight, exile and return: Mental health and the refugee.* San Francisco: Committee for Health Rights in Central America.

McFarlane, A. C. (1987). Life events and psychiatric disorder: The role of a natural disaster. *British Journal of Psychiatry, 151,* 326–367.

Penk, W. E., Robinowitz, R., Black, J., Dolan, M., Bell, W., Dorsett, D., Ames, M., & Noriega, L. (1989). Ethnicity: Post-traumatic stress disorder (PTSD) differences among black, white and Hispanic veterans who differ in degrees of exposure to combat in Vietnam. *Journal of Clinical Psychology, 45*(5), 729–735.

Pitman, R. K., Orr, S. P., Altman, B., Longpre, R. E., Poire, R. E., & Lasko, N. B. (1996a). *Emotional processing during eye-movement desensitization and reprocessing therapy of Vietnam veterans with chronic post-traumatic stress disorder.* Manuscript submitted for publication.

Pitman, R. K., Orr, S. P., Altman, B., Longpre, R. E., Poire, R. E., Macklin, M. L., Michaels, M., & Steketee, G. (1996b). *Emotional processing and outcome of imaginal flooding therapy in Vietnam veterans with chronic post-traumatic stress disorder.* Manuscript submitted for publication.

Putnam, F. W. (1992). Using hypnosis for therapeutic abreactions. *Psychiatric Medicine, 10*(1), 51–65.

Ramsey, R., Gorst-Unsworth, C., & Turner, S. W. (1993). Psychiatric morbidity in survivors of organised state violence including torture. *British Journal of Psychiatry, 162,* 55–59.

Reiker, P. P., & Carmen, E. H. (1986). The victim-to-patient process: The disconfirmation and transformation of abuse. *American Journal of Orthopsychiatry, 56,* 360–370.

Sanderson, A., & Carpenter, R. (1992). Eye movement desensitization versus image confrontation: A single session crossover study of 58 phobic subjects. *Journal of Behavior Therapy and Experimental Psychiatry, 23,* 269–275.

Scurfield, R. M., Wong, L. E., & Zeerocah, E. B. (1992). An evaluation of the impact of "helicopter ride therapy" for in-patient Vietnam veterans with war-related PTSD. *Military Medicine, 157*(2): 67–73.

Shapiro, F. (1989). Efficacy of the eye movement desensitization procedure in the treatment of traumatic memories. *Journal of Traumatic Stress, 2,* 199–223.

Shapiro, F. (1995). *Eye movement desensitization and reprocessing: Basic principles, protocols, and procedures.* New York: Guilford Press.

Sparr, L. F., Moffitt, M. C., & Ward, M. F. (1993). Missed psychiatric appointments: Who returns and who stays away. *American Journal of Psychiatry, 150*(5), 801–805.

Spiegel, D. (1989). Hypnosis in the treatment of victims of sexual abuse. *Psychiatric Clinics of North America, 12*(2): 295–305

Spiegel, D., & Cardeña, E. (1990). New uses of hypnosis in the treatment of post-traumatic stress disorder. *Journal of Clinical Psychiatry, 51*(Suppl.), 39–46.

Strupp, H. H., & Hadley, S. W. (1979). Specific versus non-specific factors in psychotherapy: A controlled study of outcome. *Archives of General Psychiatry, 36,* 1125–1136.

Turner, S. W. (1992). Therapeutic approaches with survivors of torture. In J. Kareem & R. Littlewood (Eds.), *Intercultural therapy* (pp. 163–174). Oxford: Blackwell.

van der Hart, O., Brown, P., & Turco, R. N. (1990). Hypnotherapy for traumatic grief: Janetian and modern approaches integrated. *American Journal of Clinical Hypnosis, 32*(4), 263–271.

van der Hart, O., van der Kolk, B. A., & Boon, S. (1996). The treatment of dissociative disorders. In J. D Bremner & C. R. Marmar (Eds.), *Trauma, memory and dissociation.* Washington, DC: American Psychiatric Press.

van der Kolk, B. A. (1993a). Group psychotherapy with posttraumatic stress disorders. In H. I. Kaplan & B. J. Sadock (Eds.), *Comprehensive textbook of group psychotherapy* (pp. 550–560). Baltimore: Williams & Wilkins.

van der Kolk, B. A. (1993b). The spectrum of group psychotherapies for catastrophic stress. In A. Alonso (Ed.), *Group psychotherapy in clinical practice* (pp. 289–309). Washington, DC: American Psychiatric Press.

van der Kolk, B. A. (1994). Foreword. In J. P. Wilson & J. D. Lindy (Eds.), *Countertransference in the treatment of PTSD* (pp. vii–xii). New York: Guilford Press.

van der Kolk, B. A., Michaels, M., Shera, D., Berkowitz, R., Fisler, R., & Saxe, G. (1994). Fluoxetine in post-traumatic stress disorder. *Journal of Clinical Psychiatry, 55,* 517–522.

van der Kolk, B. A., Perry, C., & Herman, J. L. (1991). Childhood origins of self-destructive behavior. *American Journal of Psychiatry, 148,* 1665–1671.

Vaughan, K., Wiese, M., Gold, R., & Tarrier, N. (1994). Eye movement desensitization: Symptom change in posttraumatic stress disorder. *British Journal of Psychiatry, 164,* 533–541.

Weisaeth, L. (1989). Importance of high response rates in traumatic stress research. *Acta Psychiatrica Scandinavica,* Suppl. 355, 131–137.

Wilson, D., Covi, W., Foster, S., & Silver, S. M. (1993, April). *Eye movement desensitization and reprocessing and ANS correlates in the treatment of PTSD.* Paper presented at the annual convention of the Calfornia Psychological Association, San Fransisco.

Wilson, J. P. (1989). *Trauma, transformation and healing.* New York: Brunner/Mazel.

Wilson, S. A., Tinker, R. H., & Becker, L. A. (in press). Efficacy of eye movement desensitization and reprocessing (EMDR). *Journal of Consulting and Clinical Psychology.*

World Health Organization. (1992). The *ICD-10 classification of mental and behavioural disorders.* Geneva: Atuhor.

Conclusions and Future Directions

ALEXANDER C. McFARLANE
BESSEL A. VAN DER KOLK

Do not go gentle into that good night . . .
Rage, rage against the dying of the light.
—DYLAN THOMAS (1953, p. 128)

In contemporary culture, the link between stress and illness has almost become a cliché. However, the complex ways in which organism and culture interact make it extremely difficult to define the exact nature of this relationship. The introduction of the diagnosis of posttraumatic stress disorder (PTSD) was an important steppingstone in helping to define how extreme environmental stress affects soma and psyche; it provided a framework for objective observation. The contents of this volume summarize the accumulated body of knowledge in this area of investigation, which is less than two decades old. During this short period, substantial advances have been made through the development of an impressive body of knowledge. This volume has provided the historical context of our recent knowledge, and has described how the study of traumatic stress is relevant to the discipline of psychiatry. The historical antecedents of contemporary studies demonstrate how fragile the unbiased study of trauma is: Various social and political factors have always interfered with honest scientific and clinical observations, usually without any awareness on the part of scientists and clinicians of what their prejudices were. Today, the same forces that have historically stood in the way of accurate scientific observation continue to exist. Our challenge is to identify the extent to which cultural prejudices continue to bias and distort our supposed truths. Future research needs to take into account not only our ignorance (what we know we do not know), but our biases (what we do not know we do not know).

MIND-BODY ISSUES

Many sociopolitical forces have shaped the study of traumatic stress. Society's responses to helplessness and victimization are at the very core of the body politic. The stakes are high for the numerous people who are ravaged by horrendous life experiences: Having caregivers who are able to grasp the impact of trauma on their lives and to respond appropriately can make the critical difference between recovering or succumbing. One of the issues that has negatively influenced the capacity of mainstream psychiatry to grasp the significance of traumatic stress in people's lives has been the nefarious persistence of a body–mind split. During the last few decades, psychiatry as a profession has made a concerted effort to make biologically based psychological problems "respectable." The basic, and seemingly logical, argument has been that people obviously cannot be held responsible for their afflictions if their problems are driven by faulty biological systems. Biologically based mental illnesses are not problems of daily living; they are real diseases, not normative adaptations to adverse life events. If people's brains are not wired properly, or if they suffer from a "chemical imbalance," they clearly cannot help the way they feel and behave. Their biology may prevent them from being able to make rational decisions, and hence decisions often need to be made for them by other people who are well trained and whose biology is not disturbed. Most likely, neurotransmitter supplements will be administered to compensate for the biological defects.

In contrast, the prevailing attitude to problems that seem to be psychologically based, such as individual reactions to terrible experiences, continues to be that their persistent reactions must be the result of a failure of courage, will, or "guts." If the problem is not biological, it is merely in people's heads; thus they should "get over it," "go on with their lives," and "stop looking back." People who merely suffer from mental problems are easily suspected of not *wanting* to function, or of trying to get something for nothing. Because so many traumatized individuals have trouble conforming their behavior to accepted social norms, and because many seem to lack the motivation to get their lives together, it is felt that they cannot expect society to compensate them for their problems. In regard to the controversies surrounding compensation, there is a surprising lack of curiosity in the psychiatric profession about what might make people willing to surrender control and mastery over their lives, in return for a pittance of financial assistance.

As documented in this volume, the study of psychological trauma shows that the Cartesian distinction between body and mind, and to some degree even between individual and society, is utterly untenable. We have tried to document that overwhelming social experiences can become indelibly etched in people's memories and set up a cascade of disturbances that can permanently alter their capacity to regulate their biological systems. This biological dysregulation, in turn, affects how these people think, feel, and act. The study of PTSD has shown that psychiatric problems cannot be easily reduced to their biological dimensions alone. However, the elucidation of the biological dimensions of PTSD has played an important role in defining it (Yehuda & McFarlane, 1995). In contrast to the original hypotheses about the disorder, PTSD does not exist on a continuum with the normative response to stressful life experiences (see Chapter 4, this volume). Several findings, such as those pertaining to hypothalamic–pituitary–adrenal axis abnormalities, suggest that PTSD has its own distinct neurobiology (see Chapter 10). The data related to the biology of PTSD will play an important role in defining the questions for future investigation. However, because of their apparent objectivity and validity, biological data have the potential to dominate the study of PTSD, just as they have done in the approach to other psychiatric disorders. It may be all too easy for us to make biological findings the metaphors for psychosocial models, and thus to disguise what we do not know.

The fact that psychosocial research is inevitably heavily influenced by the cultural and temporal context in which it occurs makes it a more fragile enterprise than research with a biological orientation. This makes it even more important to develop valid and reliable measures, while keeping in mind the degree to which findings can be generalized from one culture and victim population to another. For example, it is essential to interpret the findings from clinical samples with great care, because they inevitably do not represent a cross-section of the population. Epidemiological studies demonstrate that there is always a range of adaptations, and that both resilience and the detrimental effects of trauma are important issues to study. An excessive reliance on standardized research instruments, without attention to careful clinical observations, will lead to an increasingly constricted understanding of complex phenomena. The excessive use of such instruments will prematurely foreclose the discovery of new information and make the field a captive of the prevailing paradigms; in other words, we will tend to investigate in more and more detail what we know we know. The challenge is to value and explore the inconsistencies in our knowledge, rather than simply to confirm current definitions. This concern is further amplified by the intrusive nature of research and the vulnerable state of trauma victims. This makes it an important ethical issue to avoid simply investigating new traumas and disasters, without a clear understanding of how the expected findings will contribute to new knowledge.

Psychiatry's current reliance on phenomenological descriptions of psychopathology means that it no longer provides a conceptual basis for the traditional dynamic understanding of how the mind and the brain process information as a unit. The study of traumatic stress has become an important cultural carrier of this dynamic understanding of the relationship between current and past experience, and the relation betwen one's biology and one's way of making sense of the world. Understanding the role of trauma in people's lives is effective insurance against the tendency to rely purely on surface manifestations of mental disorders for making diagnoses and formulating treatment plans. The processing of traumatic experiences is highly individualistic, and cannot be easily captured with simple diagnostic labels. Although most of the biological underpinnings found in certain patient groups with PTSD are likely to occur in other traumatized populations as well, the ways in which any given individual adapts to his or her memories of trauma are a function of a myriad of factors: age at the time of the trauma, social support, temperament, intellectual endowment, previous life experience, societal meaning of the traumatic event, religious context, and so forth (van der Kolk et al., in press).

This complexity of both etiology and individual adaptation raises very challenging questions. The presumption behind the acceptance of PTSD is that a single disorder results from a variety of traumatic stressors, ranging from combat and rape to motor vehicle accidents. However, as we have shown, there is enormous variability in patterns of psychopathology among victims of trauma. Acute stress disorder, as defined in the fourth edition of the *Diagnostic and Statistical Manual of Mental Disorders* (DSM-IV; American Psychiatric Association, 1994), and personality change following exposure to extreme stress, as defined in the 10th revision of the *International Classification of Diseases* (ICD-10; World Health Organization, 1992), are the first two second-generation traumatic disorders to be accepted. The DSM-IV field trials for PTSD showed that there are further subtypes of reactions to traumatic stress that require independent recognition—for example, clinical presentations characterized predominantly by somatization, amnesia, and dissociative symptoms, as opposed to the conventional PTSD presentation, in which intrusions and hyperarousal are the primary features (van der Kolk et al., in press).

These different presentations of PTSD and other psychopathology following trauma require different treatment approaches, and evoke different responses from potential caregivers. If the principal issue here were merely that victims are haunted by the memories of their traumas, they would not be so troublesome to society. However, in many traumatized individuals, impairment of self-regulation causes a host of problems for themselves and those around them. Their problems in calming themselves down after being upset, and with quietly assessing what is happening and then making rational plans based on a sober evaluation of the facts, often make traumatized individuals difficult to deal with. Many victims tax our patience, our need for privacy, and our need to believe in the notion of a world that is essentially predictable and just. In fact, both the life histories and the current behaviors of victims often confront us with how irrational and unpredictable people can be.

Traumatized individuals challenge the limits of the human capacity for compassion. As long as misery occurs far away from home, we are generally able to muster considerable charity. For example, Mother Teresa regularly receives generous donations from people living in New York, just as freezing Kurds can count on substantial assistance from Swiss churches. In 1994 the U.S. Congress held hearings about the plight of the children exposed to violence in Sarajevo, but did not convene a hearing for the teenagers in its own neighborhood in the District of Columbia, who were exposed to as much daily violence as the children in Sarajevo. Prolonged misery next door seems to provoke a need to assign blame, as well as an urge to protect oneself from becoming contaminated.

NATURE AND NURTURE

Psychiatry has an important role to play in elucidating how the environment helps to shape people's psychological and biological makeup. Ever since investigators such as Jerome Kagan (1989) have shown the central role of temperament in determining people's adaptations to life, it has become obvious that the traditional literature has exaggerated the role of stressful life events in people's adjustment. This has contributed to the dismissal of the relevance of stress in people's makeup. However, the study of trauma has refocused the issue of the impact of reality on psychological, biological, and social systems, and has firmly established that exposure to overwhelming experience is an undisputed etiological factor in many psychological problems. One of the lessons learned is that there is a categorical difference between the impact of traumatic stressors and that of day-to-day life stresses. The life events field in the 1960s and 1970s did not make these categorical distinctions. In the discipline that studied stress as opposed to trauma, researchers assumed that stresses had cumulative effects, and did not take into account the fact that certain events were capable of breaking the human capacity to adapt appropriately.

For better or for worse, the concepts of traumatization have changed and have been progressively modified during the past century and a half. The study of trauma emerged from curiosity about whether the unexplainable physical symptoms seen in accident victims and hysterics could be attributed to physical or to psychic shocks to the system. Because these patients claimed to be helpless and suffered from strange symptoms that were amenable to suggestion, the genuineness of their complaints has always been the subject of vehement disputes, and they have always been suspected of malingering and of suffering from "compensation neuroses." The possibility of external causes of illness raises the thorny problem of blame and attribution. There are powerful financial and emotional reasons why finding a cause for an individual's illness could be welcomed, exaggerated, or rejected. This sets the stage for questioning not just the genuineness of these patients' symptoms, but also the significance of the traumatic events themselves.

These issues became central to the body politic during and after World War I, when there were heated debates about the nature of "shell-shock": Was it the effect of moral cowardice (the result of a combination of poor genes and bad child-rearing practices) or of the physical environment? Although poets such as Siegfried Sassoon and Wilfred Owen understood that it was the confrontation with horror, immobility, and helplessness that caused soldiers to have the same symptoms as hysterical women—memory loss, loss of speech, and loss of limb functions for no apparent reason (Barker, 1995)—psychiatrists had a great deal of difficulty giving up their medical models, and they continued to describe these men's problems as the results of either injury to brain tissue or hereditary inferiority. The emerging dominance of Freud's ideas about the pivotal role of infantile conflicts about sexuality in shaping people's responses to later stressful life events added further fuel to the fire. Testifying about the nature of war neuroses, Freud claimed (1) that every neurosis has a purpose; (2) that it constitutes a flight into illness by subconscious intentions; and (3) that after a war is over, war neuroses will disappear (Eissler, 1986). As we have seen in previous chapters, he was wrong on all three counts.

Yet external events are not the only factors that drive people over the brink. There can be no question that the mental schemata that people generate as adaptations to reality while they are young are critically important in determining how they process memories of subsequent experience, and hence whether they will or will not develop enduring problems following exposure to traumatic life experiences. The "traumatic neuroses" always have been, and are likely to continue to be, the central battlefield of the nature–nurture debate.

A number of critical factors will affect how this debate continues to play itself out. The nature of the research methods applied will have an important bearing on the findings that will be uncovered. The statistical models that are used to investigate causality have hitherto received little scrutiny. Simple regression coefficients may be insufficient to determine the precise relationships between a particular event and an individual's psychopathology (see Chapter 7, this volume). The properties of the study sample add another critical dimension: Because negative effects are overrepresented in clinical populations, studying them carries an inherent bias. Epidemiological samples will find a range of adaptations to any given type of event, not just the adverse adaptations. The fact that 20–25% of any exposed population will have met diagnostic criteria for a psychiatric disorder in the previous 6 months (see Chapter 8, this volume) is likely to have a significant influence on posttraumatic adaptation. This issue has been insufficiently acknowledged and studied. How are the posttraumatic adaptations in these individuals different from the PTSD that emerges in individuals who have never previously suffered from significant psychological symptoms?

MEMORY AND DIVIDED CONSCIOUSNESS

During the first day of the battle of the Somme in World War I, there were more British casualties than there were on the U.S. side during the entire Vietnam War. The horrors of that war were so overwhelming that it took psychiatrists more than two decades to begin to digest them. By the time Myers (1940) and Kardiner (1941) published their accounts of amnesia and reenactment of the trauma in veterans, history had already "scooped" them by demonstrating how whole societies can suffer from the same amnesia and reenactment as individuals do. As we have described earlier in this volume (see Chapter 3), the early psychiatrists who devoted themselves to the study of impact of trauma on consciousness all noted that traumatic memories are stored in a state-dependent fashion and may remain inaccessible for prolonged periods of time, only to be expressed as physical symptoms, behavioral reenactments, and vivid sensory reliving experiences (see also Nemiah, 1979; van der Kolk, 1989). Discussions about how traumatic memories are fundamentally different from the memories of ordinary experience provoked strong passions at the end of the last century (Ellenberger, 1970), just as they do today. Abram Kardiner opened the door for the eventual understanding of the phenomena of repetition and dissociation by introducing the notion that the traumatic neuroses are "physioneuroses"—psychological problems rooted in biological dysregulation and enduring hypervigilance to continuing threat. As we have noted in earlier chapters (see Chapters 10, 12, and 13), recent research has begun to clarify the biological underpinnings of these disturbances with the help of contemporary technology.

In our time, the organization of the memories of traumatic life experiences has once again emerged as the central issue in the study and treatment of trauma. This issue brings psychiatry into conflict with cherished notions about the nature of memory, about the capacity of people to bear responsibility for their actions, and about issues of justice and social control. The study of traumatic memories questions four basic notions about the nature of memory: (1) that memory is always flexible and integrated with other life experiences; (2) that memory is present in consciousness in a continuous and uninterrupted fashion; (3) that memory always disintegrates in accuracy over time; and (4) that memory is primarily declarative (i.e., that people can articulate what they know in words and symbols). A century of study of traumatic memories shows that (1) they generally remain unaffected by other life experiences; (2) they may return, triggered by reminders, at any time during a person's life, with the same vividness as if the subject were having the experience all over again; and (3) these memories are primarily sensory and emotional, frequently leaving victims in a state of speechless terror, in which they may be unable to articulate precisely what they are feeling and thinking (van der Kolk & Fisler, 1995; see Chapter 12).

Traumatic memories and their expression as physical sensations, reenactment behaviors, and intense emotional states—all of which are alien to the ordinary state of consciousness—raise critical issues about responsibility and the relationships between victims and society. The reenactment of trauma in social relationships is a major source of our collective ills. One example that we have discussed in this volume is that many violent prisoners have horrendous childhood histories of exposure to trauma (see Chapter 9). Not being consciously aware of what one is reenacting makes it difficult to take responsibility for one's actions. When individuals with histories of trauma are removed from situations that trigger their memories, their trauma-based behaviors can be expected to decrease. They may be on their best behavior in jails or hospitals, but if they have not come to terms with the origins of their disruptions, they are likely to encounter the same triggers after release and to engage in the same behaviors when they are exposed to the old triggers. Moreover, punishing these individuals for engaging in destructive acts against themselves and others, without helping them to understand the meaning of their actions, may provide some deterrent against repetition but is equally likely to reinforce it. Studies are clearly needed to demonstrate the validity of the clinical wisdom that when people are put in touch with the memories of their own trauma, they are likely to stop engaging in its repetition.

The issue of the delayed retrieval of memories for childhood abuse has become a topic for intense public debate (see Chapter 2). Interestingly, the issue of delayed recall was not controversial when Myers (1940) and Kardiner (1941) gave detailed descriptions of it in their books on combat neuroses; when Sargant and Slater (1941) reported that 144 of 1,000 consecutive admissions to a field hospital had amnesia for their trauma; or when van der Kolk noted it in Vietnam combat veterans (1989) and in a survivor of the Cocoanut Grove nightclub fire (1987). It appears that as long as men were found to suffer from delayed recall of atrocities committed either by a clearly identifiable enemy or by themselves, this issue was not controversial. However, when similar memory problems started to be documented in girls and women in the context of domestic abuse, the news was unbearable; when female victims started to seek justice against their alleged perpetrators, the issue moved from science into politics. Judith Herman (1992) has written extensively about the possible causes for this shift.

The passions raised by the issue of "false memories" have made people ignore the previously collected data and abandon customary scientific restraint. On the one hand, some laboratory researchers discarded the phenomenon of delayed memories of domestic abuse with dismissive statements such as this: "Memory is like a drop of milk in a glass of water. Who will be able to distinguish the milk from the water after the contents of the glass are spilled on the floor?" (Loftus, 1994b). In clinical circles, by contrast, a few therapists came to see a vast conspiracy of organized satanic ritual abuse that was responsible for the symptoms of their patients. How had these clinicians come to suspend their capacity for doubt and skepticism, and how had the laboratory researchers come to be so arrogant as to dismiss a century of clinical observation on the battlefield, in emergency rooms, and on psychiatric wards? Many major newspapers and magazines, such as *Time, Newsweek, The Wall Street Journal,* and *The New York Times,* threw themselves into the fray during the years 1992–1996; they featured articles that denied the existence of delayed recall for sexual abuse, and that dismissed reports of such "repressed memories" as most likely the results of "memory implantation" by "recovered memory therapists." In this debate, there was no serious discussion about the nature of suggestibility, or the complex distortions of memory that are seen as a consequence of trauma. The fact that it seems to be impossible to "implant" vivid flashbacks of imaginary events into human beings was not discussed. Laboratory experiments of ordinary events were again readily applied to extraordinary experiences that simply cannot be replicated in a laboratory, just as the life stress literature was found not to be helpful in understanding PTSD, or animal models of the stress response led to different biological models than were found in PTSD.

The issue of "false memories" has become so heated that a leading laboratory researcher on memory distortion could omit from her book *The Myth of Repressed Memory* (Loftus, 1994a)—which was dedicated to "the principles of science which demand that any claim to 'truth' be accompanied by proof"— her own study showing that 19% of a sample of sexually abused women had lost all memory of their abuse at some time in their lives, and that another 12% had large gaps in their memories (Loftus, Polensky, & Fullilove, 1994). She also failed to mention any of the numerous articles written over the last century documenting the phenomenon of delayed memories, many of which are cited in Chapter 12 of this volume. This selective attention to data has been the hallmark of the so-called "false memory" debate.

The "false memory" debate is, at least in part, a product of the adversarial environment of the courtroom. This may explain why the participants pay such selective attention to only one side of the argument, rather than acknowledging the complexity of the issues involved. This is yet another example of how the method of polarized legal argument does science and society a disservice, particularly in the field of trauma. Allegiance to truth is not the primary task in the adversarial legal environment; rather, it is devoted to defending the accused. It is a strange paradox that the courts have become the arbiters of facts, when the lawyers and judges do not have the required scientific knowledge or training. The lack of public concern about the reality of these issues may reflect the fact that generally politicians and journalists have neither scientific training nor a deep allegiance to scientific proof or argument. Scientists and clinicians who consistently become expert witnesses for one side of a legal or medical question are at risk of having a powerful financial and emotional allegiance to the issues at stake.

In the courtroom, attention to the plight of victims often conflicts directly with the need to protect the rights of the wrongly accused. Our cultures are inevitably based on the notion that when there is doubt, the rights of the accused take precedence over those of victims who seek redress. Hence the issue in the courtroom has been to promote doubt about the accuracy of the victims' testimony; this has included the reintroduction of the old issue of suggestibility in women who seek redress for their claims of past abuse. Ironically, although the problems of suggestibility and memory distortions have been vehemently argued in regard to the alleged victims in these cases, scant attention has been paid to the budding scientific literature indicating that perpetrators of crimes are prone to suffer from dissociative amnesias as well (e.g., Schacter, 1986).

The "false memory" issue illustrates that when the discoveries of psychiatry come into conflict with society's cherished beliefs, psychiatry has traditionally been vulnerable to giving up the pursuit of science and, instead, to conforming to prevailing societal attitudes. In Chapter 3 we have documented how this phenomenon has played itself out time and time again over the past century. Today we seem to be confronted with a similar cautious approach toward potentially controversial issues. For example, several leading journal editors have placed unusual restrictions on journal submissions related to the epidemiology and treatment of childhood sexual abuse (e.g., Brown, Sheflin, & Hammond, 1996). Violence, particularly of the domestic variety, continues to be an issue that is reluctantly studied and funded. In Chapter 2 we have noted that in the past decade, there were 13 controlled studies on the psychopharmacological treatment of children with obsessive–compulsive disorder, and 36 on the treatment of attention-deficit/hyperactivity disorder. In contrast, despite the facts that 2,936,000 cases of child abuse and/or neglect were reported in the United States in 1992 alone, and that homicide is the leading cause of death in children in the United States (National Victim Center, 1993), as of 1996 there was precisely one published controlled psychopharmacological study on the treatment of PTSD in children in the entire world literature. Other treatment studies of traumatized children are scarce and largely anecdotal.

This failure to collect treatment efficacy data is especially disturbing, given that the majority of children treated in psychiatric inpatient units are thought to have histories of abuse and/or neglect. Unfortunately, the lack of data collection on the treatment of abused children reflects the neglect of the issue of child maltreatment in psychiatry training programs. Obviously, the failure to conduct adequate research on effective treatments of these children has enormous costs for both individuals and society. The cultural denial of the impact of trauma is reflected in a paucity of available treatment programs and of academically based training, as well as in the ferocity with which the "false memory" debate is being pursued both in courtrooms and in academic psychiatry and psychology programs.

DEVELOPMENTAL DIMENSIONS OF TRAUMA AND NEGLECT

The developmental level at which trauma occurs has a major impact on the capacity of the victim to adapt. As we have seen in Chapter 10, there is growing evidence that trauma at an early age affects the maturation of the systems that control the fundamental regulation of biological processes. The disruption of these biological self-regulatory processes seems to be related to the chronic affect dysregulation, destructive behavior directed against self and others, learning disabilities, dissociative problems, somatization, and distortions in concepts about self and others that have repeatedly been documented in these children (e.g., Bowlby, 1969; Cicchetti, 1985; Cole & Putnam, 1991; Terr, 1991; see Chapter 14). The PTSD field trials for the DSM-IV showed that this conglomeration of symptoms tended to occur together, and that the severity of these problems was proportional to the age at onset of the trauma and to its duration (van der Kolk et al., in press).

The best scientific way to examine the specific effects of trauma and abuse on biological and psychological systems is through prospective studies, such as those currently being conducted by Frank Putnam and his group at the National Institute of Mental Health in Washington, D.C. These studies indicate that sexually abused girls develop neuroendocrine disturbances, particularly in their corticosteroid and thyroid functions (DeBellis, Burke, Trickett, & Putnam, in press), as well as major problems with attention, memory, and concentration (Putnam, in press). The ways in which early trauma disrupts the development of the ability to pay attention and to distinguish relevant from irrelevant information are further illustrated by the finding of Teicher, Glod, Survey, and Swett (in press) that histories of trauma are associated with a loss of normal synchronization of electrical activity between different cortical areas (particularly in the left hemisphere), and that this leads to impairment of the functional integration of cortical and subcortical regions. This finding may be related to the observation that abused children have significant problems in the dominant-hemisphere function of language development (Cicchetti & White, 1990). Furthermore, several studies have now shown that trauma leads to a decrease in the size of the hippocampus (e.g., Stein et al., 1994), which is likely to have an effect on the capacity to remember and to integrate incoming information into existing mental schemata.

Clearly, these emerging findings point to the profound biological disruptions caused by early adversity, whether it be abuse or neglect. Further research is needed to clarify how trauma and neglect differentially affect maturation of children's biological and psychological systems, and to what degree early intervention can prevent or even reverse some of these changes. Furthermore, prospective data are required to show how these biological and interpersonal disruptions affect personality formation at different stages of development. In this regard, the study of the impact of trauma on physical health and aging is an area of knowledge that still requires a great deal of study. The long-term effects of trauma were studied in population samples following World War II, with alarming findings regarding precipitous declines in physical and mental health, but little has been done since (see Chapters 3 and 15). The effects of trauma on aging are as important a developmental issue as its effects on development during childhood.

DISSOCIATION AND SOMATIZATION

The study of war trauma has shown how different acute and chronic reactions to trauma are. Following acute trauma, the relationships between the patients' reactions and what led up to them can still be easily understood (see Chapter 5). However, over time, the connection between the patients' symptoms and their histories can become obscured. For example, the origins of affect dysregulation and constriction of ego functioning are not easily linked to particular life experiences. Traditionally, psychiatry has had a great deal of difficulty recognizing the chronic effects of trauma. For example, when the DSM-I was created shortly after World War II, it included a "gross stress reaction" to acute trauma; however, it took another 30 years before a category was created in the DSM-III that encompassed trauma's long-term effects (see Chapter 6). This failure to formulate a category for the chronic effects of trauma can be best understood in light of the fact that World War II presented psychiatry with the observation that war can give rise to a whole range of different psychiatric disorders. Only through the formulation of the PTSD diagnosis (based on Kardiner's 1941 descriptions) was psychiatry able to reduce the posttraumatic response to some of its bare elements.

However, this diagnosis fails to take into account the heterogeneous nature of individual adaptations to trauma, as well as the complex issue of comorbidity (which to this day remains largely unaddressed). As we have seen in Chapter 9, exposure to extreme stress affects people on many levels of functioning: somatic, emotional, cognitive, behavioral, and characterological. For example, histories of childhood trauma are often found in patients who are diagnosed with borderline personality disorder, affective disorders, somatization disorder, dissociative disorders, self-mutilation, eating disorders, and substance abuse. As we have seen in Chapters 9 and 13, one central element that all these conditions have in common is the high prevalence of dissociation.

Dissociation, or the failure to integrate the cognitions, emotions, sensations, and perceptions belonging to a particular event and to synthesize them into existing mental schemata, is emerging as a critical element that predicts and probably sustains the development of chronic reactions to traumatic life experiences. The recent studies (Krystal et al., 1994) utilizing the anesthetic agent ketamine to induce derealization and depersonalization, as well as brain imaging studies of people having traumatic flashbacks (see Chapter 10), have started to open a window to the understanding of the biological substrates of these critical phenomena.

The degree to which trauma is expressed in psychosomatic problems has long been recognized, but little has been done to clarify the nature and treatment of this vexing problem. New data are just now beginning to emerge on the effects of trauma on the immune system, and these may help provide some new avenues to understanding and treating somatization. For example, a recent study found significant immunological abnormalities in women with histories of chronic sexual abuse in the ratio of CD45 "suppressor/inducer" (RA) to "memory" (RO) cells (van der Kolk, Wilson, Burbridge, & Kradin, 1996). These findings are reflections of the complex interrelationships between the brain and the immune system, which are mediated through the dysregulated hypothalamic–pituitary–adrenal axis in PTSD (Black, 1994; see Chapter 10). The work of Pennebaker and Susman (1988) and Spiegel (1993) has begun to show that being able to express one's distress verbally can have significant positive effects on immune functioning. At this time, it is hard to tell how these findings will be translated into more effective forms of treatment for traumatized patients with somatization disorder.

TREATMENT AND ADVOCACY

Enormous advances have been made in understanding and treating the effects of psychological trauma since it was rediscovered in the late 1970s. Despite the sophistication of much of the recent scientific work on PTSD, it is important to remember that this work had its origin in the social and political climate of the 1960s and 1970s: An alliance of advocates for Vietnam veterans and feminist activists provided the circumstances that made it possible to include the diagnosis of PTSD in the DSM-III. That inclusion had more to do with victim advocacy than with science, and to this day, progress in the field of traumatic stress is fueled as much by champions of trauma victims as it is by clinicians and laboratory scientists. All these groups are necessary to sustain the work of treating traumatized children and adults. After all, victims of trauma still constitute an ambivalently held segment of our societies: They are constantly at risk of being cast out of the larger community, and are also easily misused for their sensational value by the mass media and by various organizations that have an ax to grind. Moreover, because of issues related to both powerlessness and shame, it is unlikely that victims of violence will be able to organize themselves into effective lobbying organizations along the lines of the American Cancer Society or the Cystic Fibrosis Foundation.

Victims of trauma have traditionally been the subjects of intense passions in the area of therapy as well, and the various treatments proposed for PTSD have been as far-ranging and often as unsupported by good outcome data as any treatments for psychiatric conditions, if not more so. We have earlier discussed how traumatized individuals, in their desperation and their dissociation, may become "sitting ducks" for further victimization—including victimization by professionals. Many therapies have been advocated with evangelical zeal. Nevertheless, the willingness of some clinicians and researchers to try new avenues of intervention, and to subject these findings to scrutiny by their peers,

572 • Conclusions and Future Directions

has made the field of traumatic stress one of the most innovative in the area of therapeutics. In Part VI of this book we have discussed a range of psycho-therapeutic and psychobiological interventions that have shown to be helpful in alleviating and sometimes even "curing" the effects of tragic experiences on people's mind and bodies. Aside from the pharmacological interventions and the traditional psychodynamic and cognitive-behavioral techniques discussed in this book, there is great promise in some of the newer therapies that deal with the integration of traumatic memories not primarily by verbal means (i.e., having patients articulate what they remember and work through the mean-ing of the trauma), but through nonverbal techniques (such as having patients pay attention to alternative stimuli while processing trauma-related informa-tion; e.g., Shapiro, 1995). However, even with the possible paradigm shift that these newer therapies promise, professionals working in the specialty area of traumatic stress have become sufficiently sophisticated to recognize that dif-ferent treatments are needed at different stages of posttraumatic adaptation (see Chapter 18). Undoubtedly, there will always be a tension between our urge to deal, on the one hand, with both our own and our patients' sense of help-lessness, and, on the other hand, the requirement that treatment methods need to be subjected to approriate outcome studies.

THE CONUNDRUMS THAT REMAIN

Despite the explosion of new and rediscovered knowledge during the past two decades many of the questions that have always haunted the area of traumatic stress remain. How do the biological effects of trauma affect people's capacity to think and make sense out of current experience? To what degree can psy-chological interventions affect a disorder with such strong biological under-pinnings? Do patients benefit from getting compensation payments, or does it impair their recovery? What is the role of predisposition, and what are the implications of preexisting vulnerabilities for treatment? To what degree is the essence of trauma the external reality or the internal processing of that event? Should treatment focus primarily on the trauma itself, on secondary adapta-tions, or on learning to pay attention to the here and now? What is the relationship of traumatic stress to psychiatric illness other than PTSD? What is the nature of the acute reaction to trauma and its relation to chronic outcomes? To what extent do the tonic disorders of hyperarousal and memory drive the intensity and nature of traumatic memories in PTSD? What is the relationship between the capacity to protect oneself by dissociating on the one hand, and the emergence of a disorder of attention to the present and a continued embeddedness in the trauma of the past on the other? These are some of the great challenges to answer as we work toward a better understanding of the impact of trauma on people's capacities to cope, as well as the ways people find to go on with their lives.

FINAL COMMENTS

There are aspects of the experience of trauma that cannot be captured in medical and scientific models, but that go to the core of what it is like to be human—how we see ourselves and our relationships to our fellow human beings, both in our immediate environment and over time and space. How do people and societies cope with the inevitable tragedies of life, and what commitments can they make, individually and communally, beyond their immediate attention to their own survival? Trauma can have a multitude of consequences: It can produce abject misery, and make people abandon all hope; it can make the lust for revenge the center of people's lives, at the expense of the ability to rebuild; or it can be sublimated into supreme acts of artistic transformation and social action.

Scientific, empirical frameworks constitute only one way to approach human suffering. These points of view leave little room for the vital human dimensions affected by trauma: human commonality in suffering, the need to assign blame, the compulsion to take revenge, the role of faith, and a personal or communal sense of destiny. These dimensions are what fuel the intense emotions that victims stir up; the intrusive probing into people's tragedies in the mass media; and the revulsion toward their helplessness and anger that arises in political, medical, and insurance settings. Attitudes toward trauma and victimization must in important ways reflect people's basic beliefs about what it means to be human, and people's positions about the eternal questions of good and evil. In the same ways that victims tend to take extreme positions, the issue of trauma inevitably seems to provoke extreme moral judgments in bystanders. Many victims plunge into self-denial, while others become preoccupied with revenge and compensation. Many become socially withdrawn and compliant, while others alienate those around them with their persistent and unreasonable demands.

In recent years, just as after World War I, the prevailing social attitude to victims has been that they are mendacious, greedy and vengeful, even though research supports the notion that they are more often depressed, withdrawn, "spaced out," and compliant. This intolerance of victims of trauma, rather than of the circumstances that lead to those traumas, is a function of a willingness to accept the seemingly inevitable conditions that lead to traumatization: crime, wars, poverty, and family violence. Ironically, the victims who refuse to acquiesce in what happened to them are the ones who seem to provoke the most intense opprobrium from their environment. They are the ones who seem to provoke the greatest need to control them, on the assumption that otherwise their insatiable demands will get out of hand. In order to deal with victims, one needs to be able to trust their motives and to squarely confront the tragedies that have befallen them and continue to dominate their lives.

Why is the issue of suffering so important? It is the means through which both personal and social conceptions of knowledge and meaning are created.

Ideally, the capacity for empathy and shared purpose is the ultimate product of this process. The paradox is that in the process of accepting the reality of trauma, it is easy to lose one's sensitivity and to retreat into dry scientific observation or cynical capitulation. However, beneath the tidiness of emotional distancing and scientific classification lie the human vitality and energy to struggle against, and to create meaning out of, what appears to be the random cruelty of fate. This struggle to transcend the effects of trauma is among the noblest aspects of human history.

REFERENCES

American Psychiatric Association. (1994). *Diagnostic and statistical manual of mental disorders* (4th ed.). Washington, DC: Author.

Barker, P. (1995). *The ghost road.* New York: Viking.

Black, P. H. (1994). Immune system–central nervous system interactions: Effect and immunomodulatory consequences of immune system mediators on the brain. *Antimicrobial Agents and Chemotherapy, 38,* 7–12.

Bowlby, J. (1969). *Attachment and loss* (Vol. 1). New York: Basic Books.

Brown, D., Sheflin, A., & Hammond, D.C. (1996). *Memory, trauma treatment and the law.* Hillsdale, NJ: Erlbaum.

Cicchetti, D. (1985). The emergence of developmental psychopathology. *Child Development, 55,* 1–7.

Cicchetti, D., & White, J. (1990). Emotion and developmental psychopathology. In N. Stein, B. Leventhal, & T. Trebasso (Eds.), *Psychological and biological approaches to emotion* (pp. 359–382). Hillsdale, NJ: Erlbaum.

Cole, P. M., & Putnam, F. W. (1991). Effect of incest on self and social functioning: A developmental psychopathology perspective. *Journal of Consulting and Clinical Psychology, 60,* 174–184.

DeBellis, M., Burke, L., Trickett, P., & Putnam, F. (in press). Antinuclear antibodies and thyroid function in sexually abused girls. *Journal of Traumatic Stress.*

Eissler, K. R. (1986). *Freud as an expert witness: The discussion of war neuroses between Freud and Wagner-Jauregg.* Madison, CT: International Universities Press.

Ellenberger, H. F. (1970). *The discovery of the unconscious.* New York: Basic Books.

Herman, J. L. (1992). *Trauma and recovery.* New York: Basic Books.

Kagan, J. (1989). *Unstable ideas: Temperament, cognition and the self.* Cambridge, MA: Harvard University Press.

Kardiner, A. (1941). *The traumatic neuroses of war.* New York: Hoeber.

Krystal, J. H., Karper, L. P., Seibyl, J. P., Freeman, G. K., Delaney, R., Bremner, J. D., Heninger, G. R., Bowers, M. B., Jr., & Charney, D. R. (1994). Subanesthetic effects of the noncompetitive NMDA anagonist, ketamine, in humans: Psychotomimetic, perceptual, cognitive, and neuroendocrine responses. *Archives of General Psychiatry, 51,* 199–214.

Loftus, E. F. (1994a). *The myth of repressed memory.* New York: St. Martin's Press.

Loftus, E. F. (1994b, May 6). [Statement at the Harvard Conference on Memory Distortions, Boston.]

Loftus, E. F., Polensky, S., & Fullilove, M. T. (1994). Memories of childhood sexual abuse: Remembering and repressing. *Psychology of Women Quarterly, 18,* 67–84.

Myers, C. S. (1940). *Shell shock in France 1914–18.* Cambridge, England: Cambridge University Press.

National Victim Center. (1993). *Crime and victimization in America: Statistcal overview.* Arlington, VA: Author.

Nemiah, J.C. (1979). Dissociative amnesia: A clinical and theoretical reconsideration. In F. Kihlstrom & F. J. Evans (Eds.), *Functional disorders of memory* (pp. 303–323). Hillsdale, NJ: Erlbaum.

Pennebaker, J. W., & Susman, J. R. (1988). Disclosures of trauma and psychosomatic processes. *Social Science and Medicine, 26,* 327–332.

Putnam, F. W. (in press). *Dissociative disorders in children and adolescents.* New York: Guilford Press.

Sargant, W., & Slater, E. (1941). Amnesic syndromes in war. *Proceedings of the Royal Society of Medicine, 34,* 757–764.

Schacter, D. L. (1986). Amnesia and crime: How much do we really know? *American Psychologist, 41*(3), 286–295.

Shapiro, F. (1995). *Eye movement desensitization and reprocessing.* New York: Guilford Press.

Spiegel, D. (1993). Cancer and interactions between mind and body. *Journal of the National Cancer Institute, 85,* 1198–1205.

Stein, M. B., Hannah, C., Koverola, C., Yehuda, R., Torchia, M., & McClarty, B. (1994, December 15). *Neuroanatomical and neuroendocrine correlates in adulthoodof severe sexual abuse in childhood.* Paper presented at the 33rd Annual Meeting of the American College of Neuropsychopharmacology, San Juan, PR.

Teicher, M. H., Glod, C. A., Survey, J., & Swett, C. (1993). Early childhood abuse and limbic system ratings in adult psychiatric outpatients. *Journal of Neuropsychiatry and Clinical Neuroscience, 5,* 301–306.

Terr, L. C. (1991). Childhood traumas: An outline and overview. *American Journal of Psychiatry, 148,* 10–20.

Thomas, D. (1953). Do not go gentle into that good night. In D. Thomas, *The collected poems of Dylan Thomas 1934–1952* (p. 128). New York: New Directions.

van der Kolk, B. A. (1987). *Psychological trauma.* Washington, DC: American Psychiatric Press.

van der Kolk, B. A. (1989). The compulsion to repeat the trauma: Revictimization, attachment and masochism. *Psychiatric Clinics of North America, 12,* 389–411.

van der Kolk, B. A., & Fisler, R. (1995). Dissociation and the fragmentary nature of traumatic memories: Overview and exploratory study. *Journal of Traumatic Stress, 9,* 505–525.

van der Kolk, B. A., Pelcovitz, D., Roth, S., Mandel, F., McFarlane, A. C., & Herman, J. L. (in press). Dissociation, somatization, and affect dysregulation: The complex nature of adaptation to trauma. *American Journal of Psychiatry.*

van der Kolk, B. A., Wilson, S., Burbridge, J., & Kradin, R. (1996). *Immunological abnormalities in women with childhood histories of sexual abuse.* Unpublished manuscript.

World Health Organization. (1992). *International classification of diseases* (10th revision). Geneva: Author.

Yehuda, R., & McFarlane, A. C. (1995). Conflict between current knowledge about posttraumatic stress disorder and its original conceptual basis [Review]. *American Journal of Psychiatry, 152*(12), 1705–1713.

Index